T0297514

The Psychopharmacology of Herbal Medicine

The Psychopharmacology of Herbal Medicine

Plant Drugs that Alter Mind, Brain, and Behavior

Marcello Spinella

The MIT Press
Cambridge, Massachusetts
London, England

This book was set in Adobe Sabon in QuarkXPress by Asco Typesetters, Hong Kong.

Library of Congress Cataloging-in-Publication Data

Spinella, Marcello.
The psychopharmacology of herbal medicine : plant drugs that alter mind, brain, and behavior / Marcello Spinella.
p. cm.
Includes bibliographical references and index.
ISBN 978-0-262-69265-6 (pbk. : alk. paper)
1. Psychotropic drugs. 2. Herbs—Therapeutic use. 3. Psychopharmacology. 4. Medicinal plants—Psychological aspects.
RC483 .S65 2001
615′.788—dc21 00-052535

Contents

Preface

Alternative and complementary medicine have been enjoying a recent growth in popularity in the United States. People are increasingly likely to consult them in an attempt to treat their illnesses. While this may be a positive trend, there is also an enormous potential for harm, depending on what illness is being treated and the type of treatments being sought. Given the myriad of alternative and complementary treatments available, both consumers and practitioners of health care are hard pressed to select appropriate, effective, and safe treatments.

Although treating illness and creating psychological effects using plants are ancient practices, scientific developments in the past few decades allow us to now look at these phenomena in a different way. As our understanding of the nervous system advances, so does our understanding of psychoactive drugs that alter it. We can now *begin* to explain how the psychoactive effects occur, from molecular up to behavioral levels.

Whereas much of alternative and complementary medicine is criticized for a lack of empirical research, there seems to be a wealth of research done on plant medicines. In the course doing research in pharmacology and neuroscience, it became apparent that a large body of research existed concerning psychoactive herbal medicines. However, it was also apparent that few, if any, had comprehensively and thoroughly organized and integrated this research into a single source.

This text is primarily aimed to benefit researchers and health care practitioners. Since health care practitioners find many of their patients using over-the-counter herbal medicines, they need a source to help them anticipate how these herbs will interact with their patients' illnesses and treatments. Alternatively, they may wish to incorporate herbal medicines into a patient's treatment regimen whenever appropriate. Toward this end, this book details the chemical constituents, mechanisms, and physiological effects of psychoactive plant drugs. Further, information is given on any controlled clinical trials that address the safety and efficacy of psychoactive herbal medicines.

Researchers in this field will also benefit from the broad summary of data collected here, incorporating biochemistry, pharmacology, physiology, cognition, and behavior. From this perspective, future avenues for research often become apparent.

Ultimately, this book is intended to further the cause of herbal medicines. If they are properly researched and the public is properly educated about their effects and uses, herbal medicines will be an asset to us, rather than a liability.

Acknowledgments

There are several people I would like to thank regarding the creation of this book. The library staff at JFK Medical Center in Edison, New Jersey and Richard Stockton College in Pomona, NJ has been indispensable with their assistance in research. The editors and staff at MIT Press have also been extremely helpful in guiding me through the process of publishing a book.

I would like to thank my former teachers for sharing freely their knowledge and inspiration. Special thanks are extended to Richard Bodnar, Thomas Frumkes, Christopher Capuano, and John Santelli for guiding through the field of neuroscience.

Most of all, I would like to thank my family and friends for their persistent encouragement, love, and support.

Notice

Both author and publisher have tried to ensure that all information in this work concerning drug administration, doses, and schedules is accurate and in accord with the standards of the general medical community as of the time of publication. Because medical science continually advances, however, therapeutic standards may change.

Due to the possibility of human error or changes in medical sciences, neither the author nor the publisher nor any other party who has been involved in the preparation or publication of this work declares that the information herein is totally accurate or complete. They are not accountable for any errors or omissions or for the results obtained from the use of such information.

Readers are encouraged to consult with a physician who is directly involved in their care to obtain the most accurate and up-to-date information. Readers should also check the product information sheet included in the package of each drug for the most reliable information about the currently recommended doses, side effects, contraindications, etc. This recommendation is particularly important with new or unregulated drugs.

This publication is only intended to provide background information; all information on drug administration, doses, and schedules should be reconfirmed for accuracy by referring to the manufacturer's information sheet.

The Psychopharmacology of Herbal Medicine

1

Introduction

The use of psychoactive plants is practically a universal human phenomenon. Except for a few cultures lacking access to psychoactive plants, humans tend to use them routinely. The psychological and behavioral effects of such plants have long been recognized and information about their uses has been passed down through generations. However, with the advent of modern science, we are able to better understand the composition of these plants and how they specifically interact with the nervous system. Toward that end, this book has been written to compile and integrate the available information on the major psychoactive plant drugs.

Plants are the oldest and perhaps still the most commonly used medicine. A chief example is caffeine—probably the most common stimulant in the world—consumed in tea or coffee. Additionally, many modern drugs are still derived from plant sources. Despite the existence of many synthetic opioids (e.g., methadone, Darvocet), morphine and codeine are still extracted from the opium poppy because of the difficulties and economics of their chemical synthesis. Synthetic drugs are now designed for specific uses, but often their design is guided by knowledge about their plant-based predecessors.

The relationships between animals and plants date as far back as evolutionary history. Although ecological food chains necessitate that herbivorous animals eat plants to derive nutrition and energy, it is not the only reason plants are consumed. In our searches for edible plants, humans (and certain other species, arguably) have come across numerous species of plants with nonnutritive benefits.

The distinction between *drug* and *nutrient* deserves clarification. This is especially the case now with single refined nutrients (such as single amino acids), which blur the distinction. Although both nutrients and drugs are derived from external sources, they differ in their innate necessity. A nutrient is a substance that is essential to processes of life and growth. Without essential nutrients such as vitamin C, an individual suffers illness. A drug is any chemical that alters biological processes, with the connotation that it has some therapeutic or recreational use. A *poison* or *toxin*, then, is a substance with predominantly harmful effects on biological processes. However, as the sixteenth-century physician Paracelsus noted, the difference between a remedy and a poison is often a matter of dosage.

Many plant-derived drugs are common in modern medicine. For example, morphine is derived from the poppy plant and is a standard medication used to treat pain. It has also been the progenitor of many other synthetic pain killers. Digoxin and digitoxin are cardiac medicines that derive from the foxglove plant. But there are many herbal medications with reputed therapeutic value that have not gained acceptance in mainstream medicine. (For the purposes of this book, the words *herb* and *plant* will be used interchangeably.) Knowledge of such herbs has been passed down through tradition, but they have not gained mainstream acceptance due to a lack of research to support their therapeutic use. Fortunately, many such herbal medications are currently undergoing scientific study. In particular, investigations are identifying their active chemical components, physiological effects, pharmacological properties, and clinical efficacy. In the meantime, their therapeutic status is most often relegated to alternative medicine.

Herbal versus Synthetic Drugs

Herbal medications are drugs in every sense of the word. They chemically modify bodily processes and can have therapeutic or harmful effects, depending on how they are used. However, there are a few general differences between herbal and pharmaceutical drugs (Tyler 1994). Herbal drugs tend to be more dilute than pharmaceutical drugs (table 1.1). For example, caffeine is available in 200 mg tablets to produce stimulation. Coffee contains 1–2% caffeine, so in order to get the same amount of caffeine one must use 20 g of coffee bean. Similarly, aspirin is

Table 1.1
Potential pros and cons of herbal vs. refined/pharmaceutical drugs

Herbal	Refined/pharmaceutical
Pro	*Pro*
Multiple and cooperating constituents	Avoids extraneous constituents
Lower toxicity of dilute drug	Avoids antagonistic constituents
	Higher potency of concentrated drug
	Standard administration methods
Con	*Con*
Lower potency of dilute drug	Higher toxicity of concentrated drug
Variable administration methods	

derived from the bark of the willow tree. In order to get the same effects of the average dose of aspirin, one would need to consume between 3 and 20 cups of willow bark tea. This is not to say that plant drugs are necessarily weak in potency, they are simply less concentrated than pharmaceutical drugs.

This raises a second issue—the method of administration (see table 1.1). The prescribed route of administration of a pharmaceutical drug is chosen for specific pharmacological reasons. Herbal medications might be administered in a number of different ways, which greatly alter their effects. The simplest way to consume a plant is to eat it, but many medicinal plants are unpalatable, making this impractical. Instead, plants can be dried and ground and administered in capsule form. This form still supplies the entire herb. Alternately, the dried plant matter can be made into an *infusion* or *decoction.* An infusion is when hot or boiling water is poured over the herb and its chemical constituents steep into the water, which is then drunk. This is the way that tea is commonly prepared. A decoction is similar, except that the water is boiled with the plant actually in it. The length of time of steeping or boiling is significant, as it determines how much of the chemicals enter the water. Still, even with a long steeping time, only a fraction of the plant's available chemicals enter the tea.

A further step in preparing herbal medicines involves making an extract. In this method, the fresh or dried plant is allowed to soak in a solvent, which is sometimes heated to maximize the extraction. Solvents frequently used are water, alcohol (ethanol or methanol), or acetone. After soaking in the solvent, the plant matter is discarded and the solvent is allowed to evaporate so that none of it remains in the final product. All that remains is a concentration of the active constituents of the plant. The type of solvent can affect the composition of the extract. For example, aqueous preparations do not efficiently extract the lipid-soluble, hydrophobic constituents of herbs. In contrast, alcohol extracts will contain far more lipid-soluble constituents. Despite the fact that both extracts derive from the same plant, they have different compositions and can have widely varying pharmacological effects. An advantage of consuming an herbal extract instead of the whole plant is that it greatly reduces the volume of matter to be ingested. In order to get a sufficent dose of the active chemicals, in some cases, this means the difference between swallowing a few pills and consuming a bale of dried plant.

The number of different methods of application of herbal drugs means variability in the active chemicals obtained and the effects they produce. When taking or prescribing an herb, it is always necessary to attend to the type of preparation. Even pharmaceutical drugs vary from person to person in terms of how much of the ingested drug is absorbed and reaches the targeted organs. Greater variability means greater unpredictability of negative side effects. The process of *standardization* of herbs ensures that a certain percentage of the desired active constituents are present in a preparation, which allows for greater reliability in dosing.

Another significant difference between herbal and pharmaceutical drugs is that pharmaceutical drugs consist of a purified single active drug. Herbal medications, on the other hand, may have multiple active constituents. For example, the opium poppy contains more than 30 alkaloids (Robbers et al. 1996). The active chemical constituents of a plant may each have different individual effects, so that the effect of the total herb is a combination of the effects of several different constituents. In such cases, it might be preferable to purify one constituent for use, thus avoiding the extraneous effects of others. While one may desire the analgesic effects of morphine, the vasodilator effects of another poppy alkaloid, papaverine, may be unwanted. Using pure morphine, rather than opium, avoids this problem. Another scenario is when the desired effect of one constituent is antagonized or nullified by other constituents, making it even more necessary to isolate the desired constituent.

Conversely, active constituents may have cooperative effects and together act in an additive or synergistic (supra-additive) manner. In such cases, it would be better to consume the whole plant or extract, because the combination of constituents would give a greater effect than one alone. Thus, to blindly advocate either the use of whole herb or refined single constituents is naive. To fully know what is best for the desired effect, herbs must be considered on a case-by-case basis and the nature of the interactions between the chemical constituents must be carefully considered. Not only must we understand what the plant's chemical constituents do, we must also investigate how they interact.

The Use of Herbal Medicine

The Current Prevalence of Alternative Medicine

National surveys have shown the use of alternative medicines, including herbal medicine and other practices, to be prevalent (Eisenberg et al. 1998). In 1997, 42% of people in a large national sample reported consulting at least one form of alternative medicine during the previous year, increasing from 33.8% in 1990. The alternative therapies with the greatest increase in use were herbal medicine, massage therapy, megavitamins, self-help groups, folk remedies, energy healing, and homeopathy. The illnesses for which people most often consulted alternative medicine tended to be chronic conditions, such as back problems, anxiety, depression, and headaches.

The total number of visits to alternative medicine practitioners had increased by 47% across the seven-year span, and the majority of consumers (~60%) paid for these therapies at their own expense. The 1990 survey found that people made an average of 19 visits per year to an alternative medicine practitioner, with the average charge per visit at $27.60 (Eisenberg et al. 1993). A conservative estimate of the cost for all these therapies in 1997 was $21.2 billion, with $12.2 billion paid out of pocket (Eisenberg et al. 1998). To put this in perspective, this amount exceeds out-of-pocket expenditures for all U.S. hospitalizations in 1997. The authors conclude that the increase constitutes a greater number of people seeking alternative therapies, rather than just an increased number of visits per patient.

The Appeal of Herbal Medicines

Despite the developing nature of the rational use of herbal medications, many are freely available to the public as over-the-counter supplements. They have gained popularity as alternatives to traditional medicine. To some degree, their popularity may reflect a dissatisfaction with modern medicine. Another potential factor is the perception that herbal medications are more "natural" and have greater aesthetic appeal than synthetic drugs. Of course, this is not necessarily so. In many cases, herbal medications can be just as toxic or deadly as synthetic medications. There are no intrinsic benefits from a drug simply because it comes from a plant. In some cases, consuming the plant may be more beneficial, and in other cases, consuming an extract or synthetic drug is better. Such cases need to be examined on a rational basis, rather than out of blind faith to naturalist or technological dogma. All the potential risks must be weighed against the benefits.

Another possible reason for public interest in herbal medications is that they provide some autonomy from medical professionals. Multiple factors contribute to a person's satisfaction with medical care (Siahpush et al. 1999; Sixma et al. 1998; Kaptchuk and Eisenberg 1998). One cause of dissatisfaction results from the traditionally passive role of the patient. Independent of its efficacy, alternative medicine provides an individual with a greater range of explanations and treatment options for their illnesses. The psychological appeal of more options is sufficient to draw individuals to consult alternative medicine, especially in cases where modern medicine has not been effective.

Implications of Herbal Medicine for Medical Fields

A significant fact was revealed by Eisenberg and colleagues regarding disclosure and the use of herbal medicines (1993, 1998). Of the proportion of respondents who utilized alternative medicine, only about 40% had disclosed this fact to their physician. The use of herbal medications was among the most common alternative treatments, and also one of the treatments with the greatest increase in use. Further, it was estimated that during the year of the survey 15 million adults took prescription medications concurrently with herbal medications and/or high-dose vitamins. Thus, a large number of people are taking herbal medications and not disclosing the fact to their physicians. Because herbal medicines are active drugs, they present enormous potential for adverse medication interactions. Adverse interactions could be averted if people were more comfortable with informing their physicians of their use of herbal medications. Of course, physicians would need to have a greater knowledge of the actions of herbal medications to foresee such potential interactions.

The extent of knowledge among medical professionals (physician and nonphysician) about herbal medications varies across and within cultures. On the whole, American physicians are currently not very knowledgeable about herbal medications, and as a result, they tend not to prescribe them. Comparatively, the use of herbal medications by physicians is much more common in Europe and Asia (Tyler 1994).

But the American medical system is not blind to this fact, and there are some indications of change. A number of studies have appeared in medical journals reviewing the known efficacy and safety of herbs for therapeutic use (e.g., O'Hara et al. 1998; Hadley and Petry 1999; Wong et al. 1998; Cupp 1999; Onopa 1999). A good proportion (64%) of surveyed medical schools reported offering some course work in alternative or complementary medicine (Wetzel et al. 1998). A majority (68%) of these were stand-alone courses and the remaining addressed alternative medicine in the context of other courses.

The reluctance of many physicians to prescribe herbal medications is in many ways understandable. Much research needs to be done to ensure the efficacy and safety of many herbs. Few authoritative texts are available that summarize the available clinical research (see Tyler 1994). Because physicians naturally want to provide their patients with the best available care, herbal medications do not always present an attractive option due to the uncertainty that surrounds them.

The darker side to this issue concerns malpractice. Malpractice claims against nonmedical practitioners of alternative medicine are generally low (Studdert et al. 1998). Although referring a patient to another physician does not generally expose a physician to liability for malpractice, there are exceptions when the referral is negligent or when there is joint treatment. Therefore, referrals to alternative medicine can potentially carry risk.

In this context, judging the qualifications of an alternative medicine practitioner can be difficult—there are no universally accepted guidelines. Some states require licensing of alternative medicine practitioners (e.g., acupuncturists, naturopathic herbalists), and licensure is often used by courts to establish school-specific standards of care. In cases where no licensing exists, courts apply conventional medical or lay standards of care. Eisenberg (1997) has proposed strategies for physicians in guiding patients who seek alternative medical treatment.

Government Regulation of Herbal Medications

Government regulation of herbal medicines has changed appreciably over time (Tyler 1994; Ray and Ksir 1990). In the early twentieth century, the Food and Drug Act of 1906 and the Sherley amendment of 1912 were enacted to combat rampant fraud by food and drug producers. Primarily, these laws addressed mislabeling and adulteration of drugs. The Food, Drug, and Cosmetic Acts were enacted in 1938 in response to the tragic deaths of 105 people taking an untested medication (elixir sulfanilamide). These laws stipulated that drugs entering interstate commerce must demonstrate safety, while grandfathering many existing drugs. Tragedy again prompted legislation when pregnant mothers taking the sedative drug thalidomide gave birth to babies with severe limb deformities. Although this occurred outside of the United States, concern prompted the drug amendments of 1962, commonly referred to as the Kefauver-Harris amendments (Hollister et al. 1968; Tyler 1994). This legislation required that drugs marketed after 1962 be not only safe, but also effective.

The U.S. Food and Drug Administration (FDA) undertook a large study of over-the-counter drugs, releasing their results in 1990. This classified drugs and herbs into three categories: (1) effective, (2) unsafe or ineffective, or (3) insufficient evidence to evaluate effectiveness. However, this classification was criticized for overreliance on data from industry. For example, prunes were placed in category (3) as having insufficient evidence for their effectiveness as a laxative! Many herbal medications were kept on the market following this study, but the incriminating statements about their supposed use were removed. While this may have been legally feasible, it left the consumer even less informed than before.

In 1994, the Dietary Supplement Health and Education Act was passed by the U.S. Congress. This allowed herbal medications to be advertised and sold without oversight from the FDA. Specifically, it states that a substance will not legally be classified as a "drug" if it is not represented as treatment for a disease (Heiligenstein and Guenther. 1998; Dietary Supplement Health and Education Act of 1994). Thus, many herbal medicines are now sold and regulated as *dietary supplements*.

There has been some government recognition of the need for knowledge about herbal medications. European governments have traditionally been more advanced than the United States in this area. The German Federal Institute for Drugs and Medical Devices appointed a special expert committee, entitled the German Commission E, to compile scientific and clinical information regarding therapeutic herbs. Their results are published in the book, *The Complete German Commission E Monographs: Therapeutic Guide to Herbal Medicines* (English translation sponsored by the American Botanical Council, 1998). The U.S. National Institutes of Health have a branch dedicated to researching alternative and complementary medicines—the National Center for Complementary and Alternative Medicine (NCCAM). For example, in 1997 the NCCAM launched an ongoing large-scale study of Saint-John's-wort for treatment of depression.

The Evolutionary Perspective: Why Plants Make Drugs

At first glance, it seems unusually convenient that plants would be so kind as to make drugs for human benefit. What causes plants to develop therapeutic chemicals? The answer requires a slight shift of perspective, to ask why plants manufacture chemicals in general. To understand this, one must consider it in the context of natural selection.

Evolution by natural selection was first explained by Charles Darwin in his book *On the Origin of Species* (1859). Briefly stated, the theory suggests that evolution occurs through heritable propagation of adaptive traits. Nature produces a large variation in the traits of organisms. Those traits that are in some way adaptive, increasing the survival and reproductive success of the organism, are propagated to future generations. Darwin's schema is simple but powerful, having great explanatory strength; it is a cornerstone of modern biology. The context of natural selection is essential for understanding the mutual adaptations between plants and animals that led to the manufacture of drugs by plants.

Living organisms are divided into five kingdoms: Animalia, Plantae, Fungi, Protista, and Monera. Green, multicellular plants fall under the Plantae kingdom, which originated in the Silurian period (505 to 400 million years ago) (Southwood 1984). They have the shortest evolutionary history and are the only kingdom to have completely evolved on land. Also evolving around this time were insects. Insects evolving on land found an abundant source of food in plants, provided they could adapt to eating them. This probably occurred in gradual increments, beginning with insects scavenging on pollen and spores, progressing to insects feeding on the reproductive organs of plants, and eventually leaf feeding.

However, this newfound feast for insects was at a great cost to plants. Research indicates that plants protected from insect predators by pesticides live longer, produce more seeds, and propagate over a larger area. Thus, natural selection would favor plants that somehow deter predators from consuming them. The defenses plants have evolved fall into three categories: nutritional, physical, and chemical (Southwood 1984). *Nutritional defenses* involve having low nitrogen levels or balances of amino acids that are unfavorable to insect metabolism. *Physical defenses* involve the growth of external cuticles and epidermal hairs that make the plant mechanically difficult to hold, manipulate, and consume. The focus of this book is the *chemical defenses* evolved by plants, which involve the production of substances that strongly and adversely alter a predator's physiology (either by poisoning or repelling). Also, plant defenses typically are involved in life functions other than defense, so their defense advantages may well have been serendipitous. Regardless, any trait (serendipitous or not) that increases the survival and reproductive ability of a plant will propagate through natural selection. These chemical defenses alter our physiology in diverse ways. While some are outright toxic, many others can be subverted for therapeutic uses. To a large extent, this depends upon our cleverness in finding uses.

Thus, plants and predators have coevolved, reciprocally adapting to one another. Plants develop chemicals that deter predators and increase their survival advantage. Predators, in turn, adapt by developing tolerance, attractions, or even utilization of plant chemicals.

Although humans differ greatly from insects, a reciprocal relationship between humans and plants exists. In the course of foraging for food, humans have serendipitously discovered plants with therapeutic effects. Over time, traditions of knowledge about the therapeutic use of plants have accumulated within cultures, even though the rationales for why such plants are effective are often incorrect. For example, Asian systems of herbal medicine are based on the theory of balancing one's *yin* and *yang* energy. While this might have some unforeseen metaphorical value, it has no apparent basis in the actual anatomy and physiology of the human body. During the Renaissance, herbalists used the *doctrine of signatures* to guide the therapeutic use of plants. The doctrine of signatures is the belief that the shape or color of a plant indicates its therapeutic uses (e.g., if a plant contained red then it would be used to treat blood-related disorders). Although their explanations for why herbs treat an illness are inaccurate, they have still accumulated knowledge about which plants treat which illnesses, through trial and error discovery.

The therapeutic use of plants is seemingly not limited to humans. Certainly, humans are the only species with the verbal and cognitive capacity to label therapeutic plants as such and to accumulate large bodies of knowledge on their specific uses. Nonetheless, the field of zoopharmacognosy has arisen in recent years to study the therapeutic uses of plants by animals. This was prompted by the discovery of Tanzanian chimpanzees using the *Aspilia* plant (Rodrigues et al. 1985; Page et al. 1992). The chimps swallow the whole leaves of the plant without chewing them and derive no apparent nutrition. However, the plant contains a chemical called thiarubine-A, which prevents infection by certain parasites and microorganisms in the gastrointestinal tract. Chimps consuming the plant appear to be free of such infections and related illnesses.

At first glance, it may seem unlikely that chimpanzees premeditatively use such plants. However, no specific knowledge about the plant need be assumed in the chimpanzees for them to use it. From a behavioral standpoint, they would only need to ingest the plant and experience some noticeable benefit for the *Aspilia*-eating behavior to be reinforced. Simply stated, an organism (either animal or human) does not need to know *how* or *why* an herbal medication works in order to derive benefit and keep using it. The organism only needs to experience some improvement so that the plant-using behavior is reinforced. The two requirements of behavioral reinforcement are *contingency*, where the plant gives some reliable benefit, and *contiguity*, where the benefit occurs fairly close in time to the consumption. Some plants directly affect the brain mechanisms involved in behavioral reinforcement, bringing pleasure in mild cases and addiction in severe ones.

In this respect, the human use of plants with various incorrect rationales (e.g., the doctrine of signatures) is not much different than the chimpanzee use of *Aspilia*: an accurate knowledge of how the treatment works is not necessary for plant-use to be behaviorally reinforced and maintained. Human knowledge about the therapeutic uses of plants has accumulated through the millennia by trial and error. Our explanations have been secondary.

However, a new era of plant medicines began with modern science. Rather than trial and error, we can now begin to understand *how* and *why* plant medicines work. It is hoped that we can use this information to guide a more safe and effective use of medicinal plants.

Scientific Methodology in Herbal Medicine

Science is essentially a way of acquiring knowledge. It involves the formation of testable hypotheses based on observations. Further, there is a systematic collection of data to support or disprove the hypotheses. The requirement to verify one's observations through objective methods gives science enormous epistemological power. Information acquired through carefully designed experiments that are subject to repeated verification is the most reliable form of knowledge we have. This is particularly so because the misleading influences of personal bias and random chance are minimized. In order for a hypothesis to be scientific, it must not only be provable through research, but also falsifiable.

To be fair, the majority of scientific data probably do not immediately cast hypotheses into clear-cut categories of proven or disproven. There are most often multiple interpretations and conclusions to be drawn from a set of data. For this reason, scientific findings are subject to peer review and criticism. Although science is conducted by individuals, it ultimately becomes a process of interaction, discussion, and debate among a community of researchers.

The purpose of this discussion of science, clearly, is to apply it to herbal medicine. The reputed uses of drugs may not always be accurate or effective. Applying the scientific method to herbal medicine therefore allows us to test the traditional uses and to know with greater certainty what an herbal medication does and how reliably it does it. Although far from infallible, the process as a whole gives us greater confidence in our conclusions.

Scientific research has many times verified traditional remedies. It is advisable for scientists in the field who are looking for new research ideas to consult the traditional herbal literature.

Adding scientific verification to the body of traditional knowledge can only strengthen our confidence in the traditional use of herbal medicines. Delving into the chemistry and pharmacology of plants opens up a different level of understanding, which may suggest new uses of herbs never thought of before.

There are many ways in which scientific research is carried out, but there are a few essential elements. One form of scientific study is experimentation. In order for causation to be established, an experimental study must perform some kind of manipulation. When an effect is produced, it can then be attributed to the manipulation. However, in order for this to be done, one must control for extraneous influences. To the degree possible, one must keep all other conditions constant so that the experimental effect can be correctly attributed to the manipulation.

For example, if one were studying an herb to treat depression, one would want to control as many factors as possible that could influence the outcome. People already taking an antidepressant drug would have to be excluded. One might also balance the subjects in different groups for severity of depression, psychotherapy treatment, or even levels of physical exercise. Certainly, the subject groups should be balanced for number of males and females, because sex differences in depression could contaminate the results.

Table 1.2
Key methodological elements in experimental drug studies

Necessary Elements
Control groups (e.g., placebo)
Randomization
Double-blind
Useful Elements
Dose-response relationship
Comparison to an existing, established treatment

The experimental results are then analyzed using statistical methods to insure that the results are significant and not likely due to chance. A statistical technique called meta-analysis can be used to compare across several similar studies, giving greater statistical credence to replicated findings.

Experimental drug studies must have a few critical elements (table 1.2). Unfortunately, many herbal medication studies have been done that lack proper methodology controls, invalidating their potentially useful results. All experimental studies must have a *control group,* which is a group of subjects who do not receive treatment. The *experimental groups* comprise subjects who receive some form of active treatment. Thus, the experimental group(s) can be compared to the control group to gauge the effect of the drug. *Placebo control groups* are of paramount importance in a drug study. A drug *placebo* is a treatment that has no intrinsic pharmacological effects. However, the expectation that a treatment will work can have a powerful effect on subjects. Not only are placebo effects produced by inactive treatments, they are produced also by active drugs, because people expect them to have an effect. Thus, the ultimate effects produced by a drug are a combination of the actual pharmacological effects plus placebo effects. In order to sort out these two factors, one must compare the effects of the drug with those of a placebo, rather than no treatment at all.

Randomization is another critical element in experimental studies. When subjects are assigned to control groups and various experimental groups, they must be assigned randomly. This is to eliminate the effects of researcher bias (intentional or unintentional) and any self-selection effects by the subjects. As a hypothetical example, if all subjects who show up early are assigned to one group, and latecomers are assigned to another group, then the differences between groups could be a product of the subjects' personality features, and not just the effects of the drug. Randomization eliminates such a confound.

A *double-blind* control is also an essential element of drug studies. Double-blind means that neither experimenter nor subject knows who is receiving the active treatment or the placebo. Again, this is to eliminate potential bias from both parties. Otherwise, experimenters could unwittingly influence the outcome of the study by subtly treating subjects differently.

In addition to these critical elements, it is often useful to establish a *dose-response relationship* in a study. That is, to show that the size of the dose changes the magnitude of effect. This is accomplished by multiple experimental groups, each receiving a different dose. Showing a dose-response relationship supports the pharmacological nature of the effect and also helps establish the appropriate dose range for clinical treatment.

Clinical Use of Herbal Medicines: Quality of Evidence

When a treatment is considered in a clinical setting, one must evaluate the class of evidence that supports its use. In 1979, a Canadian task force developed guidelines for evaluating the quality of evidence supporting a treatment (see table 1.3). These guidelines have subsequently been adopted by a number of other regulatory panels (Canadian Task Force on the Periodic Health Examination 1979; Woolf 1992).

The Canadian Task Force categorized the quality of evidence based on the type of research study. The quality of evidence was organized into three classes: Class I evidence comes from procedures having at least one randomized controlled study to support them. Class II is divided into three subclasses, where II-1 involves a well-designed controlled study without randomization. Class II-2 evidence comes from well-designed cohort or case-control studies, preferably carried out at more than one research setting. Class II-3 involves uncontrolled research with dramatic results (e.g., penicillin trials in the 1940s). Class III evidence includes the opinions of experts and authorities in the field based on clinical

Table 1.3
Quality of evidence

Class I	At least 1 properly designed, randomized controlled trial
Class II	
II-1	Well-designed, controlled trials without randomization
II-2	Well-designed, cohort or case-control analytic studies, preferably from more than one center or research group
II-3	Comparisons between times or places without intervention; dramatic results in uncontrolled experiments
Class III	Opinions of respected authorities, based on clinical experience, descriptive studies, or reports of expert committees

Source: Canadian Task Force on the Periodic Health Examination, 1979.

experience or descriptive studies. Clearly, Class I evidence is the strongest class of evidence, and each successive class carries less empirical value.

Although the latter classes of evidence provide useful information, Class I evidence is the goal of research in herbal medication. Case studies and anecdotal evidence should be treated seriously, but they should also be followed up with empirical research.

Scientific Disciplines in Herbal Psychopharmacology

Several scientific disciplines contribute to the body of knowledge that is surveyed in this text (table 1.4). Because plants are the focus of attention, we consult *botany* to learn the structure, function, and geographical habitats of the plants in question. *Biochemistry* is necessary to understand the chemical composition of the plant, including the active constituents that give the desired psychological and physiological effects. *Pharmacology* is the study of drugs, including how they affect the body and how the body affects them. Chapter 3 is dedicated to outlining the basic principles of pharmacology, which are then applied to herbal medicines. *Psychopharmacology* is a branch of pharmacology that studies how drugs affect the mind, brain, and behavior. *Pharmacognosy* is specifically the scientific study of the medicinal uses of plants. Thus, the subject of this text could alternately be titled *psychopharmacognosy*, or the scientific study of plants that alter mind, brain, and behavior.

Table 1.4
Scientific disciplines contributing to herbal psychopharmacology

Discipline	Contribution
Botany	Structure, function, and distribution of plants
Biochemistry	Chemical composition of plants, active constituents
Pharmacology	Effects of the drug in the body, effects of the body on the drug
Psychopharmacology	Effects of the drug on mind, brain, and behavior
Pharmacognosy	Scientific study of the medicinal uses of plants
Ethnobotany, ethnopharmacology	Uses of medicinal plants/drugs in the context of culture
Neuroanatomy	Effects of drugs on large and small-scale brain structure
Neurophysiology	Effects of drugs on brain function
Neuroradiology	Imaging of the functional brain effects of drugs
Neurochemistry	Actions of drugs on brain chemistry and receptors
Clinical psychology, psychiatry, neurology	Clinical effects of drugs in the treatment of mind/brain illnesses
Neuropsychology	Characterization and quantification of the cognitive effects of drugs

Related fields are *ethnobotany* and *ethnopharmacology*, which study the use of plants and their drugs in the context of the cultures that use them. To understand the effects of a drug, one must not only look at the biological effects of the drug, but also the larger culture that employs them. The cultural context directs how plant drugs should be used, and instills beliefs about what they do. For example, the hallucinogenic drug *yage* often creates the perception in many native Amazonians that one has transformed into a jaguar. In order to understand this, one must not only describe the effects of the drug in the brain, but also the beliefs and cultural symbols of the people using it. The jaguar is a significant cultural symbol to Amazonian natives, but not to most inhabitants of North America.

Because we are examining psychoactive plants, we must consider their effects in the human nervous system. Broadly, these fields fall under the rubric of *neuroscience*. Its subdisciplines tell us about more-specific actions of the drug. For example, *neuroanatomy* and *neurophysiology* tell us the effects of drugs on the structure and function of the nervous system. Specifically, *neuroradiology* allows us to examine the functional neuroanatomical effects of psychoactive drugs through neuroimaging techniques such as single photon emission computed tomography (SPECT), positron emission tomography (PET), and functional magnetic resonance imaging (fMRI). Essentially, these methods can examine the changes in cerebral blood flow and/or glucose metabolism caused by psychoactive herbs. *Neurochemistry* describes how such drugs will interact with the various neurotransmitters and chemical messengers in the nervous system.

The disciplines of *psychiatry*, *psychology*, and *neurology* are equipped to diagnose disorders of the mind and brain and study the clinical effects of psychoactive herbs. *Neuropsychology* specializes in brain-behavior relationships and is well equipped to quantify and characterize the mental and behavioral effects of psychoactive herbs by using psychometric tests. In this text, particular attention is paid to objective testing data.

Neuropsychology: A Brief Taxonomy of Cognitive Functions

Herbal drugs can have general or specific effects on cognition. To understand the results of neuropsychological testing in drug studies, it will be useful to briefly discuss the breakdown of cognitive functions.

Attention and Concentration

Selective attention involves the ability to focus on some feature of the environment, while filtering out other extraneous features (Lezak 1995; Posner and Driver 1992). For example, when driving through an intersection, one must focus and mentally track other cars, while simultaneously filtering out distractors such as a mailbox on the corner or music on the radio. Other aspects of attention involve *sustaining* attention over a period of time, and *shifting* attention from one target to another. Attention is a limited-capacity system, so *dividing* attention among several targets reduces the amount of attention allocated to each. Also related to attention is the speed at which one is able to process information.

Colloquially, many aspects of working memory are referred to as attention or concentration. Working memory also holds information in consciousness, allowing for manipulation. An example would be remembering three numbers while adding them together. Whereas attention involves operations with present stimuli, working memory sustains activation of a percept in its absence (e.g., remembering a phone number after you looked it up).

Learning and Memory
Learning and memory refers to the ability to acquire, store, and retrieve information (Lezak 1995). A stage model posits that information first enters short-term memory, which is governed by ongoing circuits of activity in the brain. By semantic and contextual meaning, information is then consolidated into long-term memory, which is a relatively permanent store and involves synaptic changes in the brain. Information is later accessed by the process of memory retrieval. Memory is typically evaluated in two modalities: visual and verbal. There are also two very different forms of memory: explicit and implicit. Explicit memory involves personal experiences, facts, and semantic information (Schacter 1997; Verfaellie and Keane 1997). Implicit memory, on the other hand, involves skills, habits, and priming. These two forms of memory are mediated by different systems of structures in the brain.

Language
Language is a symbolic representation system that allows for sophisticated and abstract communication. Several aspects of language can be distinguished, including expression, comprehension, naming, reading, and writing. Language also incorporates our semantic store of factual knowledge and is widely distributed in the brain, typically in the left hemisphere for most people. There are specialized language areas, so that it is possible to selectively lose one aspect but not another (e.g., loss of language expressive ability while retaining comprehension).

Perception
Sensation involves the conversion of physical energy into nerve impulses (e.g., photons are converted into neural signals for vision), but *perception* involves making a meaningful representation of those signals. This includes all sensory modalities: vision (sight), audition (hearing),

somatosenses (bodily senses), olfaction (smell), and gustation (taste), but standardized tests most frequently assess visual or auditory processing. Aspects of visual perception most commonly assessed include shape discrimination, spatial location, line orientation, face perception, visual organization, and construction.

Executive Functions

Executive functions are a varied group of cognitive abilities encompassing abstract reasoning, planning, organization, mental shifting, initiation and inhibition of behavior, judgment, and social conduct. They are crucial for efficient and effective functioning in everyday life. These functions are largely governed by the frontal lobes and associated subcortical structures. To some degree, different brain structures control different executive functions, so one may have a deficit of organization and abstraction, while social conduct is preserved. Numerous experimental and clinical measures have been developed to tap into executive functions, such as the Wisconsin Card Sorting Test, Halstead Category Test, Tower of London, and go/no-go tests (Spreen and Strauss 1998).

Emotion and Personality

Emotions are subjective mood states that interact reciprocally with cognitive processes. Personality refers to traits of emotion and behavior that are more stable over time. Normal and pathological emotional states can be measured, to some degree, with objective tests to quantify changes in mood over time (or after drug treatment). Thus, several clinical scales have been developed for anxiety, depression, and mania. These measures are particularly useful for evaluating the effectiveness of psychotherapeutic herbs.

Conclusions

Psychoactive plants have been a part of human life since our beginning. Our first experiences with them probably came from foraging among plants for food. Through trial-and-error learning and behavioral reinforcement, experience has shaped our use of herbal drugs. Similarly, other nonhuman species may have acquired a limited repertoire of herbal medications through similar means.

With our capacity for language and to explain natural phenomena, humans have historically developed a number of belief systems to explain the effects of medicinal herbs. These vary across cultures and have been passed down across generations through tradition. Although many of the uses of herbs discovered by traditional means are proving to be accurate, their explanations are sometimes rooted in erroneous assumptions or archaic concepts. These traditional rationales may seem innocuous enough, but they lack heuristic value and can hinder further understanding.

Modern scientific research is providing a new analysis of traditional herbs, explaining their effects in biological terms and testing for reliability. With this biological level of understanding, science has been verifying much of traditional herbal wisdom and in some cases suggesting new uses for herbs. Thus, today's herbal medicine is an interesting combination of traditional lore and modern scientific techniques. When properly applied, they work to each other's mutual benefit.

Although our relationship with psychoactive plants is ancient, our knowledge of their uses is still developing. Numerous such plants are available in multiple forms to the general public, and all too often there is little authoritative information to guide their use. More frequently, individuals will publish books that fanatically advocate the use of herbs with overblown claims lacking empirical support. In contrast, the level of expertise among medical professionals is variable, differing across cultures and individuals. The free availability of psychoactive herbs combined with people's tendency to not disclose their use to medical personnel creates an enormous potential for adverse drug interactions. It would be unfortunate if a series of unnecessary and tragic herb-drug interactions publicly marred the enormous therapeutic potential of herbs.

There are essentially two ways to avoid such a scenario. One would be to increase government regulation of herbal medicines so that they are only available with a prescription. This solution is impractical and unfavorable for a few reasons. It would unnecessarily limit the responsible and conscientious use of herbs carried out by millions of people. Also, it would be a largely ineffective restriction because most herbal medications grow abundantly in the wild or in herb gardens. Government restriction would only effectively harm the herbal medicine industry and abolish the standardization and quality control to which we hold it.

Rather than drive herb use underground, a far more rational solution would be to further our understanding of herbs. The lack of proprietary interests in herbal medicines has limited the financial incentives that encourage research by private industry. Instead, government funds could be directed to researchers who investigate the composition of herbs, their effects in the body and brain, and their clinical efficacy. The compilation of traditional and scientific herbal knowledge could be incorporated in the education of medical professionals, guiding the responsible and effective use of herbs in the treatment of illnesses. Efforts could be directed at public education, advising on the proper use of herbs and providing information on when to consult professional medical help.

This text has been written in the spirit of the latter approach. It is hoped that the information compiled and integrated here will further our understanding and capabilities and perhaps inspire new research as well.

2

Basic Neurosciences

An understanding of the nervous system is essential to psychopharmacology. It provides the context in which the actions of drugs are understood. The effects of drugs can be compared based on the commonalities and differences of their actions on neurons. When encountering a new drug, herbal or pharmaceutical, knowing its neuropharmacological mechanisms also allows us to make predictions about its effects. Space limitations allow for only a cursory description of the nervous system here, so the reader is directed to the Recommended Reading section for a more thorough treatment of the topic.

The Neuron

A description of the nervous system probably best starts with its basic functional unit, the neuron (figure 2.1). Neurons have many features in common with other cells of the body, but there are two that make them unique. They are able to conduct electrochemical impulses and they are connected in networks suited for information processing. Their link to the senses and motor effectors allows us to monitor and operate in the environment. The adult human brain is estimated to contain 10^{11} neurons, and each may synapse with 10,000 other neurons. Despite some common core features, neurons are very heterogeneous in their morphology, with thousands of variants. The following are components of the neuron.

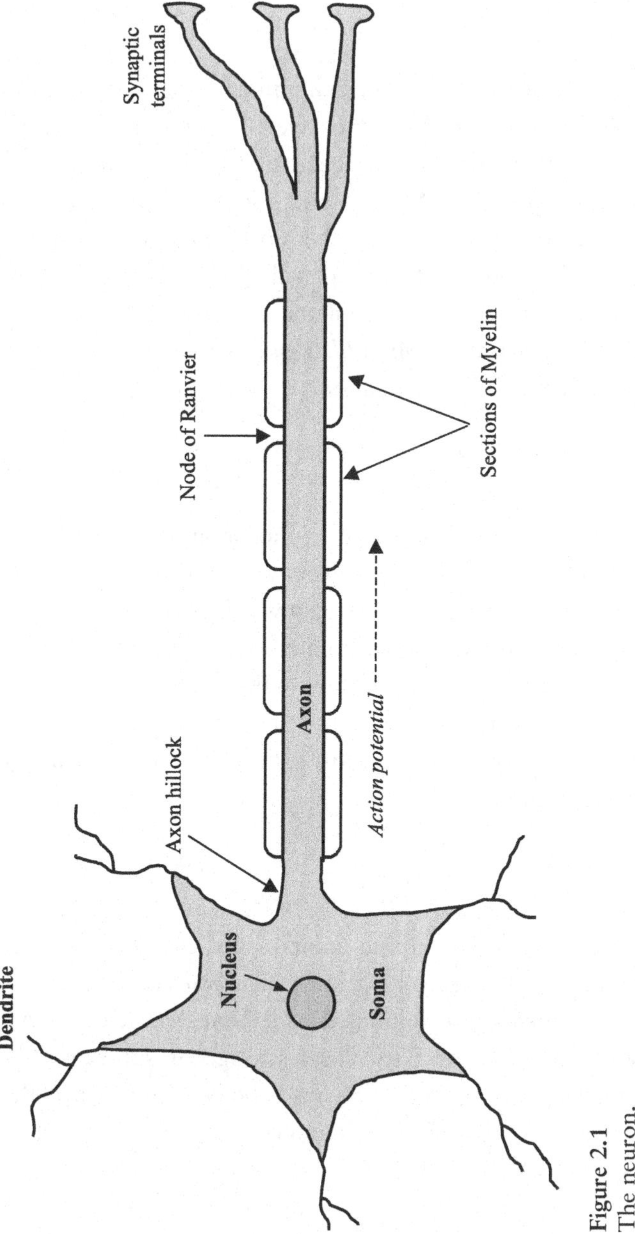

Figure 2.1
The neuron.

Cytoskeleton

The stuctural integrity of the neuron is maintained by a protein cytoskeleton. *Microtubules* are the thickest cytoskeletal elements and have an anionic polarity due to their subunit arrangement. They are composed of microtubule-associated proteins (MAPs), and provide support to the axons and dendrites. *Neurofilaments* are the most abundant cytoskeletal elements, and are composed of proteins called cytokeratins. In the pathology of Alzheimer's disease, neurofilaments are known for their characteristic tangled appearance. *Microfilaments* are the thinnest cytoskeletal elements and are composed of *actin.*

Cell Membrane

The neuronal membrane is composed of a phospholipid bilayer. The phospholipid molecules line up in two layers to form the membrane, with their hydrophobic carbon ends directed inward to the center of the membrane, and their hydrophilic heads pointed out at the extracellular fluid and cytoplasm. Several types of protein molecules are fixed in this membrane and carry out activities essential to the normal function of the neuron. For example, action potentials are propagated by protein ion channels in the membrane.

Organelles

The neuron contains several specialized components, called organelles, which are analogous to the organs of a body. The *nucleus* is approximately 3–18 μm in diameter and contains deoxyribonucleic acid (DNA). The nuclear membrane has pores to allow passage of substances in and out of the nucleus. The nucleus also has a body within called the nucleolus, which manufactures ribosomes and contains ribonucleic acid (RNA), a coating of DNA, and several enzymes.

The *endoplasmic reticulum* (ER) consists of layered membranes surrounding the nucleus. It is involved in the transport of chemicals throughout the cytoplasm. *Rough endoplasmic reticulum* is studded with ribosomes, which are the site of protein assembly from mRNA. *Smooth ER* lacks ribosomes, and provides channels for transport of molecules used in cellular processes. Smooth ER is also the site of lipid synthesis. Proteins produced in the rough ER are secreted by the cell, whereas products from the smooth ER are used within the cell. The *Golgi apparatus* is a complex of folded membranes, which is involved in the post-translational modification of proteins.

Mitochondria are found in the cell body and all processes of the neuron. They possess a double membrane and their own DNA and they play a role in cellular respiration and energy synthesis. Mitochondria contain enzymes essential for energy production in the form of adenosine triphosphate (ATP).

Cell Body

Neurons possess a cell body (also referred to as a *soma* or *perikaryon*), which consists of a nucleus surrounded by cytoplasm and membrane. The survival of the rest of the neuron is dependent upon the integrity of the cell body. Axons and dendrites are both processes that extend from the cell body. Also located in the cell body are the Golgi apparatus, smooth ER, rough ER, and mitochondria. Cytoskeletal elements—microtubules and neurofilaments—are also present.

Dendrites

Dendrites branch out from the cell body and typically form the receiving end of the neuron, although some types of neurons have bidirectional signaling. Upon closer inspection, dendrites form spines that increase the surface area of the dendrite and allow for more synaptic contacts. They contain receptor binding sites for neurotransmitters, which initiate the transmission of an action potential through the neuron. Dendrites are also known to have activity-dependent morphological changes that underly learning and memory.

Axons

The axon is a long narrow process that extends from the cell body and conveys action potentials toward the neuron's synapses. Action poten-

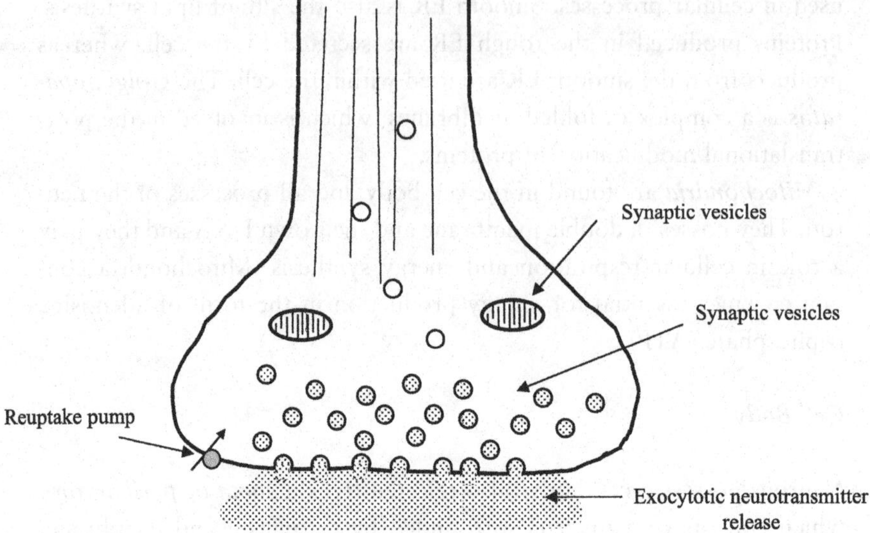

Figure 2.2
The synaptic terminal.

tials spread along the axonal membrane toward the synaptic terminals, from which neurotransmitters are released (figure 2.2). Axoplasmic transport occurs within the axon, along microtubules. Transport of substances occurs both toward and away from the terminals, referred to as anterograde and retrograde transport, respectively. Within the terminals are vesicles that contain neurotransmitters for release. The site where the cell body transitions into the axon is the *hillock*. The point of contact between the axon terminal and an adjacent neuron is called the synapse. Synapses of this type may be axo-dendritic, axo-somatic, or axo-axonic.

Glial Cells

Glial cells are thought to serve a support function in the nervous system, and are not directly responsible for information processing. Rather, they are crucial to the effective function and survival of neurons. Glia are grossly divided into *macroglia* and *microglia*. Macroglia consist of *astrocytes*, *oligodendroglia*, and *Schwann cells*. Astrocytes are present in the central nervous system (CNS), providing structural support, transporting nutrients, and phagocytizing cellular debris. They transport glucose and also perform a metabolic service by converting it to lactate before it is transported to the neurons. Astrocytes also store glucose in the form of glycogen, serving as a small metabolic reservoir.

Oligodendrocytes are present in the CNS as well and wrap around axons to form a myelin sheath. Myelin wraps into concentric layers that spiral around the axon. Gaps in the oligodendrocytes are the *nodes of Ranvier*, where the membrane maintains contact with extracellular fluid. The nodes serve to propagate the action potential in myelinated axons. Schwann cells perform an analogous function, myelinating axons in the peripheral nervous system. Not all neurons are myelinated, but myelination increases the metabolic efficiency of action potentials. Demyelination of neurons produces deficits in neuronal conduction, as is seen in multiple sclerosis.

Microglia, in contrast, serve as macrophages in the central nervous system. They are relatively inactive during normal conditions, but rapidly proliferate during inflammatory or degenerative processes.

Brain Permeability Barriers

The brain is protected from potentially toxic substances in the blood by a semipermeable barrier called the *blood-brain barrier*. This barrier is created by tight junctions between endothelial cells forming the wall of capillaries in the brain and fatty astrocytes that wrap the capillaries. Whereas in peripheral tissues the endothelial junctions contain gaps that freely allow substances to pass through, brain capillaries do not contain such gaps. Penetration of substances across the blood-brain barrier is determined by the molecular size, its lipid-solubility, and the presence of endothelial carrier transport to bring certain substances through. The epithelium of the choroid plexus and ventricles form a blood-cerebrospinal fluid (CSF) barrier, which is a small fraction of the size of the blood-brain barrier. However, it mediates a limited transport of certain circulating peptides, such as leptin.

Membrane Proteins

Ion Pumps

Present in the membrane are membrane-spanning proteins that pump ions across the membrane. The differential distribution of ions that form the membrane potential is driven by ion pumps. Despite leakage currents, the Na^+ and K^+ gradients are maintained by the Na^+/K^+ pump. Hydrolysis of one molecule of ATP allows three Na^+ ions to be carried out, and two K^+ ions to be carried in. Energy-dependent ion pumps are crucial for maintainance of steady-state ion gradients and the resting potential. Various forms of energy deprivation will hinder ion pumps, causing catastrophic neurochemical cascades and neurotoxicity.

Ion Channels

Ion channels are membrane proteins that allow the passage of ions in or out of the cell. The ion flux is a passive process and occurs down the electrical and chemical gradients. There are four general types of ion channels recognized. *Nongated channels* are continuously open, allowing a leakage current across the membrane; *voltage-gated channels* are opened and closed by their sensitivity to the local membrane potential; *chemically gated* channels are opened by the binding of a ligand to a receptor site; and *ion-gated* channels are gated by sensitivity to intracellular ion concentrations. Many ion channels may be ion-specific, selectively allowing passage of either K^+, Na^+, or Ca^+, although some are less selective. Cations such as Mg^{2+}, Mn^{2+}, Co^{2+}, and Cd^{2+} act as inhibitors of voltage-gated channels. The NMDA receptor channel is unique in that it is both chemically and voltage-gated, requiring both simultaneously for channel opening.

Membrane Potential

In a resting state, neurons maintain a negatively charged potential, referred to as the *resting potential*, that is actively maintained by energy-dependent ion pumps. Metabolic deprivation of neurons causes a breakdown of this homeostasis with neurotoxic consequences.

Membrane potentials are determined by a balance between two physical forces: *chemical diffusion* and *electrostatic pressure*. Chemical diffusion is the tendency of particles to move toward a uniform distribution throughout a volume. Electrostatic pressure is simply the tendency for like-charged particles to repel and oppositely charged particles to attract each other.

The neuronal membrane is relatively permeable to potassium (K^+). In a resting state, K^+ is in higher concentration intracellularly, due to the activity of the Na^+/K^+ pump and attraction of of intraneuronal anionic proteins (figure 2.3). However, by force of diffusion, K^+ is also drawn out of the cell by the concentration gradient. The resting potential is largely determined by the distribution of K^+ ions. The membrane is relatively impermeable to Na^+, which is pumped out of the cell and in higher concentrations extracellularly. It is drawn into the neuron by both the forces of chemical diffusion and by electrostatic pressure, due to the membrane potential set by K^+. This distribution of ions results in a resting potential of −60 to −70 mV with respect to the extracellular fluid. Chloride (Cl^-) is a negatively charged ion that is in higher concentration outisde the cell due to membrane impermeability and the Na^+/Cl^- pump. At the resting potential, Cl^- is drawn intracellularly by force of diffusion, but also repelled from the negatively charged intracellular milieu by electrostatic pressure. Finally, Ca^{2+} is another cation that, like Na^+, is concentrated outside the cell. It is drawn intracellularly by both chemical diffusion and electrostatic pressure.

The Action Potential

In response to stimulation, the neuronal membrane becomes more permeable to Na^+, which is drawn into the neuron down the electrical and chemical diffusion gradients. This depolarizes the neuron and makes the membrane further permeable to Na^+. If sufficiently depolarized, a threshold of excitation is reached (approximately −60 mV), where voltage-gated Na^+ channels open and the membrane becomes highly permeable

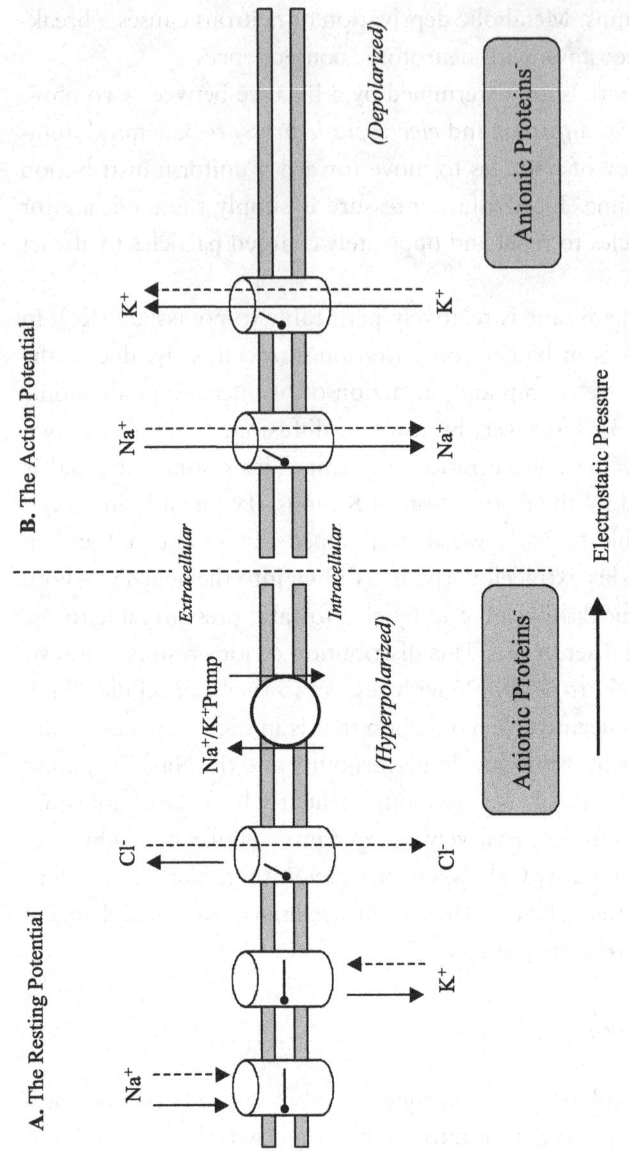

Figure 2.3
The membrane potential.

to Na^+. The critical region for triggering this event is the axon hillock. An action potential is initiated and the Na^+ influx drives the membrane potential up to approximately +55 mV. This depolarization is limited and reversed by inactivation of Na^+ channels and efflux of K^+ through delayed-opening K^+ channels. The ion pumps then restore resting-level ion gradients. The action potential is followed by a brief refractory period, during which the neuron is slightly hyperpolarized below its resting potential.

Once an action potential is initiated at the hillock, it continues in a self-propagating fashion to the end of the axon. Voltage-sensitive ion channels are opened by the depolarization, allowing further influx of Na^+ and a spread of the action potential. Thus, the action potential is a self-regenerating spread of membrane depolarization.

Myelinated Conduction

Conduction of the action potential in myelinated axons is called *saltatory conduction.* Because ion flux only occurs at the nodes of Ranvier, the action potential jumps, in effect, from node to node. This provides two advantages, speeding the rate of conduction and reducing the metabolic cost of an action potential, because energy-dependent ion transporters are not needed along myelinated segments.

Chemical Synapses

Neurotransmitter Release

Chemical messengers, or neurotransmitters, are normally released when an action potential reaches the synaptic terminals. This process is entirely Ca^{2+}-dependent. Intracellular Ca^{2+} causes movement of neurotransmitter-containing synaptic vesicles toward the membrane. Removal of Ca^{2+} will prevent this process, preventing neurotransmitter release even if an action potential arrives.

The synaptic vesicles dock with proteins on the neuronal membrane and release their contents through exocytosis. The neurotransmitters contained in the vesicles spill into the synapse and passively diffuse across.

A synaptic neurotransmitter may become inactivated by several mechanisms. It may passively diffuse out of the synapse; it may undergo enzymatic breakdown; it may be taken up into a cell through a selective reuptake pump; and, intracellularly, it may be taken back into a vesicle for future release, or it may be converted enzymatically.

In certain neurons, a different type of synapse, called a gap junction, may be formed. Gap junction transmission occurs through membrane channels made of six subunits, which directly connect with other postsynaptic gap junction channels. When the channels open, there is a continuity of cytoplasm and exchange of ions between the two neurons. This mode of transmission is faster because it does not involve the time-consuming processes of neurotransmitter release, diffusion across the synapse, and receptor binding.

Receptors

Neurotransmitters create their effects by binding to receptor proteins. These may be broadly classified by their effector mechanisms as ionotropic or metabotropic. Ionotropic receptors are located on membrane ion channels composed of five subunits, each with four transmembrane domains (figures 2.4, 2.5). The binding of a ligand to the receptor causes a conformational change in the channel, allowing ion permeability. Ions then flow passively down the concentration gradient, either depolarizing or hyperpolarizing the neuron. Other receptors on the ion channel may be allosteric, which may not itself initiate ion permeability, but instead creates effects by altering the binding of ligands to the receptor.

Metabotropic receptors, in contrast, create their effects by activating an intracellular G protein. The metabotropic receptors are monomers with seven transmembrane domains. The activated G protein, in turn, may activate an ion channel from an intracellular site. Alternately, G proteins work by activation or inhibition of enzymes that produce intracellular messengers. For example, activation of adenylate cyclase increases production of cyclic adenosine monophosphate (cAMP). Other effector mechanisms include activation of phospholipases, diacylglycerol, creation of inositol phosphates, and production of arachidonic acid products. Ultimately, these cascades can result in protein phosphorylation,

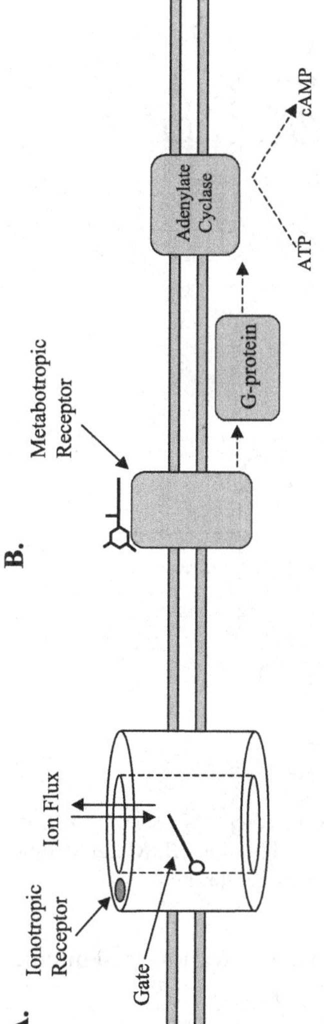

Figure 2.4
(*A*) Example of an ionotropic receptor. (*B*) Example of a metabotropic receptor.

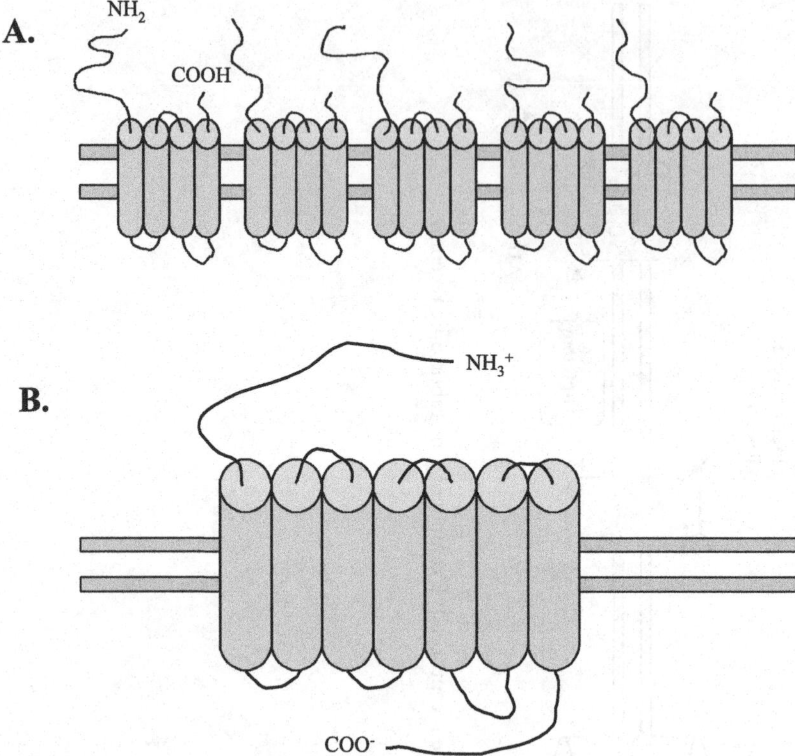

Figure 2.5
Subunit structure of receptor proteins. (*A*) Ionotropic receptors are composed of five subunits, each consisting of four transmembrane domains. (*B*) Metabotropic receptors are composed of a single unit of seven transmembrane domains.

release of intracellular Ca^{2+} from stores, enzyme activation, and altered gene transcription and protein synthesis.

Postsynaptic Potentials

Activation of ionotropic mechanisms creates postsynaptic potentials. An influx of cations or efflux of anions depolarizes the neuron, creating an excitatory-postsynaptic potential (EPSP). Conversely, an influx of anions or efflux of cations hyperpolarizes the neuron, creating an inhibitory-postsynaptic potential (IPSP). Postsynaptic potentials are summated both spatially and temporally, where they must convergently occur in the same neuron and close enough in time to amount to a larger effect and trigger an action potential.

Neurotransmitters

A variety of substances have been found to serve as neurotransmitters in the nervous system. Most of these have actions outside the nervous system as well. Classically, the term *neurotransmitter* implies ionotropic actions on neurons, while those with metabotropic actions are regarded as *neuromodulators*. This distinction is blurred, however, by the fact that many substances can have either action, depending on the receptor to which it binds. Table 2.1 summarizes the major classes of neurotransmitters and their receptor-effector mechanisms.

Acetylcholine

Acetylcholine (ACh) is a phospholipid-derived neurotransmitter. It is produced from the precursors, choline and acetyl coenzyme A (CoA), by a reaction with the enzyme choline acetyltransferase (ChAT). It is broken down in the synapse by acetylcholinesterase (AchE), and choline is taken back up into the neuron for reuse. The drug hemicholinium inhibits uptake of choline, and several drugs, including physostigmine, prevent breakdown of ACh by inhibiting AChE. ACh has both ionotropic and metabotropic receptors. Nicotinic ACh receptors are ionotropic, for which the drug nicotine is an agonist and mecamylamine is an antagonist. The nicotinic channel is cation selective and its activation results in depolarization. The muscarinic ACh receptors are metabotropic, and are subdivided into five subtypes (M_1 to M_5). Muscarinic agonists include muscarine and pilocarpine, and antagonists include atropine and scopolamine.

ACh is necessary for control of skeletal muscle in verterbrates, acting as the neurotransmitter at the neuromuscular junction. It is also involved in transmission in the autonomic nervous system (see below, under "Neuroanatomy"). Central ACh is produced in two general areas in the brain incuding the basal forebrain (medial septal nuclei, diagonal band

Table 2.1
Neurotransmitter receptor and effector mechanisms

Neurotransmitter	Subtypes	Effector mechanisms
Acetylcholine		
Nicotinic	Neuronal, muscle	Cation conductance
Muscarinic	M_1–M_5	IP_3/DAG, ↓cAMP, ↑K^+
Monoamines		
DA	D_1–D_5	cAMP (↑ or ↓), ↓K^+, ↓Ca^{2+}
NE	α_1, α_2, β_1–β_3	↓cAMP, IP_3/DAG, ↑K^+, ↓Ca^{2+}
5-HT	5-HT_1–5-HT_7	cAMP (↑ or ↓), IP_3/DAG, 5-HT_3 is ionotropic via a G-protein
Amino Acids		
Glutamate	NMDA, AMPA, kainate	Cation conductance
	$mGluR_1$–$mGluR_7$	IP_3/DAG, ↓cAMP
GABA	$GABA_A$; $GABA_B$	Cl^- conductance (A); ↓cAMP, ↑K^+, ↓Ca^{2+}
Glycine	(Strychnine-sensitive channel)	Cl^- conductance
Purines		
Adenosine	P_1 (A_1–A_3)	cAMP (↑ or ↓), IP_3/DAG, ↑K^+, ↓Ca^{2+}
ATP	P_2	Cation channel, IP_3/DAG, ↓cAMP
Selected Neuropeptides		
Opioid	μ, κ, δ, ORL	↓cAMP, ↑K^+, ↓Ca^{2+}
Tachykinin	NK_1, NK_2, NK_3	IP_3/DAG
CCK	CCK_A, CCK_B	IP_3/DAG

of Broca, and basal nucleus of Meynert) and pons (pedunculopontine tegmental nuclei, laterodorsal tegmental nuclei).

Monoamines

The monoamines are neurotransmitters derived from amino acids and are subdivided into catecholamines and indolamines.

The catecholamines are dopamine (DA), norepinephrine (NE; also referred to as noradrenaline), and epinephrine (EP; also referred to as adrenaline). They are synthesized from the amino acid L-tyrosine by a series of enzymatic steps. L-tyrosine is converted to L-dopa (dihydroxyphenylalanine) by tyrosine hydroxylase. L-dopa is then converted to DA by dopa decarboxylase. In noradrenergic neurons, DA is further converted into NE by dopamine-β-hydroxylase, and in adrenergic neurons, NE is further converted to EP by phenylethanolamine-*N*-methyltransferase. The catecholamines are degraded extracelluarly by catechol-O-methyltransferase and intracellularly by monoamine oxidase (MAO). MAO is inhibited by drugs such as phenylzine. COMT is inhibited by tolcapone. The primary metabolites of DA are 3,4-dihydroxyphenylacetic acid (DOPAC) and homovanillic acid (HVA). The primary noradrenergic metabolites are 3-methoxy-4-hydroxy-mandelic acid (VMA) and 3-methoxy-4-hydroxy-phenylglycol (MHPG).

DA receptors are classified as D_1 to D_5. Bromocriptine and pergolide act as agonists at certain subtypes, and neuroleptics such as haloperidol and thorazine act as antagonists. It is produced by several nuclei in the brain, but most notably the substantia nigra and the ventral tegmental area (VTA) of the midbrain. The substantia nigra mainly projects to the basal ganglia and the VTA supplies limbic and cortical structures.

NE and EP are agonists at α and β receptors. These are subdivided into α_{1A}, α_{1B}, α_{1D}, α_{2A}, α_{2B} α_{2C}, β_1, β_2 and β_3 subtypes. Phenylephrine is an agonist and prazosin is an antagonist at α_1 receptors. Guanabenz is an agonist at α_2 receptors, and yohimbine is an antagonist. Isoproterenol is an agonist at β receptors, and propanolol is an antagonist. NE is released by neurons originating in several brain stem nuclei, most notably the dorsolateral tegmentum and nucleus locus coeruleus. Adrenergic nuclei are located in the medulla.

Serotonin is an indolamine neurotransmitter, derived from the amino acid L-tryptophan. Tryptophan is converted to 5-hydroxytryptophan (5-HTP) by tryptophan hydroxylase. 5-HTP is converted to 5-hydroxytryptamine (serotonin, 5-HT) by aromatic amino acid decarboxylase. In the pineal gland, 5-HT may be further converted to *N*-acetyl serotonin by 5-HT *N*-acetyltransferase and then to melatonin by 5-hyroxyindole-O-methyltransferase. 5-HT is catabolized by monoamine oxidase, and the primary end metabolite is 5-hydroxyindoleacetic acid (5-HIAA).

Receptors for 5-HT are labeled 5-HT_1 to 5-HT_7. The 5-HT_1 subtype is further subdivided into 5-HT_{1A}, 5-HT_{1B}, 5-HT_{1D}, 5-HT_{1E}, and 5-HT_{1F}, and 5-HT_2 is subdivided into 5-HT_{2A}, 5-HT_{2B} and 5-HT_{2C}. 5-HT receptors work through several effector mechanisms including adenylate cyclase and phospholipases, and one subtype gates a cation channel (5-HT_3). Several 5-HT agonists exist with some subtype specificity, including sumatriptan (selective to 5-HT_{1E}, and 5-HT_{1F}) and 2,5-dimethoxy-4iodoamphetamine (selective to 5-HT_{2A}, and 5-HT_{2B}). 5-HT antagonists include spiperone (5-HT_{1A}), ketanserin (5-HT_2), and ondansetron (5-HT_3).

Nuclei of 5-HT-producing neurons are located on many parts of the brain stem, mostly consisting of the raphe nuclei. Whereas the nuclei raphe obscurus, raphe pallidus, and raphe magnus project to brain stem and spinal targets, the nuclei raphe dorsalis, raphe medianis, and raphe pontis oralis project to forebrain sites.

Amino Acids

The amino acid neurotransmitters are subdivided into primarily excitatory (glutamate, aspartate) and inhibitory (γ-aminobutyric acid, GABA, glycine) types.

The excitatory amino acids (EAA), glutamate and aspartate, are the principal excitatory neurotransmitters in the brain. They are released by neurons in several distinct anatomical pathways, such as corticofugal projections, but their distribution is practically ubiquitous in the central nervous system. There are both metabotropic and ionotropic EAA receptors. The metabotropic receptors bind glutamate and are labeled $mGluR_1$ to $mGluR_8$. They are coupled via G-proteins to phosphoinositide hydrolysis, phospholipase D, and cAMP production. Ionotropic EAA receptors have been divided into three subtypes: *N*-methyl-D-aspartate (NMDA), alpha-amino-3-hydroxy-5-methyl-4-isoxazole-proprionic acid (AMPA), and kainate receptors (Nakanishi 1992).

The ionotropic receptors, AMPA and kainate, recognize glutamate but not aspartate as a ligand. Opening the channels allows infux of both Ca^{2+} and Na^+. The NMDA receptor-channel is a cationic channel that allows influx of Ca^{2+} and Na^+, as well as efflux of K^+ when activated by glutamate or aspartate (figure 2.6). In addition to the EAA binding site, the NMDA receptor-channel has several other allosteric binding sites. Among them is the Mg^{2+} site, which is located within the channel

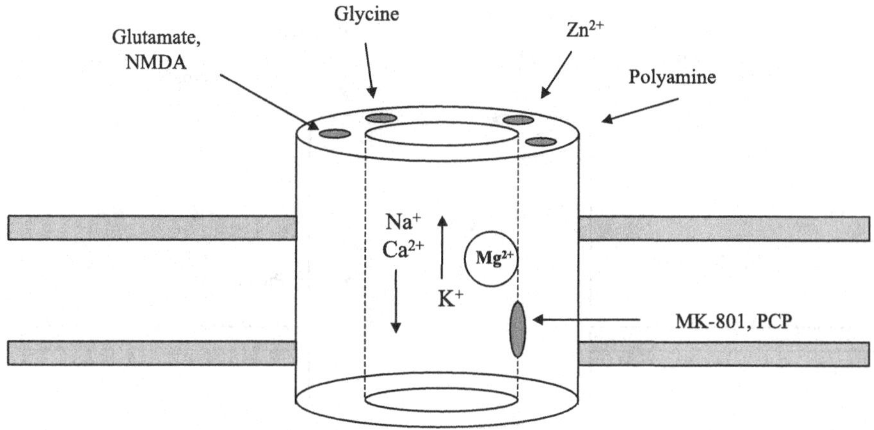

Figure 2.6
The NMDA channel.

opening and blocks the channel in a voltage-dependent manner. The Zn^{2+} site is located extracellularly and also inhibits channel opening, but in a voltage-independent manner. Thus, the NMDA receptor-channel is believed to be unique in that it is gated simultaneously by voltage and by the binding of ligands. Also within the channel opening is a binding site for MK-801, where binding inhibits ion flux as well. There is also a strychnine-insensitive glycine receptor that is essential for NMDA channel opening, so glycine is regarded as a co-agonist for the NMDA channel.

Glutamate may be converted by glutamic acid decarboxylase into GABA. GABA is the prinicpal inhibitory neurotransmitter in the brain, and is also found in the spinal cord. GABA is catabolized by GABA transaminase (GABA-T) into succinic semialdehyde. There are two GABA receptors, $GABA_A$ and $GABA_B$. $GABA_A$ is a Cl^- channel that is gated by GABA (figure 2.7). Muscimol is an agonist at this receptor and bicuculline is an antagonist. There are several allosteric sites on the $GABA_A$ channel that enhance GABA binding. These allosteric modifiers include benzodiazepines, barbiturates, ethanol, and steroids such as allopregnanolone. Picrotoxin, in contrast, inhibits $GABA_A$. The $GABA_B$ receptor is a metabotropic receptor that inhibits production of cAMP, opens K^+ channels, and closes Ca^{2+} channels via a G protein.

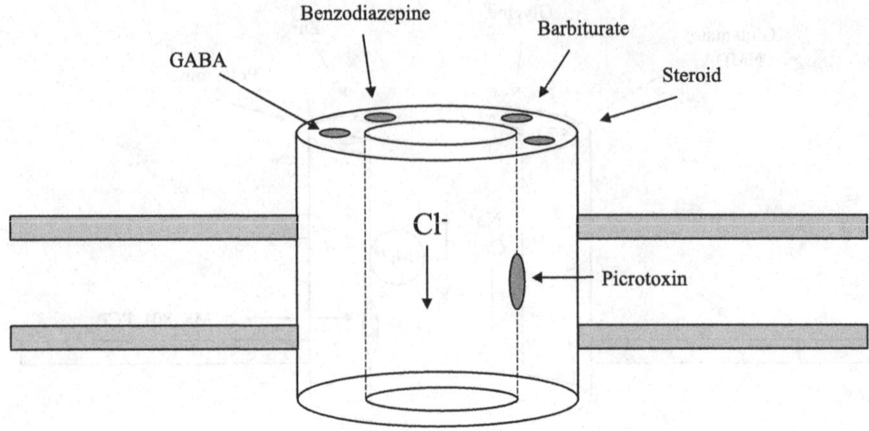

Figure 2.7
The $GABA_A$ channel.

Glycine plays an important inhibitory role in the lower brain stem and spinal cord. Little is known about the synthesis of glycine. It activates a Cl^- channel, which is antagonized by strychnine. Other endogenous amino acids may activate the glycine channel, such as taurine and *β*-alanine.

Neuropeptides

A variety of peptides are utilized in the nervous system as neurotransmitters. Unlike other neurotransmitters, which can be synthesized in various parts of the neuron like the axon terminals, neuropeptides are produced by gene transcription and translation. They may colocalize and be coreleased with ACh, monoamines, or amino acid neurotransmitters. Their receptors are metabotropic and may work through a variety of effector mechanisms. Neuropeptides are formed and degraded by a variety of peptidase enzymes.

Neuropeptides are often grouped by their structural similarity or tissue source. Among these are the hypothalamic releasing factors (e.g., corticotrophin-releasing factor [CRF], thyrotropin-releasing hormone), anteior pituitary hormones (e.g., adrenocorticotrophic hormone [ACTH], follicle-stimulating hormone [FSH]), and posterior pituitary hormones (vasopressin and oxytocin). Several gastrointestinal peptides have been found to be active in the nervous system including cholecystokinin and neurotensin. Tachykinin neuropeptides include substance P, neurokinin A, and neurokinin B. The opioid neuropeptides derive from three main families: pro-opiomelanocortin, pro-dynorphin, and pro-enkephalin (see chapter 8 for a detailed description).

Neurohormones

A number of neurotransmitter substances are used peripherally as hormones, including amines and peptides (see above). Although they are chemically identical, they represent a different pool of chemical messengers because they generally do not pass the blood-brain barrier. However, several hormones readily pass the blood-brain barrier and have direct effects in the central nervous system.

The hypothalamus releases severeal different releasing factors that travel through portal vessels to the anterior pituitary. There they initiate the release of trophic hormones, which travel through blood vessels to the various endocrine glands and trigger release of their hormones. Hormones from the adrenal, gonadal, and thyroid glands feed back to the pituitary gland and the brain, regulating releasing factors and trophic hormones. Hormones act through membrane-bound metabotropic receptors, as well as to intracellular receptors that directly initiate gene expression.

Soluble Gasses

Relatively recently, the gases nitric oxide (NO) and carbon monoxide (CO) have been found to act as neurotransmitters in the nervous system. Nitric oxide is synthesized from L-arginine via nitric oxide synthase, requiring NADPH as a co-enzyme and tetrahydrobiopterin as a cofactor. Unlike other neurotransmitters, NO is a small, very soluble molecule and cannot be stored in synaptic vesicles. Rather, it is synthesized on demand and freely diffuses through membranes. It is not broken down enzymatically because it is unstable and degrades rapidly. NO may have several actions, one of which is to increase the production of cGMP by guanylyl cyclase. It is thought to play a role in synaptic plasticity. It also serves as a chemical messenger in several other body tissues and is a vasodilator. CO is produced in the conversion of heme to biliverdin by heme oxygenase in the brain, spleen, and liver.

Purines

In addition to their role in energy metabolism, adenosine and adenosine triphosphate (ATP) serve as neurotransmitters. They are stored in synaptic vesicles and released in response to action potentials in widespread areas of the nervous system. A number of enzymes catalyze ATP and/or adenosine, including ATP diphosphohydrolase, 5′-nucleotidase, adenosine deaminase, and adenosine kinase. Membrane receptors for purine neurotransmitters are divided into P_1, which binds adenosine, and P_2, which binds ATP. The cloned P_1 receptors have been subdivided into A_1, A_{2A}, A_{2B}, and A_3, which are metabotropic receptors. The P_2 receptors are subdivided into ionotropic receptors (P_{2x1}–P_{2x7}) and metabotropic (P_{2y1}, P_{2y2}, P_{2y4} and P_{2y6}). However, P_{2x7}, P_{2y2}, P_{2y4}, and P_{2y6} subtypes are not found in the nervous system.

Neuroanatomy

The direct action of psychoactive drugs is upon neurochemical systems, but to fully appreciate their effects one must consider the neurophysiological effects they produce in the context of neuroanatomical structures. A drug may produce a spectrum of psychological and behavioral effects, each of which may be mediated by actions in different neuroanatomical structures. For example, the effects of cannabinoids on memory and cognition are through their actions in the cortex, striatum, and hippocampus. However, their behavioral reinforcing effects are likely mediated through the nucleus accumbens, and their effects on thermoregulation are mediated through the hypothalamus. These effects are dissociable through experimental intracerebral injections, but occur in concert when a drug is administered systemically.

The nervous system is divided into the central and peripheral nervous systems (CNS and PNS). The CNS consists of the brain and spinal cord, and the PNS consists of peripheral nerves and ganglia extending from the CNS. The spinal cord is functionally divided into somatic and autonomic divisions. The somatic division involves bodily sensations and skeletomotor functions, while the autonomic division controls smooth muscle, cardiac muscle, and exocrine glands.

Tissue in the nervous system is grossly classified as white or gray matter. White matter consists of tracts of axons, while gray matter consists of neuronal soma. Axons traveling in a peripheral bundle are referred to as a nerve, while central axons form a *tract* or *funiculus*. Alternately, axons that connect across the midline of the nervous system are referred to as a commissure. The largest commissure is the corpus callosum, which connects the left and right hemispheres of the brain. The cell bodies of gray matter may be organized into layers, which are referred to as cortex, such as the cerebral or cerebellar cortex. Alternately, cell bodies may be organized into a cluster, which is referred to centrally as a nucleus or peripherally as a ganglion. The exception to this is the basal ganglia, which are located deep in the brain.

Meninges

The entire CNS is covered by the meninges, which form a protective covering. The outermost is the *dura*, which is tough and leathery in consistency. It is highly vascularized and innervated, so it is sensitive to pain. The arachnoid membrane is a weblike, spongy layer beneath the dura. Beneath the arachnoid is the subarachnoid space, which is filled with cerebrospinal fluid. Beneath the subarachnoid space is a thin layer of cells called the *pia*, which covers the brain and spinal cord.

Ventricular System

Cerebrospinal fluid is produced in chambers within the brain called *ventricles*. Two lateral ventricles and a midline third ventricle are contained within the cerebrum, while the fourth ventricle exists within the brain stem. CSF is produced by the choroid plexus in the lateral and third ventricles. It flows out through the ventricles by a series of aqueducts and into subarachnoid space. CSF supports the brain and spinal cord, absorbing impact. Occlusions of the ventricular system can result in elevated intracranial pressure, or *hydrocephalus.*

Spinal Cord

The spinal cord is the major route of input and output for the central nervous system. It is covered by the meninges and sits within the vertebral column. There are 31 pairs of spinal nerves, exiting at the dorsal and ventral roots of the spinal cord. The spinal cord is divided into four levels (superior to inferior): cervical, thoracic, lumbar, and sacral. A cross section of the spinal cord shows a butterfly-shaped core of gray matter (neuronal soma), and an outer surrounding area of white matter (axon tracts).

In general, dorsal regions of the spinal cord are involved in sensory processes, while ventral regions are involved in motor functions. However, ventral roots and axonal tracts may also be involved in pain and temperature. Many simple and complex motor reflexes are well organized at the spinal level.

The cranial nerves exit directly from the brain and brain stem. They control sensory, motor, and autonomic functions for parts of the neck and head. Vision, smell, taste, balance, hearing, and sensations and movements of the face are all mediated by cranial nerves. However, one large nerve, the vagus, regulates many visceral organs including the heart and the digestive tract.

Autonomic Nervous System

The autonomic nervous system is subdivided into the sympathetic and parasympathetic nervous systems. The sympathetic branch is involved in the expenditure of energy, while the parasympathetic conserves and stores energy. The sympathetic efferent neurons are in the thoracic and lumbar spinal cord, and project ventrally out to sympathetic ganglia outside of the spinal cord. The preganglionic sympathetic neurons synapse onto postganglionic neurons, which innervate the target organs. The preganglionic neurons use ACh as their neurotransmitter, which acts on nicotinic receptors on postganglionic neurons (table 2.2). The

Table 2.2
Organization of the sympathetic and parasympathetic branches

	Sympathetic	Parasympathetic
Location of ganglia	Proximal to spinal cord	Proximal to target organs
Preganglionic fibers	ACh	ACh
Ganglionic Receptor	Nicotinic	Nicotinic
Postganglionic fibers	NE	ACh
Target organ receptor	α, β	Muscarinic

Table 2.3
Actions of the autonomic nervous system

Target	Sympathetic	Parasympathetic
Pupil	Dilation	Constriction
Salivation	Inhibits	Stimulates
Bronchi	Dilates	Constricts
Heart rate	Accelerates	Decelerates
Liver	Glycogen → glucose	Glucose → glycogen
Digestion	Inhibits	Stimulates
Adrenal	Release of NE, EP	(no effect)
Bladder	Relaxes	Constricts
Genitals	Stimulates orgasm	Stimulates arousal

postganglionic neurons, in turn, use NE as their neurotransmitter, which acts on α and β receptors on the target organs. Activation of the sympathetic branch causes pupillary constriction, inhibits salivation, dilates lung bronchi, accelerates heart rate, constricts cutaneous blood vessels, inhibits digestion, and stimulates conversion of glycogen to glucose (table 2.3).

Parasympathetic neurons are located in the brain stem and travel in the vagus nerve, although some are located in the sacral spinal cord for control of eliminative and sexual functions. The parasympathetic ganglia are distal from the spinal cord and close to the target organs. Similar to the sympathetic branch, the parasympathetic preganglionic neurons utilize ACh and nicotinic receptors at the ganglia. Unlike its counterpart, the postganglionic parasympathetic neurons use ACh and muscarinic receptors.

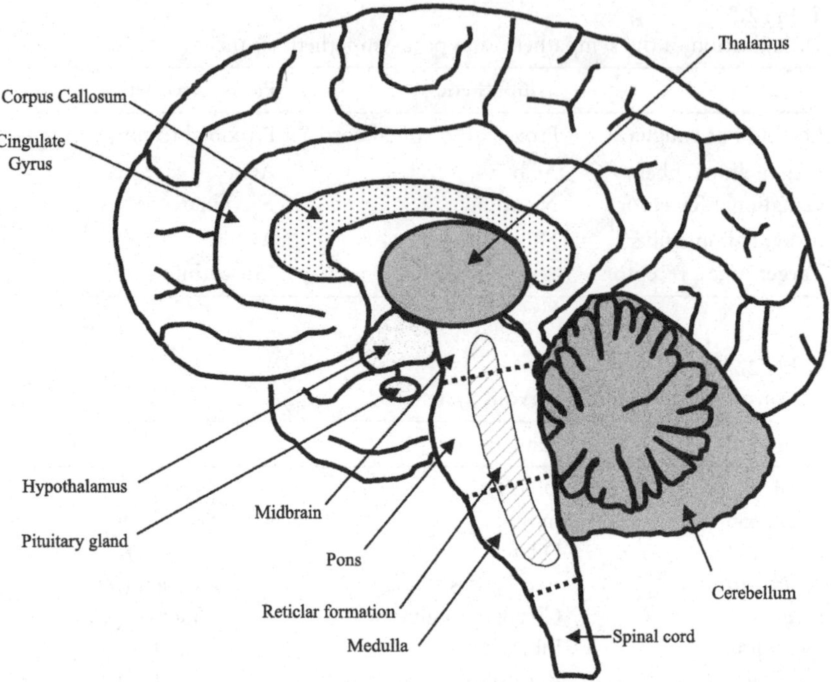

Figure 2.8
Lateral view of the brain.

Activation of the parasympathetic branch causes pupillary dilation, increases salivation, constricts lung bronchi, decelerates heart rate, increases digestion, and stimulates conversion of glycose to glycogen. Whereas the parasympathetic branch is involved in physiological sexual arousal, the sympathetic branch is involved in the physiological aspect of orgasm.

Brain Stem

The *medulla* (myelencephalon) is the most caudal part of the brain stem, and is continuous with the spinal cord. It contains several cranial nerve nuclei and part of the reticular formation, which regulates cardiovascular function, respiration, and skeletomotor tone (figure 2.8). The reticular formation consists of several nuclei that form the core of the entire brain stem, projecting rostrally to the brain and caudally to the spinal cord.

The *pons* and *cerebellum* (metencephalon) form the middle portion of the brain stem, bordered rostrally by the midbrain and caudally by the medulla. It also contains a portion of the brain stem and several nuclei important to arousal and sleep. The cerebellum branches off of the back of the brain stem. It has a cortical surface and deep nuclei imbedded in white matter. Through its connections, it has involvement in diverse functions including balance, fine motor coordination, and even cognition.

The *midbrain* (mesencephalon) is the top of the brain stem. The dorsal midbrain is the tectum, which is involved in eye movements and reflexive reactions to sensory stimuli. The mesencephalic reticular formation projects upward to the forebrain and is involved in arousal and attention. The periaqueductal gray area surrounds the cerebral aqueduct, and integrates analgesic, defensive/aggressive, sexual, and autonomic responses. The red nucleus and substantia nigra are important structures in motor function.

There are several nuclei located in the brainstem reticular formation known for their role in producing specific neurotransmitters and releasing them in the brain and/or spinal cord. As mentioned above, these are the locus coeruleus and dorsolateral tegmentum (norepinephrine), raphe nuclei (5-HT), ventral tegmental area and substantia nigra (DA), and pedunculopontine tegmental nuclei and laterodorsal tegmental nuclei (acetylcholine). These nuclei also receive projections from forebrain areas. Thus, they may be regarded as part of forebrain-brainstem circuits, providing context-dependent feedback. Through their connections, they play important modulatory roles in cognitive, emotional, motor, and homeostatic functions.

Diencephalon

The diencephalon is composed of several nuclei that are grossly grouped into the thalamus, hypothalamus, epithalamus, and subthalamic nucleus. The thalamus serves as a sensory relay, receiving projections from all of

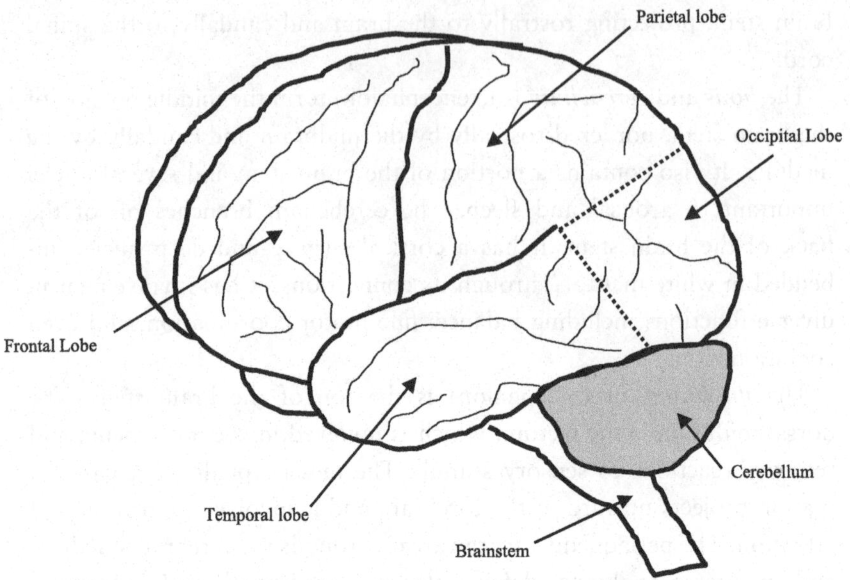

Figure 2.9
Midsagittal view of the brain.

the sensory systems except smell. It also controls forebrain arousal and participates in circuits controlling cognition, emotion, and memory. The hypothalamus monitors and regulates many homeostatic functions, including sleep, eating, drinking, sex, and body temperature. Hypothalamic control of the endocrine system is through its influence on the pituitary gland. Through its connections to other forebrain areas, it coordinates homeostatic functions with emotion, motivation, and behavior.

Also included are the epithalamus and subthalamic nucleus. The epithalamus is a collective term for the pineal gland, habenular nucleus, stria medullaris, and tenia thalami. The subthalamic nucleus is interconnected with the basal ganglia and plays a role in motor regulation.

Cerebrum

The cerebrum is composed of four lobes covered by cerebral cortex: frontal, parietal, temporal, and occipital (figure 2.9). The cortical surface is convoluted, especially in humans, allowing for maximum surface area in a limited volume (i.e., the cranium). The ridges of cortex are referred to as gyri, and the valley in between them are sulci.

The parietal lobe is involved in body sensations and the total body image, while the temporal lobe is involved in hearing. The occipital lobe is involved in basic aspects of vision. However, cortical visual processing continues into a ventral, "what" pathway in the inferior temporal lobe—which is involved in object and face recognition—and a dorsal, "where" pathway—which perceives spatial location. Higher-order cortical association areas control numerous other higher cognitive functions such as reading, arithmetic, language, and musical perception.

The frontal lobes are proportionately larger in humans than in other animals. While more posterior regions of the frontal lobe are concerned with motor function and the execution of behaviors, the more anterior portion (prefrontal cortex) is involved in cognition. In the most general sense, the prefrontal cortex is concerned with optimizing behavior by allowing for more goal-oriented and conceptually driven behavior. Thus, the prefrontal cortex is essential for such executive functions as abstract reasoning, planning, organization, goal formation, mental flexibility, initiation of behaviors, inhibition of behaviors, and social conduct.

Beneath the cortex, the brain contains white-matter tracts, which interconnect the cortex, subcortical nuclei, and lower structures. The *limbic system* is a circuit of structures surrounding the brain stem and diencephalon, which regulate emotions and memory. The *hippocampus* is a cortical structure in the medial temporal lobe, which is responsible for the formation and consolidation of long-term memories. It has reciprocal connections with the cerebral cortex, and removal of the hippocampus produces an inability to form new memories (i.e., anterograde amnesia). The amygdala is a set of subcortical nuclei that are located in the anterior temporal lobe. The amygdala is involved in determining the emotional significance of stimuli and events. Much work has been done to determine the role of the amygdala in fear and anxiety; it is also likely involved in positive emotional states. Through its connections with executive and motor systems in the brain, the amygdala allows external incentives to influence behavior.

The *basal ganglia* are a set of subcortical nuclei including the *caudate*, *putamen*, and *globus pallidus*. These structures form part of a processing loop running from the cortex to basal ganglia, and from there to parts of the thalamus and back to the frontal cortex. There are several such parallel processing loops throughout these structures, each mediating distinct cognitive and motor functions. Degeneration of the basal ganglia or its afferent inputs produces disorders of movement and cognition such as Parkinson's disease and Huntington's disease.

3

Basic Pharmacology

Herbal medicines contain active drugs, in every sense of the word. As such, the principles of pharmacology pertain to them and allow us to understand their effects. The purpose of this chapter is to outline some of these principles. For a more complete treatment of the topic, the reader is directed to the sources listed in the references. Although these principles apply to all drugs, this chapter will draw upon examples from plant drugs to illustrate them.

There are two main areas of pharmacology: *pharmacokinetics* and *pharmacodynamics*. The simplest distinction between these two is that pharmacokinetics is how the body affects a drug, while pharmacodynamics is how a drug affects the body.

Pharmacokinetics

Pharmacokinetics is specifically concerned with the transfer of a drug through the body by the processes of absorption, distribution, biotransformation, and excretion. A drug's dosage and pharmacokinetic properties will determine the concentrations that will be reached, and therefore the intensity of effect produced. Ultimately, these processes determine the *bioavailability* of a drug, or the degree to which it reaches the intended site of action.

The importance of pharmacokinetics should not be underestimated. The effects of psychoactive drugs are determined not only by their pharmacodynamic mechanisms, but also by *how much* of the drug reaches the brain, and *how fast* it does so. A cardinal example of this involves the behavioral differences between chewing coca leaves, snorting cocaine

HCl, and smoking freebase crack. All three of these deliver the drug cocaine, but each delivers progressively greater amounts to the brain at a quicker rate. The end result of this is that traditional chewing of coca leaves probably approaches the equivalence of drinking espresso coffee, while smoking crack has become an epidemic of drug addiction. Similarly, morphine and heroin may have identical mechanisms in the brain, but heroin (diacetylmorphine) gains access faster and to a greater extent.

The processes of pharmacokinetics all involve the transfer of a drug across membranes, beginning with the cell membrane, and sometimes involving single or multiple layers of cells. Drugs can cross these membranes through passive or active transport.

Passive transport is not energy dependent, and involves drugs moving along a concentration gradient, from an area of high concentration to an area of low concentration. Drugs that are nonionized generally have good lipid solubility, and thus can pass through the lipid cell membranes. Conversely, ionized drug molecules have low lipid solubility and do not pass through membranes well. Other factors influencing this process are the drug and pH concentration gradients across the membrane, where the pH gradient can influence the ionization of the drug.

Active transport of a drug is mediated by a specific carrier. This is of particular interest in neural tissues and choroid plexus. In this case, the actual molecular size and shape are important, because it involves binding to a specific carrier protein that transports it. Active transport is an energy-dependent process, and may work against a concentration gradient. It is also a saturable mechanism and may be competitively inhibited by other ligands.

Absorption

Absorption is defined as the rate and extent to which a drug leaves the site of administration. Several factors influence a drug's absorption (table 3.1). Aqueous solutions are more easily absorbed than a lipid solution or solid form. Absorption of drugs in solid form is affected by the rate at which it dissolves. Higher concentrations of a drug are more rapidly absorbed than low concentrations. The amount of blood flow to the site also influences absorption: heat and vasodilators increase absorption,

Table 3.1
Factors influencing drug absorption

Type of solution (aqueous vs. lipid)
Rate of dissolution of solid drugs
Concentrations of a drug present
Blood flow to the site of absorption
Surface area of absorption

while vasoconstrictors reduce it. The surface area of absorption is a very important factor. Drugs are very effectively absorbed by tissues with large surface areas, as in the lungs.

Routes of Administration
Absorption is greatly altered by the route of administration of a drug. These routes are broadly dichotomized as enteral or parenteral (table 3.2). Enteral administration involves absorption through the gastrointestinal (GI) tract, and parenteral refers to any other form of absorption. Each has its own respective advantages and disadvantages (table 3.3). Enteral routes are the safest, most convenient, and most economical means, and thus are the most common. However, they have the disadvantages of irregular absorption, nausea and vomiting, and enzyme degradation. They also necessitate patient cooperation, which is not possible in some instances (e.g., seizures, psychotic agitation). Parenteral routes, on the other hand, allow the drug to be absorbed in active form, in a more rapid absorption and in a predictable manner. Their disadvantages are the risk of infection, they are more difficult to perform (e.g., injections), and they produce greater discomfort.

Enteral routes of administration include oral, sublingual, and rectal. Oral ingestion of a drug results in passive absorption through the GI tract. The pH of the drug affects this process: weak acids are best absorbed from the stomach, while weak bases absorb better from the small intestine. Nonionized drugs absorb well from any part of the GI tract. *Sublingual* administration involves absorption from the oral mucosa, and avoids hepatic first-pass metabolism. *Rectal* administration involves absorption from the lower GI tract. It avoids the nausea and vomiting produced by direct stomach irritation, but also has irregular absorption.

Table 3.2
Routes of drug administration

- I. Enteral
  - A. Oral
  - B. Sublingual
  - C. Rectal
- II. Parenteral
  - A. Injection
    1. Subcutaneous
    2. Intramuscular
    3. Intravenous
    4. Intra-arterial
    5. Intraperitoneal
    6. Intrathecal
    7. Intracerebral
  - B. Noninjection
    1. Pulmonary
       - a. Smoking
       - b. Inhaler
    2. Topical
       - a. Transdermal
       - b. Intranasal

Table 3.3
Enteral vs. parenteral routes

Route	Advantages	Disadvantages
Enteral	Safer	Irregular absorption
	Easier	GI irritation, Nausea
	Economical	Metabolism of drug
		Require cooperation
Parenteral	Absorbed in active form	Risk of infection
	More rapid	More difficult
	More predictable	More discomfort

For example, rectal diazepam may be administered to people undergoing continuous seizures (status epilepticus), because other oral and parenteral routes would not be feasible.

Injection forms of parenteral administration include subcutaneous, intramuscular, intravenous, intra-arterial, intraperitoneal, intrathecal, and intracerebral injections. *Intravenous* administration (IV) involves injection of an aqueous solution into the veins, bypassing the processes of absorption. This allows accurate and rapid control of drug concentrations, and less sensitivity to irritating drugs. However, dangerously high concentrations can be easily and quickly reached this way (e.g., heroin overdose). *Subcutaneous* injection of drugs (SC) can only be done with nonirritating drugs, otherwise pain, necrosis, and slough of tissues may occur. Subcutaneous absorption depends on blood flow to the site of injection. Likewise, absorption from *intramuscular* injection (IM) depends on blood flow to the site of injection. It is performed with an aqueous solution and absorption may be very rapid. *Intra-arterial* injections are performed to highly localize the effects of a drug, but this requires great caution because hepatic metabolism and lung filtering are bypassed. *Intraperitoneal* injection (IP) involves absorption from the abdominal cavity into the portal vein. This allows a large absorbing surface, but the risk of infection to this area is serious. *Intrathecal* administration involves injection into the spinal column, bypassing blood-brain and blood-cerebrospinal fluid (CSF) barriers. This route is usually reserved for spinal anesthesia or to treat infections of the central nervous system. More directly, *intracerebral* injections may be performed surgically when a specific locus in the brain must be targeted (e.g., injection of fetal cell grafts for Parkinson's disease).

Noninjection forms of parenteral administration include pulmonary or topical absorption. Pulmonary absorption is performed with gaseous drugs (e.g., general anesthetics) and drugs aerosolized by inhalers (e.g., asthma medications) or by burning (e.g., tobacco smoking). Absorption is rapid through the large surface area of the pulmonary epithelium and respiratory tract. The disadvantages of pulmonary absorption are the difficulty in controlling the dose, inconvenient administration, and potential irritation of the pulmonary epithelium. *Topical* (or *transdermal*) administration involves absorption from mucous membranes or the

Table 3.4
Factors influencing drug distribution

Factors
Blood flow in the target organs
Lipid solubility (especially CNS)
Accumulation in drug reservoirs
Serum proteins
Fat
Muscles
Liver
Bone
Transcellular (GI, CSF)
Molecular size (especially CNS)
Specific carrier transport

skin. For example, absorption through mucous membranes is utilized when cocaine HCl is snorted, or when medieval "witches" applied hallucinogenic ointments to their vaginal membranes. Absorption through the skin is more common clinically, although few drugs absorb well this way. However, absorption is improved through an oily medium such as a cream. Nicotine patches for cessation of tobacco smoking are an example of transdermal absorption.

Distribution

Drug distribution involves its movement into the interstitial and cellular fluids. Several factors influence drug distribution, including blood flow (table 3.4). Organs with the greatest blood flow (e.g., the brain, heart, liver, and kidneys) receive most of the drug initially, while other tisses (e.g., muscle, viscera, skin, and fat) receive it more gradually. Distribtion is also influenced by a drug's lipid solubility and accumulation in *drug reservoirs.*

Certain factors determine distribution of drugs to the central nervous system. An important determinant is the drug's molecular size, because cerebral capillaries have tight junctions and only the smallest molecules can pass through unless there is a specific carrier mechanism. However, drugs that are highly lipid soluble may pass through the brain's permeability barriers. Drug distribution to the brain is limited also by the degree of cerebral blood flow. However, the blood-brain barrier is not impermeable: large doses may leak through, particularly at areas of nonuniformity (e.g., circumventricular organs).

Drug reservoirs are bodily compartments in which a drug is stored. When a portion of the drug is in a reservoir it limits the amount of free drug available, because only unbound drug is in equilibrium across membranes. On the other hand, reservoirs also prolong the action of a drug, maintaining its concentrations by releasing it gradually as blood levels decline. There are several drug reservoirs, such as plasma proteins albumin and glycoproteins. Binding to plasma proteins is usually reversible and competitive. Therefore, the plasma level of one drug will be influenced by any other drugs that bind to the same plasma proteins, displacing some of it from that reservoir. Certain intracellular reservoirs may also accumulate drugs, such as muscles and the liver, due to active transport or binding to a protein. Fat may serve as a large drug reservoir, which slowly releases the drug when plasma levels decline. Bone may also serve as a reservoir, particularly for heavy metals and chelating agents, with very slow and sustained release of the drug. Finally, drugs may accumulate in transcellular reservoirs, such as in the GI tract or CSF.

When levels of the drug decline in plasma, usually due to biotransformation and excretion, the drug then redistributes away from its site of action into other tissues (e.g., drugs may distribute across the placenta during pregnancy). This is a passive process, but lipid-soluble drugs penetrate the most. This is of special concern with psychoactive drugs, which tend to be lipid-soluble.

Biotransformation

Biotransformation involves the chemical alteration of a molecule to alter its effects. This often terminates the pharmacological effects of a drug, but active metabolites are produced in some cases. Biotransformation also changes the ease with which a drug is eliminated. This involves conversion of the drug to a more hydrophilic metabolite that enhances renal excretion. Although this process pertains to most drugs, it probably

Table 3.5
Biotransformation reactions

Phase I Reactions
- A. Oxidative Reactions
  1. N-dealkylation
  2. O-dealkylation
  3. Aliphatic hydroxylation
  4. Aromatic hydroxylation
  5. N-oxidation
  6. S-oxidation
  7. Deamination
- B. Hydrolysis Reaction

Phase II Reactions
- A. Glucuronidation
- B. Sulfation
- C. Acetylation

evolved to remove chemical constituents of ingested plants, includng flavonoids, terpenes, steroids, and alkaloids.

Biotransformation of drugs occurs in two phases (table 3.5). *Phase I* reactions involve oxidative or hydrolysis reactions. Oxidative reactions include *N*-dealkylation, *O*-dealkylation, aliphatic hydroxylation, aromatic hydroxylation, *N*-oxidation, *S*-oxidation, or deamination. Following a phase I reaction, a covalent conjugation reaction may occur, making the compound more polar, water soluble, and thus more easily excreted in urine and feces. *Phase II* reactions are conjugation reactions: glucuronidation, sulfation, and acetylation. As mentioned above, metabolic conversion of drugs can produce active metabolites, which sometimes may be more active than the drug administered. For example, although morphine is an active drug, some of its clinical effects are attributable to its active metabolite morphine-6-glucuronide (M6G). In some cases, the compound administered may itself be inactive, but becomes active after metabolic conversion.

The primary organ of biotransformation is the liver, although some other tissues have a degree of metabolic capacity, including the GI tract, kidneys, and even the skin. Depending on the route of administration, drugs may undergo *first-pass* metabolism, so that a proportion of the drug is inactivated before it reaches the target tissue.

The microsomal enzymes responsible for catalyzing oxidative and reductive reactions are the cytochrome P450 enzyme family. These are heme-containing membrane proteins that are found in the smooth endoplasmic reticulum of the cells of many tissues, but especially in the liver. Twelve gene families of the cytochrome P450 enzyme have been identified in humans, and the three families, CYP1, CYP2, and CYP3 account for most drug biotransformations. Hydrolytic reactions are carried out by the enzyme epoxide hydrolase and several amidases, esterases, proteases, and peptidases. Conjugation reactions are carried out by uridine diphosphate glucuronosyltransferases, sulfotransferases, and *N*-acetyltransferases.

Several factors may influence the processes of biotransformation. Certain drugs or toxins may induce synthesis of cytochrome P450. For drugs that are transformed into toxic metabolites, this may amount to significant hepatic or renal toxicity over time. A common example of this is with chronic alcoholism resulting in liver damage. Drugs may also inhibit cytochrome P450 enzymes, resulting in slower metabolism and prolonged drug concentrations. Unintentional interactions between diverse types of drugs may occur through competition for enzymes. For example, several studies have examined the inhibition of cytochrome P450 3A4 (CYP3A4) by grapefruit juice. Biotransformation may be reduced in cases of liver disease. It is also reduced in fetal and neonatal stages of development, and in many elderly. Genetic differences normally exist between individuals in drug metabolism capacity, which result from polymorphisms in the cytochrome P450 family.

Excretion

Excretion is the process of eliminating drugs from the body. They may be excreted as metabolites or as unchanged drug. As mentioned above, compounds that are polar and water soluble are more readily eliminated. The major routes of excretion are renal, biliary/fecal, lactational, and pulmonary.

The kidneys are the most important routes of drug excretion. This begins with filtration of a drug from the blood by renal glomeruli. Through these tiny clusters of capillaries, a filtrate is formed that has essentially the same composition of plasma, minus the larger proteins. The filtrate contains water, glucose, amino acids, urea, uric acid, creatine, creatinine, anions, and cations. Nonselective carrier systems transport organic anions and cations into the filtrate, and transport can sometimes be bidirectional, allowing for reabsorption. Organic acids and drug metabolites are transported by a carrier system that normally transports uric acid.

After glomerular filtration, fluid passes through proximal and distal tubules, and eventually collects into the ureter and bladder, where it is eliminated. However, considerable reabsorption occurs from the proximal and distal tubules. Nonionized weak acids and bases are passively reabsorbed, moving down a concentration gradient. Reabsorption of ionized substances is pH dependent. The kidneys of an average adult filter 45 gallons per 24-hour period, the majority of which is obviously reabsorbed.

Hepatic metabolites are excreted into the intestinal tract in bile. From there, the metabolites may be excreted in feces or reabsorbed into the blood. Metabolites are carried into the bile via active transport. Pulmonary excretion of drugs occurs mainly for gases and vapors, such as general anesthetic drugs. Excretion of drugs and metabolites occurs in breast milk, which is of significant concern for breast-feeding mothers. Breast milk is slightly more acidic than plasma, so basic compounds may be present in greater concentrations, while acidic compounds are in lower concentrations. Nonelectrolytes enter breast milk in a pH-independent manner. Other less-important routes of excretion are through sweat, saliva, and tears, which primarily excrete nonionized, lipid-soluble drugs. Elimination of drugs in the skin and hair is quantitatively minute, but detectable for forensic purposes.

Clinical Pharmacokinetics

There are several pharmacokinetic paramaters that are relevant to the clinical use of drugs. These help quantify a *dose-response relationship*, or

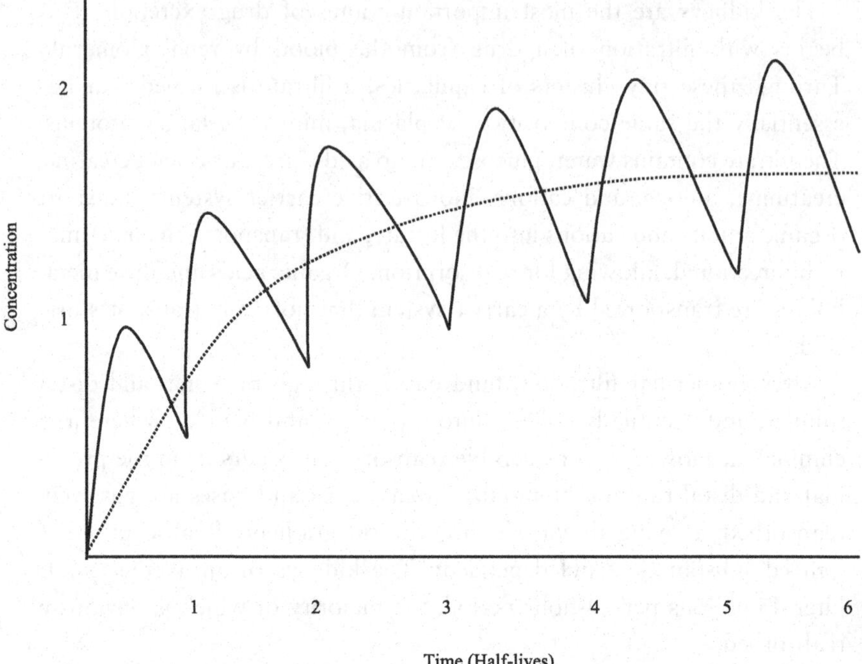

Figure 3.1
Steady-state concentration.

the relationship between the drug concentrations and its magnitude of effect. It is often desirable clinically to achieve a *steady-state concentration* of a drug to maintain a relatively constant level of effect (figure 3.1). To rapidly reach this level, a larger initial *loading dose* may be given, followed by smaller *maintenance doses* to sustain that level.

The three main parameters of clinical pharmacokinetics are clearance, distribution volume, and bioavailability. *Clearance* is the rate at which the body eliminates a drug. In order to achieve a steady-state concentration, the drug must be given so that the rate of clearance equals the rate of administration. If the drug is given as quickly as it is eliminated, a consistent level in the body will be maintained.

Clearance is constant across drug concentrations because the mechanisms are normally not saturated. Under such normal conditions, a constant *fraction* of the drug is eliminated per unit time, whereas if there is

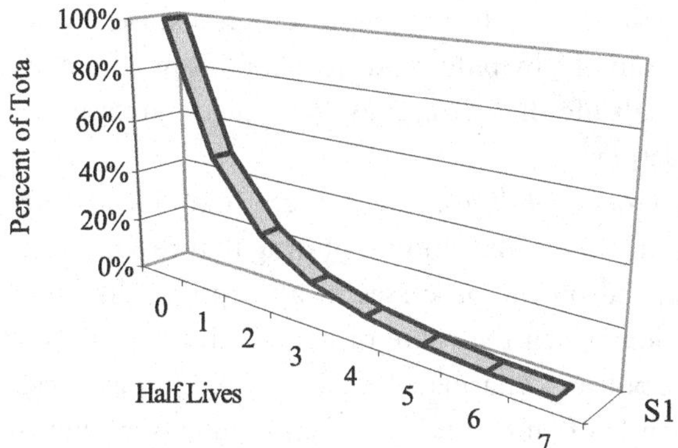

Figure 3.2
Drug concentrations after a single dose.

saturation, a certain *amount* is eliminated per unit time. This is termed *zero-order kinetics* and clearance becomes variable. Clearance is additive, equaling the sum of all the routes of elimination (i.e., renal, hepatic, etc.). Therefore, clearance is the sum of all routes of elimination proportional to the concentration of the drug, and it is expressed as a volume per unit of time.

The *volume of distribution* is the amount of drug in the body relative to the concentration of drug in blood or plasma. This value is the fluid volume that would be needed to contain all of the drug in the body at the same concentration as in blood or plasma. For drugs that bind extensively to plasma proteins, the volume of distribution approximates the plasma volume, unless the drug is significantly stored in another reservoir. A *one-compartment model* calculates the volume of distribution by assuming a single, central compartment. However, for most drugs, *multiple-compartment models* are necessary, with each compartment corresponding to a tissue reservoir.

The *half-life* of a drug is the amount of time it takes to reduce concentrations by 50%. With each successive half-life duration, drug concentrations are further reduced until it is no longer present (figure 3.2). In a one-compartment model, a single half-life may be sufficient, but in multiple-compartment models, more than one half-life may need to be calculated. Half-life varies as a function of both the volume of distribution and clearance. The half-life may be altered in certain disease states. It may be increased, for example, by reduced drug metabolism with age. On the other hand, the half-life of a drug may be reduced in cases of microsomal enzyme induction.

As mentioned above, *bioavailability* is the degree to which a drug reaches the intended site of action. The amount of drug that reaches systemic circulation will depend on the processes of absorption, distribution, and biotransformation (when the route of administration exposes the drug to first-pass metabolism). Pharmacokinetics are often linear and when they are nonlinear it is often due to a saturation of protein binding, metabolism, or active renal transport.

Pharmacodynamics

Pharmacodynamics consist of the chemical and physiological mechanisms of action of a drug. Further, it concern the relationship between drug concentrations and the magnitude of effect.

Mechanism of Drug Action

The mechanisms of most drugs involve binding of the drug to a receptor. A receptor may be any macromolecular target, but the most common receptors are proteins. These include membrane proteins, enzymes, transporters, and structural elements. Some of the main receptors of interest for psychopharmacology are receptors for neurotransmitters and hormones, which show a high degree of selectivity.

A drug may have several potential effects at a receptor target. A drug that binds to the receptor and imitates the actions of the endogenous ligand is called an *agonist*. A *partial agonist* also activates the receptor mechanism, but does not reach full efficacy. A drug that binds to the receptor and has no intrinsic effect, but instead prevents binding of other ligands, is called an *antagonist*. An *inverse agonist* is a drug that has the opposite effect of an agonist.

Drugs are thought to bind to receptors in a lock-and-key model, meaning that the molecular shape of a drug determines how well, if at all, it will attach to a receptor and what activity it will have there.

Structure-activity relationships are very important in understanding drug actions and in designing novel drugs. Seemingly small modifications in a drug's molecular structure can radically alter its effects.

Drug Receptors

Protein receptors for endogenous ligands (e.g., hormones, neurotransmitters) share some common properties. They contain a *ligand-binding domain*, where the hormone or neurotransmitter attaches, and an *effector domain*, which translates the binding into some form of action.

Receptor-effector mechanisms include (1) enzymes with catalytic activities, (2) ion channels that gate the transmembrane flux of ions (ionotropic receptors), (3) G protein-coupled receptors that activate intracellular messengers (metabotropic receptors), and (4) cytosolic receptors that regulate gene transcription. Cytosolic receptors are a specific mechanism of many steroid and thyroid hormones. The ionotropic and metabotropic receptors are discussed in relevance to specific neurotransmitters in chapter 2.

Receptor Regulation

Receptor regulation is under homeostatic control. Continuous stimulation of a receptor may lead to its desensitization (or down regulation). *Homologous densensitization* involves covalent modification, destruction, decreasesd synthesis, or relocalization of the receptor within the cell. *Heterologous densensitization*, on the other hand, occurs when a receptor is desensitized by sharing a common signaling pathway with other receptors. For example, several neurotransmitter receptors may convergently act upon adenylate cyclase synthesis of cAMP.

Conversely, understimulation of a receptor may lead to its sensitization (or up regulation). This may occur when an antagonist is administered for a long period of time, or when tissue is denervated and does not receive the normal afferent stimulation.

Quantifying Dose-Response Relationships

Under certain circumstances, the magnitude of drug effect is related to the proportion of receptors occupied, and maximal effects occur when all receptors are occupied. However, there are many exceptions and nonlinear relationships also exist. The concept of *efficacy* means that different agonists could have different intensity of activity at a receptor, and it explains why two different agonists could occupy the same proportion of receptors but have different magnitudes of effect.

Plotting the dose of an agonist against the effect produces a linear curve, and plotting the log dose versus the effect produces a sigmoidal curve (figure 3.3). A full agonist may create maximal effects at the appropriate dose. Full agonists may differ in their *potency*, where both reach maximal effects, but one does so at a lower dose (figure 3.4). In contrast, full and partial agonists differ by their maximum *efficacy*. No matter how much of a partial agonist is given, it will not achieve the same magnitude of effect as a full agonist. Combinations of agonists may produce *additive* effects, or *synergistic* effects, which are greater than the sum of the effects of each individual drug.

Antagonist drugs may reduce the potency or efficacy of an agonist, depending on the nature of their receptor binding: competitive or noncompetitive. *Competitive antagonists* can be overcome by increasing the amount of agonist, and maximum agonist effects may still be achieved. This produces a rightward shift in the dose-response curve, reflecting altered potency (figure 3.5). *Noncompetitive antagonists*, however, have irreversible receptor binding and are not overcome by agonists. This is reflected in the dose-response curve as a reduction in maximum efficacy.

Inverse agonists will not only antagonize or nullify the effects of agonists when given together, they will have the opposite effect of the agonist when administered alone (figure 3.6). This is especially true with receptors that have a basal rate of activity, which might be increased by an agonist or further decreased by an inverse agonist. For example, diazepam is regarded as an agonist at the $GABA_A$ benzodiazepine receptor and has anxiolytic effects. β-carbolines, in contrast, are regarded as inverse agonists of the benzodiazepine receptor, and are anxiogenic. (However, uncertainty over the endogenous ligand of the benzodiazepine receptor makes the assignment of *agonist* versus *inverse agonist* somewhat arbitrary. Indeed, there are endogenous β-carbolines, so they might be regarded as the actual agonists.)

Dose-response relationships may be examined in individuals or in populations. The dose-response curves discussed above (e.g., figure 3.3)

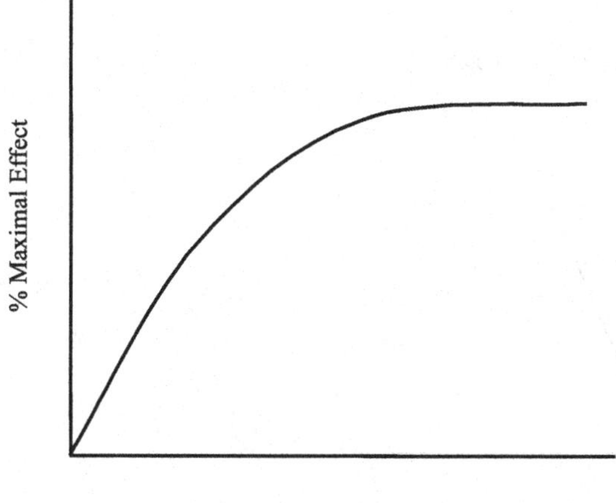

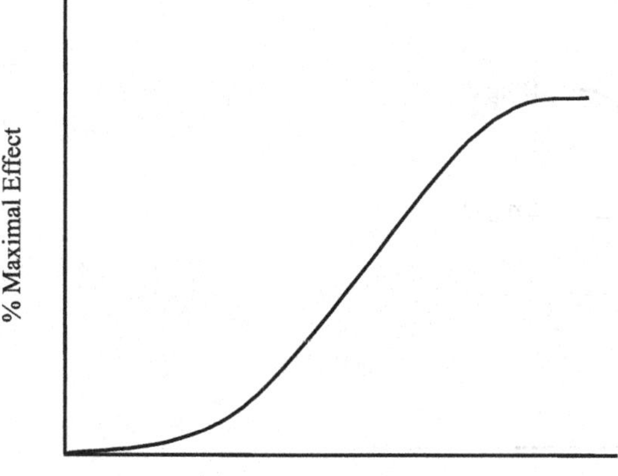

Figure 3.3
Dose-response curves.

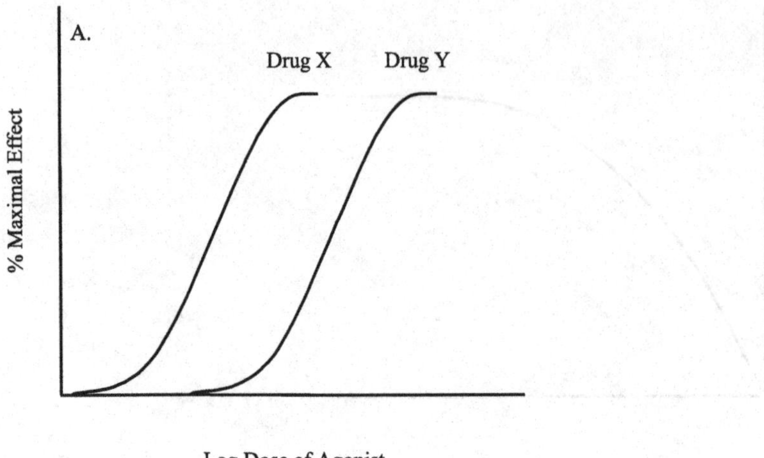

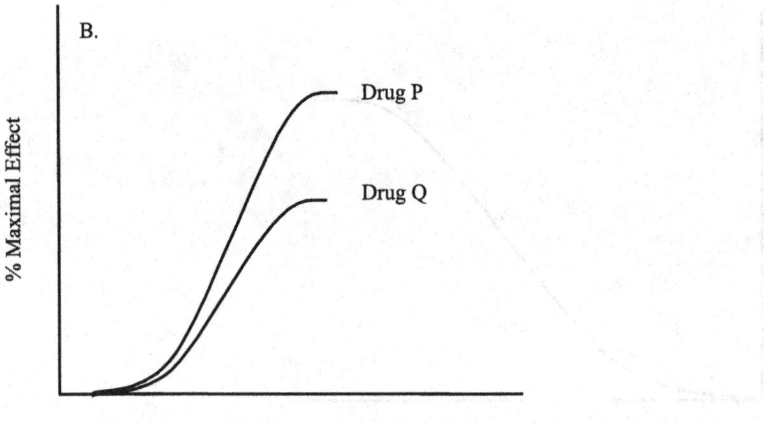

Figure 3.4
Differences in potency vs. efficacy. (*A*) Drug X and Y differ in terms of potency, but both have the same maximal effect. (*B*) Drug P and Q differ in efficacy. Drug P is a full agonist, while drug Q is a partial agonist.

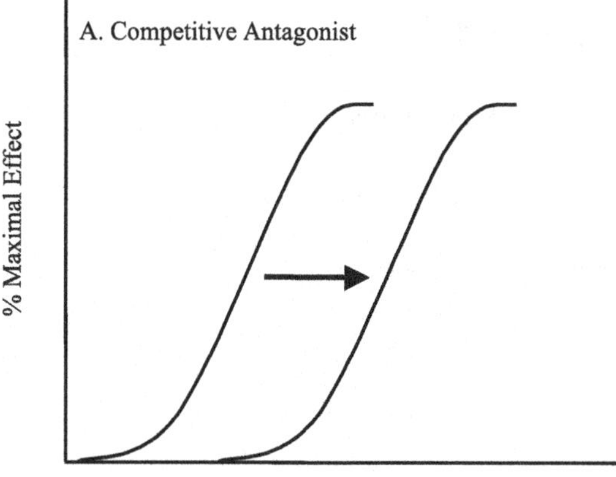

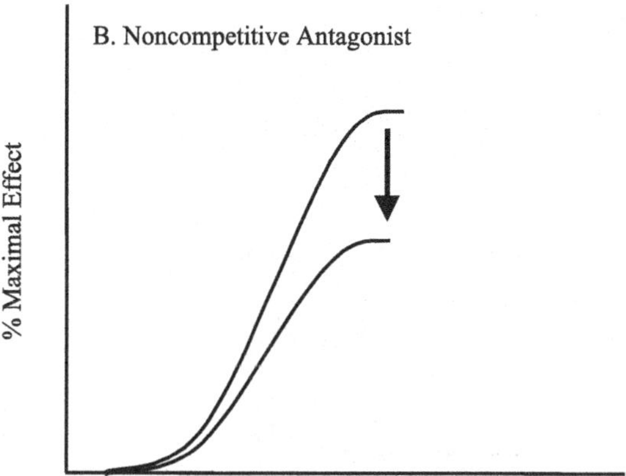

Figure 3.5
Effects of antagonist drugs. (*A*) Competitive antagonists bind reversibly, reducing the potency of the agonist and causing a rightward shift in the dose-response curve. (*B*) Noncompetitive antagonists bind irreversibly, reducing the maximum efficacy of the agonist.

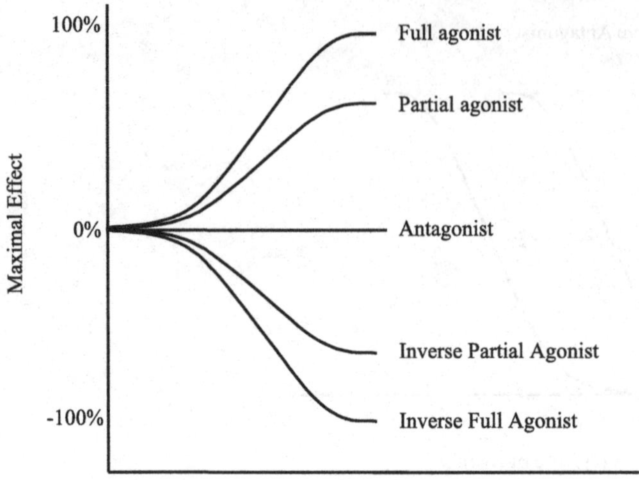

Figure 3.6
Effects of drugs on receptor activity.

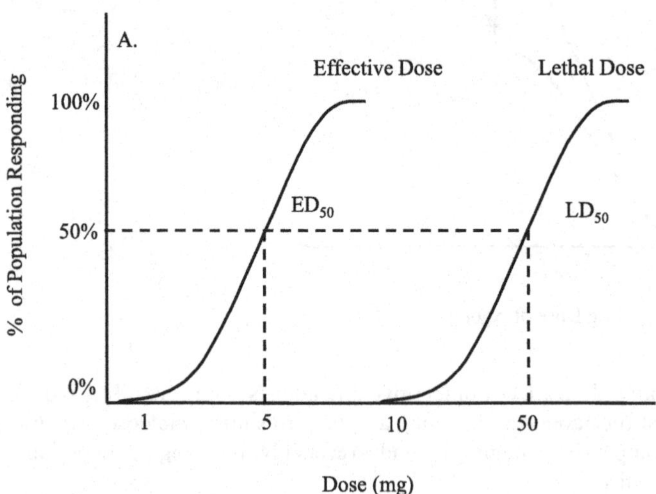

Figure 3.7
Effective and lethal doses.

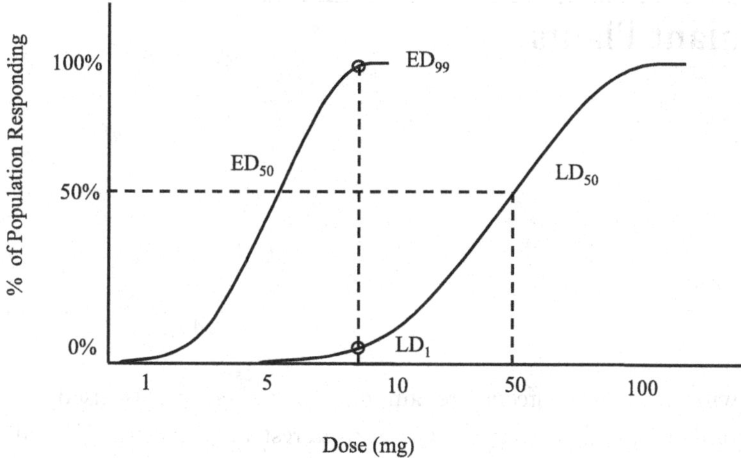

Figure 3.8
Effective and lethal doses.

refer to a *graded* dose-response curve, which represents effects in individuals. A *quantal* dose-response curve, however, refers to the proportion of a population responding to the drug. Two useful quantal curves show the *effective* and *lethal* doses (figure 3.7). The ED_{50} would represent the median effective dose, or the dose that would be sufficient for half of the population. The LD_{50} is the median lethal dose.

Naturally, as much separation as possible between these two curves is desired. Overlap of the curves would mean that the some of the higher effective doses would be killing a proportion of the population. A ratio of the median effective and lethal doses ($ED_{50}:LD_{50}$) gives a *therapeutic index*. However, this ratio does not account for the shape of the curves. In some cases, the ratio of the median doses may be adequate, but there could still be overlap. For example, figure 3.8 shows effective and lethal dose curves that partially overlap. Thus, a better ratio is $ED_{99}:LD_1$, which ensures lseparation of the curves.

4

Stimulant Plants

Plants with stimulant effects are among the earliest plants used by humankind for psychoactive effects. Our interest in them is motivated by their profound effect on mental functioning, increasing alertness, the ability to sustain effort, and in some cases, the induction of euphoria. Despite their native geographical habitats, several stimulant plants are used across the planet. A sizable portion of the world's population regularly consumes tobacco, coffee, tea, or some other form of stimulant on a daily basis (Piha et al. 1993). In some cases, these are socially accepted aspects of daily life (e.g., coffee, tea), while others are reviled for their addicting effects and socioeconmic impact (e.g., coca).

The stimulant plants are organized here by their predominant neurochemical mechanism: purinergic (coffee, tea, cocoa, maté, guarana, and kola), cholinergic (tobacco, areca, and lobelia), and monoaminergic (ephedra, coca, and khat) (see table 4.1). It is worthwhile to note that most of these plant drugs work through neuromodulatory systems. They mostly create stimulation not through direct neuronal excitation, but rather by a modulation of neuronal activity. On the other hand, drugs that directly stimulate excitatory amino acids or block inhibitory amino acids more often have excitotoxic or convulsive effects (e.g., strychnine from *Strychnos nux-vomica*, or ibotenate from *Amanita muscaria*). Rather, the stimulant plants generally act through neuromodulatory receptors linked to G-proteins and intracellular messengers.

Several synthetic stimulants have been developed for clinical use or illegal trade. Amphetamine was synthesized in 1887, but its medical applications were not investigated until the 1920s (Rudgley 1999). It was first marketed in 1932 as a treatment for asthma and nasal congestion. Since

Table 4.1
Central nervous system stimulants

Common	Botanical	Active constituents	Mechanism
Purinergic			
Coffee	*Coffea arabica*	Methylxanthines	Adenosine antagonism
Tea	*Camellia sinensis*	"	"
Cocoa	*Theobroma cacao*	"	"
Guarana	*Paullinia cupana*	"	"
Maté	*Ilex paraguariensis*	"	"
Kola	*Cola nitida & acuminata*	"	"
Cholinergic			
Tobacco	*Nicotiana tobacum*	Nicotine	Nicotinic ACh agonist
Areca	*Areca cathechu*	Arecoline, arecaidine, guvacoline guvacine	Muscarinic ACh agonist
Lobelia	*Lobelia inflata*	Lobeline	Nicotinic ACh agonist
Monoaminergic			
Ephedra	*Ephedra sinica*	Ephedrine	α, β adrenergic agonist
Coca	*Erythroxylon coca*	Cocaine	Blocks monoamine reuptake Na^{+} channel antagonist
Khat	*Catha edulis*	Cathinone	

See text for references.

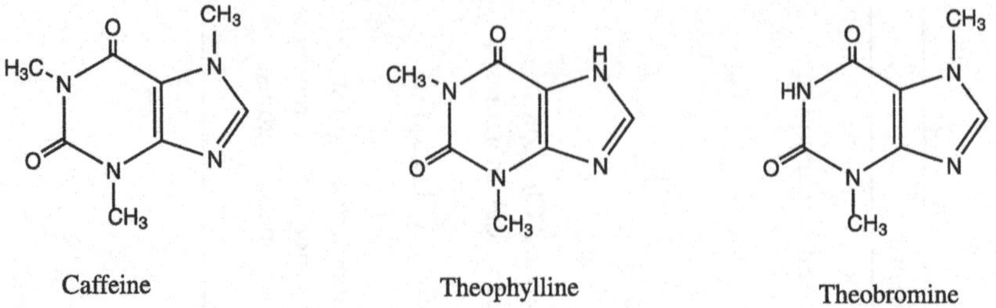

Caffeine Theophylline Theobromine

Figure 4.1
Chemical structure of the methylxanthines.

then, a number of related drugs have been developed. Methylphenidate (Ritalin) and pemoline (Cylert) have generally replaced amphetamines for treatment of attention disorders. Methylenedioxymethamphetamine (MDMA, "Ecstasy") and several other amphetamine derivatives have been labeled "entactogens," due to their prominent effect of creating feelings of interpersonal warmth and empathy. Unfortunately, they are also highly neurotoxic to serotonin neurons (White et al. 1996). Amphetamines and related drugs have long been used to reduce appetite and weight, but dependence liability, toxicity, and the tendency for rebound weight gain after drug discontinuation have made them impractical for this purpose. Despite the development of numerous synthetic stimulants, the use of plants or plant-derived drugs probably still accounts for the majority of human stimulant consumption.

Purinergic Stimulants

The purinergic stimulants are a small group of chemically and pharmacologically related drugs that are found in several different plants but commonly act on purine neurotransmitters such as adenosine. Namely, the drugs are caffeine, theophylline, and theobromine, collectively referred to as the *methylxanthines* (figure 4.1). They are probably the most commonly used stimulants in the world, and possibly the most commonly consumed of all drugs. Methylxanthines are found in several plants that are well known across the world, and in others whose use is more regional. Collectively, these plants include coffee, cocoa, guarana,

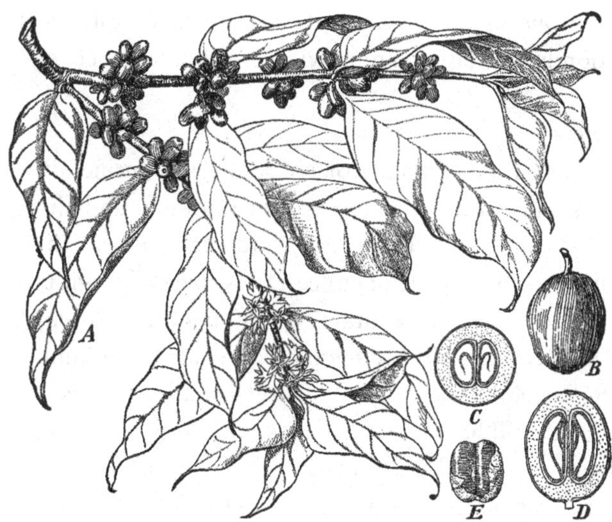

Figure 4.2
Coffee *(Coffea arabica)*. Reprinted from Culbreth DMR. (1927). *Materia Medica and Pharmacognosy*, 7th ed. Philadelphia: Lea & Febiger.

maté, and kola. Due to the common pharmacological basis of these plants, they will be briefly discussed individually for their distinct botanical and historical aspects, and then collectively addressed for their common pharmacological effects.

Coffee

History and Botany

The coffee plant *(Coffea arabica)* grows flowers in dense clusters of 10–20 (figure 4.2). The bean is elliptoid with a green color initially, changing to yellow and red with maturity. The characteristic brown color and aroma of the bean are acquired when roasted. The plant grows as a shrub or small tree, up to 8 meters in height. It is believed to be native to Ethiopia, but has long been cultivated throughout tropical regions.

The name *coffee* comes from the Turkish word *gahveh* or Arabic *gahuah*. More than a thousand years ago, Muslim mystics would drink coffee during all-night prayer sessions (Weil and Rosen 1983). When it was introduced to Europe in the seventeenth century C.E., coffee met with official opposition before later gaining widespread acceptance.

Chemical Constituents

The major pharmacological constituents of coffee are the purine alkaloids caffeine (1–2%), and to a lesser degree, theobromine and theophylline (Gruenwald et al. 1998). Also present are trigonelline, caffeic acid, and tannin. The caffeine content of coffee varies somewhat with its preparation: drip-brewed coffee may contain 60–180 mg (per 5 oz cup), while instant coffee may contain 30–120 mg (Gilbert et al. 1976; Bunker and McWilliams 1979; Lelo et al. 1986). "Decaffeinated" coffee is not completely decaffeinated, still having 5 mg or less. By comparison, over-the-counter stimulants (e.g., NoDoz, Vivarin) contain approximately 100 mg per tablet, and caffeinated soft drinks have 40–60 mg of caffeine per 12 oz serving.

Tea

History and Botany

Both black and green tea are from the plant *Camellia sinensis* (Gruenwald et al. 1998; Robbers et al. 1996). It grows white or pale pink flowers and fruit in a greenish-brown capsule, each containing one to three brown seeds (figure 4.3). Green tea is produced by simply drying the leaves and brewing them in hot water. Black tea is first fermented before drying and brewing. Tea was originally cultivated in China, but is now grown in many parts of the world including India, Indonesia, the Middle East, Africa, and Argentina. Tea has been a popular drink throughout history and, as a result, it has been a major force in trade, economics, and politics.

Chemical Constituents

The major pharmacological constituents of tea are the purine alkaloids caffeine (2.9–4.2%), theobromine (0.15–0.2%), and theophylline (0.02–0.04%). Also present are triterpene saponins (including barringtogenol C and R1-barringenol), catechins (theaflavine, theaflavin acid, thearubigine), and caffeic acid derivatives (chlorogenic acid and theogallin). A cup of brewed tea contains approximately 20–100 mg of caffeine

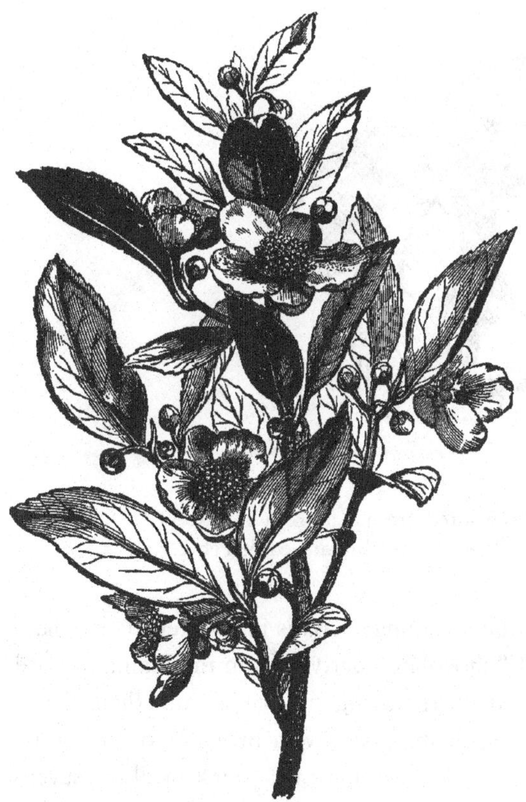

Figure 4.3
Tea *(Camellia sinensis)*. Reprinted from Culbreth DMR. (1927). *Materia Medica and Pharmacognosy*, 7th ed. Philadelphia: Lea & Febiger.

per 5 oz cup. Instant tea tends to contain somewhat less (20–50 mg per cup).

Cocoa and Chocolate

History and Botany

Cocoa is prepared by roasting the seeds of the plant *Theobroma cacao* (Robbers et al. 1996). *Theobroma* is a Greek term meaning "food of the gods," and *cacao* was the Aztec name for the plant. The tree is flowering and grows to a height of 4–6 meters. The seeds grow in grooved, ovate pods (figure 4.4).

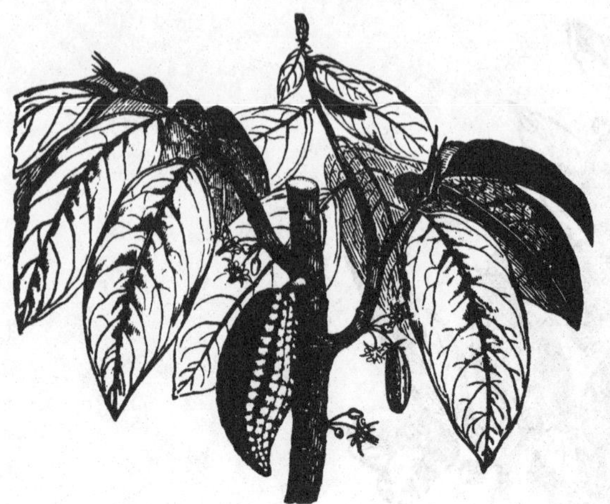

Figure 4.4
Cocoa *(Theobroma cacao)*. Reprinted from Culbreth DMR. (1927). *Materia Medica and Pharmacognosy*, 7th ed. Philadelphia: Lea & Febiger.

The most common way of consuming cocoa is in sweetened chocolate or baked goods. The word "chocolate" derives from the Nahuatl word *chocolatl*. Cocoa is prepared by removing the seeds from their shells, fermenting, and then roasting them. Cocoa was brought to Europe by Cortez in 1528, but did not become popular as a drink until the seventeenth century. It was initially consumed as a bitter drink, and was later added to milk solids and sugar to produce milk chocolate. The Swiss altered the history of candy in 1876 by marketing milk chocolate under the name Nestlé.

Chemical Constituents

Chocolate constitutes a significant dietary source of theobromine (Shivley and Tarka 1984). Hot cocoa, for example, prepared from instant mix provides approximately 60 mg of theobromine and 4 mg of caffeine per serving. Chocolate contains less caffeine per serving than coffee (0.4–1.2% of caffeine in cocoa), but may still have significant amounts, depending on the preparation. For example, milk chocolate contains up to 15 mg of caffeine per ounce, but dark chocolate can contain up to 35 mg per ounce.

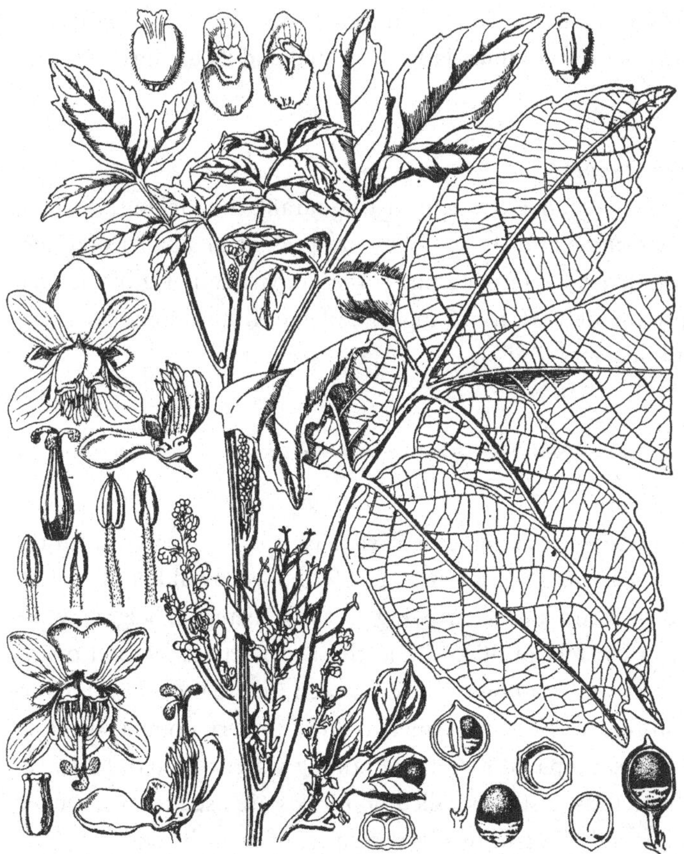

Figure 4.5
Guarana *(Paullinia cupana)*. Reprinted from Culbreth DMR. (1927). *Materia Medica and Pharmacognosy*, 7th ed. Philadelphia: Lea & Febiger.

Guarana

History and Botany

Guarana *(Paullinia cupana)* is a climbing shrub native to Brazil and Uruguay (Robbers et al. 1996; Gruenwald et al. 1998). It grows in the Amazon basin and may reach a length of 10 meters (figure 4.5). It produces a hazelnut-sized capsule, containing a purple-brown seed. The seeds are roasted over a fire, ground into a paste, molded into cylindrical sticks and dried again. Guarana is used as a stimulant by several local

Indian cultures to maintain alertness during tasks like hunting (Rudgley 1999). Guarana is now commercially cultivated and its use has increased in the West.

Chemical Constituents

The principal psychoactive constituent of guarana is caffeine (2.5–5%), although theobromine and theophylline are present in smaller amounts (Gruenwald et al. 1998). Depending on the preparation, 1 g of the seed contains approximately 35 to 55 mg of caffeine. It also contains a tannin, catechutannic acid (25%).

Maté

History and Botany

Maté (also known as yerba maté or Paraguay tea) is prepared from the plant *Ilex paraguariensis* (Robbers et al. 1996; Gruenwald et al. 1998). It is an evergreen shrub or tree, growing up to 20 meters in height. White flowers grow in clusters of 40–50, and the leaves are green and ovate. The fruit is fleshy and contains 5–8 seeds each (figure 4.6). *I. paraguariensis* grows in regions of South America and is a very popular drink in Argentina. Maté is prepared by adding boiling water to the dried leaves and stem. Characteristic straws called *bombillas* are used to drink maté. They are ornate and made of metal, with a strainer at the end.

Chemical Constituents

Maté contains both caffeine (0.4–2.4%) and theobromine (0.3–0.5%). Also found are triterpene saponins and the caffeic acid derivatives—chlorogenic acid, neochlorogenic acid, and cryptochlorogenic acid. Flavonoids in maté are rutin, isoquercetin, and kaemferol glycosides. A nitrile glycoside, menisdaurin, is also present, which is noncyanogenic.

Kola

History and Botany

Kola (also spelled cola) is a nut from the plants *Cola nitida* and *C. acuminata* (figure 4.7). It is an evergreen tree, growing 15 to 20 meters

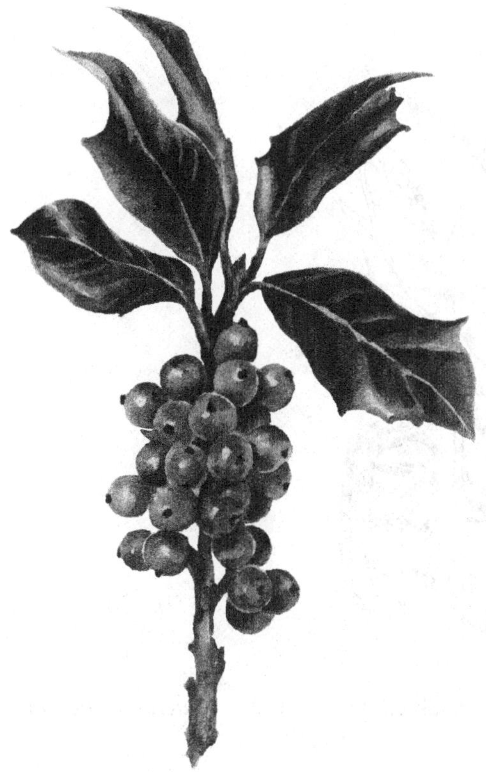

Figure 4.6
Maté *(Ilex paraguariensis)*. Reprinted with permission. Illustration by Lorraine Hara.

in height. The trunk branches as low as the base, and the dark green elliptoid leaves end in a spiraled tip. The flowers grow in small groups, and the star-shaped fruit contain 14 seeds, square to ovate in shape. The plant is indigenous to parts of West Africa, including Togo, Sierra Leone, and Angola. However, it is also cultivated in East Africa, Sri Lanka, Indonesia, Brazil, and the West Indies.

The seeds (or nuts) of the kola plant are taken from the pods and their outer coat is removed. They are chewed fresh or dried because they spoil quickly. The nuts are especially popular in Africa, where they are given as ceremonial gifts. However, kola is consumed around the world in the form of carbonated soft drinks, such as Coca-Cola. As the name implies,

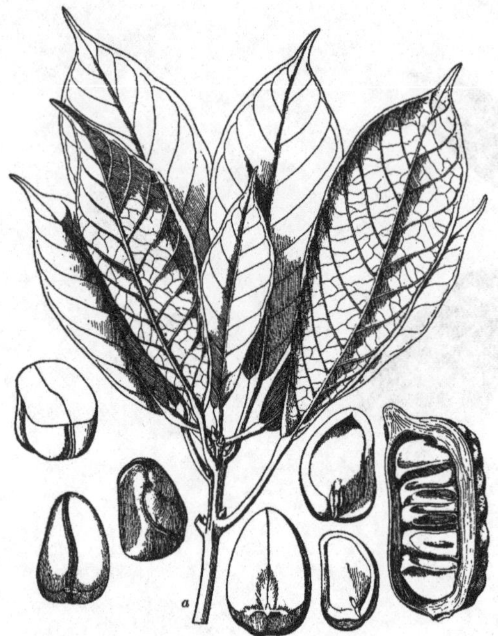

Figure 4.7
Kola *(Cola nitida)*. Reprinted from Culbreth DMR. (1927). *Materia Medica and Pharmacognosy*, 7th ed. Philadelphia: Lea & Febiger.

the original Coca-Cola contained extracts from the coca shrub *(Erythroxylon coca)* and the kola nut, thus making a small but potent combination of caffeine and cocaine. The drink, initially green in color, was first sold in 1887. However, cocaine was eliminated from the drink around the turn of the century. Decocainized coca extract is still used by the Coca-Cola company for flavoring.

Kola is not to be confused with gotu kola *(Centella asiatica)* (Gruenwald et al. 1998). Gotu kola is indigenous to Southeast Asia, and shows some antidepressant and sedative-like effects in animals, but has not yet been thoroughly researched.

Chemical Constituents

Kola nuts contain up to 3.5% caffeine. Theophylline and theobromine are present in smaller amounts (i.e., less than 1% theobromine). Also contained are (+)-catechin, (–)-epicatechin, catechin tannins and oligomeric proanthocyanidins. The fresh nut contains the tannin kolacatechin, which is split into caffeine and theobromine in the drying process. This process also gives kola the characteristic red-brown color, which is imitated by caramel coloring in cola soft drinks.

The Pharmacology of Purinergic Stimulants

Pharmacokinetics

Caffeine is highly bioavailable, being rapidly absorbed from the digestive tract (Serafin 1996). Absorption of oral theophylline is somewhat slower, peaking at 2 hours in the absence of food. Food generally slows, but does not limit, the absorption of methylxanthines. They are readily distributed to all body tissues and cross the placental barrier to enter breast milk. Caffeine and theophylline have similar volume distributions. Blood and brain concentrations of caffeine and theophylline in commonly consumed doses are 10–50 μM (Snyder and Sklar 1984). The half-life of caffeine is 3 to 7 hours, which increases in women using oral contraceptives or in late-stage pregnancy. The elimination of caffeine is variable, as much as fourfold, among individuals. The elimination half-life in adults is usually 8 to 9 hours.

Caffeine pharmacokinetics are nonlinear. For example, when comparing a 500 mg dose to a 250 mg dose, the clearance is reduced and elimination half-life is prolonged with the higher dose (Kaplan et al. 1997). Thus, larger doses prolong the action of the drug. Active metabolites of caffeine are paraxanthine, and to a lesser degree, theobromine, and theophylline. Urinary metabolites are l-methylxanthine, l-methyluric acid, and an acetylated uracil derivative.

Mechanisms of Action

Adenosine

The chief direct mechanism of the methylxanthines is the antagonism of adenosine receptors (Snyder and Sklar 1984). Adenosine is an inhibitory neurotransmitter, acting at inhibitory presynaptic autoreceptors. At micromolar concentrations, methylxanthines occupy 50% of adenosine receptors. Low micromolar concentrations of adenosine inhibit the release of most neurotransmitters, both excitatory and inhibitory. Chronic administration of caffeine elevates the number of adenosine receptors, likely reflecting a compensatory supersensitivity. So, by antagonizing adenosine receptors, methylxanthines cause a disinhibitory release of neurotransmitters.

Indirect Mechanisms

Several indirect neurochemical effects of methylxanthines contribute to their effects. Micromolar concentrations of caffeine enhance release of acetylcholine (Pedata et al. 1984). However, this effect is biphasic, augmenting release at 50 μM, but decreasing it at 0.5 μM. This effect is also modulatory, affecting stimulated, but not basal, release. Caffeine enhances acetylcholine release in the hippocampus, which is due to adenosine A_1 receptor subtypes (Carter et al. 1995). Conversely, chronic caffeine reduces the excitatory effect of acetylcholine in the cerebral cortex (Lin and Phillis 1990).

Adenosine inhibits the evoked release of excitatory amino acids glutamate and aspartate (Poli et al. 1991). So, methylxanthines cause a disinhibited release of excitatory amino acids. Caffeine also has a net disinhibitory effect on GABA neurotransmission (Kardos and Blandl 1994). It enhances GABA release in the spinal cord through nonbenzodiazepine mechanisms (Berti and Nistri 1983).

Caffeine increases extracellular serotonin levels in the hippocampus (Okada et al. 1999). Enhanced release of dopamine and norepinephrine occurs at higher doses (Morgan and Vestal 1989). An inhibition of monoamine reuptake occurs, but only in the millimolar range, which would not matter at normal oral doses (Reith et al. 1987).

Methylxanthines are inhibitors of the enzyme phosphodiesterase, preventing breakdown of and increasing intracellular levels of cAMP (Serafin 1996; Snyder and Sklar 1984). However, this action also only occurs in the millimolar range, at concentrations 100 times greater than those normally achieved (10–50 μM).

Caffeine induces a release of stored intracellular calcium (Snyder and Sklar 1984; Garaschuk et al. 1997). It augments twitching in skeletal muscle, but this effect is found in the millimolar range. Ca^{2+} effects alone do not explain caffeine's psychoactive effects, which occur at normal doses, but they could contribute to enhancement of neurotransmitter release (Avidor et al. 1994).

General Effects

Smooth Muscle

Methylxanthines relax smooth muscle, and have a bronchodilating effect in the lungs. Theophylline is used as a treatment for asthma. Methylxanthines dilate coronary arteries, increasing cardiac blood flow, but an opposite effect occurs on cerebral blood vessels (see below).

Diuretic Effects

Methylxanthines increase urine production. Increases are also seen in renal blood flow and glomerular filtration rate.

Cardiovascular Effects

Methylxanthines have complex effects on circulation (Serafin 1996). They mildly reduce peripheral vascular resistance, and were used to treat congestive heart failure until more selective drugs were developed. But the net cardiovascular effect of methylxanthines is due to a diverse mix of influences. Methylxanthines influence vagal and vasomotor areas in the brain, vascular, and cardiac tissues, and hormonal systems such as plasma catecholamines and renin-angiotensin. Caffeine generally increases blood pressure (Smith et al. 1994). Higher doses of caffeine can cause tachycardia and arrhythmias.

Neuroendocrine

High doses of caffeine produce a stresslike neuroendocrine response (Spindel 1984; Spindel et al. 1984). This includes increased levels of corticosterone, β-endorphin, and decreased serum growth hormone and thyrotropin-stimulating hormone in the rat. However, similar effects are not observed in humans until approximately 500 mg is consumed, the equivalent of 5 cups of coffee. At this dose in humans, elevations are seen in adrenocorticotrophic hormone, β-endorphin, and cortisol.

Metabolic clearance of caffeine is altered according to menstrual phase and hormonal status in women (Lane et al. 1992). Clearance is slower during the late luteal phase compared to the follicular phase, prior to the onset of menstruation. However, the size of the effect and significance in everyday activity remains in question.

Skeletal Muscle

Caffeine increases the capacity of skeletal muscle. This effect is probably due to the release of intracellular Ca^{2+}, and is observable in human performance. The contribution of central effects is also likely. Whether caffeine actually benefits exercise is contested (Spriet 1995; Dodd et al. 1993). Research does not consistently support caffeine enhancement of performance during high-intensity, short-term exercise. There is some evidence to suggest benefit during prolonged, moderate-intensity exercise.

Motor and Behavioral Effects

Caffeine improves psychomotor performance. For example, improvements are seen in manual dexterity (Bernstein et al. 1994). Enhancement of psychomotor performance is most evident when subjects are fatigued (Snyder and Sklar 1984).

Although perhaps counterintuitive, caffeine does not increase disruptive behavior in preschool children when objectively assessed (Baer 1987). A meta-analysis of 12 studies failed to show any adverse cognitve or behavioral effects in children (Stein et al. 1996).

The effect of caffeine in children may depend on physiological predisposition (Rapoport et al. 1984). Children who are normally high habitual consumers of caffeine (500 mg/day or more) show higher anxiety and lower autonomic arousal when not receiving caffeine. Habitually low caffeine consumers are more emotional, inattentive, and restless when receiving 10 mg/kg of caffeine, while the high habitual users are rated as unchanged. Low doses of caffeine added to methylphenidate produce greater improvement in attention deficit disorder than methylphenidate alone (Garfinkel et al. 1981). Although some people ingest caffeine in an attempt to "sober up" after drinking ethanol, research does not support this. While caffeine may increase arousal and reverse deficits in reaction time caused by alcohol, it does not affect other variables such as standing steadiness, manual dexterity, numerical reasoning, perceptual speed, or verbal fluency (Franks et al. 1975).

Sleep and Arousal

Caffeine has potent psychostimulant effects, increasing the general level of arousal (Rogers and Dernoncourt 1998). Along with increasing alertness, caffeine increases the sleep latency (Zwyghuizen-Doorenbos et al. 1990). Coffee and caffeine have insomnia-like effects on sleep, shifting the onset of REM sleep and stages 3 and 4 to later in the night (Karacan et al. 1976).

Emotional

Caffeine has mixed effects on mood and emotion. Low doses improve feelings of energy and mood (Warburton 1995; Rogers and Dernoncourt 1998). However, progressively higher doses also increase subjective feelings of anxiety, tension, and nervousness (Loke 1988; Bernstein et al. 1994). For example, positive mood effects are generally obtained with a 250 mg dose, and negative effects occur at a 500 mg dose (Kaplan et al. 1997). People with anxiety or panic disorders are even more susceptible to the anxiogenic effects of caffeine (Shear 1986). Caffeine also increases the autonomic response to novel situations (Davidson and Smith 1991).

Electrophysiological Effects

As might be expected, caffeine produces an activation effect on the EEG, reducing theta and delta power (Dimpfel and Schober 1993). Caffeine reverses the EEG slowing brought on by nicotine abstinence (Cohen et al. 1994). ERP studies of the effects of caffeine on visual attention suggest that it depends on the number of relevant visual targets, and not the overall number of targets (Lorist et al. 1996). On the other hand, caffeine withdrawal causes a decrease in P300 amplitude or latency (Reeves et al. 1999). Caffeine improves performance on a visual search task, with increases in the amplitude of the N1, N2b, and P3b waves (Lorist et al. 1995). The effect of caffeine on the P300 is more pronounced in fatigued than well-rested subjects performing a visual search task (Lorist et al. 1994).

Cerebral Blood Flow and Glucose Metabolism

PET and ^{133}Xenon SPECT show significant decreases (~30%) in whole-brain cerebral blood flow after a dose of 250 mg of caffeine (Cameron et al. 1990; Mathew et al. 1983). Local cerebral blood flow is decreased after administration of caffeine, mostly in motor and auditory areas, but no regional differences are seen in humans (Nehlig et al. 1990; Cameron et al. 1990). Decreases in cerebral blood flow persist at least 90 minutes after ingestion (Mathew and Wilson 1985). Despite decreased cerebral blood flow, caffeine causes widespread increases in brain metabolism and glucose utilization (Schroeder et al. 1989; Nehlig et al. 1984).

In subjects who experience anxiety and unpleasant physiological arousal from caffeine, it can cause an incease in brain lactate (Dager et al. 1999). This is significant in light of the association between lactate and anxiety in general (Dager et al. 1990).

Cognitive Effects

Caffeine has been found to quicken reaction time and enhance vigilance, increase self-rated alertness, and improve mood (Rogers and Dernoncourt 1998). Even though some tolerance might develop to the cognition-enhancing effects of caffeine, improvements are sustained with chronic consumption (Jarvis 1993). Conversely, caffeine withdrawal has adverse effects on cognition (James 1998; Lane and Phillips-Bute 1998). For example, several psychometric measures of managerial performance suffer upon withdrawal (Streufert et al. 1995). Some have contended that caffeine-induced improvements are partly due to reversal of withdrawal-associated deficits (Rogers and Dernoncourt 1998).

However, caffeine still shows improvements in mood, attention, problem solving, and memory, which are distinct from alleviating abstinence (Warburton 1995). Cognitive effects are somewhat more associated with coffee than tea, but the stimulant and cognitive effects of black tea and coffee are similar on several cognitive measures (Hindmarch et al. 1998; Jarvis 1993). Several studies indicate sex differences in the cognitive effects of caffeine, with generally greater effects in females (Smith et al. 1993). However, this effect varies with the menstrual cycle, so it has been suggested that estrogen levels may play a role (Arnold et al. 1987). For unknown neurochemical reasons, a combination of caffeine with aspirin further improves vigilance and mood, more so than caffeine or aspirin alone (Lieberman et al. 1987).

Caffeine reverses deficits in alertness produced by sleep deprivation (Penetar et al. 1993). It also improves performance in sustained attention tasks (Smith et al. 1994; Warburton 1995). Some studies show non-significant effects on attention, but improvement is evident in more complex attention tasks, like complex cancellation (involving addition and multiplication) as compared to simple digit cancellation (Loke 1988). But this may depend on the nature of the task. Caffeine also reduces subjective fatigue, making exertion of concentration less effortful. This effect differs across sexes, decreasing subjective effort in men and increasing it in women performing a complex mental task (e.g., Raven's progressive matrices) (Linde 1995). On the other hand, caffeine may have some adverse effects on attention as well. Some have shown poorer accuracy with caffeine in vigilance tasks (Smith et al. 1992). Men given caffeine perform more poorly on a numerical version of the Stroop task, which requires suppression of automatic responses to conflicting stimuli (Foreman et al. 1989). However, other studies (using 125 or 250 mg) have not shown any effect of caffeine in the Stroop test (Edwards et al. 1996).

Although caffeine increases response speed in some visual attention tasks, it is apparently not due to decreased distractibility or suppression of irrelevant responses (Kenemans and Verbaten 1998). Cognitive decline is evident during withdrawal from caffeine, primarily on measures of response time and sustained attention (Bernstein et al. 1998). The degree of habitual caffeine use is the strongest variable predicting the response to caffeine in a visual attention task (Loke and Meliska 1984). Similar to caffeine, theophylline produces improvement on sustained attention tasks (Bryant et al. 1998), but caffeine appears to be a more potent CNS stimulant (Yu et al. 1991). Caffeine improves the accuracy of reaction time tasks in hyperkinetic children (Reichard and Elder 1977).

Caffeine improves performance on tests of semantic memory, free recall, and recognition memory (Smith et al. 1994; Warburton 1995). However, the effects are both dose and task dependent. In some studies, higher doses produced greater improvement, while in others subjects receiving caffeine performed slightly worse than placebo (Loke 1988;

Terry and Phifer 1986). Caffeine reduces the impairments caused by scopolamine in short- and long-term free recall memory in humans (Riedel et al. 1995). It also reverses scopolamine-induced decrements in visual search, reading speed, and fine motor speed (e.g., finger-tapping). These effects are interesting in light of caffeine's effect on cerebral acetylcholine activity. Indirect cholinergic mechanisms may be involved in the mnestic effects of caffeine, because scopolamine reverses caffeine's effect in animal maze tasks (Roussinov and Yonkov 1976). However, dopamine may also be involved because the beneficial effects of caffeine on memory consolidation in mice are also blocked by a D_2 antagonist (sulpiride) (Cestari and Castellano 1996).

Caffeine improves performance on tests of logical reasoning and problem solving (Smith et al. 1994; Warburton 1995). However, this varies with the task, because no effects are objectively seen on Raven's Progressive Matrices, a test of nonverbal reasoning (Linde 1995)

Addiction and Dependence

Some individuals use caffeine in a manner that could arguably be classified as abuse. Tolerance is evident with chronic use, and discontinuation can produce an aversive withdrawal syndrome. Cessation of even low to moderate use (the equivalent of 2.5 cups of coffee per day) causes fatigue, headache, increased anxiety, and decreases in mood. Physiological changes such as altered adenosine receptors may accompany dependence, and caffeine affects the release of dopamine. Certainly, caffeine dependence is not as intense and consuming as that produced by cocaine or heroin. Severe withdrawal is avoidable by gradual tapering of the dose, and clinical treatment is generally not necessary. However, combined cigarette and coffee abstinence in regular consumers can cause more severe symptoms such as mental cloudiness, irritability, and muscular tension, (Cohen et al. 1994).

Toxicity

Consumed in normal doses, caffeine generally does not have any acute toxicity. Fatal poisoning with caffeine is rare, occuring with doses between 5 and 10 g. Adverse effects are seen with doses of 1 g or lower, due primarily to circulatory and central effects. Overdoses initially present with behavioral excitation and insomnia, progressing to delirum and convulsions. Tachycardia and vomiting are common at these doses.

Chronic use of large amounts of caffeine has been associated with an increased risk of cardiovascular disease. However, this finding is debated because statistically adjusting for other risk factors shows a minimized added risk for caffeine (Grobbee et al. 1990). Nonetheless, a lipid fraction of boiled coffee dose-dependently elevates cholesterol and low density lipoproteins, which is prevented by the filtered preparation of coffee (Pirich et al. 1993). Another potential influence on cardiovascular disease is an elevation of homocysteine levels, which also occurs in drinkers of filtered coffee (Nygård et al. 1997).

Genotoxicity

Genotoxic effects of caffeine have been reported, but they only occur in large doses (>1 mM), far exceeding what could be obtained by oral dosing (D'Ambrosio 1994).

Pediatric and Prenantal Toxicity

Caffeine is likely the most commonly used drug among pregnant women, but whether or not it is safe during pregnancy is still a matter of debate. Caffeine intake during pregnancy is not related to infant height, weight, or head circumference, or to measures of IQ and attention at 7 years of age (Barr and Streissguth 1991). On the other hand, there are associations with reduced fertility, miscarriage, growth retardation in utero, and sudden infant death syndrome (Golding 1995; Ford et al. 1998). Unlike the adult brain, fetal brains may accumulate theophylline and theobromine when exposed to doses reached during normal consumption (Wilkinson and Pollard 1993). Definitive prospective studies on the safety of caffeine during pregnancy have not yet been done (Golding 1995; Barr and Streissguth 1991).

Seizures and Epilepsy

Very high doses of caffeine can induce seizures in those with no preexisting seizure disorder. Caffeine also prolongs seizures induced by electroconvulsive treatment in humans (Shapira et al. 1987). Given the known neurochemical actions of methylxanthines, they are probably best avoided by people with epilepsy.

Cholinergic Stimulants

Tobacco

History and Botany

The tobacco plant *(Nicotiana tabacum)* is an annual or biennial plant growing 1–3 meters in height (Gruenwald et al. 1998). The leaves range from ovate in shape to narrow and tapering, and grow up to 50 cm in length. Its pinkish flowers grow in branched pedicels (figure 4.8). The tobacco plant originated in tropical regions of America, but is now cultivated in China, Turkey, Greece, Holland, France, Germany, and many countries in subtropical regions. The leaves are harvested and dried for consumption by smoking or chewing.

The tobacco plant was long used by Native Americans before the arrival of Europeans. The word *tobacco* derives from *tabacum*, the Indian name for the pipe they used to smoke it. Nicotine, the principle psychoactive chemical in tobacco, was named after Jean Nicot de Villemain, a French diplomat who advocated its use in Europe in the late 1500s (Rudgley 1999). It is less commonly known that tobacco grew wildly in the interior of Australia, and was used by inhabitants there before Europeans arrived.

Chemical Constituents

The primary psychoactive alkaloid in tobacco is nicotine (figure 4.9), occuring between 0.6 and 9.0% (Robbers et al. 1996; Gruenwald et al. 1998). Other alkaloids include nornicotine, *N*-formylnornicotine, cotinine, myosmin, *β*-nicotyrine, anabasine, and nicotellin. Nicotine alone can produce the effects commonly associated with tobacco use, but other tobacco alkaloids are likely to contribute.

Mechanisms of Action

Acetylcholine Nicotine is an agonist at nicotinic acetylcholine receptors, which were named after the drug (Taylor 1996). Nicotine opens the

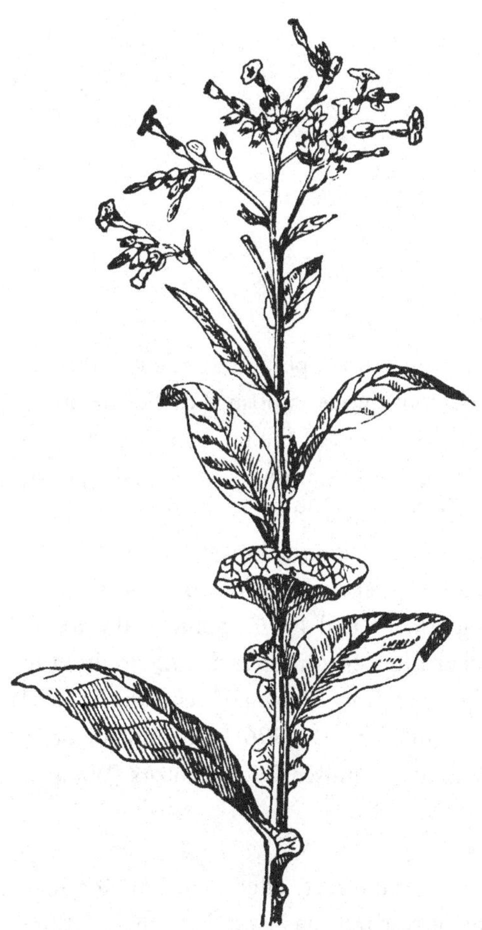

Figure 4.8
Tobacco *(Nicotiana tabacum)*. Reprinted from Culbreth DMR. (1927). *Materia Medica and Pharmacognosy*, 7th ed. Philadelphia: Lea & Febiger.

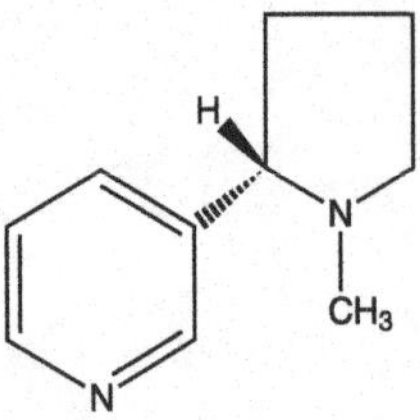

H
N
N
CH_3

Figure 4.9
Chemical structure of nicotine.

ion channel, allowing influx of cations and depolarizing the membrane. However, to complicate matters, continuous exposure of the nicotinic receptor to an agonist causes desensitization of the receptor, resulting in an inactivation of the channel. Thus, the drug initially acts as an agonist, and then as an antagonist (Reitstetter et al. 1999).

Nicotinic receptors are widely distributed in the brain and are involved in a number of physiological processes. The prefrontal cortex is a major site for the cognitive effects of nicotine (Vidal 1996). Some of the cognitive benefits of nicotine may occur after chronic treatment, resulting in part from nicotinic receptor up-regulation in frontal, entorhinal, and dorsal hippocampal regions (Abdulla et al. 1996). Chronic nicotine treatment also increases the sensitivity of muscarinic receptors (Wang et al. 1996).

Indirect mechanisms Nicotine has indirect effects on monoamine systems. A considerable amount of research has examined the relationships between nicotine and dopamine activity in the brain, in light of dopamine's role in reinforcement and nicotine's addictive properties. Nicotine increases dopamine turnover in the striatum and cerebral cortex (Clarke and Reuben 1996; Tani et al. 1997; Nanri et al. 1998). It also increases burst activity in dopamine neurons of the ventral tegmental area (VTA), a primary source of dopamine to the forebrain (Nisell et al. 1995; Fisher et al. 1998). Such a firing pattern in the VTA is associated with processes of reinforcement, learning, and cognitive activity. Nicotine actions on dopaminergic neurons occur at both somatodendritic sites and synaptic terminals. Further, both systemic nicotine and direct administration into the VTA increase dopamine release in the nucleus accumbens. Nicotine sensitizes mesoaccumbens dopamine neurons, which is related to enhanced burst firing (Balfour et al. 1998).

Nicotine causes a release of norepinephrine from the locus coeruleus and facilitates release of norepinephrine in the hippocampus (Gallardo and Leslie 1998; Mitchell 1993; Sershen et al. 1997; Fu et al. 1999). The norepinephrine released by nicotine, in turn, modulates raphe neurons (Li et al. 1998).

More complicated effects are seen on 5-HT turnover, with increases at low doses but decreases at higher doses (Smith et al. 1991). Systemic nicotine increases release of serotonin in frontal cortex, beginning within 20 minutes and lasting approximately 2 hours (Ribeiro, et al. 1993) Smokers show a 40% decrease in the level of MAO_B and 28% decrease in MAO_A compared to nonsmokers or former smokers (Fowler et al. 1996a, 1996b, 1998). This difference is likely to be pharmacological and not genetic because former smokers do not differ from nonsmokers in this respect. Chronic nicotine increases tyrosine hydroxylase activity in noradrenergic and dopaminergic cell bodies (Smith et al. 1991).

Nicotine also has effects on amino acid neurotransmitters. Presynaptic nicotinic receptors enhance transmission at glutamate and GABA synapses (McGehee et al. 1995; Gray et al. 1996; Léna and Changeux 1997). Nicotine dose-dependently increases glutamate release in rat prefrontal cortex, and facilitates activity in projections from the thalamus to prefrontal cortex (Gioanni et al. 1999). In the hippocampus, nicotinic stimulation enhances synaptic transmission of glutamate in a Ca^{2+}-dependent manner (Radcliffe and Dani 1998). This enhancement lasts for minutes, and could alter the time span during which incoming signals could elicit synaptic plasticity. Nicotine modulates excitatory neurotransmission through NMDA receptors in prefrontal cortex (Vidal and Changeux 1993). It also increases production of nitric oxide and cyclic GMP in the hippocampus through NMDA receptors (Fedele et al. 1998).

Pharmacokinetics

When smoked, nicotine is very rapidly and efficiently (90%) absorbed into the bloodstream. When chewed, absorption is slower but the duration of effect is longer. The average cigarette contains approximately 12 mg of nicotine and delivers approximately 1 mg to the smoker (Fukumoto et al. 1997; Gori and Lynch 1985). Changing the intensity of puffing can greatly alter the delivery of nicotine. Behavioral studies using reduced-nicotine cigarettes show that people increase their consumption to compensate for the lower nicotine levels (Rusted et al. 1996).

Absorption occurs through the respiratory tract, oral membranes, and skin (Taylor 1996). Absorption from the stomach is limited, unless the acidity is reduced, because nicotine is a strong base. Between 80 and 90% of nicotine is metabolized, mainly in the liver but also the kidneys and lungs. Cotinine is the primary metabolite of nicotine, and the half-life of nicotine is about 2 hours. Elimination occurs by the kidneys, but it is also present in the breast milk of lactating women.

General Effects

Nicotine affects nearly every physiological system of the body (Le Houezec and Benowitz 1991). However, the effects are complex and unpredictable due to actions on multiple sites, and the stimulation-desensitization of nicotinic receptors.

Cardiovascular Nicotine increases heart rate, heart contractility, and blood pressure by activation of the sympathetic ganglia and inactivation of parasympathetic ganglia (Haass and Kubler 1997; Grassi et al. 1994). Nicotinic receptors are present on postganglionic sympathetic nerve endings and the adrenal medulla. Effects also occur through receptors on the aortic and carotid bodies, and central medullary areas regulating heart rate. Cessation in smoking is associated with notable improvements in exercise capacity (Albrecht et al. 1998).

Gastrointestinal Tobacco has gastrointestinal effects that result from parasympathetic stimulation, with a net effect of increased bowel activity (Taylor 1996). Initial exposure to nicotine typically causes nausea, vomiting, and occasionally diarrhea.

Neuroendocrine Tobacco smoking is acutely related to elevations in plasma arginine vasopressin, neurophs I, β-endorphin, and β-lipotropin (Pomerleau et al. 1983). Cigarette smoking elevates plasma cortisol levels via a central mechanism in the hypothalamus or brain stem

(Targovnik 1989). Smoking cessation causes a decrease in plasma cortisol and epinephrine levels. However, effects on the adrenal medulla are biphasic, with small doses evoking release of plasma catecholamines and large doses inhibiting it (Talyor 1996).

Nicotinic receptors are present in the pineal gland (Stankov et al. 1993). Although there appear to be no direct effects of nicotine on the release of melatonin, it indirectly reduces the accumulation of melatonin stimulated by norepinephrine. Nicotine increases circulating levels of norepinephrine and epinephrine (Pomerleau et al. 1983).

Neuromuscular Nicotinic receptors are responsible for transmission at the neuromuscular junction. While briefly causing stimulation, this phase is rapidly obscured by desensitization and neuromuscular blockade. Thus, nicotine has muscle-relaxant effects.

Behavioral and emotional Nicotine has a number of behavioral and emotional effects. It increases locomotor activity, which is mediated by increased dopamine in the nucleus accumbens (Mirza 1996). Nicotine suppresses appetite and decreases weight gain in rats (Grunberg et al. 1986). Conversely, cessation of smoking causes increases in body weight. Nicotine increases sexual receptivity in female rats, but whether this occurs in humans has not been studied—or at least not formally (Fuxe et al. 1977).

Nicotine reduces anxiety in humans, more so in females than males (Stewart et al. 1997). Similar to nicotine, the nicotinic channel activator ABT-418 has anxiolytic effects (Brioni et al. 1994). Nicotine reduces anxiety and right hemisphere EEG activation in subjects watching a stress-inducing movie (Gilbert et al. 1989). Conversely, smoking cessation is commonly associated with increases in anxiety and dysphoria (West and Hajek 1997).

Electrophysiological Tobacco smoking produces cortical activation on the EEG. Broadly, it reduces slow-wave activity (theta and delta) and increases activity in alpha and beta frequency bands (Knott et al. 1998; Pritchard et al. 1999). Other studies have found more isolated effects in alpha frequencies (Domino and Matsuoka 1994; Foulds et al. 1994).

Nicotine gum similarly increases alpha and beta activity on the EEG and decreases theta activity (Pickworth et al. 1986). In contrast, denicotinized cigarettes do not have any EEG effects (Pritchard et al. 1999).

Nicotine increases the occurrence of the hippocampal theta rhythm in rabbits (Yamamoto 1998). The hippocampal theta activity is closely associated with learning and memory (Bennett 1973). Nicotine also induces theta activity in the rat hippocampus and activates functionally related neurons in the posterior cingulate gyrus (Colom et al. 1988). Similar effects are found in nicotine replacement (Newton et al. 1983). Conversely, smoking abstinence causes an increase in theta power and decreases in alpha and beta activity (Pickworth et al. 1989, 1996). This effect appears as early as 29 hours after cessation and may persist for a week. The nicotinic antagonist mecamylamine causes decreases in alpha frequency and increases in delta frequency, and exacerbates EEG signs of tobacco abstinence in smokers (Pickworth et al. 1997). This is accompanied by cognitive decrease in peformance on tests of vigilance, distractibility, and delayed recall.

The anxiolytic effects of nicotine are evident in EEG changes. While subjects watched a stress-inducing movie, higher doses of nicotine reduced anxiety and reduced right hemisphere EEG activation (Gilbert et al. 1989).

When abstaining smokers resume smoking, a beneficial reduction in P300 latency occurs for visual, but not auditory, oddball tasks (Houlihan et al. 1996). Using ERPs and a recognition memory task, smokers show enhanced P300s to both targets and distractors (Pineda et al. 1998). Abstinent smokers, however, show less of a discriminating difference in reactions to targets versus distractors. Further, abstinent smokers have greater latencies relative to nonsmokers.

Cerebral blood flow and glucose metabolism Nicotine increases cerebral blood flow (Hara et al. 1993; Yokoi et al. 1993). Functional MRI of smokers who were administered intravenous nicotine shows increases of cerebral blood flow in several areas of the brain. Corresponding to feelings of mood elevation, nicotine activates the nucleus accumbens, amygdala, cingulate cortex, and frontal lobes. This activation is very consistent with functional systems subserving arousal and reinforcement.

Increases in cerebral blood flow elicited from stimulation of the basal forebrain are mediated by nicotinic and not muscarinic receptors (Linville et al. 1993). During an attention task, nicotine increases cerebral blood flow to the the anterior cingulate cortex, cerebellum, and occipital cortex, supporting its role in activating attentional systems (Ghatan et al. 1998).

Nicotine dose-dependently increases regional glucose metabolism in the rat brain (McNamara et al. 1990). The regional specificty also depends on dosage used, where low doses (0.1 mg/kg) have no effect, moderate doses (1.0 mg/kg) have region-specific effects in multiple areas, and high doses (10 mg/kg) produce generalized activation. Moderate doses increase glucose metabolism in primarily subcortical areas: thalamic nuclei, cerebellum, superior colliculus, median raphe, reticular formation, and the habenulointerpeduncular pathway. Similar to other abused drugs, nicotine increases glucose utilization and dopamine activity in the shell of the nucleus accumbens (Pontieri et al. 1998).

Dependence and Addiction

Few, if any, clinicians or scientists would argue with the position that tobacco is addicting. It has addictive properties in both animals and in humans (Dougherty et al. 1981). Regular smokers who undergo abstinence show a common withdrawal syndrome consisting of craving, mood changes, overarousal, cognitive deficits, and sleep disturbance (Shiffman et al. 1995). Light occasional smokers, however, do not seem to experience this syndrome. Although the physical withdrawal symptoms of nicotine are mild compared to those of ethanol or opioid withdrawal, they are still unpleasant and there is a high rate of long-term relapse (Nil 1991).

Emotional factors play a significant role in quitting tobacco use (Carmody 1989). Depression is overrepresented among smokers (Hall et al. 1993). Depressed smokers experience more intense withdrawal symptoms, have less success at quitting, and a greater chance of relapse. They report higher levels of dependence than nondepressed smokers and are more likely to use nicotine as self-medication to reduce depression and gain stimulation (Lerman et al. 1996). There may be some sex differences in the pattern of smoking: women report smoking more in emotional and social situations, whereas men smoke more in situations requiring close attention to a task. In both sexes, the trait of sensation seeking is related to being a former or current smoker.

The habit-forming property of tobacco occurs through a combination of positive and negative reinforment. Nicotine effects of mood elevation and cognitive enhancements serve as positive reinforcers for smoking. The rewarding effects of tobacco are related to nicotine's stimulation of the mesolimbic dopamine system (Balfour 1994; Stolerman and Shoaib 1991; Clarke 1990). This is similar to other drugs of abuse and occurs through nicotinic receptors in the ventral tegmental area, although the stimulus properties of nicotine do not depend on dopamine alone, and involve multiple neuroanatomical areas (Corrigall et al. 1992; Leshner and Koob 1999; Schilstrom et al. 1998; Shoaib 1998). Nicotine increases burst activity in mesolimbic areas, which is associated with motivational processes in reinforcement, learning, and cognition (Nisell et al. 1995). Chronic exposure to levels achieved by smokers desensitizes nicotinic receptors that modulate mesolimbic dopamine activity (Benwell et al. 1995; Pidoplichko et al. 1997). This correlates with the fact that inital exposures are reinforcing or pleasurable, which subsequently decrease over repeated exposures.

Negative reinforcement of tobacco use occurs in the form of anxiety reduction and avoidance of the unpleasant nicotine withdrawal syndrome. Nicotine withdrawal is aversive, involving depressed mood, irritability, and drug craving. It also increases anxiety, which abates approximately after one week of abstinence (West and Hajek 1997; Hughes et al. 1991). Other withdrawal symptoms include increased appetite, sleep disruption, difficulty concentrating, restlessness, and irritability (Jorenby et al. 1996). Most symptoms return to baseline level by 1 month, but weight gain, appetite increases, and drug craving continue for 6 months in many smokers (Hughes et al. 1991). Cravings may particularly contribute to relapse in the long term. Prevention of the weight gain that ensues after tobacco cessation may serve as a further source of negative reinforcement. Reinstatement of nicotine alleviates the withdrawal symptoms. Nicotine withdrawal is also accompanied by elevations in brain reward thresholds for several days (Epping-Jordan et al. 1998).

Dependence on nicotine does not necessarily begin immediately, but rather may develop over time (Nelson and Wittchen 1998). Among a sample of adolescent and young adult smokers in Germany, the lifetime prevalence of nicotine dependence (using DSM-IV criteria) was 19% and rose to 52% over time. No gender differences are seen in the progression of occasional use to dependence. A dose-response relationship is found between the number of cigarettes smoked daily and unsuccessful cutback attempts. Despite one's desire and repeated attempts to quit, smoking is a behavior that is resistant to change.

Pharmacological Treatment of Nicotine Dependence

Several pharmacological approaches have been developed to treat tobacco dependence (Sachs and Leischow 1991). Optimally, they should be integrated with psychotherapeutic or behavior modification programs.

Replacement strategies One strategy to treat tobacco addiction is nicotine replacement. This allows one to alter the behavioral habit of smoking while keeping nicotine levels constant, which can eventually be tapered. Nicotine replacement is achieved through transdermal and oral (gum) approaches. The primary difference between nicotine delivery from cigarettes versus nicotine gum and transdermal nicotine is the rate of absorption (Pomerleau 1992). Smoking allows high levels to build up in the blood stream, whereas the other methods allow more gradual absorption across the skin or mucosal membranes. Thus, the gum and patch have a slower onset of action and less reinforcing effects. Nonetheless, controlled studies of nicotine replacement show that it reduces the severity of withdrawal symptoms such as anxiety, irritability, increased appetite, and weight gain (Jorenby et al. 1996).

Alternative pharmacological approaches Clonidine, an α_2 adrenergic agonist, has been employed as adjunctive therapy to assist in smoking cessation. However, results have been mixed or the effects small (Gourlay et al. 1994; Hilleman et al. 1993; Franks et al. 1989). Buspirone (BuSpar) is a 5-HT_{1A} partial agonist with anxiolytic effects. It has been tested as a treatment for smoking cessation because anxiety is a prominent feature of nicotine withdrawal (Farid and Abate 1998). To date, results have been mixed and more controlled research is needed.

Bupropion is another alternative pharmacological approach to tobacco abstinence. It is an antidepressant drug that blocks reuptake of norepinephrine and dopamine, and also blocks nicotinic receptors in the low to intermediate micromolar range (Fryer and Lukas 1999). Thus, the effects of bupropion on nicotine addiction may be through dual effects on dopaminergic and nicotinic systems. Further, it has been an effective treatment in controlled studies, both alone and in combination with the nicotine patch. Bupropion alone or in combination with a nicotine patch was more effective than placebo or the nicotine patch alone.

Toxicity

Acute Nicotine is a very toxic drug in acute high doses (Taylor 1996). The lethal dose in adult humans is approximately 60 mg. Symptoms of acute poisoning include headache, dizziness, salivation, cold sweats, abdominal pain, nausea, vomiting, and diarrhea. Sensory disturbances, confusion, and convulsions also occur. Blood pressure drops, the pulse becomes weak and irregular, and respiration becomes difficult. Death usually results from respiratory failure.

Chronic Several illnesses are associated with long-term chronic tobacco use. Over 435,000 deaths in the United States and 2.5 million deaths worldwide are annually attributed to tobacco smoking (U.S. Department of Health and Human Services 1989; Barry 1991). These associated illnesses are primarily cancer, pulmonary, and cardiovascular disease. Cigarette smoking is a primary cause of lung cancer, which results from carcinogenic products in cigarette smoke. One identified carcinogen damages the cancer suppressor gene P53 (Denissenko et al. 1996).

Respiratory problems caused by chronic cigarette smoking include labored breathing, wheezing, chest pain, congestion, and increased susceptibility to respiratory infections. Tobacco smoking is also the leading cause of emphysema (Thurlbeck 1984). Smoking can increase blood pressure and heart rate, and both nicotine and the carbon monoxide in tobacco smoke increase the incidence of atherosclerosis and thrombosis. Chronically, smoking is associated with a 3 to 19 times greater rate of death by coronary artery disease.

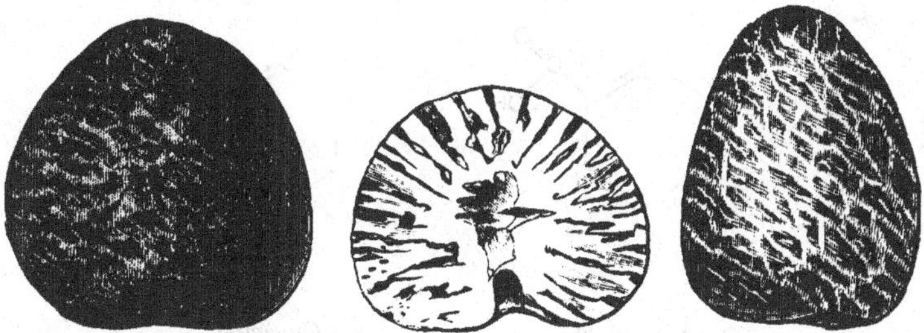

Figure 4.10
Areca *(Areca catechu)*. Reprinted from Culbreth DMR. (1927). *Materia Medica and Pharmacognosy*, 7th ed. Philadelphia: Lea & Febiger.

Prenatal and neonatal toxicity Although nicotine may provide cognitive benefits in adulthood, particularly in dementia, there is evidence that developmental exposure to tobacco or nicotine is detrimental. Prenatal exposure to nicotine in rats causes subtle changes in choice accuracy and response latency during learning (Levin et al. 1993). Further, such rats show an exaggerated impairment when challenged with nicotinic antagonists. Neonatal exposure to nicotine causes impairments in the electrophysiological responses of the hippocampus to novel auditory stimuli (Ehlers et al. 1997).

In humans, smoking during pregnancy is associated with reduced size during the fetal stage and infancy, and a greater tendency toward obesity at age 5 (Vik et al. 1996). Passive exposure to smoke is associated with reduced pulmonary function in children, especially in those with respiratory illnesses such as asthma (Bek et al. 1999; Di Benedetto 1995). Prenatal cigarette smoking, and perhaps postnatal passive exposure, also increases the risk for sudden infant death syndrome (Schellscheidt et al. 1997; Malloy 1988; Alm et al. 1998).

Areca

History and Botany

Areca *(Areca catechu)* is a palm tree that grows up to 30 meters in height (Gruenwald et al. 1998; Robbers et al. 1996). It is cultivated in India, southeast Asia, the East Indies, and East Africa. It grows green leaflets and numerous flowers. The fruit of the areca palm is a nut that contains a single seed and a thin seed coat (figure 4.10). Areca is chewed alone or

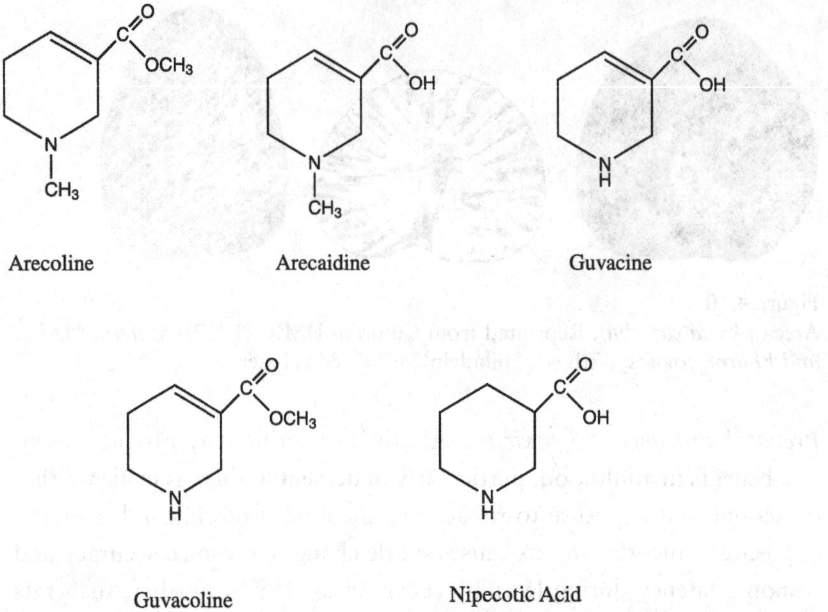

Arecoline Arecaidine Guvacine

Guvacoline Nipecotic Acid

Firgure 4.11
Chemical structure of areca alkaloids.

in a quid by over 200 million people around the world for its stimulating effects. It is most popularly consumed in central, southern, and southeast Asia. Areca is the fourth most popular drug in the world, following nicotine, ethanol, and caffeine (Norton 1998).

The areca nut is sometimes erroneously referred to as the betel nut (Trivedy et al. 1999). *Betel* refers to a combined preparation of the areca nut *(Areca catechu)* and lime (calcium hydroxide), rolled into the leaf of the betel pepper *(Piper betle)* (Morton 1998).

Chemical Constituents

Areca contains several alkaloids that are derived from pyridine (Robbers et al. 1996; Gruenwald et al. 1998). These include arecoline, arecaidine, guvacoline (or norarecoline), and guvacine (figure 4.11). Arecoline is the most abundant alkaloid, and total alkaloid content can reach 0.45%. Arecoline and arecaidine are up to 15 times more potent than guvacoline and guvacine (Wolf-Pflugmann et al. 1989). Areca also contains nipecotic acid and tannins (Johnston et al. 1975; Gruenwald et al. 1998).

Pharmacokinetics
Limited data are available on the pharmacokinetics of arecoline. Intravenously administered arecoline in subjects with Alzheimer's disease shows variation in the optimal dose (between 4 and 16 mg/day) due to differing plasma kinetics (Asthana et al. 1996). The mean plasma half-lives for these doses were 0.95 ± 0.54 and 9.3 ± 4.5 minutes, respectively. However, the mean plasma concentrations that optimized cognitive effects were 0.31 ± 0.14 ng/ml. Drug clearance was 13.6 ± 5.8 L/min and the volume of distribution was 205 ± 170 L.

Oral administration of arecoline is ineffective for clinical purposes due to first-pass metabolism (Hussain and Mollica 1991). The nasal route is an alternate possibility, with 85% bioavailability compared to intramuscular administration.

Mechanisms of Action

Acetylcholine All four alkaloids derived from areca (arecoline, arecaidine, guvacoline, and guvacine) act as full agonists at muscarinic acetylcholine receptors (Wolf-Pflugmann et al. 1989). Peripherally administered arecoline (10 mg/kg) subtly reduces cortical and subcortical acetylcholine levels (Molinengo et al. 1986).

Monoamine Arecoline has indirect effects on catecholamine levels (Molinengo et al. 1986). Significant reductions occur in norepinephrine levels, but increases occur in dopamine levels in both cortical and subcortical areas.

Amino acid Nipecotic acid is a potent inhibitor of GABA uptake, effective in the low micromolar range (Johnston et al. 1975; Liachenko et al. 1999). Nipecotic acid is structurally related to the antiepileptic drug tiagabine (Gabatril), which also blocks reuptake of GABA in the micromolar range. Arecaidine and guvacine also inhibit GABA uptake in micromolar concentrations, but do not inhibit glycine or taurine (Lodge et al. 1977; Johnston et al. 1975). This effect is observed in the cat spinal cord and cerebellum, enhancing the activity of Purkinje cells. However, the relevance of arecaidine in chewing areca is questionable because arecaidine was active only when applied centrally, and not systemically.

General Effects

Autonomic effects Areca produces autonomic effects through actions at cholinergic receptors. It causes sweating, facial flush, and a superficial warm sensation (Chu 1995). Skin temperature may rise up to 2 degrees Celsius, through both sympathetic and parasympathetic mechanisms. Heart rate increases during areca chewing (Sekkadde et al. 1994). Arecoline, isoarecoline, and arecaidine cause a brief depressor and bradycardic response, followed by an increase in arterial blood pressure and heart rate, which are mediated through muscarinic M_1 receptors (Wess et al. 1987).

Neuroendocrine In human subjects with Alzheimer's disease, intravenous infusion of arecoline caused elevations of adrenocorticotrophic hormone, cortisol, and β-endorphin, indicating an activation of the hypothalamic-pituitary-adrenal axis (Asthana et al. 1995).

Cerebral blood flow and glucose metabolism Increases in cerebral glucose metabolism are produced by arecoline, as seen in autoradiography with 2-deoxy-D-glucose (Soncrant et al. 1985). Lower doses produced selective increases in areas such as the hippocampus and nucleus raphe medianis, but higher doses produced more generalized elevations. More specifically, hippocampal metabolism is increased in layers that receive cholinergic innervation. Elevations in metabolism in extrapyramidal motor areas were related to the intensity of tremor. The increases in cerebral glucose utilization are accompanied by increases in cerebral blood flow during both acute and chronic treatment (Maiese et al. 1994). However, glucose utilization increases to a greater degree than blood flow in the hippocampus.

Electrophysiological effects Areca chewing in experienced users creates EEG activation (Chu 1994b). Increases are seen in beta and alpha activity, and decreases in theta activity. Topographically, alpha increases are seen in the occipital region, while the beta and theta effects are widespread. These effects are consistent with those of other cholinergic stimulant and cognitive enhancing drugs.

Cognitive effects Animal studies have found some beneficial effects of arecoline on memory, varying with the task employed, dose, and degree of tolerance. Areca chewing in human subjects increases the speed of mental processing. Mixed results have been found in subjects with Alzheimer's disease. The cognitive effects of areca are discussed at greater length in chapter 5.

Addiction and Dependence

A dependency syndrome occurs in many who chew areca (Trivedy et al. 1999). This is not entirely suprising because other cholinergic stimulants (e.g., tobacco) also have addictive properties, and arecoline causes a release of dopamine like many other abused drugs. Use of areca persists despite adverse health effects—one of the criteria for addiction.

Toxic Effects

Chewing of areca nuts causes a reddish-brown discoloration of the oral mucosa and a tendency for the epithelial surface to peel (Reichart and Phillipsen 1998). This has been called *betel chewer's mucosa*, and other oral lesions such as leukoedema, leukoplakia and ulceration may occur. The teeth also become stained reddish-brown or even black in more extreme cases (Morton 1992). Chewing areca is also associated with oral submucous fibrosis and squamous cell carcinoma (Warnakulasuriya et al. 1997; Kuo et al. 1999; Jeng et al. 1999). Several carcinogenic *N*-nitrosamines are formed during areca chewing (Hoffman et al. 1994). Tannins are another source of potential carcinogenicity in areca (Morton 1992).

Associations have also been made between areca and cardiovascular disease, diabetes, and asthma (Winstock et al. in press). Areca may affect cardiovascular disease by increasing homocysteine concentrations and/or through areca copper concentrations and interaction with the lysyl oxidase enzyme (Trivedy et al. 1999). Areca chewing has been associated with cardiac dysrhythmias in a few cases and a case of myocardial infarction was temporally associated with areca use (Hung and Deng 1998; Chiang et al. 1998).

Approximately 61% of people with asthma report that areca aggravates the condition. Clinical studies show that areca causes bronchoconstriction, as evidenced by decreases in forced expiration volume (Sekkadde et al. 1994; Taylor et al. 1992).

Areca may interact adversely with antipsychotic medications (Deahl 1989). Two cases have been reported of schizophrenic patients who were taking neuroleptics and developed severe extrapyramidal symptoms after areca chewing. Given the functional antagonism between dopamine and acetylcholine in the striatum, it is likely that arecoline amplified the dyskinetic effect of neuroleptic medications.

Lobelia

History and Botany

Lobelia *(Lobelia inflata)*, also referred to as Indian tobacco, is an annual or biennial herb that grows from 30 to 60 cm in height (Gruenwald et al. 1998). Its leaves are green or yellowish and range from ovate to lanceolate in shape (figure 4.12). Its flowers are a pale violet-blue and the fruit is an ovoid capsule containing many small brown seeds.

Lobelia was named after a Flemish botanist, Matthias L'Obel (Robbers et al. 1996). *Inflata* refers to the hollow, distended fruit. It was also used by Native Americans as a substitute for tobacco. It was used medicinally by a group of physicians during the nineteenth century C.E. (Tyler 1994). However, due to toxicity and better treatments for tobacco dependence, lobelia is now rarely, if ever, indicated.

Chemical Constituents

Lobelia contains 14 alkaloids, of which lobeline is the most significant (figure 4.13). Other alkaloids include lobelanine, lobelanidine, norlobelanine, and isolobinine. Another relevant chemical that is isolated from the leaves of lobelia is beta-amyrin palmitate.

Pharmacokinetics

Lobeline is somewhat soluble in water, but not soluble in alcohol (Robbers et al. 1996). It is no longer used medicinally, but has been put in lozenges to assist in breaking the tobacco habit. Unfortunately, it has not been successful in this regard. Lobelia derivatives may cross the blood-brain barrier by passing through basic amine transporters

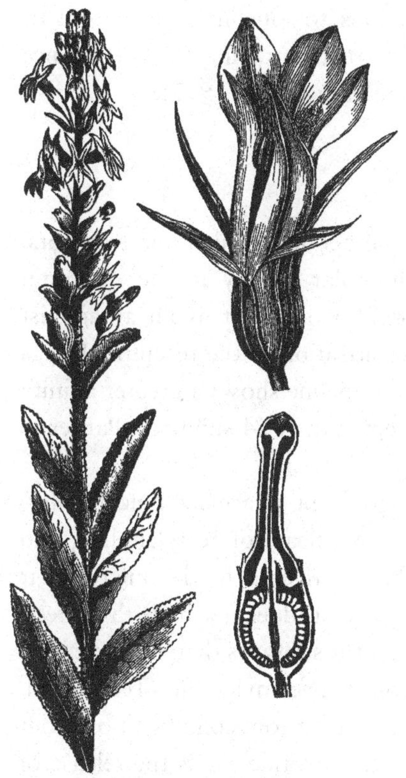

Figure 4.12
Lobelia *(Lobelia inflata)*. Reprinted from Culbreth DMR. (1927). *Materia Medica and Pharmacognosy*, 7th ed. Philadelphia: Lea & Febiger.

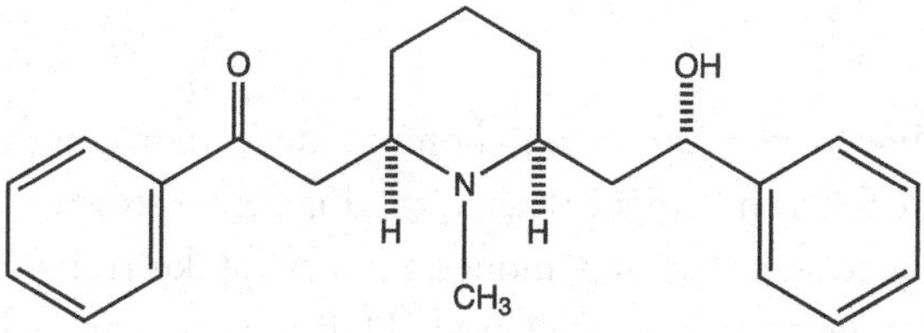

Figure 4.13
Chemical structure of lobeline.

(Metting et al. 1998). Tolerance develops to lobeline's behavioral or analgesic effects by 10 days of daily treatment, and cross-tolerance develops between lobeline and nicotine (Damaj et al. 1997).

Mechanisms of Action

Acetylcholine Lobeline acts as a partial agonist at nicotinic receptors. It displaces nicotine with a low nanomolar affinity in the rat brain (Damaj et al. 1997). Similar to nicotine, it may act as an antagonist through persistent activation and desensitization of the receptor (Briggs and McKenna 1998; Tani et al. 1998). Lobeline shows a greater affinity for the $\beta 2$ subunit of the nicotinic receptor than $\beta 4$ subunits (Parker et al. 1989).

However, lobeline shows several significant pharmacological differences from nicotine. It decreases the basal release of acetylcholine, and also reduces NMDA-evoked acetylcholine release in the micromolar range (Rao et al. 1997). Nicotine, in contrast, does not have this effect. Lobeline binds to different nicotinic receptor subtypes than nicotine, and it is unaffected by the nicotine antagonist mecamylamine (Terry et al. 1998). Lobeline activates nicotinic channels at low concentrations, but inhibits at higher concentrations. Whereas nicotine elicits the release of acetylcholine in the hippocampus and frontal cortex, lobeline does not (Tani et al. 1998). Additionally, lobeline displaces methylscopolamine in the micromolar range, suggesting activity at muscarinic receptors, and it is a weak AChE inhibitor—several hundred times less potent than physostigmine (Terry et al. 1998).

Monoamines Lobeline has direct effects on monoamine systems, independent of cholinergic effects. It alters presynaptic dopamine storage in the striatum by binding to the vesicular monoamine reuptake transporter and preventing uptake (Teng et al. 1998). Half-maximal inhibition occurs in the submicromolar range (20 times lower than that of *d*-amphetamine). Lobeline inhibits dopamine uptake more potently than it evokes release, but low micromolar concentrations still cause the spontaneous and evoked release of dopamine (Teng et al. 1997; Clarke and Reuben 1996; Rao et al. 1997; Sakurai et al. 1982). This dopamine release is independent of calcium and mecamylamine, suggesting that it is caused by inhibiting the uptake of dopamine into vesicles. Lobeline does not alter levels of dopamine or DOPAC in the nucleus accumbens (Benwell and Balfour 1998).

Lobeline also increases basal release of norepinephrine, but norepinephrine release may be reduced at higher lobeline concentrations (Rao et al. 1997). Unlike acetylcholine, lobeline does not reduce the release of dopamine or norepinephrine by NMDA receptors, but it does block nicotine-induced release of norepinephrine from the locus coeruleus (Gallardo and Leslie 1998). Lobeline also evokes release of serotonin, which is mediated by uptake transporters and unaffected by mecamylamine (Lendvai et al. 1996).

Another psychoactive constituent of lobelia, beta-amyrin palmitate, causes a release of norepinephrine in mouse brain synaptosomes, possibly releasing it from newly synthesized pools (Subarnas et al. 1993b).

Ca^{2+} channels Lobeline acts as an antagonist at neuronal Ca^{2+} channels (Toth and Vizi 1998). Micromolar doses of lobeline block Ca^{2+} currents in superior cervical ganglia neurons, and are not altered by G-protein manipulations.

General Effects

Physiological effects Humans given intravenous microgram doses of lobeline experience sensations of choking and pressure in the throat and upper chest, and eventually a dry cough (Raj et al. 1995). Reflex changes in breathing occur shortly before the onset of the sensations. Chronic three-week treatment with lobeline in rats induced no changes in weight, rectal temperature, or motor coordination (Sopranzi et al. 1991). Lobeline dose-dependently decreases body temperature in mice (Damaj et al. 1997). Gastrointestinal symptoms may occur with larger doses, resembling nicotine's effects.

Behavioral and cognitive effects Lobeline appears to be reinforcing in a similar manner to nicotine. Despite weak nicotinic effects, drug-naive animals will self-administer lobeline, as they would with other reinforcing drugs (Rasmussen and Swedberg 1998). However, unlike nicotine, lobeline does not induce a conditioned place preference nor stimulate locomotor activity (Benwell and Balfour 1998; Fudala and Iwamoto 1986; Stolerman et al. 1995). Lobeline's effects are also distinguishable from nicotine's effects on animals in drug discrimination paradigms (Reavill et al. 1990). Beta-amyrin palmitate also dose-dependently decreases locomotor activity in mice (Subarnas et al. 1993c). Pharmacological evidence suggests that this is through α_1 adrenergic and not dopamine receptors.

An acute dose of lobeline impairs attention in one animal model, but not as much as mecamylamine (Turchi et al. 1995). Lobeline improves memory when administered after a passive avoidance paradigm (Decker et al. 1993). Pretreatment with lobeline improves performance in rats with septal lesions on a spatial discrimination water maze. Lobeline is about one-tenth as potent as nicotine in the passive avoidance memory task, but equivalent to nicotine in the water maze.

Electrophysiology Studies of the electrophysiological effects of lobelia are scant. In one study, increases were seen in low-frequency activity in the hippocampus but in higher-frequency activity in the amygdala (Sopranzi et al. 1991).

Antidepressant Some animal models show antidepressant effects of lobelia extract (Subarnas et al. 1992). Similar to imipramine and mianserin, beta-amyrin palmitate shows antidepressant-like effects in the forced-swimming test (Subarnas et al. 1993a). Whereas mianserin and beta-amyrin palmitate reduce locomotor activity induced by methamphetamine, imipramine increases it. It potentiates sodium pentobarbital-induced sleep more potently than imipramine, but less than mianserin. Collectively, the effects of beta-amyrin palmitate in behavioral and physiological assays suggests it may work in a manner more similar to mianserin than imipramine. However, the mechanism of antidepressant-like effects of lobelia is uncertain. It may be through the beta-amyrin palmitate's ability to release norepinephrine (Subarnas et al. 1993b). An antidepressant effect of lobelia has not been established in humans.

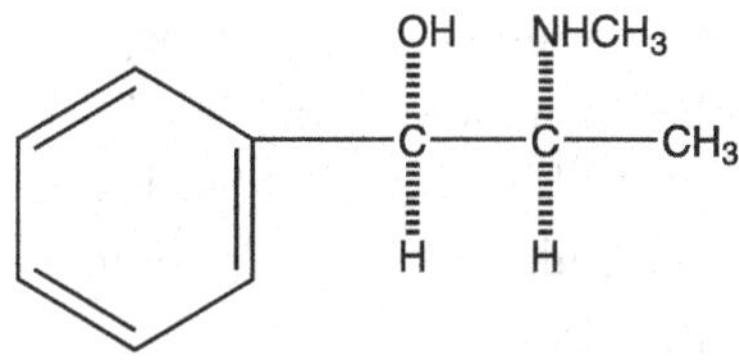

Figure 4.14
Chemical structure of ephedrine.

Monoamine Stimulants

Ephedra

History and Botany

Ephedra is a group of related plant species that have long been used for their stimulant effects. *Ephedra sinica* is a shrub that grows 60–90 cm in height (Robbers et al. 1996; Gruenwald et al. 1998). It has long cylindrical branches 1–2 mm in diameter, which terminate in a sharp point. The branches are green and have very small leaves, which sometimes are reduced to pointed scales. The fruit is red and berrylike. *Ephedra sinica* is native to Asia, growing mostly in Mongolia and neighboring parts of China.

Ephedra is also known by the Chinese name *ma huang,* which translates as "yellow astringent." It has been used medicinally by the Chinese for more than five thousand years. A related species, *Ephedra nevadensis,* grows in North America and is sometimes referred to as Mormon tea (Rudgley 1999). The Mormons were introduced to ephedra by Indians when they arrived in Utah. They used it as an alternate to tea and coffee, ironically, because their religious views prohibited use of those stimulants. Ephedra might be the oldest known human stimulant, because remains of the plant were discovered in a fifty thousand-year-old Neanderthal grave in Iraq. Modern medical use of ephedra began with the identification of the alkaloid ephedrine in 1923.

Chemical Constituents

Several alkaloids are present in Ephedra, with ephedrine being the most significant (Gruenwald et al. 1998). *Ephedra sinica* contains approximately 1.25% ephedrine (figure 4.14). Also present are pseudoephedrine, methylephedrine and norpseudoephedrine, or cathine, which is also a major alkaloid of khat *(Catha edulis)* (Robbers et al. 1996; Kalix 1991). Different ephedra species may vary considerably in their content of alkaloids (Robbers et al. 1996; White et al. 1997).

Pharmacokinetics

Commercial samples containing approximately 400 mg of ephedra per capsule yield roughly 5 mg of ephedrine, 1 mg of pseudoephedrine, and less than 1 mg of methylephedrine (White et al. 1997). For a dose of four capsules, yielding approximately 20 mg of ephedrine, the elimination half-life is 5.2 hours. The time to reach maxium concentration is 3.9 hours. Compared to pure ephedrine tablets, the elimination kinetics of ephedra are comparable. However, ephedra showed somewhat different absorption kinetics (e.g., lag time, area under the concentration-time curve, and maximum plasma concentration). So, ephedra tablets may vary from pure ephedrine in the onset of action, but the durations of action are grossly equivalent.

Mechanisms of Action

Ephedrine is an agonist of α and β adrenergic receptors (Meston and Heiman 1998; Robbers et al. 1996). However, it does not bind to β_3 adrenergic receptors (Shannon et al. 1999). It also increases release of norepinephrine from sympathetic neurons.

General Effects

Ephedrine increases heart rate and increases systolic blood pressure (Kuitunen et al. 1984). Stimulation of β receptors in the lung by ephedrine promotes bronchial dilation. Accordingly, ephedra has been used historically to treat asthma, and pseudoephedrine is commercially available as an over-the-counter decongestant. Stimulation of α adrenergic receptors on smooth muscle increases resistance to urine flow. Although ephedrine facilitates the neuromuscular endplate potential by increasing the quantal release of acetylcholine, this only occurs at high concentrations unlikely to be reached with oral dosing (10^{-4} M). Ephedrine increases the physiological aspect of sexual arousal in women

Table 4.2
Relative doses for stimulus generalization of psychostimulants (ED50)

Drug	ED_{50}
(−)ephedrine	0.8 mg/kg
S(+)amphetamine	0.4 mg/kg
cocaine	2.7 mg/kg
methylphenidate	1.2 mg/kg
S(−)methcathinone	0.3 mg/kg
caffeine	36.7 mg/kg

Source: Young and Glennon 1998.

viewing erotic material, as measured by vaginal pulse amplitude (Meston and Heiman 1998). Insomnia, anxiety, cardiovascular, and other sympathomimetic effects limit the clinical use of ephedrine (Kalix 1991). Chronic doses may be associated with a toxic psychosis.

Ephedrine causes a potent stimulation of the central nervous system, resulting in increased arousal and activity. On neuropsychological tests, ephedrine does not have any effects on finger-tapping, sign-recording, or digit-span tests (Kuitunen et al. 1983). It does reverse impairments in auditory vigilance and serial-choice performance produced by the sedating antihistamine chlorpheniramine, but does not affect simple reaction speed (Millar and Wilkinson 1981). Ephedrine counteracts some of the deficits produced by scopolamine in sensory processing (critical fusion flicker) (Nuotto 1983).

Animal drug discrimination paradigms show stimulus generalization between ephedrine and other CNS stimulants such as amphetamine, methylphenidate, methcathinone, cocaine, and caffeine (see table 4.2; Young and Glennon 1998). However, it does not generalize to MDMA. Pseudoephedrine substitutes for amphetamine, but only at high doses (40 mg/kg in rats) (Tongjaroenbuangam et al. 1998).

Toxicity

Normal doses range from 15 to 30 mg of actual alkaloid (ephedrine), and the lethal dose is in the 1–2 g range. Side effects from ephedra use include headache, irritability, restlessness, anxiety, insomnia, tachycardia, urinary disorders, and vomiting.

Recently, ephedra preparations have been sold with misleading names alluding to the drug ecstasy (MDMA) (Blumenthal and King 1997). Several deaths have resulted from cardiac toxicity because hypertension and cardiac arrhythmia are chief problems with higher doses of ephedrine. Use of ephedra is thus contraindicated in people with existing high blood pressure. Cases have been reported of intracerebral hemorrhage and vasculitis in association with ephedrine (Forman et al. 1989; Kaye and Fainstat 1987; Wooten et al. 1983). The risk of cerebral hemorrhage is even greater when combining ephedrine with other catecholamine stimulants such as the over-the-counter stimulant phenylpropanolamine (Stoessl et al. 1985). Pseudoephedrine may be safer than ephedrine in some respects (Porta et al. 1986). In a large sample ($n > 100{,}000$) of pseudoephedrine users, there were no reports of cerebrovascular disorders within 15 days after administration. The incidence of myocardial infarction, seizures, and neuropsychiatric disorders were no greater than base rates in the general population.

Other conditions in which ephedra is contraindicated are anxiety disorders, angle-closure glaucoma, prostate adenoma with residual urine volume, pheochromocytoma, and thyrotoxicosis (Gruenwald et al. 1998). Known medications that may interact adversely with ephedrine include heart glycosides, halothane, guanethidine, MAO inhibitors, secale alkaloids, and oxytocin.

Addiction and Dependence

Use of ephedrine is sometimes associated with dependence (Gruber and Pope 1998). One study reported a high incidence of eating and body-image disorders among ephedrine users, but this is likely confounded by the fact that the sample consisted entirely of female weightlifters and is likely not to represent the greater population.

Coca

History and Botany

Coca *(Erythroxylon coca)* is a small shrublike tree that grows to 5 m in height. The leaves are oval, green, and tough, growing 5 cm in length and 2.5 cm in width (Robbers et al. 1996; Gruenwald et al. 1998). The

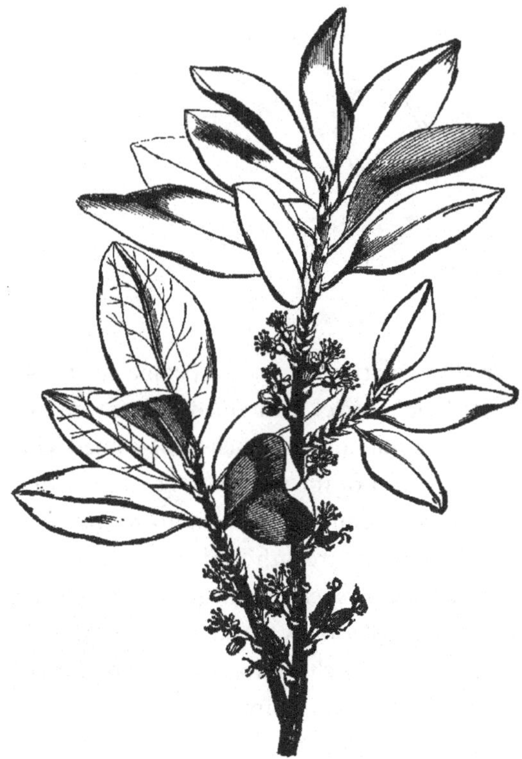

Figure 4.15
Coca *(Erythroxylon coca)*. Reprinted from Culbreth DMR. (1927). *Materia Medica and Pharmacognosy*, 7th ed. Philadelphia: Lea & Febiger.

flowers are small and greenish-white and grow in axillary clusters (figure 4.15). It produces a red fruit with one seed. The coca plant is native to the Andes region of South America, but it is also cultivated in Indonesia, India, and Sri Lanka.

Coca is arguably the most infamous of the stimulant plants. The number of Americans who have tried cocaine rose from 5.4 million in 1976 to 21.6 million in 1982. In 1995, an estimated 1.5 million Americans used cocaine, and 500,000 used it on a weekly basis (Bolla et al. 1998).

Coca has long been known to the Indians of the Andes region, who chewed the leaves for stimulation and increased endurance (Rudgley 1999). The coca leaf was an important part of the Inca culture. Knowledge of the plant spread to western cultures with colonialism, but wide-

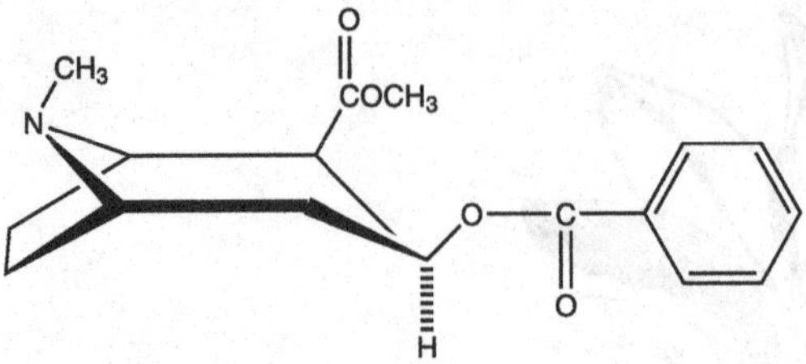

Figure 4.16
Chemical structure of cocaine.

spread use really began after the isolation of pure cocaine in 1884 (Musto 1991). Coca-Cola (see kola above) contained a mixture of extracts from the coca plant and kola nut, and a French wine named Vin Mariani also contained coca. At the turn of the twentieth century in the United States, the euphoric effects of cocaine led people to mistakenly assume it was a health tonic, increasing strength and well-being and reducing appetite. After a few years, however, the negative effects became more evident, and government legislation was enacted to control it. Cocaine has local anesthetic effects also, which led to the development of several modern synthetic local anesthetics (see chapter 8).

Cocaine is prepared by mixing the leaves with an organic solvent and mashing them. When the solvent evaporates, a coca paste remains. In South America, this paste is sometimes mixed with tobacco and smoked. Alternately, the paste can be further refined into cocaine hydrochloride. This is a stable salt form that is hydrophilic. In this form it can be snorted and absorbed through the nasal mucosa. Cocaine HCl can also be made into a "freebase" or alkaloidal form by mixing it with the organic solvent ether. In freebase form it can be smoked, but the flammability of ether makes this a dangerous practice. It was later discovered that cocaine freebase could be made by mixing it with baking soda and water—commonly known as *crack*.

Chemical Constituents

Cocaine is the principal psychoactive alkaloid from the coca plant (figure 4.16). Other tropine alkaloids include *cis*-cinnamoyl cocaine, *trans*-cinnamoyl cocaine, α-truxillin, and β-truxillin (Gruenwald et al. 1998).

Pharmacokinetics

Cocaine is administered in several ways. When the leaves are chewed, the drug absorbtion is slow and prolonged (Homstedt et al. 1979). Snorting or smoking cocaine allow for rapid absorption through the nasal mucosa or the lungs, respectively. Absorption is poor through the nasal mucosa (20–30% absorption), which is further limited by the vasoconstriction it causes. Cocaine is less frequently injected intravenously, but it is sometimes combined with heroin to make an especially addictive concoction called a *speedball*. While the euphoric effects of heroin and cocaine are additive, they also counteract each other's negative side effects of sedation and overstimulation. Smoking crack is probably the fastest and most direct means of delivering cocaine to the brain, and thus probably the most addictive (Hatsukami and Fischman 1996). When equivalent doses are given through smoked and intravenous routes, the smoked method produces greater behavioral responses (Cone 1995). Absorption is rapid and complete through the lung surfaces, with onset occuring in seconds and the effect lasting about 30 minutes.

Once in the blood stream, cocaine levels quickly rise in the brain, faster than plasma levels, which then redistribute to other tissues. Cocaine is rapidly metabolized in the blood and liver, with a half-life of 30 to 90 minutes. The major metabolites have a half-life of approximately 8 hours. Although cocaine itself is detected in urine for only 12 hours, the metabolite benzoylecgonine can be detected in urine for at least 48 hours and sometimes up to 2 weeks. Concurrent use of cocaine and ethanol produces an ethyl ester of benzoylecgonine called cocaethylene. Cocaethylene is an active metabolite, blocking dopamine reuptake, and potentiating the effect of cocaine. Thus, concurrent use of cocaine and ethanol can further increase the additional effects of the drugs and the risk of dependency.

Mechanisms of Action

Monoamine The primary psychoactive mechanism of cocaine is blocking reuptake of the monoamine neurotransmitters dopamine, norepinephrine, and serotonin, leading to increased available synaptic transmitters (O'Brien 1996). Chronic use is associated with changes in monoamine metabolites, receptors, and uptake transporters (Belej et al. 1996; Perret et al. 1998; Baumann and Rothman 1998). A decreased availability of D_2 receptors is seen, possibly reflecting a compensatory down-regulation of the postsynaptic receptors in response to increased stimulation (Volkow et al. 1993). Evidence of low dopamine function after chronic cocaine use is supported by concurrent hyperprolactinemia (Dackis and Gold 1985). Neuroimaging studies show decreased dopamine activity in cocaine withdrawal, when comparing cocaine users to nonusers (Wu et al. 1997). Collectively, evidence strongly suggests that alterations in monoamine systems and their targets mediate the acute effects of cocaine, and that changes in these systems mirror the addiction, cravings, and withdrawal symptoms.

Na^+ channels Cocaine is an antagonist of voltage-gated Na^+ channels, reducing axonal conduction and acting as a local anesthetic. This effect will be discussed at greater length in chapter 8. Cocaine's blockade of Na^+ channels as a contribution to its psychotropic effects is possible but has not been examined.

General Effects

Cocaine causes profound mental stimulation, behaviorally evidenced by increased talkativeness and activity, flight of ideas, euphoria, and inflated self-esteem. Fatigue is offset and there is a reduced need for sleep. Supression of appetite also occurs.

Autonomic Cocaine has stong sympathomimetic effects due to inhibition of norepinephrine reuptake, and perhaps central mechanisms as well. Effects include those typical of sympathetic autonomic activation. Cardiovascular and cerebrovascular effects are prominent.

Vascular effects Cocaine causes increases in blood pressure and heart rate, which fall to normal levels between doses (Foltin et al. 1995). Tachyphylaxis develops to the cardiovascular effects, even within a single session. Concurrent use of ethanol, cannabis, and cocaine causes even greater cardiovascular effects than those of each drug alone. Interactions can also occur with antidepressant drugs like desipramine.

Cerebral blood flow and glucose metabolism Several studies have examined the effects of cocaine using neuroimaging techniques. In humans and nonhuman primates alike, cocaine decreases cerebral glucose metabolism (Volkow et al. 1991). This includes areas such as the nucleus accumbens, ventral striatum, orbitofrontal cortex, prefrontal cortex, and hippocampus, suggesting a pronounced effect of cocaine on corticostriatal circuits. When methylphenidate (Ritalin) is given to cocaine users, increases in metabolism are seen in the orbitofrontal cortex and striatum, which correspond to reports of cravings. On the other hand, increases in other prefrontal areas correspond to enhanced mood (Volkow et al. 1999). In cocaine users, decreased metabolism in the prefrontal cortex (including cingulate and orbitofrontal regions) is associated with decreases in D_2 receptors (Volkow et al. 1999).

Decreases are also seen in cerebral blood flow in cocaine users (Volkow et al. 1988). This may be due, in part or wholly, to the vasoconstrictor effects of cocaine. Indeed, greater deficits are seen in cerebral blood flow compared to glucose metabolism, even within the same individual.

Cognitive Cognitive studies of cocaine users have produced conflicting results. Deficits have been found in cocaine users in mental processing speed, visual and verbal memory, and executive functions (O'Malley et al. 1992; Easton and Bauer 1997; Berry et al. 1993; Hoff et al. 1996; Selby and Azrin 1998). Executive deficits have been seen in measures such as the Category test, the Trail Making Test B, and the Shipley Abstraction Subtest. Yet improvements are seen in some studies on tests of nonverbal reasoning (Wisconsin Card Sorting Test—categories achieved) and verbal fluency (Controlled Oral Word Association). Others have found improvement on other tests like the Finger Tapping Test and visuospatial memory.

Methodological issues are paramount in the cognitive studies of cocaine users. Primary concerns surround preexisting cognitive deficits or a self-selection effect among subjects (Bolla et al. 1998). Other confounding factors include duration of use, duration of abstinence, sample size, control groups, premorbid depression, and personality factors such as antisocial personality disorder. Still, the available neuropsychological and neuroimaging data convergently support executive deficits resulting from altered frontostriatal function. It remains to be shown how long it takes for these deficits to develop (and at what doses), how long they persist, and to what degree they recover.

Addiction and Dependence

Addiction is a prominent problem with cocaine use. Cocaine is highly reinforcing to both animals and humans, probably through inhibition of dopamine reuptake in mesolimbic systems and stimulation of brain areas known to subserve behavioral reinforcement (Kiyatkin and Stein 1995; Woolverton and Johnson 1992; Ritz et al. 1987). Although sensitization to the stimulant effects occurs in animals, humans do not sensitize to the euphoric effects of cocaine but develop a tolerance (O'Brien 1996). In animals and humans alike, self-administration often follows a binge pattern, consisting of repeated use over a period of hours or days until the supply is used up.

A cocaine withdrawal syndrome is recognized that generally mirrors the acute effects of intoxication. It includes depression, sleepiness, fatigue, increased appetite, bradycardia, and craving cocaine. Treatment of cocaine addiction is a stubborn problem resulting from the intense euphoria and reinforcement caused by the drug (O'Brien 1996). Treatments include psychosocial support (e.g., Narcotics Anonymous) and behavioral reinforcement of abstinence, often monitored with serial urine tests. Pharmacological treatments of cocaine addiction have been attempted with antidepressants (e.g., fluoxetine), dopamine agonists (e.g., amantadine), and opioids (e.g., buprenorphine). The benefits of any pharmacological treatment to date for treatment of cocaine addiction have been modest at best. A novel approach to treatment involves catalytic or monoclonal antibodies for cocaine (Mets et al. 1998; Fox et al. 1996). Rather than replace the neurochemical effects of cocaine, this strategy seeks to neutralize cocaine in the blood stream, making future administration of cocaine less effective or ineffective.

Toxicity

Cardiovascular and cerebrovascular Cocaine has cardiotoxic effects, sometimes resulting in arrhythmia, ventricular fibrillation, or cardiac arrest (Nanji and Filipenko 1984; Sherief and Carpentier 1991). Vasoconstriction caused by cocaine greatly increases the risk for ischemic or hemorrhagic stroke (Levine et al. 1991). Vasoconstriction is also caused by benzoylecgonine, and norcocaine, in addition to cocaine (Bolla et al. 1998). Whereas freebase alkaloidal cocaine (crack) is equally likely to cause either kind of stroke, cocaine HCl is more likely to cause a hemorrhagic stroke.

Neonatal Cocaine freely crosses the placental barrier, and prenatal exposure to cocaine alters neurobehavioral development in rat pups (Sobrian et al. 1990). The effects on humans exposed prenatally to cocaine is a complicated matter, because so many other concurrent factors contribute to development. Common confounds are prenatal care and maternal polydrug use. Prenatal cocaine use is associated with reduced gestational age, birth weight, body length, and head circumference (Richardson et al. 1999). In children exposed prenatally to cocaine, some studies have shown behavioral differences evident at 1 to 3 years of age (Richardson et al. 1993; Richardson 1998). Associations are also made with impulsivity and attention deficits at age 6 (Leech et al. 1999).

Toxic psychosis Several monoamine stimulants including cocaine are known to produce a temporary or even a lasting psychotic state after heavy use. Reviews of numerous clinical case reports have shown amphetamine to produce a chronic psychotic state, sometimes persisting for months after cessation. There appears to be a sensitization effect in this regard, because after recovery, psychotic states may recur with minimal use of amphetamine or alcohol. When compared to schizophrenic patients, people with amphetamine-induced psychosis demonstrate fewer negative symptoms (Boutros and Bowers 1996).

Chronic cocaine use can cause a syndrome of insomnia, hallucinations, delusions, and apathy. This syndrome develops around the time when the euphoria turns to a paranoid psychosis, which resembles paranoid schizophrenia. Further, after cessation of cocaine use, the hallucinations may stop, but the delusions can persist. Still, the incidence of a persistent cocaine-induced psychosis appears to be rare. One study found only 4 out of 298 chronic cocaine users receiving a diagnosis of psychotic disorder (Rounsaville et al. 1991). This incidence is approximately the same as the base rate of schizophrenia in the general population, so cocaine may be precipitating paranoid psychosis in individuals who had predisposing factors.

Khat

History and Botany

Khat *(Catha edulis)* is a small shrub or tree native to East Africa (Robbers et al. 1996; Gruenwald et al. 1998). It is cultivated in the highlands of Ethiopia as well as Yemen and South Africa. Khat is alternately referred to by different regional names such as *qat*, *tschat*, and *miraa*. Medieval Arabic writings mention khat as far back as 1237 C.E. (LeBras and Fretillere 1965; Kalix 1992; Wilder et al. 1994). In some Muslim cultures it is regarded as a more acceptable alternative to alcohol. Khat is often used in social settings in some cultures, such as Yemen, where users gather in private homes and chew the leaves while conversing (Kalix 1994). At times khat is used by laborers and students to offset fatigue.

Chewing leaves of the khat shrub is practiced in parts of East Africa and the Arabian peninsula (Kalix 1988; Widler et al. 1994). Some estimate daily use at 5 million portions. Use in the West is less common, but has increased somewhat. More common in the United States has been use of the synthetic drug methcathinone (or "cat"), which is derived from khat alkaloids. Only the fresh khat leaves are pharmacologically active, so for some time use was limited to local areas that grew the plant. However, with air transportation, use has spread with emigrants in Europe and the United States. Because of its pharmacological similarities to amphetamine and its addictive properties, khat has been listed on Schedule I of the United Nations Convention on Psychotropic Substances.

Chemical Constituents

There are more than 40 alkaloids, glycosides, tannins, and terpenoids in khat (Elmi 1983). Two phenylalkylamines, namely, cathine (norpseudoephedrine) and cathinone [S(−)-alpha-aminopropiophenone] well account for the CNS stimulant effects (Kalix 1988) (figure 4.17). The

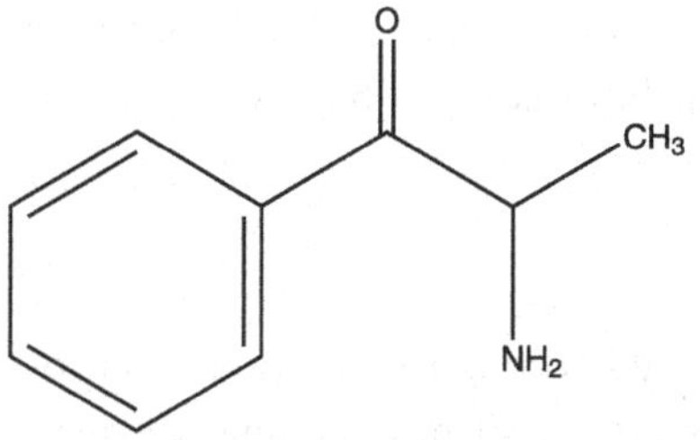

Figure 4.17
Chemical structure of cathinone.

S(−) enantiomer occurs naturally, and the R(+) enantiomer is synthetic (Kalix 1992).

Pharmacokinetics
In its natural form, fresh khat leaves are chewed because the drug is perishable. Young leaves from the tip of the branch are more potent. While the leaves are chewed, the juices are swallowed and the residue is rejected. During a session, one may ingest 100 to 200 grams of leaves.

When khat is chewed, absorption of cathinone is slow, with maximal plasma concentrations occurring at approximately 2 hours (Widler et al. 1994; Halket et al. 1995). The terminal elimination half-life is approximately 4.3 hours. Similar effects are achieved with orally administered pure cathinone. Cathinone is the keto-analog of cathine and because it is more lipophilic it penetrates the blood-brain barrier more easily.

The plasma half-life of cathinone is 1.5 hours. The primary metabolites are norpseudoephedrine, norephedrine, 3,6-dimethyl-2,5-diphenylpyrazine, and 1-phenyl-1,2-propanedione (Szendrei 1980; Brenneisen et al. 1986; Guantai and Maitai 1983). However, norpseudoephedrine and norephedrine also originate directly from the leaves, as well as being metabolic products (Widler et al. 1994). Maximal plasma concentrations of norephedrine and norpseudoephedrine are reached at about 3.3 and 3.1 hours, respectively. These two drugs have a much longer duration of action than cathinone, where terminal half-lives could not be calculated after 10 hours.

Animal drug discrimination paradigms show cross-tolerance between cathinone, cathine, and amphetamine (Schechter 1990). S(+)methcathinone is about twice as potent as S(+)amphetamine, and five times as potent as R(+)methcathinone, although both isomers have CNS stimulant effects (Glennon et al. 1995).

Mechanisms of Action

The stimulant effects of khat are mediated through monoamine neurotransmitter systems. Cathinone induces release of monoamines through membrane transporters (Kalix 1984, 1992). It causes release of dopamine in the striatum and nucleus accumbens, with similar potency to amphetamine in low micromolar concentrations (Kalix 1980, 1982; Pehek et al. 1990). Consequently, increases are seen in extracellular levels of the metabolite DOPAC in the caudate nucleus, nucleus accumbens, and frontal cortex (Mereu et al. 1983). Norpseudoephedrine also induces release of catecholamines (Kalix 1983).

Cathinone decreases firing of substantia nigra neurons, similar to amphetamine. Animal discrimination of cathinone is dependent on dopamine release, but is independent of 5-HT_3 modulation or Ca^{2+} influx through L-type channels (Schechter 1992). High doses of cathinone result in depletion of dopamine and also have neurotoxic effects on dopaminergic neurons (Wagner et al. 1982). In contrast, long-term administration of cathinone does not deplete norepinephrine or serotonin (Wagner et al. 1982). Cathinone and cathine may also have monoamine oxidase inhibition effects (Nencini et al. 1984).

General Effects

Khat produces effects similar to those of other monoamine stimulants, (i.e., increases in mental stimulation, physical endurance, elevated mood) (Widler et al. 1994; Kalix 1994; Brenneisen et al. 1990). Stimulus generalization occurs between cathinone, amphetamine, and cocaine, suggesting similar subjective effects (Huang and Wilson 1986). Similar to other monoamine stimulants, cathinone causes dose-dependent reductions in eating and body weight (Islam et al. 1990; Zelger and Carlini 1980). Oral cathinone increases sexual arousal in rats, but does not affect erectile or ejaculatory responses (Taha et al. 1995).

Khat may cause irritability, but in the cultural context, sociability is generally increased. Users may increase in talkativeness, sometimes to the point of logorrhea. Elevated self-esteem occurs, sometimes to a manic degree. As with other monoamine stimulants, psychosis is possible with chronic heavy use. There have been a few reported cases of khat-induced psychosis, which are treated with phenothiazines or haloperidol (Pantellis et al. 1989). Persistent hypnagogic hallucinations have been reported in chronic khat chewers, possibly through chronic suppression of REM sleep (Granek et al. 1988).

Khat produces sympathomimetic effects, increasing heart rate and blood pressure. When khat is chewed, the increases are gradual, maximizing at about 2 hours and lasting for 4 hours. However, tolerance develops to blood pressure and heart rate effects in habitual users. Mydriasis and increases in respiration also occur. Cathinone induces thermogenesis in brown adipose tissue, which is mediated by β-adrenergic receptors (Tariq et al. 1989).

Cathinone and norpseudoephedrine have antagonist effects at the neuromuscular junction (Guantai et al. 1987). This is likely a direct blocking effect, independent of cholinergic and adrenergic innervation. However, motor effects are not reported at doses commonly used.

Addiction and Dependence

The similarities between cathinone and amphetamine raises the possibility of abuse potential (Kalix 1994). Amphetamine and cathinone both appear to produce their stimulus-discrimination effects through the dopamine system (Kalix and Glennon 1986).

Animals self-administer cathinone in a pattern common to abuses of monoamine stimulants such as cocaine (Woolverton and Johanson 1984). Cathinone can induce a conditioned place preference in rats (Schechter 1991). Withdrawal symptoms of khat include lethargy, depression, nightmares, and mild tremor (Kalix 1994). *N*-methylated cathinone (methcathinone) is more potent, and has become available on the illegal market. It was subsequently scheduled as a controlled substance (Glennon et al. 1995).

Use of cathinone in the form of chewing khat may have some features that limit its addictiveness (Kalix 1994). The large bulk of the material and the effort required to chew khat limits the amount that can be ingested in a given time. Absorption in this manner is slow and gradual, and the short half-life of cathinone also limits the amount that can accumulate over time. Thus, the addictive potential of khat is likely minimized by a combination of pharmacokinetic factors.

Toxic Effects

As would be expected, khat overuse produces symptoms similar to those of other monoamine stimulants, such as cocaine or amphetamine, including signs of sympathetic overarousal. In the extreme this can involve a toxic psychosis. Disorders more frequently associated with chronic khat use in males are headaches, anorexia, insomnia, constipation, and respiratory illnesses (Kennedy et al. 1983). Females report higher incidences of acute gastritis, jaundice, bronchitis and hepatic diseases. Also, cathinone has toxic reproductive effects in humans and experimental animals (Islam et al. 1990). It decreases sperm count and motility, and increases the number of abnormal sperm cells. It also decreases plasma testosterone in rats.

Summary

As reviewed in this chapter, a number of plants are recognized for their stimulant effects on the central nervous system. Although they work through a variety of neurochemical mechanisms, they all convergently alter neuromodulatory systems to produce a common effect.

All of the stimulants discussed have some potential for abuse, varying with environmental factors, context of use, and individual predispositions. Still, pharmacology plays a major causal role: drugs with direct or indirect actions on dopamine systems are more likely to be used compulsively. Stimulants have important roles in the cultures that use them. Whether used for positive or negative purposes, it is likely that our relationships with stimulant plants will long continue.

5

Cognitive Enhancers

Humans draw heavily on cognitive abilities to survive and flourish. Compared to other species we rely far less on instinctual and environmentally driven behaviors, and instead have a greater capacity for behavior driven by internal goals and abstract representations. This strategy for survival depends on more complex cognitive ability and has coincided phylogenetically with enlargement of the cerebral cortex and frontal lobes. Consequently, in the search for plant medications, attention has been paid to those that improve mental ability. Some individuals are interested in cognitive-enhancing drugs, or *nootropics*, in an attempt to optimize their mental functioning. However, their potential use in treating dementia is of paramount interest. Whatever the impetus, several herbs have been identified with benefical cognitive effects.

Dementia

Dementia is a general term for loss of cognitive functions and behavioral impairment. It may arise from several etiologies and may present with a large variety of manifestations. The financial cost in health care engendered by dementia is enormous, because individuals with dementia require progressive amounts of supervision, eventually needing total care. The human and emotional costs are unquantifiable. Several forms of dementia exist, which will be briefly classified and described here.

Dementia generally involves an impairment in (1) memory and other cogntive abilities and (2) social and occupational functioning. The *Diagnostic and Statistical Manual of Mental Disorders* (DSM-IV) defines dementia as a persistent deficit in memory and at least one other area of cognitive function: language, praxis, object recognition, or executive functions (organization, planning, abstract thinking, sequencing, etc.) (American Psychiatric Association, 1994). In addition to cognitive difficulties, impairments occur in social and occupational functioning. Other classification systems do not require memory to be present to diagnose dementia, because several progresssive dementias, such as frontotemporal dementias, may not show marked memory loss (Neary et al. 1998). The onset of dementia is usually slow and other conditions that could mimic its symptoms (e.g., metabolic disorder) must be ruled out. However, the onset may be rapid in a vascular dementia, resulting from compromised cerebral blood flow. A diagnosis of vascular dementia requires neuroimaging evidence or focal neurological signs, such as limb weakness or abnormal reflexes.

Dementia may be dichotomized into degenerative and nondegenerative types. Degenerative dementia involves progessive cell loss due to pathological processes. Each subtype of dementia may have characteristic neuropathological signs, although there is much overlap in some cases. There is also specificity in the neuroanatomical distribution of pathology, which determines the functional brain changes and constellation of clinical symptoms. For example, dementias arising from the basal ganglia typically have pronounced motor symptoms, while a cortical dementia such as Alzheimer's disease may have little motor involvement until end stages.

Two neurodegenerative diseases will be considered in greater detail here, Alzheimer's disease and Parkinson's disease, due to the pertinence of herbal medications to their treatment. Also discussed in some detail are vascular dementia and normal aging. Other degenerative conditions may benefit from herbal medications, but have not received the amount of attention in research that the above conditions have. Of particular interest to many degenerative conditions are herbal medications with demonstrated antioxidant and neuroprotective effects.

Degenerative Dementias: Cortical and Mixed Cortical/Subcortical Types

Alzheimer's Disease

The most common form of dementia is *Alzheimer's disease*, constituting 20% of psychiatric hospitalizations (Adams et al. 1997). In a European sample, the prevalence was 0.02% for ages 30–59, 0.3% for ages 60–69, 3.2% for ages 70–79, and 10.8% for ages 80–89. Progression of the disease follows three general stages, which last approximately 2 years each (Boller and Duyckaerts 1997). The earliest stage is characterized by deficits of episodic and semantic memory and language. Following this stage is a frank dementia, in which other cognitive functions decline and one's ability to function in daily activities is impaired. There may be a considerable amount of interindividual variation and even intraindividual fluctuation during this period. The final stage is a vegetative state in which the person is bedridden and unable to perform basic self-care. Death results from health complications and not directly from the disease itself, per se.

Risk factors for Alzheimer's disease The incidence of Alzheimer's disease increases with age, but it is a specific disease process and not a part of normal aging. A hereditary component of the disease is evident, with an autosomal dominant mode of transmission. Genetic studies have identified an association between Alzheimer's disease and a gene on chromosome 19 encoding alipoprotein E (Boller and Duyckaerts 1997). There are four alleles of the gene, and the Apo ε4 allele codes for the Apo E4 phenotype. Apo E4 is associated with both familial and sporadic incidences of the disease. Another risk factor for Alzheimer's disease appears to be lower levels of education. One explanation for this finding is that education increases cerebral development and synaptic connections, providing a greater cognitive reserve.

Neuroanatomical and neuropathological basis of Alzheimer's disease Histological features of Alzheimer's disease include neuritic plaques and neurofibrillary tangles (Boller and Duyckaerts 1997). Neuritic plaques are composed of extracellular deposits of β-amyloid protein and apolipoprotein E and are found primarily in neocortex. β-amyloid is derived from an amyloid precursor protein, and is suspected to be a chief causal factor in Alzheimer's disease pathology (Samuel et al. 1997). Neurofibrillary tangles are clusters of protein fibers found in the cell body and composed of tau protein, which normally serves as a cytoskeletal element. Neurofibrillary tangles progress from entorhinal cortex to hippocampus, and then to neocortical areas.

There is clear gross atrophy in the brains of people with Alzheimer's disease, but whether this involves overall neuronal death or volume loss is debated. Structural neuroimaging shows widened sulci and ventricles, and functional neuroimaging shows hypoactivity, beginning with bilateral temporoparietal areas. Significant pathology in Alzheimer's disease occurs in the basal forebrain nuclei (Samuel et al. 1997). These nuclei are the primary source of cholinergic innervation to the forebrain (Lawrence and Sahakian 1998). Alzheimer's disease is associated with a loss of cortical choline acetyltransferase and acetylcholinesterase, the synthesizing and degrading enzymes for acetylcholine. Also seen are neurofibrillary tangles, neuritic plaques, and synaptic and neuronal loss in the basal forebrain.

Several neurotransmitter and receptor changes are observed in Alzheimer's disease (Nordberg 1992). Losses occur in nicotinic receptors, but muscarinic receptors are relatively preserved. Reductions are also seen in serotonin 5-HT_1 and 5-HT_2 receptors. Glutamate NMDA receptors decrease, while kainate receptors increase. β-adrenergic and dopamine receptors are preserved. Decreases occur in receptors for somatostatin and neuropeptide Y, but corticotrophin-releasing factor receptors increase. Across all receptor subtypes for which there is a loss, the number of receptors decrease but the affinity constant remains unchanged.

Cognitive deficits in Alzheimer's disease Attention deficits are a core feature of Alzheimer's disease (Lawrence and Sahakian 1995). Problems arise primarily from divided and disengaging/shifting attention and less from focusing of attention (Nebes 1997). Language deficits are seen early in the course of Alzheimer's disease. While grammar is relatively intact, there is a deficit in expression and comprehension of semantic meaning.

Memory deficits are typically the first to appear in Alzheimer's disease. There is a pronounced impairment of explicit long-term memory. This involves subjective memory for events (episodic) and for factual information (semantic). Remote memories are impaired, but less so than recent ones. Later stages of Alzheimer's disease show a spread of decline to other areas of cognitive functioning such as visuospatial and executive abilities.

Other Cortical Dementias

Frontotemporal dementia involves an early and primary degenerative process of frontal and/or temporal cortex. Several disorders fall under this rubric, such as *Pick's disease* and the dementia associated with *amyotrophic lateral sclerosis* (ALS). ALS is a degenerative disease of upper motor neurons that is sometimes accompanied by a frontal lobe dementia (Vercelletto et al. 1999; Abe et al. 1997). ALS has been associated with mutations in the free radical scavenging enzyme superoxide dismutase 1 (Price et al. 1997). Pick's disease is associated histologically with a loss of neurons and cytoplasmic Pick bodies in surviving neurons.

Frontotemporal dementias are characterized by gross structural changes in the frontal and anterior temporal lobes, metabolic disturbances, and involvement of certain subcortical structures as well (Ishii et al. 1998). Whereas in Alzheimer's disease the early cognitive disturbances are in memory, in frontotemporal dementias the early manifestations are in executive and behavioral function (Pfeffer et al. 1999; Varma et al. 1999). This relative cognitive distinction persists throughout the course of the two disorders (Pachana et al. 1996). Disinhibition and disorganization are common, and psychotic symptoms may be prominent in frontotemporal dementia.

Corticobasal degeneration involves degeneration in frontal and anterior parietal cortex along with projections to subcortical nuclei. Alien hand syndrome, involuntary limb posturing, and parkinsonism are frequent accompanying motor signs. *Lewy body dementia* is a form of dementia involving neuritic plaques and spherical inclusion bodies entitled Lewy bodies. Although it is Alzheimer's-like in cognitive presentation, hallucinations and parkinsonian features may be prominent. *Primary progressive aphasia* and *semantia dementia* are focal forms of progressive dementia, characterized by relatvely isolated language deficits with insidious onset and gradual progression. The language deficit may be the only noticeable deficit for two years or longer. Other deficits in praxis and arithmetic calculation may also occur.

Pharmacological Treatments for Alzheimer's Disease

Several drugs are available or under consideration for the treatment of Alzheimer's disease. They may be broadly characterized under neurotransmitter replacement strategies or neuroprotective drugs. Whereas neurotransmitter replacement strategies attempt to compensate for what is already missing, neuroprotective strategies aim to halt or slow the progression of the disease.

Neurotransmitter replacement strategies Inhibitors of acetylcholinesterase, and in some instances butyrylcholinesterase, have been put to clinical trials for treatment of cognitive decline in Alzheimer's disease (Krall et al. 1999). Collectively, they produce statistically significant but modest-sized effects on measures of cognitive function. Three cholinesterase inhibitors are available for clinical use in the United States: tetrahydroacridine or tacrine (Cognex), donepezil (Aricept) and rivastigmine (Exelon) (Nordberg and Svensson 1998). Several other cholinesterase inhibitors are under clinical evaluation. Donepezil and several other newer drugs are more selective to cerebral acetylcholinesterase and have few peripheral effects. Tacrine has also been associated with liver and cardiovascular toxicity in a number of patients, while donepezil does not appear to have this problem (Shintani and Uchida 1997).

Chronic treatment with tacrine produces improvements in cerebral blood flow, EEG activation, and cognitive performance (Nordberg et al. 1998; Shigeta et al. 1993). Increases are seen in nicotinic receptors, but decreases in muscarinic receptors occur in temporal cortex (Nordberg et al. 1997). Tacrine also indirectly induces an increase in turnover of serotonin, norepinephrine, and dopamine. It may also reduce levels of β-amyloid protein (Lahiri et al. 1998). A meta-analysis of controlled tacrine studies in Alzheimer's disease confirmed improvements in cognitive performance and global clinical functioning (Qizilbash et al. 1998). However, behavioral changes were mild and there were no changes in functional autonomy. Cholinesterase inhibitors may also have benefits for Lewy body dementia (Lebert et al. 1998).

Neuroprotective strategies Antioxidants have been considered as therapeutic agents for Alzheimer's and other neurodegenerative diseases. Their mechanism of action is scavenging free radicals and providing protection from cellular damage. High blood levels of antioxidants correlate with better performance in the elderly (Perrig et al. 1997).

Two drugs proposed for Alzheimer's disease are α-tocopherol, or vitamin E, and selegiline (Eldepryl). Selegiline is also an inhibitor of MAO_B and may provide additional benefit through monoamine mechanisms. Vitamin E has neuroprotective effects in several models and reduces apoptosis (Tagami et al. 1999; Yatin et al. 1999). It prevents β-amyloid-induced neurotoxicity and memory deficits in rats (Yamada et al. 1999). Conversely, vitamin E levels are reduced in the cerebrospinal fluid of people with Alzheimer's disease, and postmortem temporal cortex samples from Alzheimer's disease patients show increased susceptibility to free radical damage (Jimenez-Jimenez et al. 1997; McIntosh et al. 1997). On the other hand, those who had taken antioxidants showed a reduction in damage. A controlled study of selegiline (10 mg/day) and vitamin E (2000 IU/day) in patients with Alzheimer's disease of moderate severity was undertaken (Perrig et al. 1997). Those taking both drugs showed a slowing of disease progression and a delay of the necessity for nursing home placement.

Another neuroprotective strategy is with nonsteroidal anti-inflammatory drugs (NSAIDs). People regularly taking NSAIDs have a 50% lower chance of developing Alzheimer's disease (Stewart et al. 1997). The mechanism of this effect is uncertain, but anti-inflammatory and platelet mechanisms have been proposed (Karplus and Saag 1998). The cognitive effect of NSAIDs is significant: they reduce decline on tests of visual memory, object naming, verbal fluency, spatial recognition, and orientation in patients with Alzheimer's disease (Rich et al. 1995).

Finally, estrogen may preserve cognition in Alzheimer's and non-Alzheimer's conditions. Possible mechanisms are trophic effects on cholinergic neurons, altered expression of apolipoprotein E, antioxidant effects, and altered processing of β-amyloid (Inestrosa et al. 1998). Females taking estrogen have a reduced risk of developing Alzheimer's disease (Kawas et al. 1997).

Subcortical Dementias

Parkinson's Disease

Parkinson's disease is a neurological disorder with marked motor, cognitive, and emotional sequelae (Adams et al. 1997). It affects approximately 1% of the population over age 50. Although it typically affects ages 40 to 70, it has been known to occur at younger ages. The etiology of idiopathic Parkinson's disease is not certain, but there are manifold causes of parksinsonism, including exposure to various toxins, viral encephalitis, and stroke.

The motor symptoms of Parkinson's disease consist of difficulty initiating movement, slowed movement (bradykinesia), and muscle rigidity (Adams et al. 1997). A resting tremor is frequently the initial motor sign, and occasionally may manifest as a pill-rolling motion of the thumb and fingertips. Cogwheel rigidity also occurs, where there is a ratchet-like rhythmic resistance to passive opening of a limb. Stooped posture results from axial muscle hypotonus and a festinating gait is characteristic, where the person leans forward and executes a rapid, shuffling gait to prevent from falling. A poverty of facial expression or a mask-like face becomes evident.

Along with the motor symptoms, a host of cognitive and emotional symptoms accompany Parkinson's disease. Depression is prominent, occuring in 45% of cases. People with Parkinson's disease also have a higher incidence of dementia compared to age-matched controls, occurring in 30–50% of cases (Jacobs et al. 1997). This seems to involve additional and extranigral neuropathology compared to nondemented cases. However, a number of cognitive deficits have been found in nondementia cases of Parkinson's disease (Raskin et al. 1992; Taylor et al. 1986; Brown et al. 1991). These occur in executive, visuospatial, and short-term memory functions, with preservation of global intellectual function. Memory deficits are limited to immediate recall, while long-term semantic knowledge is preserved. Executive deficits are seen in tasks requiring planning, working memory, set shifting, and dual task performance. These deficits are thought to arise from alteration of frontostriatal processing loops by the nigrostriatal dopamine deficiency (Jagust et al. 1992; Owen et al. 1998).

It is widely accepted that Parkinson's disease primarily results from degeneration of pigmented neurons in the substantia nigra (Gibb 1998). This causes a loss of nigrostriatal projections and lack of dopamine modulation in the striatum. In addition to loss of neurons, many of the remaining neurons contain Lewy bodies.

Table 5.1
Pharmacological treatment of Parkinson's disease

Class	Drug	Trade name
Anticholinergic	trihexyphenidyl	Artane
	benztropine mesylate	Cogentin
Dopamine precursor	L-DOPA/Carbidopa	Sinemet
Dopamine agonists	Bromocriptine	Parlodel
	Amantadine	Symmetrel
	Pergolide	Permax
Enzymatic inhibition		
MAO_B	Selegiline	Eldepryl
COMT	Tolcapone	Tasmar
Antioxidants	Selegiline	Eldepryl
	Vitamin E	

See text for references.

Pharmacological Treatment of Parkinson's Disease
Parkinson's disease results from loss of striatal dopamine from degeneration of nigrostriatal dopaminergic neurons (Standaert and Young 1996). The therapeutic pharmacological strategy is to replace or otherwise functionally compensate for the loss of dopamine (table 5.1). The earlier drug treatment for Parkinson's disease was with anticholinergic drugs, because there is a functional antagonism between dopamine and acetylcholine in the striatum (Mendis et al. 1999; Standaert and Young 1996).

The anticholinergic drugs used for Parkinson's disease are muscarinic antagonists and related to atropine. The more common pharmaceutical drugs in this category are trihexyphenidyl (Artane) or benztropine mesylate (Cogentin). As with other anticholinergic drugs, they have the side effects of dry mouth, blurred vision from pupil mydriasis, constipation, and urinary retention. Cognitive side effects result as well, such as mental slowing and impairment of attention and memory. In higher doses, they may cause hallucinations and frank confusional states.

A more recent strategy developed for Parkinson's disease is dopamine replacement, which began with L-dihydroxyphenylalanine (L-DOPA or levodopa). L-DOPA is converted from tyrosine by the enzyme tyrosine hydroxylase. In turn, L-DOPA is converted to dopamine by dopa decarboxylase either in the capillary endothelium or in dopaminergic neurons. Thus, administration of L-DOPA increases the substrate for dopamine and results in increased dopamine synthesis and release. Although L-DOPA passes the blood-brain barrier, L-DOPA is rapidly converted into dopamine in the blood when administered orally. This renders approximately 95% of it unable to enter the CNS, while the remaining 5% penetrates and is then converted to dopamine. Although this was enough to alleviate parkinsonian symptoms, the large amounts of circulating dopamine created the side effect of nausea. The next step of progress came with the drug carbidopa, which inhibits peripheral DOPA decarboxylase. Thus, conversion of L-DOPA to dopamine is supressed in circulation, but continues unhindered centrally because carbidopa does not cross the blood-brain barrier. This effectively reduces the necessary dose of L-DOPA by 75%. L-DOPA and carbidopa are sold in combination under the name Sinemet. Two-thirds of patients given L-DOPA tolerate it well initially, while others may experience nausea, hypotension, or in some cases, depression. But more frequently, mood tends to improve with L-DOPA, and other changes such as excitement, aggressiveness, or increased libido may occur.

One of the drawbacks of L-DOPA/carbidopa treatment is that it loses effectiveness over time. Greater fluctuations are seen between doses due to the short half-life of the drug (1–3 hours), so a sustained-release preparation of Sinemet (Sinemet CR) has been developed to improve the stability of blood L-DOPA levels. As the effectiveness of L-DOPA wanes, the dose must be increased. With higher doses, the therapeutic margin decreases and there is greater incidence of dyskinesia. Common dyskinesia seen in high doses of L-DOPA are facial grimacing, head wagging, dystonia of the limbs and neck, choreoathetosis, and general restlessness. Psychoses consisting of delusional thinking and/or hallucinations also occur in 15–25% of people taking L-DOPA.

As an adjunct or alternate to L-DOPA, dopamine agonists are employed. Because they are direct receptor agonists, these have the advantage of not relying on the integrity of presynaptic nigrostriatal neurons, which are necessary for the synthesis and release of dopamine. Bromocriptine

(Parlodel) is an ergot alkaloid and a potent agonist of D_2 receptors located on corticostriatal terminals. It has a longer duration of action (3–7 hours) than L-DOPA and tends to produce less nausea. Pergolide (Permax) is another ergot derivative that is an agonist at both D_1 and D_2 receptors. Lisuride is a third dopamine agonist ergot-derivative and is a D_2 agonist. However, its usefulness may be limited by its side-effect profile. Amantadine (Symmetrel) was developed as an antiviral agent but was later found to have antiparkinsonian effects. It is not a dopamine receptor agonist, but rather seems to work by releasing dopamine in the striatum. Amantadine is also an antagonist of NMDA receptors, by binding at the phencyclidine (PCP) site within the channel (Kornhuber et al. 1995). NMDA antagonism prevents release of ACh in the striatum, thus providing a potential second mechanism for amantadine's antiparkinsonian effects (Stoof et al. 1992).

A final pharmacological strategy for treatment of Parkinson's disease comes from enzyme inhibition. This was initally done with an MAO inhibitor, L-deprenyl (selegiline, Eldepryl), but more recent drugs have become available that are COMT inhibitors. L-Deprenyl is an inhibitor of MAO_B, which is the form of MAO selective to dopamine. Thus, it may increase the amount of available dopamine for release. Second, it may protect dopamine neurons by reducing the oxidative stress concomitant with dopamine metabolism (Olanow 1997). Third, L-deprenyl is metabolized into amphetamine and methamphetamine, which may contribute to their antiparkinsonian effects. Unlike other treatments for Parkinson's disease, L-deprenyl seems to slow the progression of the disease. Tolcapone (Tasmar) is a COMT inhibitor, which prevents extracellular breakdown of dopamine.

Other Subcortical Degenerative Diseases

Wilson's disease (or hepatolenticular degeneration) is a autosomal recessive parkinsonian condition resulting from abnormalities of copper metabolism. Degeneration is most prominent in the putamen and globus pallidus, and it is treatable with chelating agents. *Progressive supranuclear palsy* (PSP) is characterized by supranuclear ophthalmoplegia (resulting in an impairment of vertical gaze), pseudobulbar palsy, and dysarthria (Jacobs et al. 1997; Adams et al. 1997). Parkinsonian symptoms are seen but axial rigidity is more predominant than the limb rigidity seen in Parkinson's disease, and dopaminergic medications are of limited benefit. Cognitive changes in PSP include forgetfulness, slowed information processing, emotional changes, and working-memory deficits.

Striatonigral degeneration is another parkinsonian syndrome involving loss of projections from the striatum to the substantia nigra. *Olivopontocerebellar atrophy* (OPCA) is a degenerative condition involving the inferior olivary complex, pontine nuclei, middle cerebellar peduncle, cerebellar cortex, and dentate nucleus. Motor deficits consist of typical cerebellar motor signs of ataxia, dysmetria, and tremor. Mild to moderate cognitive deficits occur in attention, memory, and executive function. *Huntington's disease* is a hereditary disorder involving degeneration of the caudate and putamen, with moderate atropy in frontal and temporal cortex. Motor manifestations are characterized by choreiform movements. Psychiatric and cognitive disturbances are also prominent.

Nondegenerative Dementias

Vascular Dementia

Vascular dementia results from several etiologies, all resulting in compromised cerebral blood flow and pathological changes (Nyenhuis and Gorelick 1998). The severity, volume, and location of the vascular lesions all contribute to the clinical picture. Risk factors for vascular dementia include hypertension, atherosclerosis, high alcohol consumption, stress, lower formal education, and occupational toxic exposure (Skoog 1979; Konno et al. 1997). *Binswanger's disease* is a form of vascular dementia with characteristic changes in periventricular white matter, as seen on structural neuroimaging (Olsen and Clasen 1998). Clinical manifestations include cognitive disturbance, depression, gait abnormalities, motor rigidity, and neurogenic bladder incontinence.

Frontal and subcortical lacunar infarcts typically affect attention, language, visuospatial function, and motor programming (Babikian et al. 1990). Compared to patients with Alzheimer's disease, those with vascular dementia show better orientation, recall, and language ability. On the other hand, Alzheimer's patients show better attention, executive function, and fine motor control (Bowler and Hachinski 1997).

Traumatic Brain Injury

Although not a neurodegenerative disorder, traumatic brain injury is another condition where dysfuntional cholinergic transmission may play a major role, and thus cholinergic medications may be useful. Memory is a cardinal cognitive problem after traumatic brain injury, and concurrent alterations in cerebral cholinergic systems have been found. Postmortem examination of humans after fatal traumatic injuries shows choline acetyltransferase activity to be reduced in several cortical areas including inferior temporal gyrus, cingulate gyrus, and superior parietal cortex (Murdoch et al. 1998). Nicotinic receptors are unchanged, but synaptophysin immunoreactivity is reduced by 30% in the cingulate gyrus, suggesting a loss of presynaptic cholinergic terminals.

Normal Aging

Normal aging involves some degree of cognitive decline and neuropathological changes (Boller and Duyckaerts 1997). There is a reduction in gross volume and weight in the aged brain, approaching 15% of total weight. After the age of 60, there is an average loss of 2% of brain weight per decade, primarily due to reduction of white matter. Neuritic plaques and neurofibrillary tangles occur, but their distribution and degree is different than that seen in Alzheimer's disease. On functional neuroimaging, there is a trend toward decreased metabolism in frontal areas during old age, but this is distinct in degree and progression from patterns seen in dementia (Mielke et al. 1998). Age-related memory changes are also apparent on electrophysiological measures, but still distinct from dementia (Joyce et al. 1998; Stevens and Kircher 1998).

Age-related changes in many cognitive functions are seen in healthy elderly adults. Most notable are changes in processing speed and short-term memory (Sliwinski and Buschke 1999; Unger et al. 1999; Keefover 1998). While difficulties occur in the formation of new memories, memory for familiar information and skills is well preserved (Burke and Mackay 1997). Mild cognitive complaints are fairly common in

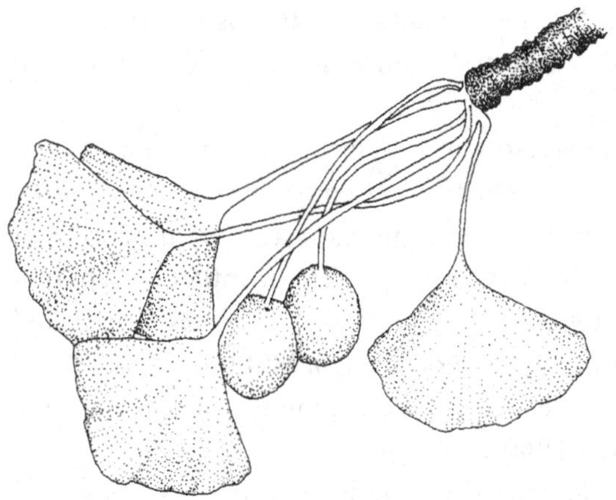

Figure 5.1
Ginkgo *(Ginkgo biloba)*. Reprinted with permission from Sturdivant and Blakely. (1999). *Medicinal Herbs in the Garden, Field, and Marketplace.* Friday Harbor, WA: San Juan Naturals. Illustration by Peggy Sue McRae.

community-dwelling elderly, but these are accounted for by age-related effects and depression (Schroder et al. 1998). Literacy and education play a role in preserving cognitive function and providing the neural basis for cognitive reserves to be drawn upon later in life (Manly et al. 1999).

Herbal Nootropics

Ginkgo

History and Botany

Ginkgo biloba, also known as the kew or maidenhair tree, is a species of gymnosperm that has been in existence for 200 million years. Some living specimens are estimated to be more than 3,000 years old (Field and Vadnal 1998). Ginkgo is a seed-bearing tree that typically grows to a height of 35–80 feet. Its leaves are green and fan shaped, and produce an acid that is resistant to insects (figure 5.1). Ginkgo trees do not reproduce until 20 years of age, but may continue to reproduce past 1,000 years of age (Major 1967). The seeds (sometimes referred to as fruit) are round, fleshy, and have a yellow or green color (Gruenwald et al. 1998). At present, approximately fifty million ginkgo trees are in cultivation for preparation as herbal supplements, yielding 4,000 tons of dried leaves annually from the United States and France alone (Field and Vadnal 1998).

The name *ginkgo* is a Japanese word derived from the Chinese *yin-shing*, meaning "silver apricot." The Chinese emperor Shen Nung wrote in his medical text *Pen T'sao Ching* that ginkgo leaves are used to treat memory loss and breathing ailments. Liu Wen-Tai in 1505 C.E. reported uses of ginkgo for skin sores and diarrhea due to parasites (Fields and Vadnal 1998). The ginkgo tree was not brought to Europe and North America until the eighteenth century, and common use of ginkgo in the West did not occur until the 1960s.

Today, ginkgo extracts are marketed under a variety of registered trade names including Ginkgobene, Ginkgold, Ginkoba, Kaveri, Rokan, Tanakene, Tramisal, Valverde Vital, and Vasan. Although brands may vary in their bioequivalence, no one to date has examined the implications of this variance on cognitive function (Itil and Martorano 1995). Ginkgo is among the most commonly prescribed drugs in France and Germany, making up 1% and 4% of their prescriptions, respectively.

Chemical Constituents

Ginkgo's active chemical constituents are classified into flavonoid glycosides, biflavones, and terpene lactones (table 5.2) (Field and Vadnal 1998; Oken et al. 1998). Flavonoid glycosides include kaemferol, quercetin, apigenin, luteolin, and myricetin. Biflavones include amentoflavone, bilobetin, ginkgetin, isoginkgetin, sciadopitysin, and 5′-methoxybilobelin. Terpene lactones in ginko are the ginkgolides A, B, C, M, and J, and bilobalide (figure 5.2). The ginkgolides are diterpenes and bilobalide is a sesquiterpene (Gruenwald et al. 1998). Ginkgolides are unique twenty-carbon terpenes, occurring naturally only in the roots and leaves of the ginkgo tree (Braquet and Hosford 1991). Other constituents of interest are alkylphenols such as ginkgolic acid (Satyan et al. 1998; Jaggy and Koch 1997). Proanthocyanidins are also present, and may create vasoactive and antioxidant effects. Ginkgo extracts are standardized by their flavonoid glycoside and terpene content (Li and Wong 1997).

Preparations include dried leaf, tinctures, and several extracts (Field and Vadnal 1998). Different extracts of ginkgo are used in research, which produce different relative compositions of its chemical

Table 5.2
Chemical constituents of ginkgo

Flavonoid glycosides	Kaempferol Quercetin Apigenin Luteolin Myricetin
Biflavones	Amentoflavone Bilobetin Ginkgetin Isoginkgetin Sciadopitysin 5′-methoxybilobelin
Terpene lactones	Ginkgolides A, B, C, M, and J Bilobalide
Alkylphenols	Ginkgolic acid
Proanthocyanidins	

See text for references.

constituents. The most common standardized extraction process, termed EGb 761, uses water and acetone extraction in the initial stage. The lipophilic and condensed polyphenolic compounds are then removed (Itil and Martorano 1995; Kleijnen and Knipschild 1992a). This produces an extract containing 24% ginkgo-flavone glycosides and 6% terpenoids, and has been marketed in Europe under several trade names. Another extract, LI 1370, has 25% ginkgo-flavone glycosides and 6% terpenoids. Preparation of ginkgo as a tea is ineffective because it would only contain small amounts of active constituents (Tyler 1990).

Mechanisms of Action

Ginkgo has effects on several neurotransmitter and physiological systems, which are addressed here separately (table 5.3).

Acetylcholine Ginkgo enhances release of acetylcholine and alters cholinergic receptors. Both direct in vitro application and long-term oral administration increases presynaptic uptake of choline in hippocampal synaptosomes (Kristofikova et al. 1992). The effective concentrations for

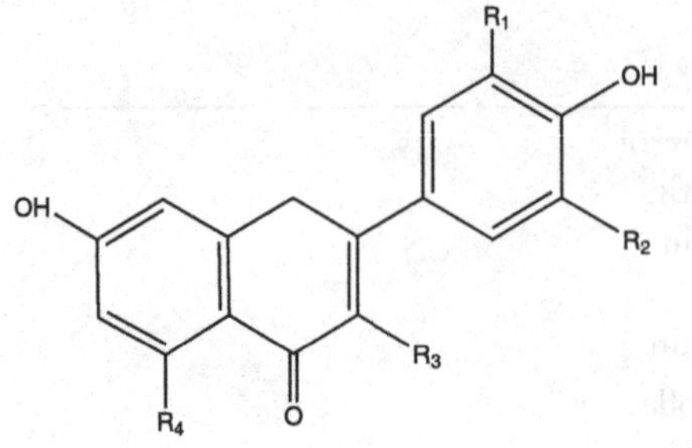

	R_1	R_2	R_3	R_4
Kaempferol	H	H	OH	OH
Rutin	OH	H	O-Rha-Glu	OH
Quercetin	OH	H	OH	OH
Myricetin	OH	OH	OH	OH

Flavonols

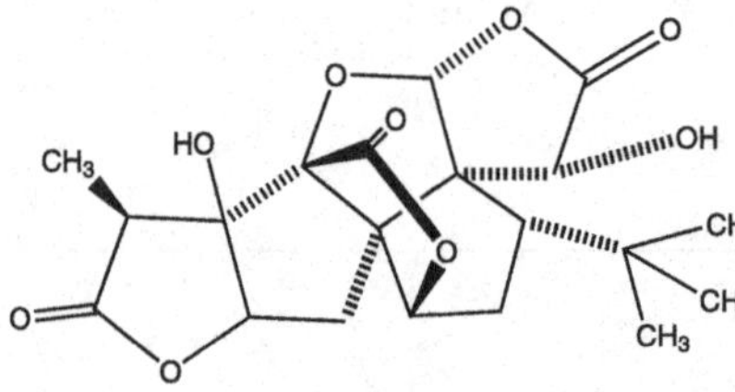

Ginkgolide A

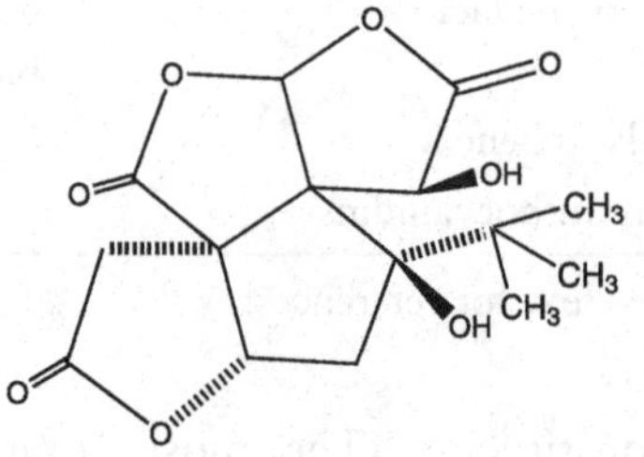

Bilobalide

Terpene Lactones

Figure 5.2
Chemical structure of ginkgo constituents.

this effect are 100 mg/ml in vitro or 20–30 mg/g of brain tissue, which could be achieved with chronic dosing. The increase in choline uptake is due to an increase in the number of choline uptake transporters and/or rate of transport (Kristofikova et al. 1997). Chronic oral treatment with extract also increases the number of muscarinic receptors in the hippocampus (Taylor 1986).

Short-term memory tasks increase high-affinity uptake of acetylcholine, whereas long-term reference memory tasks cause an acute increase followed by a long-lasting decrease and inhibition (Decker et al. 1988). In contrast, the drug scopolamine creates amnestic effects by blocking muscarinic receptors and decreasing acetylcholine levels. Thus, at

Table 5.3
Mechanisms of action of ginkgo

Cholinergic	Increases uptake of choline and release of acetylcholine Increases the number of muscarinic receptors
Monoamine	Increase uptake of 5-HT Inhibition of MAO_A and MAO_B Prevents desensitization and age-related reduction of $5\text{-}HT_{1A}$ Alters norepinephrine turnover Reduced β-adrenergic binding and activity Reverses age-related decline in α_2 adrengic receptors
GABA	Elevation of GABA levels Increased glutamic acid decarboxylase activity
Vasoactive	PAF inhibition NO-dependent vasodilation

See text for references.

normal oral doses in humans, perhaps slightly higher than those commonly used, ginkgo extracts enhance cholinergic transmission by increasing uptake and release. The nootropic drugs tacrine and donepezil similarly enhance cholinergic transmission by preventing breakdown of acetylcholine by acetylcholinesterase. Although not the only effect of ginkgo, cholinergic mechanisms could well account for its cognitive effects.

Monoamines Ginkgo extracts and commercial preparations inhibit MAO_A and MAO_B in vitro, achieving total inhibition, but it has yet to be demonstrated that this occurs in the brain and at normal oral doses (White et al. 1996). Although EGb 761 increases uptake of 5-HT (but not dopamine), chronic administration to aged rats increases serotonin in frontal cortex, hippocampus, striatum, and hypothalamus (Ramassamy et al. 1992). Chronic treatment reverses an age-related reduction in the maximal binding sites of $5\text{-}HT_{1A}$ receptors (Huguet et al. 1994). Chronic oral administration of EGb 761 prevents stress-induced desensitization of $5\text{-}HT_{1A}$ receptors, without altering their density or affinity (Bolanos-Jimenez et al. 1995). Accordingly, drug discrimination paradigms suggest effects at $5\text{-}HT_{1A}$, but not $5\text{-}HT_2$ receptors (Winter and Timineri 1999).

A biphasic effect of ginkgo is seen over time on norepinephrine turnover (Brunello et al. 1985). An initial decrease in the norepinephrine metabolite normetanephrine occurs at 45 minutes, followed by a marked increase that was present after 14 days. Chronic treatment reduces β-adrenergic binding and β-adrenergic-stimulated adenylate cyclase activity. Thus, an increase in norepinephrine levels is inducing β-adrenergic receptor regulation and functional activity. Ginkgo chronically administered also reverses the age-related decline in binding density of α_2 adrenergic receptors (Huguet and Tarrade 1992).

GABA Flavonoids present in ginkgo may endow it with benzodiazepine actions but it remains in question whether they cross the blood-brain barrer (Lobstein-Guth et al. 1988; Baureithel et al. 1997). However, oral doses of bilobalide elevates GABA levels in the hippocampus (Sasaki et al. 1999). Increases occur in the activity and amount of glutamic acid decarboxylase. Glutamate levels are not affected by bilobalide, nor are the number or dissociation constants of the $GABA_A$ receptor. Such effects were suggested to mediate the antiseizure effects of bilobalide.

Intracellular messengers A biphasic effect of ginkgo extract is seen on cAMP phosphodiesterase under in vitro and ex vivo conditions (Saponara and Bosisio 1998; Macovschi et al. 1987). Whereas low concentrations (0.25–4.0 mg/L) activate the enzyme, higher concentrations (5–250 mg/L), dose-dependently inhibit it. However, tolerance develops to this effect because it is undetectable after daily administration for 4 days. Thus, ginkgo may initially produce effects by inhibiting enzymatic breakdown of cAMP. This mechanism is similar to the stimulant caffeine, but it is not likely to explain any long-term effects of ginkgo because it disappears after chronic daily treatment. The responsible constituent for this effect has not been identified.

Pharmacokinetics

Ginkgo extracts show rapid absorption after oral administration of capsules, tablets, and drops (Li and Wong 1997; Wójcicki et al. 1995). The pharmacokinetics for the ginkgo terpene lactones have been determined

Table 5.4
Pharmacokinetics of ginkgo terpene lactones

Constituent	Oral bioavailability	Time to peak concentration	Half-life	Elimination half-life
Ginkgolide A	>98%	1–2 hrs	4–6 hrs	4.5 hrs
Ginkgolide B	>80%	1–2 hrs	4–6 hrs	10.5
Bilobalide	70%	1–2 hrs	3 hours	3.2

See text for references.

(table 5.4) (Kleijnen and Knipschild 1992a). Ginkgo flavone glycosides have an oral bioavailability of >60%, and reach peak concentrations in 1.5–3 hours. Their half-life is between 2 and 4 hours. Ginkgolides A or B have an oral bioavailability of greater than 80% (>98% for A, >80% for B). They reach peak concentrations in 1–2 hours and have a half-life of 4–6 hours. Bilobalide has an oral bioavailability of 70%, reaches peak concentrations in 1–2 hours, and has a half-life of approximately 3 hours. Elimination half-lives for ginkgolides A, B, and bilobalide are, respectively, 4.5, 10.5, and 3.2 hours. Similar results were confirmed by others (Biber and Koch 1999).

Another study showed high bioavailability of ginkgolides and bilobalide, and was suggestive of twice-daily dosing (Fourtillan et al. 1995). Concurrent food intake did not alter the total effect, but increased the time to reach peak concentrations. Different extraction processes can enhance the bioavailability of ginkgo constituents (Li and Wong 1997). The brain bioavailability of ginkgo has been shown indirectly with electrophysiological studies of oral dosing in humans (Itil and Martorano 1995; Itil et al. 1998).

Pharmacokinetic parameters have been determined for the ginkgo flavonoid glycosides quercetin, kaempferol, and isorhamnetin (table 5.5) (Wójcicki et al. 1995). Rapid absorption occurs and peak concentrations are reached in approximately three hours for all three flavone glycosides. Elimination follows a typical exponential function and the volume distribution suggests extensive tissue penetration. A short elimination half-life and total body clearance suggest that ginkgo flavone glycosides are rapidly eliminated. Futher, bioequivalence is found for these constituents across capsule, drops, and tablet formulations, based on FDA guidelines.

Table 5.5
Pharmacokinetics of ginkgo flavonoid glycosides

Parameter	Quercetin	Kaemferol	Isorhamnetin
AUC [ng/ml*h]	67.3±12.71	138.43±28.42	34.63±8.47
C_{max} [ng/ml]	12.16±2.55	26.73±5.03	7.26±1.56
T_{max} [h]	2.55±0.43	2.53±0.45	2.49±0.42
V_d [l]	170.01±38.03	190.92±38.12	208.13±46.91
K [h^{-1}]	0.24±0.05	0.25±0.06	0.25±0.05
T_2 [h]	2.98±0.56	2.89±0.52	2.84±0.55
Cl_T [h]	39.07±8.45	45.86±10.28	44.72±10.14

See text for references.
Key: AUC Area under the curve, C_{max} maximal serum concentrations, T_{max} time to reach peak concentrations, V_d volume distribution, K rate constant for elimination, T_2 Elimination half-life, and Cl_T Total body clearance time. (Wójcicki et al. 1995)

Ginkgo extract has no effect on the hepatic microsomal drug oxidation system, as measured by antipyrine elimination, even at doses of 400 mg per day (Duche et al. 1989). Ginkgo metabolites, the substituted benzoic acids (4-hydroxybenzoic acid conjugate, 4-hydroxyhippuric acid, 3-methoxy-4-hydroxyhippuric acid, 3,4-dihydroxybenzoic acid, 4-hydroxybenzoic acid, hippuric acid and 3-methoxy-4-hydroxybenzoic acid [vanillic acid]), are excreted in urine (Pietta et al. 1997).

General Effects

Vascular and hematologic effects Ginkgo exerts vascular effects through at least two mechanisms: inhibition of platelet-activating factor (PAF) and nitric oxide mechanisms. Ginkgo extract relaxes the porcine basilar artery in a concentration-dependent and partly endothelium-dependent manner (Chen et al. 1997). It also enhances vasorelaxation created by transmural nerve stimulation in arteries with and without the endothelium intact, and is prevented by nitro-L-arginine, indicating that the effect is mediated by nitric oxide.

PAF is a lipid-derived chemical messenger with many biological roles, including aggregation of blood platelets. Ginkgolides A, B, and C antagonize PAF, by preventing its enzymatic formation from PAF-acether

(Lamant et al. 1987). Ginkgolide B is the most potent, followed by Ginkgolides A and C. Half maximal inhibition occurs for all three in the low micromolar range. Nonginkgolide, nonflavonoid fractions of ginkgo extract have a potent vasorelaxing effect, producing a dose-dependent relaxation of rabbit and human cavernosal smooth muscle (Paick and Lee 1996). A subfraction (304U-1) shows the most potent effects, which are mediated by cAMP and perhaps adrenergic effects. Thus, gingko may improve microcirculation by inhibiting platelet-aggregation by PAF.

Ginkgo has a number of other hematologic effects. Acute administration of the ginkgo extract, Kaveri, does not alter blood pressure or heart rate in humans (Jung et al. 1990). Chronic treatment with ginkgo extract (120 mg/day for 3 months) lowered diastolic blood pressure (Winther et al. 1998). However, no changes were seen at a higher dose (240 mg/day for 3 months). Also unchanged by ginkgo are haematocrit, plasma viscosity, erythrocyte rigidity, thrombocyte and leukocyte count, and thrombocyte aggregation. However, ginkgo does reduce erythrocyte aggregation by 15.6% (Jung et al. 1990). Ginkgo reduces pulmonary hypertension induced by chronic isobaric hypoxia (Cheng et al. 1996). In human platelets, ginkgolides reduce phospholipase C activation and the mobilization and influx of Ca^{2+} (Simon et al. 1987). This action is not observed with thrombin, suggesting that ginkgolides act through the membrane receptor of PAF-acether. Ginkgolides also reduce thromboxane B_2 levels (Becker et al. 1988).

EGb 761 has both antiplatelet and antithrombotic effects when administered orally, prolonging bleeding time in experimental models (Kim YS et al. 1998; Bourgain et al. 1987). Ginkgolide B prevents thrombus formation in experimentally injured arterial segments (Bourgain et al. 1986). It also inhibits specific binding of PAF to eosinophils and neutrophils in a concentration-dependent manner (Kurihara et al. 1989). Intravenous EGb 761 significantly reduces arteriolar spasm in rat cremaster muscle, effective when vasospasm is induced by serum and a thromboxane analog, but not by serotonin or thrombin (Stœcker et al. 1996). Ginkgolides and proanthocyanidins are believed to mediate this effect.

A systematic literature review showed ten controlled studies of ginkgo for treatment of intermittent claudication (Ernst 1996). Many studies had methodological flaws, but the consensus is that gingko is an effective therapy for intermittent claudication. This effect is most likely mediated by ginkgo's effects on vessel dilation and microcirculation through inhibiting platelet activation. A meta-analysis found ginkgo to have a significant effect in treating peripheral arterial diseases, with a global effect size of 0.75 (Schneider 1992).

Sexual effects Ginkgo was serendipitously found to improve sexual function in an elderly patient taking it for memory effects. A subsequent open trial of ginkgo extract was performed to assess its effect on antidepressant-induced sexual dysfunction (SSRI, SNRI, MAOI, and tricyclics) (Cohen and Bartlik 1998). Ginkgo had a positive effect on sexual function in 84% of subjects. Both male and female subjects participated, and a larger proportion of females reported benefit (91% female, 76% male). Improvement was noted across all four phases of the sexual cycle: desire, excitement, orgasm, and resolution. The dosages used for this effect were in the range of 240 mg. A controlled study is needed to confirm these findings and determine magnitude of effect.

Penile erection occurs by relaxation of the smooth muscle of the corpus cavernosum, increasing blood flow into the penis and producing erection and rigidity. In a parallel fashion, vaginal pressure stimulation increases blood velocity and flow into clitoral arteries (Lavoisier et al. 1995). Cavernosal vasodilation is accomplished by neurotransmitters released from the cavernosal nerve and endothelial cells. One of the most important transmitters in this cascade is nitric oxide (NO), which induces synthesis of cyclic GMP from guanylate cyclase (Rajfer et al. 1992). Thus, ginkgo's vascular mechanisms could be responsible for some of the putative sexual effects.

Vestibulocochlear effects Ginkgo has positive effects on vestibulocochlear function in animal models, primarily through vasoactive and antioxidant mechanisms. EGb 761 dilates the cochlear vasculature and prevents flow reduction caused by sodium salicylate (Didier et al. 1996). Oral EGb 761 reduced tinnitus induced by sodium salicylate in rats (Jastreboff et al. 1997). The recovery of balance after unilateral vestibular neurectomy is accelerated by postoperative treatment with EGb 761, most likely due to cerebral plasticity mechanisms involved in vestibular compensation (Tighilet and Lacour 1995; Smith and Darlington 1994). Effects are dose-dependent and involve nonterpene constituents. EGb 761 has a direct excitatory effect on the lateral vestibular nuclei and decreases gain of the horizontal vestibulo-ocular reflex without altering phase (Yabe et al. 1995). Functional improvements in balance are accompanied by morphological neural correlates, such as faster synaptic reoccupation in the deafferented medial vestibular nucleus (Lacour et al. 1991). Oral and parenteral ginkgo extract morphologically preserve the vestibular epithelia, probably due to improved capillary permeability and microcirculation (Raymond 1986).

Ginkgo also improves tinnitus and dizziness in human studies, but this effect may occur later than improvements in memory and concentration (Soholm 1998). Ginkgo extract reduces tinnitus and vertigo in humans associated with vertebrobasilar insufficiency (Cano-Cuenca et al 1995). Sizable multicenter controlled studies indicate that ginkgo is effective in treating tinnitus, irrespective of prognostic factors such as the site and periodicity of the disease (Meyer 1986a, 1986b).

In humans, chronic (3 month) treatment with EGb 761 reduces vertigo and dizziness, with efficacy comparable to betahistine dihydrochloride (Cesarani et al. 1998). Oculomotor improvements are seen in a slight decrease of saccadic delay and significantly increased saccadic velocities, improved smooth pursuit gain, and reduced nystagmus. Also noted are improvements of the sinusoidal vestibulo-ocular reflex and visuovestibular ocular reflex. Other multicenter, controlled studies have supported ginkgo in the treatment of vertigo (Haguenauer et al. 1986).

Neuroprotective effects Ginkgo has a number of significant antioxidant effects. EGb 761 protects against oxidative damage induced by peroxyl radicals (Maitra et al. 1995; Lugasi et al. 1999). It reduces oxidative-induced morphological changes in mitochondria, glutathianone oxidation, and peroxide formation (Sastre and El-Fattah 1998; Seif-El-Nasr et al. 1995). Terpenoid constituents of ginkgo show anti-ischemic effects in the myocardium, due to inhibition of free radical synthesis, but not by direct free radical scavenging (Pietri et al. 1997). The ginkgo flavonoids myricetin and quercetin reduce oxidative metabolism at nanomolar concentrations (3 and 10 nM, respectively) (Oyama et al. 1994). Ginkgo and methylprednisolone both reduced injury in a spinal cord compression injury model in rats, probably by antioxidant actions (Koc et al. 1995). EGb 761 has dual effects on the free radical nitric oxide (Kobuchi et al. 1997; Marcocci et al. 1994). It scavenges nitric oxide as well as inhibits its synthesis in lipopolysaccharide/interferon-gamma macrophages. Ginkgo extract protects neurons against oxidative stress produced by hydrogen peroxide (Oyama et al. 1996). Also reduced are apoptosis and DNA fragmentation induced by oxidative stress (Ni et al. 1996). This is accomplished by flavonoids and other constituents of EGb 761, but not terpenoids (Chen et al. 1999). EGb 761 protects against oxidative free radical damage in the retina, as evidenced by electrophysiological changes (Droy-Lefaix et al. 1995). Ginkgo extract and ginkgolide B reduce glutamate excitotoxicity after peripheral administration by preventing increases in Ca^{2+} flux (Zhu et al. 1997). Ginkgo also protects dopaminergic neurons from the neurotoxic agent *N*-methyl-4-phenyl-1,2,3,6-tetrahydropyridine (MPTP) (Ramassamy et al. 1990).

Ginkgo shows some anti-ischemic effects, although results depend highly on methodology. EGb 761 prevents reduction of Na,K-ATPase after cerebral ischemia (Pierre et al. 1999). PAF has been implicated in hypoxic damage during cerebral ischemia. Hypoxic/ischemic injuries in neonatal rats are mediated by PAF, and are reduced by EGb 761 (Akisü et al. 1998). Ginkgolides reduce the cerebral damage produced by ligature of the common carotid artery in adult Mongolian gerbils (Spinnewyn et al. 1987). A methodologically controlled study of ginkgo extract was carried out in adults with acute ischemic stroke (Garg et al. 1995). Although results were negative, this may relate to a relatively low dosage and/or administration time post-injury (>48 hours). The authors also conclude that there appear to be no adverse effects of ginkgo in acute ischemic stroke.

Ginkgo alters lipid metabolism created by electroconvulsive shock treatments. EGb 761 reduced accumulation of free fatty acids and removal of diacylglycerol, which is more pronounced in the hippocampus than cerebral cortex (Rodriguez de Turco et al. 1993). Ginkgo also has protective effects on lipid membranes under hypoxic conditions. Bilobalide, but not ginkgolides, suppressed hydrolysis of choline induced by hypoxia (Klein et al. 1997). This effect is seen in the low micromolar range, both in vitro and ex vivo by oral doses (6 mg/kg). EGb 761 had the same effect at 200 mg/kg. EGb 761 and bilobalide both inhibit the hypoxia-induced drop in ATP release from endothelial cells (Janssens et al. 1995). Bilobalide increases glucose transport under normal oxygen conditions but not under hypoxia.

Ginkgo may speed recovery from neurological injury. EGb 761 accelerates recovery from hemiplegia induced by ablation of motor cortex (Brailowsky and Montiel 1997). This effect required chronic treatment (10 days) in aged rats. Histologically, treated rats showed less glial fibrillary acid protein and ex vacuo hydrocephalus. Bilobalide also has trophic and protective effects on neurons and Schwann cells in nerve injuries (Bruno et al. 1993). In rats treated with bilobalide, a faster reinnervation of the extensor digitorum longus muscle was observed following traumatic nerve damage.

Neurophysiological effects PAF decreases b-wave amplitude on the electroretinogram, which is reversed by ginkgo extract and ginkgolide B (BN 52021) (Doly et al. 1987). This effect is interpreted in terms of direct effects on PAF membrane receptors in the retina. Membrane receptors for PAF receptors act through intracellular messengers, activating the phosphatidylinositol cycle and forming inositol-triphosphate (Doly et al. 1987).

PAF enhances excitatory amino acid release in the hippocampus and may serve as a retrograde messenger in long-term potentiation (Bazan and Allan 1996). On the surface, this might seem at odds with ginkgo's pro-mnestic effects because ginkgolides inhibit PAF. However, the role of PAF in long-term potentiation occurs at low concentrations and it is not essential for its induction, so ginkgo may not significantly inhibit this process (Wieraszko et al. 1993; Kobayashi et al. 1999). On the other hand, ginkgolides may impair long-term potentiation, but other pro-mnestic effects of ginkgo may overshadow this.

Chronic treatment with EGb 761 in mice created histological changes in the hippocampus (Barkats et al. 1995). Increases are seen in the projection field of hippocampal mossy fibers and a reduction in the area of the stratum radiatum. These changes are hypothesized to result from neuroprotective or neurotrophic actions of ginkgo. Other researchers have also found histological changes in the hippocampus after treatment with ginkgo (Cohen-Salmon et al. 1997).

Cerebral blood flow and glucose utilization Local cerebral blood flow is increased by ginkgo extract in multiple regions of the brain in conscious rats (Krieglstein et al. 1986). Ginkgo increases cerebral blood flow in humans as well (Heiss and Podreka 1978).

Although ginkgo causes an increase in cerebral blood flow, it can decrease cerebral glucose utilization. An autoradiographic study of chronic oral EGb 761 showed decreases up to 18% in frontoparietal somatosensory cortex, the nucleus accumbens, cerebellar cortex and pons (Duverger et al. 1995). Another study, using higher doses, showed greater decreases (20%) of glucose utilization in the hippocampus, globus pallidus, neostriatum, ventral thalamus, inferior colliculus, and inferior olive (Lamour et al. 1992). Changes in several of these neuroanatomical areas could account for the cognitive therapeutic effects of ginkgo. Studies on the effects of individual ginkgo constituents on glucose metabolism are needed to discern their respective effects (Duverger et al. 1995). The reasons for decreases are uncertain, but one author suggests that it is a factor of route and duration of administration as well as the physiological state of the organism (Duverger et al. 1995). Although ginkgo raises the blood glucose level dose-dependently, perfusion studies show that cortical glucose concentration is reduced, suggesting that ginkgo may inhibit glucose uptake (Krieglstein et al. 1986).

Neuroendocrine effects In both young and old rats, chronic treatment with oral ginkgo extract reduces stress-induced impairments in learning and elevation of stress hormones (Rapin et al. 1994). Ginkgolide B reduces the binding and expression of peripheral-type benzodiazepine receptors in the adrenal cortex (Amri et al. 1996; Amri et al. 1997; Papadopoulos et al. 1998). This reduces the production of corticosterone in response to adrenocorticotrophic hormone (ACTH). Thus, gingkolide B causes a reduction of glucocorticoid production. Additionally, there is a reduction of progesterone production in pregnant rats. Ginkgo constituents may also act at the hypothalamic level, reducing expression and secretion of corticotrophin-releasing hormone under certain conditions (Marcilhac et al. 1998).

Chronic elevation of corticosteroids has been shown to impair cognitive processes and have neurotoxic effects (Sheline et al. 1996; de Kloet et al. 1999). The cumulative effects of elevated cortisol levels are associated with cognitive impairments in human aging (Lupien et al. 1999). Thus, the cognitive and neuroprotective effects of ginkgo may be partly mediated through its neuroendocrine effects.

Electrophysiological effects Several studies have looked at the electrophysiological effects of ginkgo. Short-term chronic (3 day) oral doses of ginkgo extract produces electrophysiological effects in many frequencies and topographical areas, and on several EEG power measures (Kunkel 1993). Effects are seen across widespread cerebra regions, but are maximal in frontotemporal areas. Further, different fractions of the ginkgo extract produced similar effects. Other studies consistently show activation effects or decrease in slow-wave activity (Kanowski et al. 1996; Pidoux 1986).

Other researchers report a more specific cognitive activation effect both in young healthy subjects and elderly subjects suffering from mild dementia. The activation effects are characterized by relative increases in alpha activity (7.5 to 13 Hz) and decreases in delta and theta activity (1.3 to 7.5 Hz) (Itil et al. 1998). Ginkgo extract has electrophysiological effects similar to tacrine, donepezil, and other nootropic drugs (piracetam and oxiracetam). In the study by Itil and colleagues (1998), more subjects showed the cognitive activation response to ginkgo extract (240 mg; 44% responders) than tacrine (40 mg; 18% responders). This was an open study, so controlled studies are now needed to confirm these results. They also used a single test dose, so a study of chronic dosing is needed to see if these effects sustain or increase over time.

The differences found by these two EEG studies may be due to methodological factors. Kunkel (1993) prescreened subjects for high alpha activity (70% or more of the recording period), whereas Itil and colleagues did not. Kunkel also used lower doses (40, 80, and 160 mg) than Itil and colleagues (240 mg).

One study of chronic ginkgo extract found no differences in EEG between ginkgo and placebo in elderly subjects with age-related decline. However, subjects with the more severe baseline EEG findings showed the most improvement in vigilance with ginkgo (Gessner et al. 1985). This study used a smaller dose of extract than others who found positive results (120 mg).

Ginkgo extract shortens stimulus evaluation time in an ERP paradigm (auditory oddball) (Semlitsch et al. 1995). Subjects with age-related memory decline show a shortening of the latency P300, while no effects are seen on the latency of N1, P2, or N2, nor the amplitudes of N1, P2, N2, and P300. Chronicity of dosage does not affect the P300 latency, because similar results were found for both acute and chronic administration.

Cognitive effects: Animal studies A few studies have examined ginkgo extracts on cognition in animal models. An aqueous ginkgo extract shortens sleeping time induced by anesthetics in mice (hexobarbital, a-chloralose, and urethane) (Wada et al. 1993). The terpene lactones bilobalide and ginkgolide A accomplished this effect. Improvements in maze learning are noted in mice after ginkgo treatment (Gajewski and Hensch 1999). Similarly, acute administration to rats produces improvement in working memory (delayed nonmatch to position) as well as learning and error rate in maze tasks (Winter 1998). Also noted in this study was a greater longevity of rats administered ginkgo versus placebo. The mechanism of this effect is uncertain, but it did not appear to involve caloric restriction. Antioxidant mechanisms are hypothesized by the author to be the responsible agents. Ginkgo extract improves short-term memory in a passive avoidance task in mice (Stoll et al. 1996). Although it also improved lipid membrane fluidity, it did not correlate with improvements in short-term memory.

A ginkgo extract (GK 501) produces improvement on four animal models of learning (shuttle box, step down, step through, and Morris water maze) (Petkov et al. 1993). In some cases, combined administration of ginkgo and ginseng showed a potentiation of effects. Ginkgo extract protects against stress-induced learning deficits in older rats (Rapin et al. 1994). Finally, ginkgo attenuates amnesia induced by scopolamine, a muscarinic antagonist, in rats (Chopin and Briley 1992). At higher doses, effects are comparable to those of tacrine.

Cognitive effects: Humans with dementia Several studies have looked at the effects of ginkgo extracts on cognitive function in people with dementia. German health authorities approved a ginkgo extract in 1994 for treatment of primary degenerative and vascular dementias (Itil et al. 1998). Ginkgo has been examined in a number of clinical populations, including Alzheimer's disease, vascular dementia, and age-associated cognitive decline. Most studies employed the extracts EGb 761 or LI 1370. Many have methodological flaws including limited sample size or insufficient description of randomization, patient characteristics, measurement techniques, or result presentation, but there are a number of well-controlled studies available for drawing preliminary conclusions (Field and Vadnal 1998).

Ginkgo's cognitive effects are examined using a number of measures, but the focus has been on memory and attention/processing speed. Subjects presenting with mild memory complaints show improvement on measures such as the digit copying (Kendrick battery) and a computerized classification task, indicating underlying improvements in processing speed (Rai et al. 1991). Short-term memory improvements are produced by ginkgo on the Sternberg memory test (Hindmarch 1986). The Sternberg test measures short-term retention of 4–6 digits, assessed with yes/no discrimination responses. Benefits are seen in subjects with age-related memory loss using a dual-coding task that involves rapid encoding of visual and verbal material into memory (Allain et al. 1993). Ginkgo extract improves performance when given in one acute dose one hour before testing. Improvements are also seen in subjects with Alzheimer's disease and vascular dementia using the German syndromkurztest, a battery measuring attention and memory (Maurer 1997). Changes have not been seen in the Trail Making Test in subjects with Alzheimer's disease taking ginkgo extract. Other studies have shown improvement in cognitive measures designed to grossly gage cognitive function in Alzheimer's disease, such as the ADAS (Alzheimer's Disease Assessment Scale), which samples memory, language, praxis, and orientation (LeBars et al. 1997).

Ginkgo treatment also produces improvements in ratings by examiners and caregivers (clinical global impressions scale, geriatric evaluation by relative's rating scale) as well as self-assessment of activities of daily living (Nürnberger Alters-Beobachtungsskala) relative to placebo (Maurer 1997; Kanowski et al. 1996; Haase et al. 1996; Taillandier et al. 1986). Improvements are also noted in several studies on subjects' self-ratings versus placebo (Kleijnen and Knipchild 1992b).

A meta-analysis of studies using rigorous methodological inclusion criteria was carried out by Oken and colleagues (1998). Collectively, the studies reviewed support a real effect of ginkgo extracts on cognition in people with Alzheimer's disease. A small effect size (0.4) was found, but this may be partly due to the fact that effects were averaged over ten outcome measures, some of which were less sensitive to improvement. Another reason may be the variable dosages used in the studies, ranging from 120 to 240 mg. Studies using 240 mg showed greater effect sizes. However, the effect size is substantial when compared to the prescription nootropic donepezil (Aricept), for which effect sizes are between 0.42 to 0.48 (Rogers et al. 1998). Other review of the literature reached similar conclusions about ginkgo's cognitive effects in dementia (Soholm 1998). Also mentioned is a therapeutic lag period of 4–6 weeks after initiation of treatment, which likely corresponds with receptor regulation and functional changes.

Although the meta-analysis by Oken and colleagues examined efficacy in Alzheimer's disease only, improvements have been seen in other conditions such as age-related memory decline and vascular dementia (Kanowski et al. 1996; Haase et al. 1996; Allain et al. 1993). More research is needed to establish the quantitative clinical significance of ginkgo extract.

Cognitive effects: Normal subjects Two studies to date have examined the cognitive effects of an acute dose of ginkgo in normal subjects. Similar to studies in memory-impaired subjects, benefits occurred in the Sternberg memory test, but not in critical flicker frequency and choice reaction time (Subhan and Hindmarch 1984). Although preliminary, this methodologically controlled study indicates that one need not have severe memory deficits to derive benefit from ginkgo. A replication of this study only found benefits on a free-recall measure (Warot et al. 1991). More studies are needed to establish the beneficial effects of ginkgo in young healthy subjects, perhaps using chronic dosing.

Cognitive effects: Conclusions A number of studies have shown cognitive benefits from ginkgo extracts. The majority of studies have been done in subjects with some form of dementia (Alzheimer's disease, vascular dementia, or age-related memory impairment), and primarily focus on memory, speed of information processing, and clinical and functional ratings. Meta-analyses indicate a modest but consistent benefit from ginkgo in methodologically-controlled studies. Cognitive improvement is not found in all measures administered, and results may depend on several methodological factors. One factor is the dosage used, where studies have used between 120 and 600 mg in a single dose. A second factor is the chronicity of the dosage. Although many studies show improvement with a single acute dose, greater benefit may be derived from chronic doses. Congruently, ginkgo has both immediate and chronic neuropharmacological effects. Another possible factor determining the cognitive benefits of ginkgo is the cognitive task employed. Benefits may be specific to certain cognitive operations while not affecting others.

Future studies should employ stringent methodology, as several have done, with ample descriptions of their methods to allow comparison with the existing body of literature. They also might use more standard neuropsychological measures. Some studies have exemplified this approach (Winther et al. 1998). These would allow for easier replication, generalization to clinical populations, and comparison to other cognitive-enhancing medications.

Toxicity

No serious side effects are reported by large clinical studies of ginkgo (Field and Vadnal 1998). Adverse effects resulting from improper dosage have also not been reported (Gruenwald et al. 1998). Mild gastrointestinal symptoms may occur or allergic skin reactions, albeit rarely. Other potential side effects are headaches, dizziness, and palpitations. However, some studies have reported adverse effects to be the same as that of placebo (Le Bars et al. 1997). Ginkgo appears well tolerated even in doses many times higher than usual recommended levels (Warburton 1986).

The most concerning side effect of ginkgo probably relates to its hematologic effects. Given that it potently inhibits platelet-activating factor, such side effects should be closely examined in those at risk for bleeding disorders. Four cases of bleeding have been reported in people taking ginkgo. A case of spontaneous bilateral subdural hematomas was reported, but the role of ginkgo was later disputed (Rowin and Lewis 1996; Odawara et al. 1997). A second case involving hyphema was reported in a person concurrently taking aspirin (325 mg/day) (Rosenblatt and Mindel 1997). A third case was reported of a 72-year-old man taking ginkgo extract. Finally, a fourth case developed parietal intracerebral hemorrhage with concurrent use of warfarin. Given the large number of people taking ginkgo and the small number of reported cases, it is not likely that ginkgo poses a major risk. However, the possibility of cases being underreported makes the magnitude of the problem unknown. Individuals with blood-clotting disorders or taking blood thinner medication should be monitored by medical professionals, or may avoid ginkgo altogether.

An injectable form of ginkgo extract was removed from the market due to adverse effects, and use of ginkgo seed kernels rather than leaves is more associated with toxicity.

Summary and Conclusions

The ginkgo tree has a long history of medicinal uses, which include cognitive actions. The chief active chemical constituents are flavonoid glycosides, biflavones, and terpene lactones, which have effects on cholinergic, monoamine, and amino acid neurotransmitters and adrenocortical hormones. Additionally, ginkgo has vasodilating effects through PAF and nitric oxide systems. Its effects on blood flow in the cavernosum probably account for reputed benefits in sexual performance. Benefits are seen in the vestibulocochlear system through increased peripheral blood flow, antioxidant effects, and perhaps central mechanisms. The neuroprotective effects of ginkgo are mediated by its antioxidant free radical-scavenging effects, and it may speed recovery from neurological injury.

Table 5.6
Species of ginseng

Colloquial name	Botanical name
Asian ginseng	*Panax ginseng*
American ginseng	*Panax quinquefolius*
Japanese ginseng	*Panax japonicus*
Vietnamese ginseng	*Panax vietnamensis*
"San qui"	*Panax notoginseng*
Non-Panax "ginseng" Species	
Siberian ginseng	*Eleutherococcus senticosus*
Brazilian ginseng	*Pfaffia paniculata*

See text for references.

Additional cognitive and neuroprotective effects may occur through attenuation of stress-induced release of glucocorticoids. Ginkgo increases cerebral blood flow, decreases glucose utilization, and produces activation effects in electrophysiological studies.

Improvements are seen in memory across animal and human studies of ginkgo. A meta-analysis of controlled studies showed modest but consistent beneficial effects in Alzheimer's disease. Further, the effects are comparable in size to the pharmaceutical drugs such as donepezil (Aricept). Given the common cholinergic mechanisms, concurrent use of ginkgo with cholinesterase inhibitors may be contraindicated until formally studied. Ginkgo may also have benefits in vascular dementia and normal aging. It has relatively low incidence of toxicity and side effects. Some cases of spontaneous bleeding have been reported, underscoring the need for caution when combining ginkgo with blood thinners such as aspirin or warfarin.

Ginseng

History and Botany

Ginseng is a plant with a long history of use across several cultures (Hobbs 1996). The name *ginseng* is used traditionally to refer to several related species of plants (table 5.6). To further confuse the picture, it is also used to refer to several other unrelated species with similar effects.

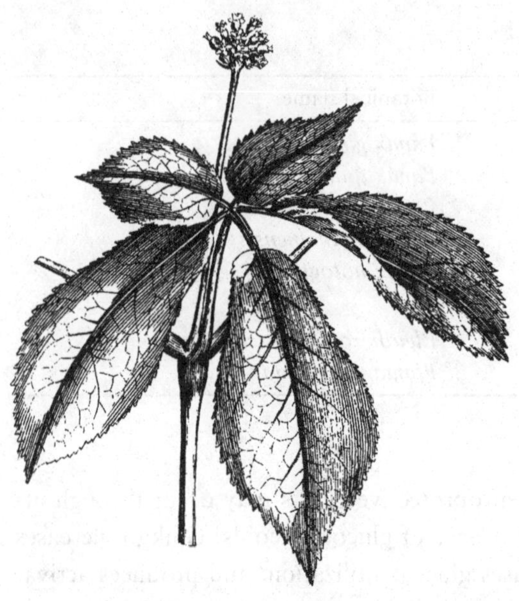

Figure 5.3
Asian ginseng *(Panax ginseng)*. Reprinted with permission from Hobbs, C. (1996). *Ginseng: The Energy Herb*. Loveland, CO: Botanica Press.

Most ginsengs belong to the genus *Panax* and the family Araliaceae. Chinese or Korean ginseng refers to *Panax ginseng* (figure 5.3). This is also referred to as "true ginseng" and the most studied form of ginseng in the scientific research literature. *Panax ginseng* is indigenous to China, but is also cultivated in Korea, Japan, and Russia (Gruenwald 1998). Unless otherwise specified, the word "ginseng" will be used to refer to *Panax ginseng* throughout this text. *Panax* is a Latin term derived from the Greek words *pan*, "all," and *akos*, "cure." As the name implies, it has been used in traditional herbal medicine to treat a wide variety of ailments. *Panax ginseng* may be either "white" or "red," depending on its preparation. White ginseng is the peeled and dried root, while red ginseng is steamed with the root intact, and then dried. This distinction has potential pharmacological implications because different chemicals are produced in the process.

American ginseng is the species *Panax quinquefolius* (figures 5.4 and 5.5) (Tyler 1994; Gruenwald et al. 1998). It grows in several parts of the

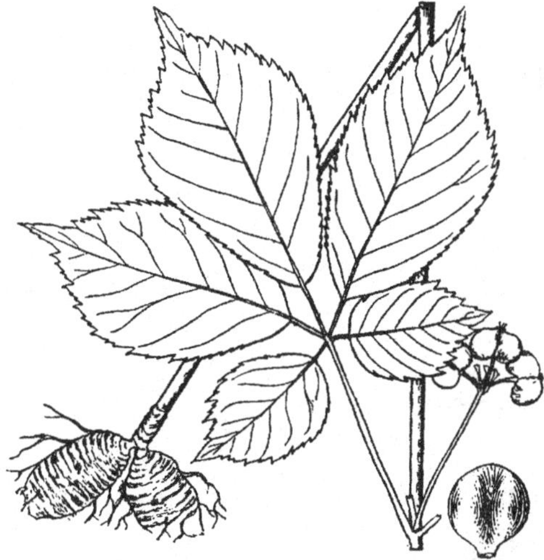

Figure 5.4
American ginseng *(Panax quinquefolius)*. Reprinted with permission from Hobbs, C. (1996). *Ginseng: The Energy Herb*. Loveland, CO: Botanica Press.

United States, but approximately 80% of it is produced commercially in Wisconsin (Kowalchik and Hylton 1987).

Japanese ginseng is *Panax japonicus*, and Vietnamese ginseng is *Panax vietnamensis*. Another variety of ginseng, also called *san qui*, is *Panax notoginseng*. Two non-Panax species are Siberian ginseng *(Eleutherococcus senticosus)* and Brazilian ginseng *(Pfaffia paniculata)*. To avoid confusion, many now simply refer to Siberian "ginseng" by its scientific name *eleuthero* (Tyler 1994).

Panax ginseng is a perennial plant, growing 30–80 cm high. It has a round stem and bears terminal whorls of 5–8 palmate leaves (Gruenwald et al. 1998). The flowers have greenish-yellow corollas and grow in 1–3 umbels of 15–30 flowers. The fruit are red, pea-sized, and round. The rhizome is fusiform and is the principal part for medicinal interest.

Ginseng is expensive to produce, requiring more than $20,000 to plant and harvest one acre (Kowalchik and Hylton 1987). Its seeds have a low rate of germination and grow slowly, and it is ideally harvested after 6 years of cultivation (Hobbs 1996). As a result, the price of ginseng is high. Pure American ginseng can sell for $400–600 per pound. Ginseng

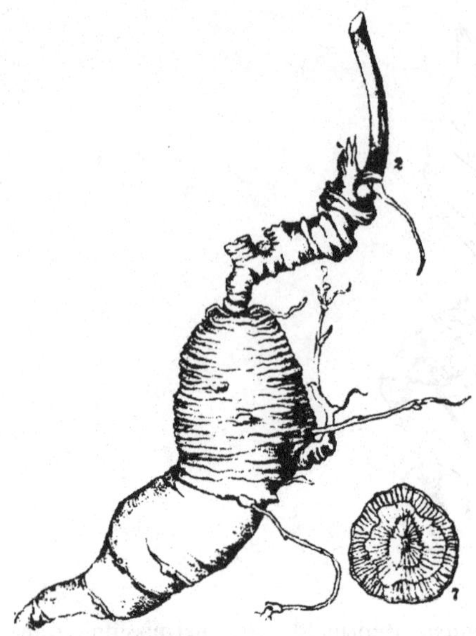

Figure 5.5
Root of American ginseng *(Panax quinquefolius)*. Reprinted with permission from Hobbs, C. (1996). *Ginseng: The Energy Herb*. Loveland, CO: Botanica Press.

sales in the United States amount to over $300 million annually (Gillis 1997). The United States is a major exporter of ginseng as well, and has exported it to Asia since the eighteenth century. Not surprisingly, ginseng is an endangered species in the United States. Ginseng has a longstanding reputation for numerous health benefits, seeming to treat any ailment one could name. Perhaps the effects are best summarized as adaptogenic and aphrodisiac, but cognitive effects were noted in ancient Chinese medical texts. The term *adaptogen* refers to an agent that increases ones biological and mental resistance to stress (Tyler 1994).

Chemical Constituents
Ginseng has a mix of chemical constituents that are classified as steroidal saponins (table 5.7) (Robbers et al. 1996; Attele et al. 1999). These are glycosides that have been categorized into ginsenosides, panaxosides, and chikusetsusaponins. The major pharmacologically active constituents

Table 5.7
Chemical constituents of ginseng

Saponins	Ginsenosides Malonylginsenosides
Polysaccharides	Panaxanes
Acetylenic compounds	Panaxynol Panaxydol Panaxtryol

of ginseng are the ginsenosides (Gillis et al. 1997; Robbers et al. 1996). Based on their chemical structure, the ginsenosides fall into two major subgroups: panaxadiols and panaxatriols (Attele et al. 1999) (figure 5.6). Ginsenoside nomenclature consists of a capital R followed by a lowercase letter or lowercase letter and number. Identified ginsenosides are: Ro, Ra1, Ra2, Ra3, Rb1, Rb2, Rb3, Rc, Rd, Re, Rf, Rg1, Rg2, Rg3, Rh1, Rh2, Rs1, and Rs2. Ginsenosides Rg2, Rg3, Rh1, and Rh2 are products of Rb1, Rb2, Rc, and Rd, formed when white ginseng is steamed to produce red ginseng (Hobbs 1996). Unlike the rest, however, ginsenoside Ro is nonsteroidal in structure. Three acidic malonylginsenosides are identified as mRb1, mRb2, and mRc. Ginseng species vary in their saponin content. *Panax ginseng* contains 1.5–4.4% saponins, *Panax quinquefolius* contains 4.3–4.9%, *Panax notoginseng* contains 8.2–20.6%, and *Panax japonica* contains approximately 9.34% (Huang 1998; Wang 1982).

Other chemical constituents include water-soluble polysaccharides, designated as panaxanes (Gruenwald et al. 1998). Acetylenic constituents include panaxynol, panaxydol, and panaxtryol (Matsunaga et al. 1995).

Mechanisms of Action

The several mechanisms of action of ginseng are summarized in table 5.8.

Acetylcholine Ginsenoside Rb1 facilitates acetylcholine release in the rat brain (Benishin 1992). This increase is not associated with increased Ca^{2+} uptake, but rather with increased uptake of choline into synaptic

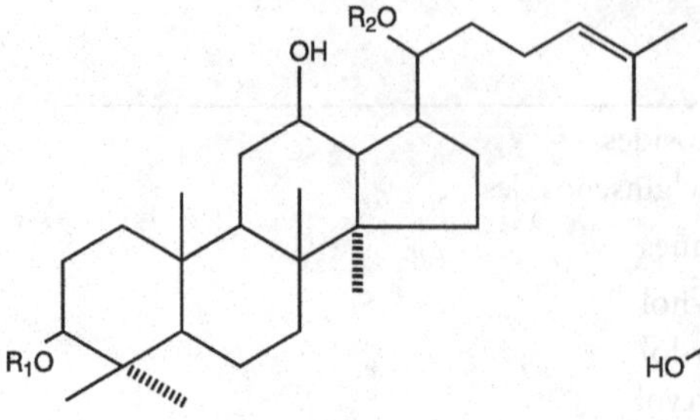

Panaxadiols

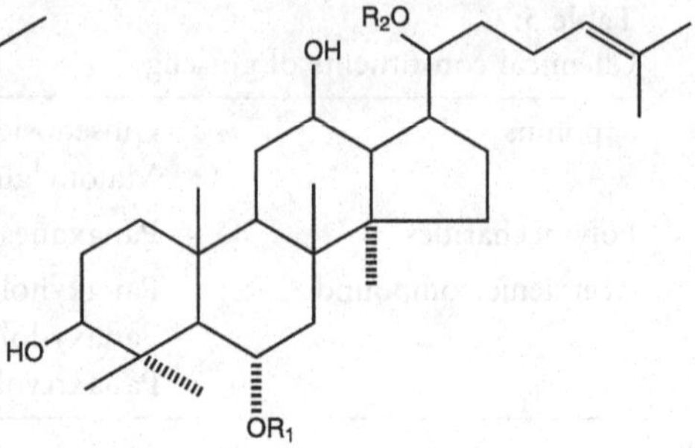

Ginsenoside	R_1	R_2
Rb$_1$	-glc(2-1)glc	-glc(6-1)glc
Rb$_2$	-glc(2-1)glc	-glc(6-1)arap
Rc	-glc(2-1)glc	-glc(2-1)araf
Rd	-glc(2-1)glc	-glc
Rg$_3$	-glc(2-1)glc	-H
Rh$_2$	-glc	H
Rh$_3$	-glc	

Panaxatriols

Ginsenoside	R_1	R_2
Re	-glc(2-1)rha	-glc
Rf	-glc(2-1)glc	-H
Rg$_1$	-glc	-glc
Rg$_2$	-glc(2-1)rha	H
Rh$_1$	-glc	-H

Figure 5.6
Chemical structure of ginsenosides.

terminals. Ginsenoside Rb1 increases velocity of choline uptake without altering the affinity of the choline uptake transporter. Acute treatment does not alter the number of uptake sites, but chronic (3 day) treatment did in the hippocampus and cortex. Ginsenosides have no effect on quinuclidinyl benzilate binding or on acetylcholinesterase activity, nor do they bind to muscarinic receptors (Benishin et al. 1991; Zhang et al. 1990). Ginsenoside Rb1 does increase the expression of mRNA for choline acetyltransferase and trkA in the basal forebrain (Salim et al. 1997). Functionally, ginsenoside Rb1 prevents memory deficits induced by the muscarinic antagonist scopolamine. Recently, it has been shown that extracts of *Panax ginseng* and *Panax quinquefolius* have affinity for nicotinic receptors, and to a lesser degree, muscarinic receptors. The responsible chemical was not identified, but it is not due to ginsenosides (Lewis et al. 1994).

Table 5.8
Mechanisms of action of ginseng

Cholinergic	Increased acetylcholine release	Ginsenoside Rb1
	ChAT expression	Ginsenoside Rb1
	Nicotinic binding	Non-ginsenoside (*PQ*)
Amino acid	$GABA_A$	Ginsenoside Rg2 (*PQ*)
	$GABA_A$ neurosteroid site	Majonoside-R2 (*PV*)
Monoamine	Complex effects on turnover	Ginsenosides Rb, Rg1
Nitric oxide	Enhanced epithelial synthesis	Ginsenosides
Neurotrophic	Increased NGF expression	Ginsenosides Rb1, Rg1 malonylginsenoside Rb1
Ca^{2+} flux	Inhibits Ca^{2+} channels	Ginsenosides Rc, Re, Rf, Rg1, & Rb1

See text for references.
Key: PQ *Panax quinquefolius*, PV *Panax vietnamensis.*

Amino acid neurotransmitters *Panax quinquefolius* extracts reduce the discharge rate of neurons in the medial nucleus solitarius with microgram doses and reversed by muscimol, indicating actions at $GABA_A$ receptors. There is no direct binding of ginsenosides Rb1 or Rg1 to GABA receptors (Zhang et al. 1991). In adrenal chromaffin cells, ginsenoside Rg2 putatively blocks GABA receptors (Tachikawa et al. 1999). Majonoside-R2, from Vietnamese ginseng, creates behavioral effects though the neurosteroid site on the $GABA_A$ receptor (Nguyen et al. 1997).

Monoamines Ginseng has complex effects on endogenous monoamines. After two weeks of treatment, turnover of dopamine and norepinephrine is increased in the cerebral cortex, and serotonin turnover is increased in the striatum and cerebellum (Itoh et al. 1989). However, dopamine turnover in the striatum is reduced, as is serotonin in the hypothalamus and midbrain. After seven weeks of treatment, on the other hand, serotonin turnover in the cerebellum is increased, but turnover of dopamine, norepinephrine, and serotonin is reduced in all other areas studied. Ginsenosides Rb1 and Rg1 decrease 5-HT levels or reduce 5-HT turnover (Zhang et al. 1991). There is no specific binding observed of Rg1 and Rb1 adrenergic (α_1, α_2, or β), dopamine, or 5-HT receptors.

In contrast, some studies have reported elevations in monoamines by chronic doses of ginseng through an unspecified mechanism (Wang et al. 1995). Ginseng prevents the heat stress-induced reduction in brain norepinephrine and serotonin (Yuan et al. 1998). Ginseng saponins also reverse κ-opioid analgesia through serotonergic mechanisms (Kim HS et al. 1992).

Chronic (5 day) oral ginseng extract alters striatal D_2 receptors in aged rats, but acute administration does not affect either D_1 or D_2 receptors (Watanabe et al. 1991).

Nitric oxide Ginsenosides enhance nitric oxide synthesis, with effects in the endothelium of the lungs, heart, and kidneys and in the corpus cavernosum (Kim H et al. 1992; Ko et al. 1996). This is a potential mechanism of ginseng-associated vasodilation. Effects on neuronal nitric oxide have not been specifically investigated.

Neurotrophic factors Some ginsenosides enhance neuronal survival in culture and interact with nerve growth factor. Ginsenoside Rb1 increases the expression of mRNA for nerve growth factor in the hippocampus (Salim et al. 1997). However, the brain-derived neurotrophic factor and neurotrophin-3 are not affected. In micromolar doses, malonylginsenoside Rb1 potentiates neurite growth induced by nerve growth factor in dorsal root ganglion cells (Nishiyama et al. 1994). Potentiation was also seen between ginsenoside Rg1 and nerve growth factor in cultured cortical neurons (Himi et al. 1989).

Neuropeptides Ginsenosides have no apparent effect on neuropeptide precursors (preproenkephalin, preprotachykinin) or amyloid protein precursor (Salim et al. 1997).

Ca^{2+} channels Ginseng extract rapidly and reversibly inhibits high-threshold, voltage-dependent Ca^{2+} channels in micromolar doses (Nah and McCleskey 1994; Nah et al. 1995). This effect is mediated by a receptor linked to a pertussis toxin-sensitive G protein, but it is not through α_2 adrenergic, $GABA_B$, muscarinic, or opioid receptors (Nah and McCleskey 1994). Several ginsenosides inhibit Ca^{2+} currents by 16 to

37%, depending on the ginsenoside (Kim HS et al. 1998). The order of potency for this effect is: Rc > Re > Rf > Rg1 > Rb1.

Pharmacokinetics
Ginsenosides are rapidly absorbed from the upper gastrointestinal tract, varying with different ginsenosides, doses, preparation, and stomach acidity (Odani et al. 1983). Between 2 and 30% of ginsenoside Rg1 is absorbed within 30–60 minutes, but little of ginsenoside Rb1 is absorbed. Above doses of 3–9 g, absorption is reduced (Han 1986). Peak blood concentrations are reached in 30 minutes, and tissue levels peak at 90 minutes. Differences between ginsenoside pharmacokinetics may be due to differences in protein binding (Chen et al. 1980). Tinctures and extracts allow for more rapid absorption than whole root. Ginsenosides are excreted in urine mostly unmetabolized (Huang 1998).

General Effects

Physiological There is an extensive literature that deals with the effects ginseng on CNS function, but effects are also seen in neuroendocrine function, carbohydrate and lipid metabolism, the immune system, and cardiovascular function (Gillis 1997). Ginsenosides induce a decrease in heart rate and have biphasic effects on blood pressure, with decreases preceded by a slight increase (Kaku et al. 1975). Ginsenoside Rg1 had the most potent effects on blood pressure. Little or no effect is observed on respiration.

Vascular and sexual effects Ginseng saponin has demonstrated vasoactive effects. It activates the release of NO from bovine aortic endothelium, and from the endothelial cells and perivascular nerve of the rabbit corpus cavernosum (Kim HS et al. 1998; Ko et al. 1996; Choi and Seong 1995; Chen and Lee 1995). Nitric oxide synthesis is also observed in the endothelium of the lung, heart, and kidney (Gillis 1997).

Ginseng's mechanism of vasorelaxation and nitric oxide release is probably by conversion of L-arginine to L-citrulline (Kim H et al. 1992). Ginseng saponin induces relaxation of the corpus cavernosum smooth muscle in a dose-dependent manner (Kim HJ et al. 1998). This effect is reduced by anticholinergic and nitiric oxide inhibitors, and restored by addition of L-arginine. These findings convergently suggest that ginseng facilitates penile erection via a nitric oxide pathway.

One study indicated beneficial effect of ginseng on sexual behavior in male rats, increasing the frequency of copulation in a 45 minute period, but also decreasing the latency to ejaculation (Kim et al. 1976). Another study found a decrease in sexual behavior in male rats acutely administered ginseng, but increases when it was chronically given (Murphy et al. 1998). In humans, ginseng was more effective than placebo and trazodone for treatment of erectile dysfunction (Choi and Seong 1995). Although objective measurement, placebo control, and randomization were employed in this study, there is no explicit mention of a double-blind element.

Neuroendocrine and stress effects Ginseng activates the hypothalamo-pituitary-adrenal axis. Combined ginsenosides elevate plasma ACTH and corticosterone up to 90 minutes after injection in rats, by actions in the hypothalamus and/or pituitary (Hiai et al. 1979). The ginsenosides Rg1 and Rb1 alone increase plasma levels of ACTH (Zhang et al. 1990). Ginsenoside Rg1 is a functional ligand at the glucocorticoid receptor (Lee YJ et al. 1997). It competes with dexamethasone and binds with low micromolar affinity. However, ginsenosides inhibit the stress-induced elevation of plasma corticosterone in mice (Kim DH et al. 1998). The effect is central, occuring in low microgram intracerebral doses, and is dependent on nitric oxide synthesis.

Plasma prolactin levels are reduced with acute treatment and remain suppressed after 28 days of chronic treatment (Murphy et al. 1998). With acute treatment, no effects are seen on plasma luteinizing hormone or testosterone levels. However, chronic dietary 5% ginseng increases testosterone levels in male rats (Fahim et al. 1982). Chronic ginsenosides do not alter posterior pituitary hormones oxytocin and vasopressin (Zierer 1991). Similarly, human males administered ginseng extract showed an increase in plasma testosterone, dihydrotestosterone, follicle-stimulating hormone, and luteinizing hormone, but a decrease in prolactin (Salvati et al. 1996).

Neurophysiological and neuroprotective effects Two ginsenosides have been found to affect long-term potentiation (Abe et al. 1994). While ginsenoside Rb1 attenuates it in the hippocampus, malonylginsenoside Rb1 facilitates it. This effect of malonylginsenoside Rb1 is dose dependent, facilitating it in the low nanomolar range (5 nM), but not at higher nanomolar doses (50 nM).

Decreased c-fos mRNA and fos protein are observed in the hippocampus during aging, and ginsenoside Rg1 increases the expression of c-fos mRNA and protein in both young and aged rats (Liu and Zhang 1996). Also increased are levels of cAMP in the hippocampus. The expression of c-fos serves as a marker for neuronal activity and is likely to be involved in neuronal plasticity. Thus, ginsenoside Rg1 may improve cognitive function by altering c-fos and cAMP in cerebral structures.

Ginseng may have neuroprotective effects. An ischemia paradigm in gerbils showed that ginseng improves response latency in a step-down passive-avoidance task (Wen et al. 1996). Loss of pyramidal neurons in the hippocampal CA1 region is prevented in a dose-dependent manner. While ginsenoside Rb1 was effective, Rg1 and Ro were ineffective. Central administration of ginsenoside Rb1 after cerebral ischemia protects hippocampal neurons. The likely mechanism of this effect is antioxidant scavenging of free radicals (Lim et al. 1997). Oral red ginseng powder reduces the learning impairment produced by ischemia in a passive-avoidance test, and preserves hippocampal neurons and synapses (Wen et al. 1996). Ginsenosides have a similar neuroprotective effect. Nonginsenoside constituents are also effective, but less potent in this regard.

Behavioral and emotional effects In animal studies, ginseng does not prolong pentobarbital-induced sleep, nor does it affect spontaneous locomotion (Mitra et al. 1996). It does potentiate amphetamine-induced locomotion, but it reduces the stereotypy and lethality caused by amphetamine. Ginseng has analgesic effects, which are discussed at greater length in chapter 8. Catalepsy induced by haloperidol is potentiated by ginseng, while the hyperthermic effect of 5-HTP is attenuated. No antiseizure effects have been observed.

Although a single dose of ginseng has little acute effects, chronic dosing (twice daily, 5 days) reduces anxiety in behavioral models (open-field and elevated plus-maze) (Bhattacharya and Mitra 1991). Also reduced by ginseng are aggressive behavior in water-deprived rats and foot-shock-induced fighting in mice.

Majonoside-R2, a saponin found in Vietnamese ginseng restores the deficit in pentobarbital sleep caused by the stress of social isolation (Nguyen et al. 1997). This effect appears to be mediated by the neurosteroid receptor on the $GABA_A$ receptor.

The effects of ginseng on motor activity are highly variable. An oral dose of 1.8% ginseng extract decreases spontaneous activity in young rats, but increases it in aged rats (Watanabe et al. 1991). The increase in activity in aged rats corresponds with reduced striatal D_2 receptors. Thus, results vary across ginsenosides, the age of subjects, and chronicity of administration.

The effects of two ginsenosides on ingestive behavior have been investigated in animal paradigms. Ginsenoside Rg1 reverses the supression of water intake by interleukin-1 β when administered intracerebroventricularly (Kang et al. 1995). However, this effect was observed at the millimolar range, and no effects on feeding were observed. Rg1 did reverse anorexia induced by heat and surgical implantation, again only at millimolar doses (8 mM). On the other hand, low micromolar doses (0.01 μM) of ginsenoside Rb1 decreases food intake when injected into the ventromedial hypothalamus (Etou et al. 1988). Drinking behavior is also decreased with doses in the low micromolar range (0.2 μM). No effects were observed in the lateral hypothalamus. Ginseng extract stabilized fluctuations in wakefulness and slow-wave sleep in food-deprived rats (Lee et al. 1990).

Ginseng extract has reported anti-aggresive effects in animals, although results vary depending on administration and which ginsenoside is used (Mitra et al. 1996). Ginsenoside Rb1 and Rg1 suppress resident aggression in a resident-intruder paradigm using mice (Yoshimura et al. 1988a). In the same paradigm, Rb1, but not Rg1, suppresses aggression in the intruder. In a maternal aggression paradigm, crude ginseng saponins and Rb1 suppress aggression when administered acutely, but Rg1 is ineffective. During chronic administration, crude ginseng saponins again reduce maternal aggression, while Rg1 facilitates it (Yoshimura et al. 1988b). Slightly different results are found in mice, where

Rg1, Rf, and Rd suppress foot-shock-induced aggression, but Rb1 and Rb2 have little effect (Kaku et al. 1975). Aggression is also reduced by ginseng between water-deprived rats and in foot-shock-induced conflict in mice (Bhattacharya and Mitra 1991).

Cognitive effects: Animal studies There is an extensive literature that deals with the effects of ginseng on memory, learning, and behavior (Gillis 1997; Wang et al. 1995). However, ginseng extract (G115) failed to show anxiolytic effects in an animal model (Petkov et al. 1987)

Ginseng extract improves the spatial learning performance of aged rats in an eight-arm radial maze and operant discrimination task (Nitta et al. 1995). It also improves memory performance in active-avoidance (shuttle-box) and passive-avoidance (step-down) tasks, and reinforces staircase-maze learning in both young and aged rats. (Petkov and Mosharrof 1987; Petkov et al. 1990; Petkov et al. 1992). The effects were also very dose dependent, with inverted U-shape dose-response curves.

The effects of ginsenoside Rg2 on learning and memory in rats were evaluated using a two-way active-avoidance method. Memory impairments induced by scopolamine and cycloheximide are reversed by ginsenoside Rg2 (Ma et al. 1991; Ma and Yu 1993). Ginseng extract (G115) reduces the memory impairment produced by electroshock treatment on a passive-avoidance (step-down) task (Lasarova et al. 1987). Adult rats given lesions of medial prefrontal cortex show cognitive deficits in a position-reversal task, which is improved by chronic (30-day) treatment with ginseng.

Several studies have looked at the effects of combined preparations that include ginseng. A preparation of *Biota orientalis*, *Panax ginseng*, and *Schisandra chinensis* (S-113 m) improved memory retention in a passive-avoidance task with senescence-accelerated mice (Nishiyama et al. 1996). This combination also reduced memory impairments induced by ethanol and scopolamine in the step-down test and electroconvulsive shock-induced memory impairment (Nishiyama et al. 1995). Gincosan is a combination of extracts from *Panax ginseng* (G115) and *Ginkgo biloba* (GK501) (Petkov et al. 1993). Chronic oral pretreatment with

Gincosan improved learning in some animal models. Effects between ginseng and ginkgo were comparable, and effective in combination.

While promising, the use of multiple herbs in studies makes their results of limited generalizability. However, studies such as the one by Petkov and colleagues (1993), which examine both the individual and combined effects, have conscientiously avoided this methodological problem.

Cognitive effects: Human studies Few studies of the effects of ginseng on cognitive function have been performed on humans. One controlled study assessed the effect of chronic (12 week) administration of a ginseng preparation (G115) on cognitive function in healthy volunteers (D'Angelo et al. 1986). Several functions were measured: visual attention (with a cancellation task), auditory reaction time, processing speed (choice reaction time, digit symbol substitution), fine motor speed (tapping test), mental arithmetic, and logical deduction. However, significant improvements were only seen in the mental arithmetic test.

A controlled study of chronic (8 week) ginseng and multivitamin complex in elderly adults showed no apparent benefits on tests of attention or memory, as measured by the Trail Making Test and Kendrick Object Learning Test. No differences were seen in the length of hospital stay, objective measures of emotional and somatic symptoms, or activities of daily living. Although this study produced negative results, a greater variety of cognitive measures with more sensitivity could have been used. In contrast, another study of ginseng extract (G115) in adults showed improvement in all 11 items of a standardized quality of life index (Caso Marasco et al. 1996).

Toxicity

Ginsenosides show low toxicity in pharmacological studies (Chen et al. 1980). A "ginseng abuse syndrome" was reported as consisting of hypertension, irritability, nervousness, and sleeplessness (Siegel 1979). However, the types of ginseng that produced this syndrome are unknown. The people in this study were also taking enormously high doses, such as 15 g per day, whereas conventional doses are 1 to 2 g per day (Gruenwald et al. 1998). Conventional doses of ginseng are not usually associated with serious adverse effects (Tyler 1994; Gruenwald et al. 1998).

Summary and Conclusions

Ginseng has an ancient reputation for treating several illnesses, including memory loss. A variety of species are colloquially labeled as "ginseng," requiring attention to the exact species used for experimental trials and clinical preparations. Several members of the *Panax* genus are appropriately labeled ginseng, and have similar chemical and neuropharmacological effects. The chief chemical constituents are the ginsenosides, which have actions on cholinergic, GABA, monoamine, and neurotrophic systems. Additionally, ginseng blocks Ca^{2+} channels and is a vasodilator through nitric oxide mechanisms.

Vasodilating effects probably enhance cerebral blood flow and increase sexual performance, although elevations in dopamine and testosterone function may also contribute. Other neuroendocrine effects include elevation of plasma ACTH and supression of prolactin. Ginseng has neuroprotective effects that likely relate to its antioxidant properties. Effects are seen on analgesia, anxiety, motor activity, ingestive behavior, and aggression. Benefits in memory and learning are seen in several animal studies. However, most of the empirical research in ginseng has been done on animals. There are some preliminary results with humans, but much more is needed to establish its effects. In reasonable doses, ginseng has shown little toxicity.

Ergot Derivatives: Hydergine

History and Botany

Ergot alkaloids (or ergoloids) are derived from the ergot fungus *Claviceps purpurea* (van Dongen and de Groot 1995). As a toxic fungus that grows on rye and other grains, it has gained infamy throughout the history of civilization. Ergot is discussed at length in chapter 9 because of its potent hallucinogenic chemical lysergic acid diethylamide (LSD). However, its other nonhallucinogenic constituents have been tried in clinical trials to treat dementia conditions, peripheral vascular disease, hypertension, angina pectoris, and tinnitus. Currently, the primary proposed use for

Table 5.9
Natural and semisynthetic ergot alkaloids (ergoloids)

Amine alkaloids and Congeners	d-Lysergic acid
	d-Isolysergic acid
	d-Lysergic acid diethylamide
	Ergonovine (ergometrine)
	Methylergonovine
	Methysergide
	Lisuride
	Lisurol
	Lergotrile
	Metergoline
Amino acid alkaloids	Ergomatine
	Ergotine
	Ergostine
	Ergotoxine:
	Ergocristine
	Ergocornine
	α-Ergokryptine
	β-Ergokryptine
	Bromocriptine

Source: Adapted from Peroutka 1996.

Hydergine is for treatment of dementia. It has been approved by the Food and Drug administration for treatment of "idiopathic decline in mental capacity."

Chemical Constituents
Two general classes of alkaloids are distinguished in ergot: amine alkaloids and amino acid alkaloids (table 5.9) (Peroutka 1996). While the amine alkaloids are selective for antagonist effects on serotonin receptors, the amino acid alkaloids are less selective and act upon other monoamine receptors. The constituents of interest for cognitive enhancement are predominantly the amine alkaloids.

The chemical constituents of interest for cognitive effects are the ergotoxine derivatives, otherwise referred to as *ergoloid mesylates* (Schneider and Olin 1994). Ergotoxine was isolated in 1906, but later discovered to be a mix of four alkaloids: ergocristine, ergocornine, α-ergokryptine,

Table 5.10
Mechanisms of action of Hydergine

Cholinergic	Site-specific alteration of acetylcholine levels
	Reverses age-related decline in choline acetyltransferase
	Reverses an age-related decline in muscarinic receptors
	Stimulates learning-related cholinergic activity
Monoamine	Facilitates release of norepinephrine (through α_2)
	Agonist/antagonist effects on serotonin receptors
	Time-dependent increases/decreases on dopamine and norepinephrine
	Age-dependent effects on MAO
	Increased firing of locus coeruleus neurons

See text for references.

and β-ergokryptine. Co-dergocrine (referred to here by the trade name, Hydergine) was introduced clinically in 1949, and is a combination of four dihydro derivatives of ergotoxine (Peroutka 1996).

Mechanisms of Action

Hydergine's mechanisms of action are summarized in table 5.10.

Acetylcholine A few studies have shown Hydergine to augment central cholinergic transmission. In vivo microdialysis shows that Hydergine decreases concentrations of acetylcholine in the striatum, while dose-dependently increasing it in the hippocampus (Imperato et al. 1994). Treatment with Hydergine reverses age-related decline in choline acetyltransferase activity in the hippocampus and striatum (Dravid 1983). It also reverses an age-related decline in the number of muscarinic receptors in rats (Amenta et al. 1989). Greatest change in muscarinic receptors is seen in CA1 and CA2 of the hippocampus, and in the dentate gyrus to a lesser degree. Hydergine stimulates learning-related increases in central cholinergic activity in rats (Le Poncin-Lafitte et al. 1985).

Monoamines Hydergine has effects on the monoamines dopamine, norepinephrine, and serotonin. It facilitates electrically-evoked norepinephrine release though antagonism of α_1 and presynaptic α_2 adrenergic receptors (Markstein 1985). Mixed agonist/antagonist effects are seen at postsynaptic D_1 receptors, and at pre- and postsynaptic D_2 receptors. Mixed agonist/antagonist effects are also seen at serotonin receptors in the hippocampus and cortex. Collectively, these results indicate a dual effect of Hydergine on monoamine receptors, possibly compensating for deficits in transmitter function and reversing overactivity.

Hydergine shows time-dependent effects on monoamines in various brain regions. Dopamine and norepinephrine levels in the midbrain and diencephalon increase at 90 minutes and then sharply decrease up to 120 minutes (Copeland et al. 1981). A similar pattern is seen with norepinephrine in the pons and medulla, and with dopamine in the caudate nucleus. Hydergine alters MAO activity to varying degrees with age: increases in MAO are greater in the hypothalamus and cerebellum of aged rats, while increases are more pronounced in the hippocampus of adult rats (Büyüköztürk et al. 1995).

Systemic administration of Hydergine significantly increases the firing rate of noradrenergic neurons in the locus coeruleus in rats (Olpe and Steinmann 1982). At a dose of 1 mg/kg, a mean increase in firing rate of 70% is observed. Given the role of the locus coeruleus and norepinephrine in cognition, this could account in part for Hydergine's effects (Aston-Jones et al. 1994).

Pharmacokinetics

After intravenous administration, dihydroergotoxine alkaloids show maximal uptake in visceral organs (10^{-5} M) and the central nervous system (10^{-7} M), and concentrations increase with repeated administration (Iwangoff et al. 1978). Maximal plasma concentrations of ergoloids occur approximately 2 hours after oral administration (Aellig and Nuesch 1977). Elimination half-life varies from 1.4 to 6.2 hours for the alpha phase and from 13 to 50 hours for the beta phase.

General Effects

Neuroprotective effects Hydergine may have some neuroprotective effects. It protects neurons in hippocampal CA1 following ischemia (Izumiyama et al. 1988). Hydergine also increases the activity of the antioxidant enzymes superoxide dismutase and catalase, most prominently in the hippocampus and striatum (Sözmen et al. 1998).

Cognitive effects: Animal studies A few studies have been done on the cognitive effects of Hydergine in animal models. Hydergine elicits increases in spontaneous motor activity and self-stimulation of the ventral tegmental area, peaking at 80–120 minutes (Copeland et al. 1981). In mice, systemic and central doses of hydergine improve recall and retrieval memory in a T-maze and step-through apparatus, with an inverted-U dose-response curve (Flood et al. 1985). No benefits were seen in the acquistion phase of active-avoidance tasks. Memory is improved in rats learning maze navigation, but paradoxically none of the components of Hydergine individually had a similar effect (Jaton and Vigouret 1985). Hydergine reverses the amnestic effects of the muscarinic antagonist scopolamine and a protein synthesis inhibitor. Although effective against scopolamine-induced memory deficits, Hydergine is ineffective against hypoxic memory disturbance in rats (DeNoble et al. 1986). Higher doses (10 mg/kg PO) impaired motor function.

Cognitive effects: Human studies A meta-analysis was performed of methodologically controlled trials of Hydergine in treatment of dementia (Schneider and Olin 1994). The studies examined had both inpatient and outpatient subject pools, with a mean age of subjects varying from 59 to 84 across studies. The mean treatment duration was of 17.1 weeks, and the mean dose of Hydergine per subject was 4.5 mg per day. Several studies examined effects in populations with Alzheimer's disease or vascular dementia. Outcome measures used included clinical global rating scales or neuropsychological measures (among them were subtests of Wechsler Adult Intelligence Scale, the Trail Making Test, and measures of orientation). Overall, studies showed a modest but consistent effect of Hydergine in the areas assessed. The effect size varied with the type of measure used: 0.47 for comprehensive ratings, 0.56 for clinical global ratings, and 0.27 for combined neuropsychological measures. Analysis of just the studies of Alzheimer's disease subjects found an effect only in combined neuropsychological testing (0.30). Despite the modest size of the effect, it is generally consistent with the effects obtained with other antidementia drugs (e.g., Aricept, ranging from 0.42 to 0.48) (Rogers et al. 1998).

Toxicity

Hydergine has been approved by the U.S. Food and Drug Administration as a treatment for cognitive decline. No serious side effects are reported. Those reported include transient nausea and other gastrointestinal effects. Hydergine does not have the vasoconstrictive effects of other ergoloids. Hydergine may be contraindicated in people suffering from chronic psychoses. Depending on the dosage, overdoses of Hydergine can produce mild symptoms such as nasal stuffiness, flushing of the face, and headache, or more serious effects such as nausea, vomiting, tremulousness, spasticity, hypotension, circulatory collapse, and coma.

Summary and Conclusions

Hydergine is composed of four ergot alkaloids derived from the fungus *Claviceps purpurea*. Other constituents have vasoconstrictive or hallucinogenic effects, but Hydergine is now considered primarily as treatment for cognitive decline. Its mechanism of action appears to be through cholinergic and/or monoamine mechanisms, and there is also evidence for antioxidant effects. Cognitive effects are seen in several animal models looking at memory. Human studies show Hydergine to provide a modest but consistent benefit. Despite this, Hydergine seems to have fallen out of favor for treatment of dementia. Perhaps this is due to the promise of more recent cholinesterase inhibitors.

Tobacco

Although tobacco *(Nicotiana tabacum)* is widely known for its stimulant and addictive properties, its principal psychoactive constituent, nicotine, has become a candidate drug for improving cognition (Le Houezec 1998; Lawrence and Sahakian 1998; Newhouse et al. 1997). Clearly, the health risks associated with smoking tobacco preclude its clinical use, but nicotine delivered in other forms may be useful.

Nicotine is the principal psychoactive alkaloid from tobacco and has effects on cognition in animal and human studies. This is not surprising given its direct effects on central cholinergic systems, and indirect effects on many other neurochemical systems. When considering research on the cognitive effects of nicotine, one must not only take into account the species (e.g., human, nonhuman), but also the degree of exposure and tolerance in research subjects. Chronic administration of nicotine induces neurochemical and functional compensatory mechanisms that alter the neural milieu. Thus, chronic tobacco smokers and nicotine-naive subjects are not equivalent, physiologically or on cognitive measures. The differences found between them are informative of effects of nicotine withdrawal.

Mechanisms of Cognitive Enhancement

Nicotine acts as an agonist at the nicotinic cholinergic receptor (Cooper et al. 1996). It binds to a subunit of the nicotinic receptor, creating a conformational change in the receptor and allowing influx of cations. Cholinergic receptors are widespread in the forebrain, rich in many anatomical areas thought to underlie cognition. The prefrontal cortex is a major site for the cognitive effects of nicotine (Vidal 1996). Cognitive effects may result from immediate receptor activation and/or chronic effects. For example, the cognitive effects of nicotine result, in part, from nicotinic receptor up-regulation after chronic treatment (Abdulla et al. 1996). It increases the number of nicotinic receptors in frontal, entorhinal, and dorsal hippocampal regions. Chronic nicotine also increases the sensitivity of muscarinic receptors (Wang et al. 1996). Nicotine interacts with other neurochemical systems, including dopamine, norepinephrine, serotonin, and glutamate (Levin and Simon 1998). Nicotine's cognitive effects may be due in part to monoamine mechanisms. Depletion of monoamines reduces the cognitive benefit of nicotine (Riekkinen et al. 1996). See chapter 4 for a more detailed description of nicotine's neuropharmacological mechanisms.

Cognitive effects: Animals Cognitive effects of nicotine have been observed in several species, including humans. Experimental studies have focused primarily on the effects on attention and memory. Cognitive benefits are seen after both acute and chronic administration (Levin et al. 1992). In experimental animals, nicotine improves learning and memory on a variety of tasks. Conversely, the nicotinic antagonist mecamylamine impairs memory. Nicotine facilitates memory in a passive-avoidance task in mice with accelerated senescence; aged rats administered nicotine have a better rate of learning in an active-avoidance pole-jumping test (Arendash et al. 1995a; Meguro et al. 1994). Errors are also reduced in maze tests (Lashley III, 17-arm radial maze), affecting reference but not working memory. In the Morris water maze, chronic (3 day) nicotine improves the learning acquisition of aged rats and the memory retention of young adult rats (Socci et al. 1995). Nicotine also augments choice accuracy in the radial-arm maze (Levin and Rose 1991).

Memory impairments produced by choline deprivation in rats are improved by nicotine (Sasaki et al. 1991). It reduces memory deficits due to septohippocampal lesions or aged animals (Levin 1992). Nicotine's effect on memory not only appears after acute administration, but may persist for at least 4 weeks after the end of chronic administration (Levin et al. 1992).

Nicotine increases sensory gating, as measured in an acoustic startle paradigm, although results have varied with subject strain (Acri et al. 1994; Faraday et al. 1998). Also improved is sustained attention in rats, depending on task parameters (Mirza and Stolerman 1998). In choice reaction-time paradigms there is improved accuracy and decreased omission errors under weak signal and low event-rate conditions. No benefits are seen under high event-rate conditions. Improvements are also seen in reaction time.

Working-memory enhancement by nicotine is seen using delayed matching-to-sample tasks in monkeys (Terry et al. 1993). This benefit is reversed by scopolamine, suggesting that nicotine's beneficial effect is due to increased central acetylcholine release and subsequent actions at muscarinic receptors. Nicotine appears to shift female rats toward a male-typical navigational strategy, using spatial cues rather than landmarks (Kanit et al. 1998).

Other nicotinic agonists show similar cognitive benefits. GTS-21 is as effective as nicotine in aged rats for improving memory performance in a one-way active-avoidance task, Lashley III maze, and 17-arm radial maze testing (Arendash et al. 1995b). ABT-418 is a recently developed drug that activates nicotinic channels (Buccafusco et al. 1995; Anderson et al. 1995). Peripheral doses (2–30 nM/kg) improve performance in a delayed matching-to-sample task in macaques. Over an 8 day period, no tolerance is seen in this mnestic effect, and similar cognitive benefits have been observed in rats. ABT-418 may represent a more attractive alternative to nicotine because it shares many of its beneficial effects, but not dose-limiting side effects.

Cognitive effects: Human nonsmokers Administration of nicotine to tobacco nonusers produces small cognitive enhancements. Studies in tobacco nonusers have primarily measured attention, information processing speed, and memory. Nicotine improves perceptual speed, choice reaction time, and digit recall (Stough et al. 1995; Le Houezec et al. 1994; Foulds et al. 1996). Improvements also occur in digit symbol substitution and continuous performance tests without reducing accuracy (Petrie and Deary 1989; Levin et al. 1998).

A stimulus-filter model of nicotine reinforcement has been proposed that suggests that it helps screen irrelevant stimuli from awareness (Kassel 1997). An alternative explanation asserts that nicotine induces attentional narrowing and facilitates perceptual processing. Human nonsmokers given an acute dose of nicotine (adminstered in gum) showed dose-related trends toward decreased accuracy and increased response time (Heishman et al. 1993).

Cognitive effects: Smokers and abstinence Nicotine abstinence in chronic tobacco users creates a mild cognitive impairment (Snyder et al. 1989). Abstinent cigarette smokers performed comparably to nonsmokers on cognitive tasks when administered nicotine, but the abstinent smokers had poorer performances before the nicotine was given (Foulds et al. 1996). Abstinent smokers show mental slowing on complex cognitive tasks that is beyond any reduction in simple reaction time or motor performance (Shiffman et al. 1995). Smoking cessation causes a reduction in digit recall and serial addition/subtraction (Sommese and Patterson 1995). A decrease in performance on the trail-making test B is seen as soon as 4 hours after tobacco discontinuation (Hatsukami et al. 1989). At 24 hours after cessation, changes occur in increased reaction time and decreased accuracy on a vigilance task.

Reinstatement of nicotine reverses the cognitive deficits produced by withdrawal. Tobacco smoking after short-term (overnight) abstinence improves processing speed in smokers on the Stroop color and color-word tasks (Pomerlau et al. 1994). Speed is reduced in a modified Stroop task using smoking-related words as compared to neutral words, suggesting that abstinence produces a content-specific shift in attentional focus (Gross et al. 1993). Improvements are seen in complex visual-reasoning tasks as well (Raven's advanced progressive matrices) after tobacco reinstatement (Stough et al. 1994). Improved driving skills such as brake reaction times and tracking accuracy are evident when smokers receive nicotine (Sherwood 1995). Withdrawal deficits are also reversed by replacement with nicotine gum (Snyder and Henningfield 1989). On measures of choice reaction time, memory scanning, tracking, and flicker fusion threshold, smokers showed increased improvement with nicotine gum after smoking (Hindmarch et al. 1990).

The cognitive and behavioral changes brought on by tobacco abstinence are worsened by quitting both caffeine and tobacco simultaneously. Combined cigarette and coffee abstinence in regular users reduces performance on serial arithmetic and digit recall tasks, and decreases reports of feeling clear headed and quick witted (Cohen et al. 1994). Conversely, reports of feeling irritability, muscular tension, headache, and drowsiness, are increased.

Cognitive effects: Dementia Nicotine has been considered as a therapeutic agent for indivduals with Alzheimer's disease (Warburton 1992). People with Alzheimer's disease show modest cognitive improvements when given nicotine (Sunderland et al. 1988). Cognitive effects are seen in doses lower than those required in normal controls, suggesting increased sensitivity to cholinergic agents in Alzheimer's disease. Learning improvements persist for a period of time after the drug is stopped (Wilson et al. 1995). However, behavior and global cognitive function are not markedly improved. Chronic transdermal nicotine improves attention in Alzheimer's patients, as assessed by a continuous performance test (White and Levin 1999). However, another study of transdermal nicotine did not show improvement over a 4-week period (Snaedel et al. 1996).

Summary and Conclusions

Nicotine, the principal psychoactive alkaloid in tobacco, has cognitive-enhancing effects. It directly activates nicotinic acetylcholine receptors in brain areas critical for cognition, creating both acute and chronic effects.

Nicotine also indirectly interacts with a number of other neurotransmitter systems including monoamines and excitatory amino acids. Cognitive benefits are seen in attention and memory across many animal and human experiments, partially depending on the test methodology used. Modest effects are produced in nonsmokers administered nicotine, and larger effects are seen in abstinent smokers. A limited number of studies have been performed in Alzheimer's disease. Again, effects have been modest, but further research is warranted. It is not certain what the long-term benefits of nicotine or nicotinic drugs will be to Alzheimer's disease or other dementias, whether the improvements sustain or whether it will result in daily functional changes.

The harmful effects of smoking and chewing tobacco (e.g., cancer, emphysema) make it an impractical form of drug delivery, but other delivery systems such as gum and transdermal patches may circumvent this problem. Alternatively, other nicotinic drugs are under development, such as ABT-418, which may create the desired clinical effects and minimize side effects.

Areca

Areca *(Areca catechu)* is a tall palm tree that yields a nut, commonly chewed in Asia for its stimulant effects. It is discussed at greater length in chapter 4, but is mentioned here briefly for its cognitive effects. Areca's psychoactive constituents (arecoline, arecaidine, guvacoline, and guvacine) are agonists at muscarinic acetylcholine receptors. They also directly inhibit reuptake of GABA.

In addition to autonomic effects, areca produces mental stimulation, increases cerebral blood flow and glucose metabolism, and creates electrophysiological activation as seen on the EEG.

Cognitive Effects

Studies on the cognitive effects of areca are scarce, but its known cholinergic mechansims have led some researchers to formally investigate the effects. Arecoline improves memory on a staircase test in rats, but effects were dose dependent (Molinengo et al. 1995). A low dose (0.5 mg/kg) improves performance, but a large dose (3.5–8 mg/kg) causes impairment. However, the beneficial effect diminished with tolerance. The memory effects of a single administration are also time dependent, where improvements occur at 3 and 24 hours, but no effect was seen at 168 hours (Flood et al. 1988). Some studies have found a time lag for the onset of cognitive benefits, suggesting that receptor regulation is partly responsible for the effects (Mondadori et al. 1994). Arecoline and other cholinergic agonists reverse memory and working-memory deficits induced by scopolamine (Hironaka and Ando 1996; Quartermain and Leo 1988). However, arecoline does not reverse scopolamine-induced deficits in mice learning a maze, and may actually potentiate the deficit (Bratt et al. 1996). Arecoline also partially offsets cognitive deficits induced by chronic ethanol intake (Arendt 1994). A synergistic effect occurs between tacrine and arecoline, independent of route of administration (Flood and Cherkin 1988).

A few formal studies have been done on cognitive effects of areca chewing in humans (Chu 1994). Although no differences are seen on simple reaction time, areca facilitates choice reaction time. It is interesting to note that some improvement is produced by the chewing movements themselves (i.e., chewing gum), but higher significance is found with areca, indicating effects of cholinergic mechanisms. No effects are seen in early-stage visual processing, as measured by the critical flicker fusion test (Frewer 1990). A limited study of betel quid showed an increase in reaction time latency. Whether this is an experimental effect or interactive effect of other chemical constituents (e.g., *Piper betle* and/or calcium hydroxide) was not discerned. Human studies have also shown arecoline to reverse scopolamine-induced deficits in serial learning tasks (Sitaram et al. 1978).

Given its cholinergic activity, some have suggested arecoline as a treatment for Alzheimer's disease, although the benefits have not been investigated nearly as much as other cholinergic agents (Asthana et al. 1996). People with Alzheimer's disease show improvement in verbal ability at low doses, but improvements in attention and visuospatial ability at higher doses (Raffaele et al. 1996). Significant improvements occur in verbal memory, with the average number of words recalled nearly doubling (11.8–20.1 words) at a dose of 4 mg/day. However, two of the eight subjects in one study did not respond to the drug.

However, another controlled study in Alzheimer's disease patients found only marginal improvements in picture recognition and ratings of word-finding ability (Tariot et al. 1988). No benefits were seen in semantic or episodic memory. Biphasic effects were found on psychomotor activation, with improvements at lower doses and impairments at higher doses.

Solanaceae

The fruit of a number of solanaceous plants, including tomato *(Lycopersicon esculentum)*, potato *(Solanum tuberosum)* and eggplant *(Solanum melongena esculentum)*, have cholinesterase-inhibiting effects (Krasowski et al. 1997). They contain solanaceous glycoalkaloids α-solanine and α-chaconine, which are triglycosides of solanidine, a steroidal alkaloid derived from cholesterol. They are the only plant chemicals known to inhibit both acetlycholinesterase and butyrylcholinesterase, both in vitro and in vivo.

Levels of solanaceous glycoalkaloids can be significant, occasionally causing toxicity in humans and livestock. Symptoms of potato poisoning include gastrointestinal disturbances, apathy, drowsiness, mental confusion, visual disturbances, dizziness, hallucinations, and trembling. Symptoms may perist 2–24 hours after consumption, and one recent outbreak showed reduced butyrylcholinesterase levels six days later, which then returned to normal in 4 to 5 weeks.

Apart from rare toxic-level exposures to solanaceous glycoalkaloids, there is evidence that normal dietary consumption still contains physiologically significant levels. An indivudual consuming a normal portion of potatoes can ingest 20 to 60 mg of solanaceous glycoalkaloids. Meals combining other common solanaceae such as tomatoes and eggplant may further increase the levels ingested. Krasowski and colleagues (1997) have elucidated how dietary solanaceae can alter metabolism of anesthetic drugs by blocking butyrylcholinesterase. Given the role of cholinesterase inhibitors in human cognitive function, it is speculative whether dietary consumption of solanaceae has a measurable effect on cognition. Perhaps of greater practical concern are potential interactions for those taking pharmaceutical cholinesterase inhibitors such as tacrine or donepezil.

Fava Beans

Fava beans (broad beans, *Vicia faba*) contain a significant amount of L-DOPA. Anecdotal reports have noted improvement of Parkinson's disease after the consumption of fava beans (Spengos and Vassilopoulos 1988). Rabey and colleagues (1992, 1993) have demonstrated the efficacy of fava beans in this respect.

Six patients with Parkinson's disease were withdrawn from their antiparkinsonian medications (L-DOPA/carbidopa, bromocriptine, or lisuride) (Rabey et al. 1992, 1993). After 12 hours off medication, the subjects ate 250 g of cooked fava beans. Significant improvements in motor symptoms were noted, comparable to those seen with 125 mg of L-DOPA and 12.5 mg of carbidopa. In fact, three subjects developed severe dyskinesias after fava ingestion, akin to those seen after larger doses of pharmaceutical L-DOPA. Plasma levels of L-DOPA increased after fava ingestion in a manner comparable to that seen with administration of oral L-DOPA. These results suggest that the L-DOPA contained in fava beans was transported into the CNS and converted to dopamine. In five nonparkinsonian, healthy volunteers, a similar increase in plasma L-DOPA was observed after fava ingestion, although much lower. The difference in plasma L-DOPA between normal volunteers and parkinsonian patients is apparently due to a residual effect of carbidopa in the subjects with Parkinson's disease. Without carbidopa, the L-DOPA from fava is rapidly converted to dopamine in the blood stream and never crosses the blood-brain barrier.

The therapeutic usefulness of fava beans in Parkinson's disease is unlikely because of the variable content of L-DOPA in available fava beans. In addition, the palatability of indefinitely eating fava beans several times daily to maintain therapeutic concentrations makes it impractical. Rabey and colleagues suggest that fava beans may serve as a complementary source of L-DOPA for Parkinsonian patients (Rabey et al. 1993). Conversely, they should also be regarded with caution, if not avoided altogether, by individuals already taking L-DOPA/carbidopa because additive effects would occur. Thus, fava beans pose a source of unanticipated toxicity to a casual consumer. Nonparkinsonian people, on the other hand, would not meet with this degree of toxicity because most of L-DOPA is rapidly converted to dopamine in the blood and never reaches the brain. One peripheral effect of fava beans, which would be experienced by all those consuming them, is increased natriuresis and diuresis through renal dopamine receptors (Vered et al. 1997).

Nootropic Herbs: Summary and Conclusions

The need for medications to improve cognitive function is rooted in the desire of healthy people to optimize their performance, and to preserve function in those with dementia conditions. Of the several forms of dementia, the ones given most attention here are Alzheimer's disease, Parkinson's disease, and vascular dementia. The two general strategies for treatment of dementia include replacement/augmentation of neurotransmitter and neuroprotective drugs to slow the loss of neuronal function. To varying degrees, herbal treatments such as ginkgo offer both of these.

Of the herbal medications reviewed here, ginkgo, ginseng, Hydergine, nicotine, and areca all have prominent effects on cholinergic and monoamine systems. Ginseng and ginkgo also have direct effects on increasing cerebral blood flow. Similarly, ginkgo, ginseng, and Hydergine also have significant antioxidant effects and neuroprotective effects in several models. Ginkgo has received the most attention recently for treatment of dementia, with cognitive effects in animal and human trials comparable to pharmaceutical cholinesterase inhibitors tacrine and donepezil. Hydergine shows similar modest effects across trials. Ginseng has some common neuropharmacological mechanisms with ginkgo, but has only been studied in animals for the most part. Nicotine produces measurable improvements, but carries the problems of dependence and tolerance. Newer nicotinic medications may provide the same cognitive benefits with a more tolerable profile. Areca provides mixed cognitive benefits, and does not seem to offer any clear advantage over other available medications.

It is unlikely that any herbal medications will replace the pharmaceutical drugs for dementia at present. However, ginkgo makes a compelling case because it is similar in efficacy to the available cholinesterase inhibitors, has additional antioxidant effects, and is relatively inexpensive.

The chief unresolved issue with ginkgo is the concern of bleeding when combined with anticoagulant medications. The possibility of combining herbal and/or pharmaceutical medications for a greater cognitive effect has not yet been addressed.

Solanaceous vegetables (tomato, potato, and eggplant) might contribute to cognitive function due to their cholinesterase-inhibiting constituents. Similarly, fava beans could contribute significant amounts of L-DOPA to people with Parkinson's disease. However, this would necessitate daily intake, leading to a rather mundane diet. A more critical problem would be the unpredictable varying levels of the active constituents. To ensure reliability in their effects, herbal extracts need to be standardized. A more practical concern with solanaceous vegetables and fava beans is that they may interfere with ongoing therapeutic regimens.

6

Herbal Sedatives and Anxiolytics

Functioning in a complex and dangerous environment requires one to possess effective mechanisms of arousal, both arousal to consciousness and emotional arousal, in order to meet the demands on behavior. For example, an organism needs to be able to arouse behaviorally in order to deal with predators and other environmental threats. As is often the case with disorders of the mind and brain, normal and adaptive mechanisms can be overactivated and thus become maladaptive. A common outcome of this overactivation is anxiety and insomnia.

Anxiety is a subjective feeling of unease and discomfort, and is accompanied by a host of autonomic and somatic manifestations. It correlates with activity in neuroanatomical structures, including the amygdala and other related limbic structures (Davidson et al. 1999). Anxiety is discussed in greater detail in chapter 7. Insomnia is the inability to sleep or obtain a good quality sleep. This frequently manifests as difficulty falling asleep, awakening at night or early morning, and daytime fatigue (American Psychiatric Association 1994; Eddy and Walbroehl 1999). Insomnia may be a primary disorder, but frequently it is a symptom of another neurologic or psychiatric disorder, such as anxiety.

Central Nervous System Depressants

Herbal sedatives and anxiolytics are a diverse group of plant drugs that commonly act as depressants of the central nervous system (CNS) (table 6.1). Pharmaceutical CNS depressants are used as anxiolytics, anti-epileptics, sedatives, sleep-inducers (sedatives or hypnotics), general anesthetics, and recreational drugs (e.g., ethanol) (table 6.2). CNS

Table 6.1
Herbal CNS depressants

Herb	Active principle(s)	Mechanisms
Catnip	*Cis-trans*-nepetalactone	Unknown
Chamomile	Apigenin	Benzodiazepine agonist Inhibition of Ca^{2+} channels MAO inhibition, blocks NE uptake
Hops	2-methyl-3-butene-2-ol	Unknown
Kava	Kavalactones	Facilitation of GABA binding Inhibition of Na^{+}, Ca^{2+} channels Inhibits NE uptake MAO inhibition Inhibits TXA_2 synthesis
Passionflower	Chrysin	Benzodiazepine partial agonist
Valerian	Sesquiterpenes	GABA release and reversal of uptake Inhibition of GABA breakdown

depressants produce a continuum of effects starting with reduction of anxiety (or anxiolysis) (table 6.3). With larger doses, the effects progress to behavioral disinhibition, sedation, sleep, general anesthesia, coma, and death. Death from an overdose of CNS depressants typically results from respiratory suppression.

In many cases, a single drug can accomplish all of these effects depending on the dosage administered. For example, very low doses of a barbiturate may relieve anxiety, larger doses will induce sleep, and still larger doses will create general anesthesia, where the person will not arouse even to a surgical procedure. Although this is dose-dependent, some drugs tend to work more favorably in a certain range. For example, benzodiazepines work well for anxiolysis and sleep-induction, whereas halothane would be used for general anesthesia only.

Although sedation is the general effect of CNS depressants, behavioral disinhibition can occur at some dose ranges. Although this may seem paradoxical, it reflects early effects of the drug on brain regions that monitor and inhibit behavior (e.g., orbitofrontal cortex). Less benignly, sedative drugs may also induce an agitated confusional state under certain conditions, such as when a person is moderately sedated but in extreme pain.

Table 6.2
Pharmaceutical CNS depressants

Class	Generic name	Trade name	Mechanism
Barbiturate	Amobarbital	Amytal	Barbiturate receptor ($GABA_A$)
	Phenobarbital	Luminal	"
	Pentobarbital	Nembutal	"
	Thiopental	Pentothal	"
Benzodiazepine	Alprazolam	Xanax	Benzodiazepine receptor ($GABA_A$)
	Clonazepam	Klonopin	"
	Chlorazepate	Tranxene	"
	Chlordiazepoxide	Librium	"
	Diazepam	Valium	"
	Flunitrazepam	Rohypnol	"
	Lorazepam	Ativan	"
	Triazolam	Halcion	"
Alcohol	Ethanol		$GABA_A$ channel, NMDA antagonist
Antiseizure	Carbamazepine	Tegretol	Na^+ channels, NMDA antagonist
	Ethosuximide	Zarontin	Ca^{2+} channels
	Felbamate	Felbatol	NMDA glycine site, GABA potentiation
	Gabapentin	Neurontin	GABA release
	Lamotrigine	Lamictal	Na^+ channels (slowed recovery)
	Phenytoin	Dilantin	Na^+ channels (slowed recovery)
	Tiagabine	Gabatril	GABA uptake inhibition
	Topiramate	Topamax	GABA pot., AMPA antagonism
	Vigabatrin	Sabril	GABA transaminase inhibition
General anesthetic (inhalational)	Chloroform		Uncertain (multiple mechanisms)
	Halothane	Fluothane	Uncertain (multiple mechanisms)

Table 6.3
Continuum of effects of CNS depressants

Anxiolysis
Behavioral disinhibition
Sedation
Sleep
General anesthesia
Coma
Death

Pharmacological Issues in CNS Depressants

Several pharmacological issues pertain to most CNS depressant drugs (Hobbs et al. 1996; Julien 1997). Depending on their pharmacological mechanisms, combinations of CNS depressants can produce additive or synergistic effects, when the total effect is equal to or greater than the sum of their individual effects, respectively. For example, in doses that would be safe individually, combinations of alcohol and barbiturates can be lethal.

Many CNS depressants have some liability for dependence. This is typically greater with barbiturates, but lesser with benzodiazepines, and perhaps nonexistent in many antiseizure medications. CNS depressants produce tolerance when administered chronically, where increasingly larger doses are required to sustain the same level of effect. Further, a cross-tolerance often develops, where the tolerance is generalized to other CNS depressants. For example, a person with an ethanol tolerance will also display some tolerance to barbiturates. The therapeutic index tends to decrease as tolerance increases, so that the difference between an effective and toxic dose diminishes. Thus, tolerance to CNS depressants is accompanied by a smaller safety margin.

Once tolerance develops, acute cessation of CNS depressants creates a withdrawal syndrome. Tolerance is associated with neural adaptations to the continued inhibitory influence of the drug. Suddenly removing the drug and its inhibitory influence creates a rebound excitation, due to neuronal disinhibition. Depending on the degree of tolerance, subjects may experience anxiety, irritability, delirium, and seizures. Withdrawal from CNS depressants is a serious medical issue, and must be controlled carefully. Typically, people are switched to a safer CNS depressant drug such as a benzodiazepine, and the drug is slowly tapered over a number of weeks. This allows for gradual neural adaptation and minimizes withdrawal symptoms.

General Mechanisms of Action for CNS Depressants

In order for a drug to induce CNS depression it must either facilitate neuronal inhibition or inhibit the neuronal excitation. There are a few mechanisms by which these may occur, and CNS depressant drugs may possess one or more of these mechanisms.

Many CNS depressants work by facilitating the activity of the inhibitory neurotransmitter GABA (table 6.1). The $GABA_A$ receptor is an ion channel with several receptor sites (Cooper et al. 1996). There is a binding site for the endogenous neurotransmitter GABA, which opens the channel and allows Cl^- flux into the neuron. This hyperpolarizes the neuron, making it less likely to reach the threshold of excitation. In addition to the GABA receptor, there are several separate allosteric binding sites for benzodiazepines, barbiturates, certain steroids, and ethanol. Agonists at these sites have no intrinsic inhibitory effects, but instead potentiate and facilitate the the Cl^- conductance induced by GABA. Other means of enhancing GABA activity include blocking its reuptake (e.g., tiagabine), or increasing its release (gabapentin). The net result of all of these actions is a facilitation of neuronal inhibition by GABA.

A second mechanism of action of CNS depressants is the inhibition of an excitatory neurotransmitter. Several of the drugs in this class (ethanol, barbiturates, Tegretol) block the actions of the excitatory amino acid (EAA) neurotransmitter glutamate at the *N*-methyl-D-aspartate (NMDA) receptor. The NMDA channel requires both receptor activation and membrane depolarization to open, allowing Ca^{2+} influx. An intracellular chemical cascade follows, inducing synaptic changes thought to be the cellular basis of memory formation (Kandel et al. 1991). Congruently, drugs that inhibit the NMDA channel prevent the formation of memories while the drug is in effect. This would explain, in part, why a common side effect of some CNS depressants is memory impairment.

However, it is not the only mechanism, because drugs that do not work at NMDA receptors can impair memory (e.g., benzodiazepines). Other EAA receptors include the ionotropic AMPA and kainate receptors, and the metabotropic glutamate receptors (mGluR).

The third mechanism of CNS depressants is the blocking of voltage-gated ion channels (Hille 1992). These are typically Na^+ or Ca^{2+} channels, which are located in the neuronal membrane. Na^+ channels are responsible for conveyance of the action potential along the membrane, and Ca^{2+} entry is necessary for release of neurotransmitters from synaptic terminals. Thus, drugs that block either or both of these channels will reduce the neuronal output. The CNS depressant drugs that have this mode of action are predominantly antiseizure drugs, although many local anesthetics are antagonists of the Na^+ channel (see chapter 8).

Herbal CNS Depressants

Valerian

History and Botany

Valerian is native to Europe and Asia, but now grows in most parts of the world. *Valeriana officinalis* is the most commonly known and studied, but approximately 200 species are known (figure 6.1) (Kowalchick and Hylton 1987). Unless otherwise specified, the name valerian will be used here to refer to *V. officinalis*. Valerian grows 50 to 100 cm in height, with an erect stem with pinnate leaves and numerous small pink-white flowers at the top. The parts of the plant used medicinally are the roots and rhizome (figure 6.2).

The use of valerian extends back at least 1000 years, and it gained a reputation in sixteenth-century Europe as a treatment for epilepsy (Tyler 1994; Temkin 1971). Its reported uses are broad (digestive aid, muscle relaxant, antipyretic, etc.) but it is commonly known to treat insomnia and anxiety (Gruenwald et al. 1998; Kowalchick and Hylton 1987). Valerian has a distinct, unpleasant odor. Perhaps appropriately, it is believed to be an herb in the writings of Galen and Dioscorides, called *phu* (Leyel 1994).

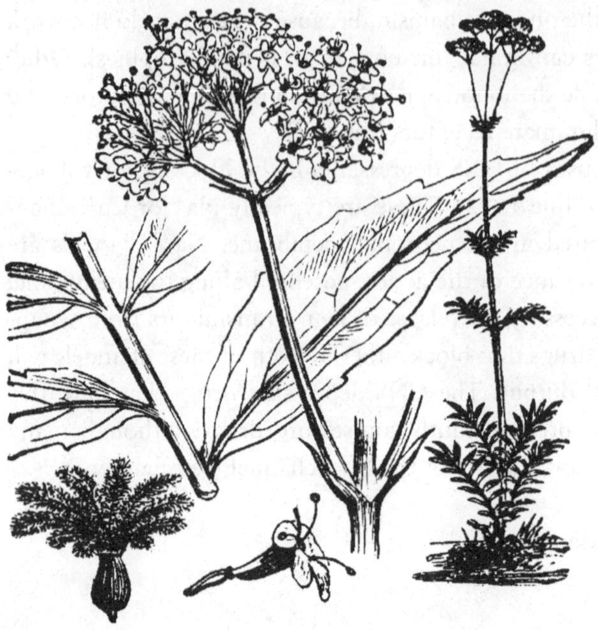

Figure 6.1
Valerian *(Valeriana officinalis)*. Reprinted from Culbreth DMR. (1927). *Materia Medica and Pharmacognosy*, 7th ed. Philadelphia: Lea & Febiger.

Chemical Constituents

Valerian's main chemical constituents fall into three categories: monoterpenes, sesquiterpenes, and alkaloids (table 6.4). The monoterpenes include bornyl acetate, l-borneol, valenol, and valmane (figure 6.3). A subgroup of the monoterpenes are the valepotriates, which include valtrate and its derivatives, baldrinal, and homobaldrinal (Houghton 1988; Cott 1995). Of the four other Valerianaceae examined *(V. pulchella, V. prionophylla, V. condamoana,* and *V. micropterina)*, rhizomes of *V. prionophylla* had the highest concentration of valepotriates (Chavadej et al. 1985). However, valepotriates rapidly decompose in the stored herb, so their content in valerian preparations is very low (Tyler 1994).

The sesquiterpenes present in valerian include isovaleric acid, valerenic acid, valerenal, valeranone, and valerenol. The alkaloids found in valerian include valeranine and actinidine.

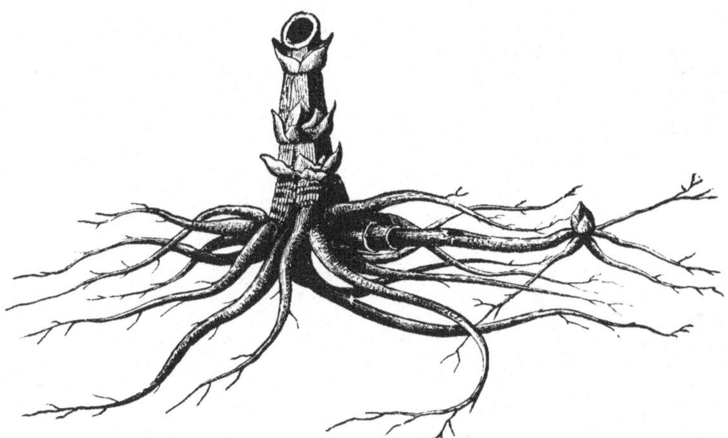

Figure 6.2
Valerian root and rhizome *(Valeriana officinalis)*. Reprinted from Culbreth DMR. (1927). *Materia Medica and Pharmacognosy*, 7th ed. Philadelphia: Lea & Febiger.

The content of valepotriates and sesquiterpenes varies across species of the *Valeriana* genus. For example, *Valeriana officinalis* has relatively high content of sesquiterpenes and low content of valepotriates, while *Valeriana edulis* has a high proportion of valepotriates and low content of sesquiterpenes (Lindahl and Lindwall 1989).

Mechanisms of Action
The mechanisms of action of valerian are uncertain, but they likely involve a facilitation of GABA transmission (see table 6.1). Low microgram concentrations of an aqueous valerian extract inhibits uptake and stimulates release of GABA from synaptosomes (Santos et al. 1994a, 1994b). GABA release by the valerian extract is independent of Ca^{2+} and membrane depolarization, and thus not from vesicular stores. Further, the GABA release is dependent on Na^+ concentrations, suggesting that valerian inhibits and reverses the GABA reuptake transporter. Thus, valerian extract appears to reverse GABA uptake and release it from the cytosolic pool.

However, further investigation found that the actual GABA content of the extract can partially account for the reversal of GABA uptake

Table 6.4
Chemical constituents of valerian

Monoterpenes
Bornyl acetate
l-Borneol
Valenol
Valmane
Valepotriates:
Valtrate
Isovaltrate
Homovaltrate
Acevaltrate
Homacevaltrate
Diavaltrate
Dihydrovaltrate
Isovalerylhydovaltrate
Seneciovaltrate
Baldrinal
Homobaldrinal
Sesquiterpenes
Isovaleric acid
Valerenic acid
Acetylvalerenic acid
Valerenal
Valeranone
Valerenol
Kessane
Bornyl acetate
Bornyl isovalerate
Elemol
Alkaloids
Valeranine
Actinidine
Naphtyridylmethylketone
Valtroxal
Epoxylathyral 3,5 dibutrate

See text for references.

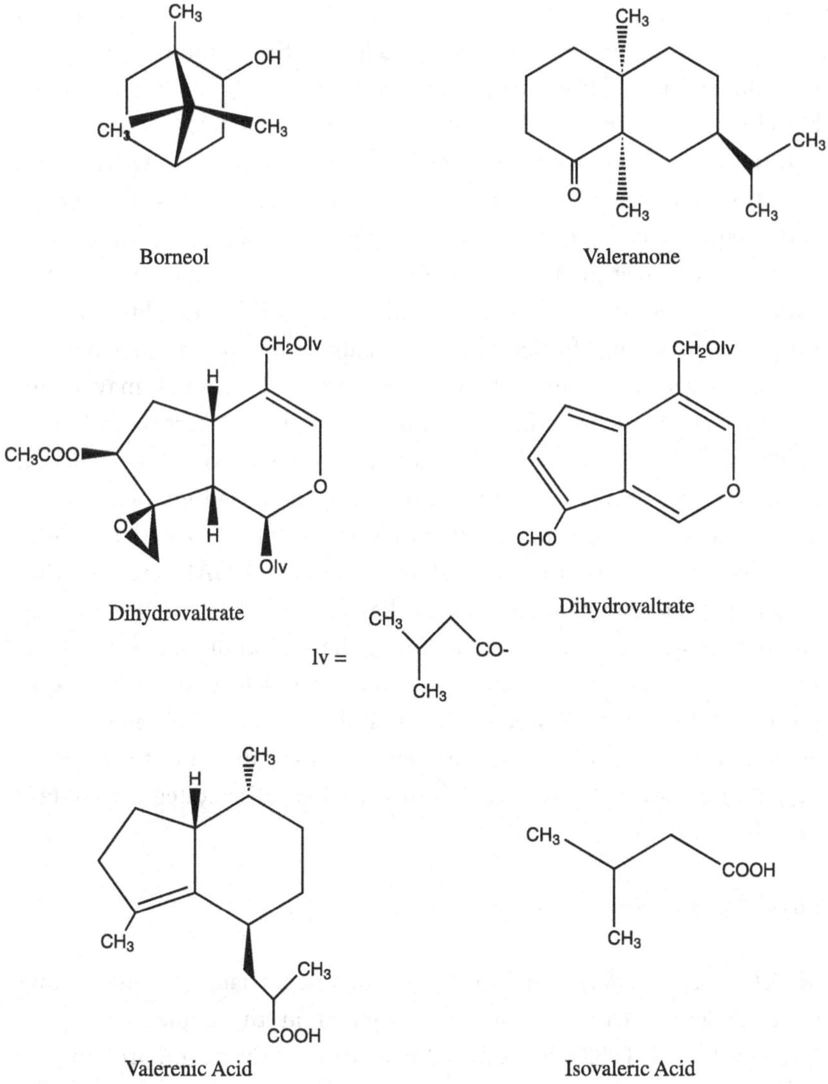

Borneol

Valeranone

Dihydrovaltrate

Dihydrovaltrate

lv =

Valerenic Acid

Isovaleric Acid

Figure 6.3
Chemical structure of valerian constituents.

in vitro (Santos et al. 1994c). Alternately, because GABA does not pass the blood-brain barrier well, it is possible that the glutamine content of valerian extract contributes to this effect because it both crosses the blood-brain barrier and serves as a precursor for GABA.

Although some binding of valerian extract occurs at $GABA_A$ receptors, this has been attributed to the amino acid content of the extract and deemed insufficient by itself to explain valerian's CNS depressant effects (Cavadas et al. 1995). Valerenic acid has been shown to inhibit enzymatic breakdown of GABA (Riedel et al. 1982; Houghton 1999). Low concentrations of valerian extracts enhance benzodiazepine binding ([^{3}H]flunitrazepam) (Ortiz et al. 1999). The valepotriates may themselves have CNS depressant effects through in vivo conversion to homobaldrinal (Houghton 1999). Further, an ethanol extract of valerian potentiates the effects of a barbiturate (thiopental) and inhibits seizures induced by the $GABA_A$ antagonist picrotoxin (Hiller and Zetler 1996).

Collectively, valerian extracts show a variety of GABAergic mechanisms. The predominant mechanism has yet to be determined, but an additive or synergistic interaction among the several mechanisms is possible. Future research on valerian extracts needs to address any compositional differences between aqueous and nonaqueous extracts, and to determine the responsible active constitutents. For some time it was thought to be the valepotriates, but this was later discredited due to their unstable nature.

Physiological Effects

Muscle relaxant effects In vitro effects of valepotriates (isovaltrate and valtrate) and valeranone were investigated in the guinea pig ileum (Hazelhoff et al. 1982). It produced relaxation of the ileum, probably by a direct muscular action and not by action on autonomic receptors. The GABAergic effects of valerian may provide central muscle relaxant effects through spinal actions, but this has yet to be explicity investigated.

Behavioral effects Several behavioral effects of valerian have been noted in animals. These include suppression of the orienting response in an open-field paradigm, decreasing spontaneous and caffeine-induced motor activity, and potentiation of the behavioral actions of barbiturates (Dunaev et al. 1987). Oral and intravenous doses of valtrate and acetoxyvaltrate, more specifically, were found to reduce locomotor activity (Hölzl and Fink 1984).

Valerian extracts show sedative and anxiolytic effects. Whereas passionflower and chamomile have relatively specific anxiolytic effects, valerian shows more general sedative effects, but all effects occur in a dose-dependent manner (Della Logia et al. 1981; Leuschner et al. 1993). The sedative effects of valerian extract are moderate when compared to diazepam and the neuroleptic chlorpromazine (Leuschner et al. 1993). However, valepotriates reverse the anxiogenic effects of diazepam withdrawal in rats in the elevated plus maze. This effect is dose dependent, effective at 12 mg/kg but not 6 mg/kg. Interestingly, the fragrant valerian compound bornyl acetate has sedative effects in mice, but only when inhaled (Buchbauer et al. 1992).

In a manner similar to imipramine, an ethanol extract of valerian root was found to prevent immobility induced by a forced-swimming test in rats, suggesting a potential antidepressant effect of valerian (Sakamoto et al. 1992).

Antiseizure effects Valerian extracts were found to have weak antiseizure effects in mice (Dunaev et al. 1987; Leuschner et al. 1993). This would be consistent with its putative GABAergic mechanisms. So the traditional use of valerian to treat epilepsy is perhaps an empirical reality. However, no studies have been done to date that compare valerian to modern antiseizure medications.

Sleep electrophysiology To date, four studies have been published that examine the effects of valerian on human sleep and its electrophysiology, which have produced variable results. An early study (Muller-Limmroth and Ehrenstein 1977) showed that a combined preparation of valerian and hops in sleep-disturbed subjects increased the amount of slow-wave and REM sleep. Another study using an aqueous extract (400 mg) of valerian did not show significant EEG effects, but suggested a relation between the EEG effects and subjective effects, that is, shortened sleep latency and increased latency to first waking (Leathwood and Chauffard 1982–3, 1985). Another study using aqueous extracts showed no effects on sleep stages or EEG spectra (Balderer and Borbely 1985).

A methodologically controlled study of valerian in sleep was published that utilized both double-blind and placebo controls, as well as randomization (Gessner and Klasser 1984). Also employed were two doses of valerian (60 and 120 mg), computerized EEG power spectral analysis and psychometric mood questionnaires. Valerian increased sleep stages 1, 2, and 3 and reduced stage 4 and REM. Dose-dependent effects were noted, where the 120 mg dose produced greater sedative effects. Peak effects occurred 2–3 hours after administration. Mood ratings did not differ, positively or negatively, between the experimental and control conditions.

The effects of valerian in poor sleepers was studied comparing it to placebo controls (Schulz et al. 1994). Valerian showed an increase in slow-wave and a decrease in stage 1 sleep. K-complex density was increased, but REM was unaltered, and no effects were reported on subjective sleep quality.

The physiological effects of valerian across animals and humans are consistent with its sedative properties. The human electrophysiological findings are somewhat incongruent, but the methodology must be taken into account. Earlier studies used less-rigorous controls, and one used aqueous extract vs. the entire herb, so that hydrophobic constituents were likely excluded. Such differences have been observed with other sedative herbs such as kava (Jamieson et al. 1989). Another difference between the two latter studies that may account for differing results is the different populations used (normal versus sleep-disturbed) (Gessner and Klasser 1984; Schulz et al. 1994). Indeed, poor-quality sleepers of various etiologies are noted to have sleep EEG patterns that differ from normals (Kupfer et al. 1976; Bourdet and Goldenberg 1994; Morisson et al. 1998; Adam et al. 1986).

The EEG effects of valerian are most concordant with those of tiagabine, a GABA uptake inhibitor used to treat epilepsy. Tiagabine also increases slow-wave sleep, but unlike valerian has little or no effect on REM (Lancel et al. 1998). $GABA_A$ agonists also tend to have this effect, in contrast to $GABA_B$ and benzodiazepine agonists (Faulhaber et al. 1997; Lancel and Faulhaber 1996; Lancel et al. 1996; Juhász et al. 1994).

Sleep quality A randomized, placebo-controlled, and double-blind crossover study was employed using a commercially available valerian preparation (Lindahl and Lindwall 1989). The preparation used contained primarily sesquiterpenes, and very low amounts of valepotriates. The subjects were 27 adults who were seen in a medical clinic for sleep difficulties. Those receiving valerian experienced improvements in sleep quality (89% of subjects), with a proportion (44%) rating highest quality sleep. No differences were seen between those who received either valerian or placebo first. An absence of adverse side effects, including nightmares, was reported. Although these results are promising, this study unfortunately used a preparation that included two other herbs (lemon melissa and flores humuli), which limit the conclusions that can be exclusively drawn with valerian. Another methodologically well-controlled study was performed, which had a much larger ($n = 128$) number of subjects (Leathwood et al. 1982). Improvements were seen in sleep quality and decreases in sleep latency. Furthermore, sleep quality was most improved in poor sleepers and tobacco smokers.

Thus, the above two studies plus the one conducted by Gessner and Klassner (1984; see above) constitute three methodologically controlled studies of valerian on human sleep. By established guidelines, this constitutes Class I evidence for valerian in the treatment of insomnia (Woolf 1992).

Cognitive effects Studies of the cognitive effects of valerian are scant. One study compared the effects of valerian to those of the benzodiazepine flunitrazepam, and to a combined preparation of valerian and hops (Gerhard et al. 1996). Whereas flunitrazepam produced significant impairment the morning after administration, valerian (alone or in combination with hops) did not. However, 1 to 2 hours after administration, valerian produced a slight but statistically significant decrease in vigilance and processing of complex information. Although mild, this effect may contraindicate valerian use in situations where peak cognitive performance is required (e.g., driving).

Toxicity

Because of their chemical structure, there has been concern over liver damage resulting from valepotriates. Baldrinal and homobaldrinal were noted to have some mutagenic effects in vitro (von der Hude et al. 1986). However, *Valeriana officinalis* has a low valepotriate content—they decompose rapidly in the stored herb and they are not well absorbed. Liver toxicity in animals or humans has never been demonstrated (Tyler 1994; Lindahl and Lindwall 1989). Thus, the valepotriate content of valerian is not likely to cause toxicity. No health hazards have been reported with normal use of valerian, and it has been approved by the German Commission E as a treatment for anxiety and sleep (Gruenwald et al. 1998).

High doses of valerian are reported to produce headache, vomiting, stupor, dizziness, and cardiac dysfunction (Kowalchick and Hylton 1987; Gruenwald et al. 1998). A case was reported of a single overdose (approximately 20 times the "recommended" therapeutic dose) that produced reportedly mild symptoms, which resolved in 24 hours. One other study published the results of overdoses of "Sleep-Qik," an over-the-counter herbal sedative (Chan et al. 1995). However, in addition to valerian, the preparation included cyproheptadine hydrochloride and hyoscine hydrobromide, a potent anticholinergic drug. Given its CNS depressant effects and putative GABAergic mechanisms, concurrent use of valerian with other CNS depressants, including ethanol, should be avoided.

Summary

There is preliminary but promising empirical evidence that valerian is a useful medication for improving sleep (tables 6.5, 6.6). Although the responsible constituents are uncertain, valerian likely acts through facilitation of central GABAergic transmission. Further, its pharmacological mechanisms suggest it may be useful in treating anxiety or other mood disorders, but there have not been any controlled studies to support this.

Table 6.5
Evidence for the effects of herbal sedatives and anxiolytics

	Sedative	Anxiolytic	Antiseizure	Analgesic	Antidepressant
Kava	Pharmacol. Animal beh. Human beh.	Pharmacol. Animal beh. Human beh.	Pharmacol. Animal beh.	Pharmacol. Animal beh.	Pharmacol. Animal beh.
Valerian	Pharmacol. Animal beh. Human beh.	Pharmacol. Animal beh.	Pharmacol. Animal beh.	Pharmacol.	Animal beh.
Passionflower	Pharmacol. Animal beh.	Pharmacol. Animal beh.	Pharmacol. Animal beh.	Pharmacol. Animal beh.	
Chamomile	Pharmacol. Animal beh.	Pharmacol. Animal beh.	Pharmacol.		Pharmacol.
Lemon Balm	Animal beh.			Animal beh.	
Hops	Pharmacol.	Pharmacol. Animal beh.	Pharmacol.		
Catnip	Pharmacol. Animal beh.	Pharmacol.			
Skullcap					
Geranium					

Key:
Pharmacol.—Chemical contituents identified which could possibly afford it with the effect.
Animal beh.—Demonstration of statistically significant effects in an animal behavioral paradigm.
Human beh.—Demonstration of statistically significant effects in a human behavioral paradigm.
See text for references.

Table 6.6
Quality of clinical evidence for herbal sedatives and anxiolytics

	Sedative	Anxiolytic	Antiseizure
Kava	untested	Class I	untested
Valerian	Class I	untested	untested
Passionflower	untested	untested	untested
Chamomile	untested	untested	untested
Skullcap	untested	untested	untested
Geranium	untested	untested	untested
Hops	untested	untested	untested
Lemon balm	untested	untested	untested
Catnip	untested	untested	untested

Toxicity has not been reported with proper use, and one case has shown that it is relatively nonfatal in overdoses.

Kava

History and Botany

Kava *(Piper methysticum)* is a plant native to the South Pacific islands, including Hawaii, Fiji, Samoa, Tonga, the Marshall and Solomon islands, Vanuato, New Guinea, Tahiti, and New Zealand (figure 6.4) (Lebot et al. 1997). It is also known by the names *kava kava*, *awa*, *waka*, *lawena*, or *yaquona*. The botanical name, *Piper methysticum*, is translated as "intoxicating pepper," because it belongs to the pepper family Piperaceae. It is thought that *Piper methysticum* is a cultivated variant of the wild relative *Piper wichmannii* (Lebot et al. 1997). Kava, (used here to refer to *Piper methysticum*) is a bush that grows 2–3 m in height, with large heart-shaped leaves (Gruenwald et al. 1998). The large rhizome is the part of the plant used medicinally, weighing 2–10 kg. When harvested, the root is pounded, chewed, or grated and then drunk in a cold-water infusion. In the West, it is typically sold in dried, ground encapsulated form or may be prepared as a tea.

In South Pacific cultures, kava has been primarily used as a ceremonial or recreational herb. It has been in use at least since the eighteenth century when Europeans first traveled to Polynesia, but its use probably extends back into prehistory. Kava may also be given reciprocally as a

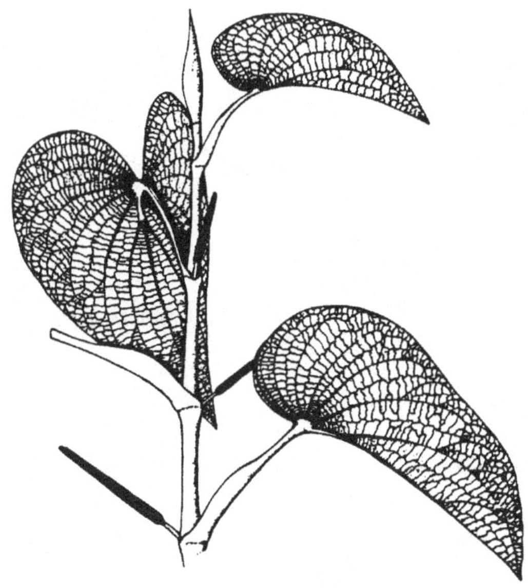

Figure 6.4
Kava *(Piper methysticum)*. Reprinted with permission from Lebot V, Merlin M, Lindstrom L. (1997). *Kava—the Pacific Elixir: The Definitive Guide to Its Ethnobotany, History, and Chemistry*. Rochester, Vt.: Healing Arts Press.

gift in the resolution of a social conflict, or partaken as an after-work drink to relax. It is known traditionally for producing relaxation (Lebot et al. 1997). In contrast to many other sedative herbs and pharmaceutical drugs that commonly cause sleepiness, kava is reputed to produce an alert, relaxed mental state. Other reported effects have been for sleep (in higher doses than those for relaxation), analgesia, anticonvulsant, and muscle relaxant.

Chemical Constituents
The pharmacologically active chemicals most studied from the kava plant are collectively called kavapyrones or kavalactones (referred to here as kavalactones) (figure 6.5). Some of the principal kavalactones are: kavain, dihydrokavain, yangonin, 11-methoxy-yangonin, methysticin, and dihydromethysticin (Lebot et al. 1997; Boonen et al. 1997). The concentrations of kavalactones vary across different parts of the plant: kavain and dimethoxyyangonin are more concentrated in the rootstalk, but dihy-

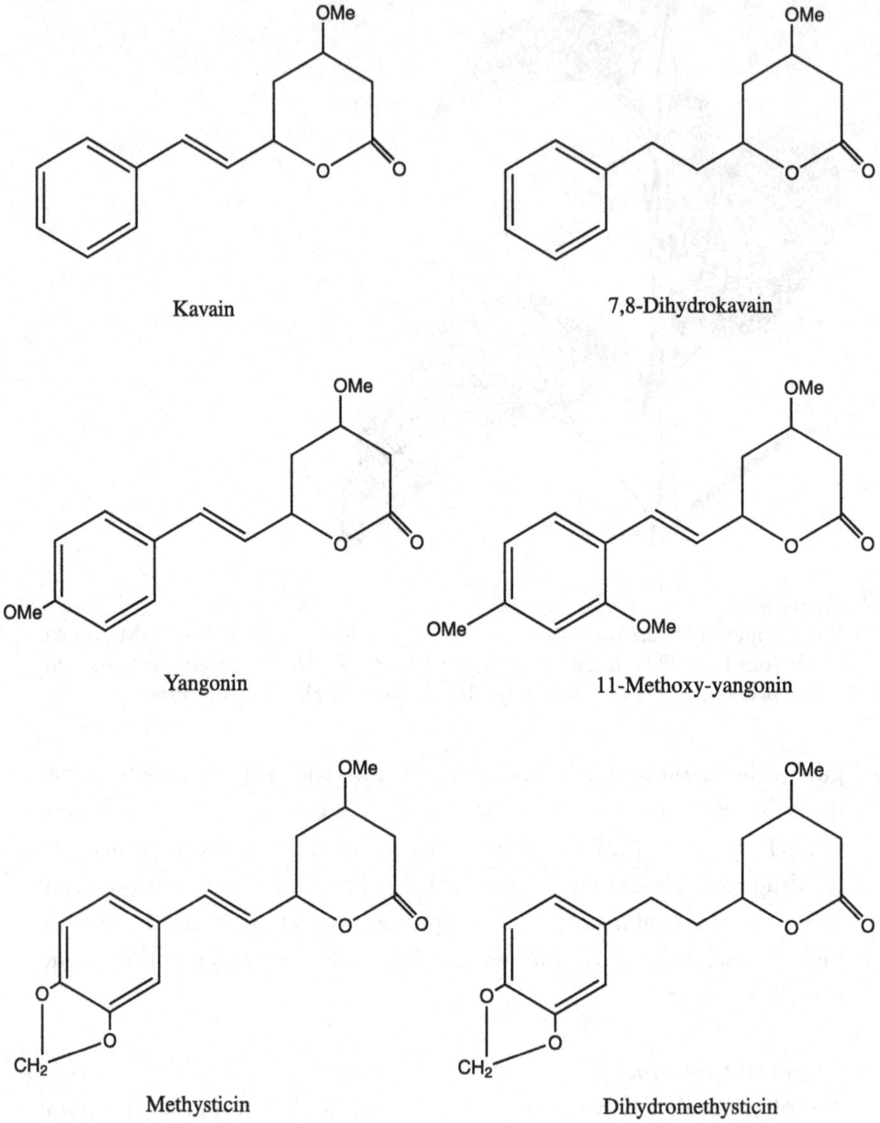

Kavain

7,8-Dihydrokavain

Yangonin

11-Methoxy-yangonin

Methysticin

Dihydromethysticin

Figure 6.5
Chemical structure of the kavalactones.

drokavain and dihydromethysticin are found in higher concentrations in the stalks and leaves (Cass and McNally 1998). Kavain and dihydrokavain are reportedly the most permeable to the blood-brain barrier.

Mechanisms of Action

Like many psychotropic herbs, Kava seems to create its effects by a combination of effects that are mediated by several of its constituents. To date, at least four mechanisms have been identified that appear to mediate the effects of kava.

GABA Kava appears to facilitate GABA transmission. Low micromolar (0.1–1 μM) concentrations of kavalactones [(+)-kavain, (+)dihydrokavain, (+)-methysticin, and (+)-dihydromethysticin] enhance the binding of ligands to the $GABA_A$ receptor (Boonen and Heberlein 1998; Jussofie et al. 1994). This facilitation would potentiate binding of GABA and increase Cl^- influx. Some structure-activity relationships were noted to increase the efficacy of kavalactones, such as the addition of an aromatic methoxy group and angular lactone ring. Kavalactones do not alter the binding of flunitrazepam, so their effect on $GABA_A$ is not through the benzodiazepine receptor (Davies et al. 1992). Therefore, kavalactones and benzodiazepines similarly facilitate $GABA_A$ activity, but apparently through different mechanisms. Convergently, kavalactone displacement of the $GABA_A$ agonist muscimol is highest in the hippocampus and amygdala (Jussofie et al. 1994). Combination with pentobarbital caused synergistic effects on binding.

Voltage-gated ion channels A second mechanism by which kava produces CNS depression is by inhibition of voltage-gated ion channels (Gleitz et al. 1995; Gleitz et al. 1996a; Magura et al. 1997; Schirrmacher et al. 1999). Kavain has a fast and specific inhibitory action on Na^+ channels. (+)-methysticin was 4–5 times more potent than (±)-kavain in this respect (Magura et al. 1997). Kavain, dihydrokavain, and dihydromethysticin act as noncompetitive inhibitors of the Na^+ channel (Friese and Gleitz 1998). It has been proposed that (+)-methysticin and (±)-kavain bind to the Na^+ channel in its inactivated state and prolong the inactivation (Magura et al. 1997). Kavain blocks the [^{3}H]batrachotoxin binding, but not [^{3}H]saxitoxin binding (Gleitz et al. 1996a).

This suggests an action at receptor site 2 of the Na^+ channel, a site common to local anesthetic drugs.

It was further shown that kavain inhibits L-type Ca^{2+} channels as well, and the subsequent release of glutamate (Gleitz et al. 1996b; Ferger et al. 1998; Schirrmacher et al. 1999). At concentrations of 70 μM/L, glutamate release was reduced by 70%. The effects of kavain and dihydromethysticin were found to be additive when both were administered in vitro (Walden et al. 1997). These effects on voltage-gated ion channels are obtained in the micromolar range, and are consistent with concentrations reached in the brain by peripheral administration (Keledjian et al. 1988). Further, many of these studies examined individual kavalactones, which does not account for the additive or synergistic effects of combined kavalactones.

Monoamine Kavalactones block the reuptake of norepinephrine with the following order of potency: (±)-kavain = (+)-kavain > (+)-methysticin (Seitz et al. 1997). However, neither acute nor chronic doses of kavalactones alter turnover of serotonin. The effects of kavalactones were far less potent than desipramine, and only occurred at concentrations of less than 10 μM. However, this study only used a single kavalactone in vitro, ruling out additive and synergistic actions of combined administration. Another potential monoamine mechanism of kavalactones is inhibition of MAO_B (Uebelhack et al. 1998). Kavalactones reversibly inhibited platelet MAO_B in the micromolar range (IC_{50} 1.2–24 μM). The order of potency for MAO_B inhibition is: desmethoxyyangonin > (±)-methysticin > yangonin > (±)-dihydromethysticin > (±)-dihydrokavain > (±)-kavain. The two most potent, desmethoxyyangonin and (±)-methysticin, both showed competitive inhibition and mean Ki of 0.28 μM and 1.14 μM, respectively. This would be consisent with a slow onset of MAO inhibition by kavalactones. In three subjects given 120–240 mg of kavalactones for 3–4 weeks, a 26–34% reduction of MAO_B in platelet-rich plasma was observed (Uebelhack et al. 1998).

Neither an acute dose of dihydromethysticin (100 mg/kg) or chronic doses of (±)-kavain altered levels of dopamine, serotonin, or their metabolites in the striatum and cortex of rats (Boonen et al. 1998). However, kavalactones have complex and mixed effects on monoamine levels in the nucleus accumbens, depending both on which kavapyrone was used and at what dose (Baum et al. 1998). D,L-kavain had biphasic effects on dopamine, decreasing it at low doses (20 mg/kg), and increasing or not altering it at high doses (120 mg/kg). Similarly, desmethyoxyyangonin caused increases in dopamine levels in the accumbens. In contrast, yangonin potently decreased dopamine levels to below the limits of detection. Other kavalactones (dihydrokavain, methysticin, and dihydromethysticin) had no effect on dopamine levels. Kavain also caused a decrease in serotonin levels. Baum and colleagues suggest that the elevations in dopamine by kavain are due to blocking reuptake of cytoplasmic dopamine into vesicles, because large amounts of DOPAC were excreted. This proposed mechanism is similar to that of the drug reserpine, except that unlike reserpine the actions of kavalactones are reversible.

The interactions of kava with monoamines are complex, apparently varying with which dose, which kavalactone is used, and which neuroanatomical region is examined. Isolated findings with individual kavalactones in isolated brain regions are insufficient to explain the actions of kava unless they are integrated in a larger picture. The neurophysiological and neurochemical effects of kava extract need to be further investigated when administered to the whole organism. For example, although increases in dopamine levels in the accumbens have been found with certain kavalactones, other lines of evidence point to a sum antagonistic effect on central dopamine. Cases of dyskinesia suggestive of dopamine antagonism have been reported (Schelosky et al. 1995). Kava extracts also antagonize apomorphine-induced stereotypies in mice (Jamieson et al. 1989).

Thus, although the mechanism of interaction with monoamine is uncertain, peripheral doses of kava do have functional effects on central monoamine systems (Baum et al. 1998).

Eicosanoid Finally, (+)-kavain was reported to inhibit cyclooxygenase, suppressing synthesis of thromboxane A_2 in the high micromolar range (Gleitz et al. 1997). Thromboxanes are prostaglandins synthesized from arachidonic acid (see chapter 7). Although they are more commonly known for their hemodynamic effects, they are also present in the brain. Their function in the CNS has not been well delineated, but they have been shown to inhibit $GABA_A$ receptors. So, suppression of thromboxane A_2 synthesis would increase $GABA_A$ function (Schwartz-Bloom et al. 1996). Again, because only one kavalactone was examined, whether combined kavalactones or extract could create a physiologically signifi-canct effect remains to be determined. In order for central eicosanoid effects to be relevant, it would likely require additive or synergistic effects of combined kavalactones.

Summary of mechanisms of action Of the above-mentioned mechanisms, GABA facilitation and blockade of voltage-gated cation channels would best account for the sedative properties of kava. Other drugs that facilitate GABA transmission (e.g., benzodiazepines, barbiturates) are well known for their sedative and anxiolytic effects. Such activity in the amygdala could particularly account for anxiolytic effects (Jussofie et al. 1994; Sanders and Shekhar 1995; Davis et al. 1994). Inhibition of voltage-gated cation channels depresses neuronal function and can create sedation as well. Indeed, many antiseizure medications (e.g., hydantoins, carbamazepine) have such actions, and are known for their sedating side effects. In contrast, the blocking of norepinephrine reuptake by kava would be expected to have alerting effects, based on animal and human studies of noradrenergic function (Aston-Jones et al. 1994; Rajkowski et al. 1994). This effect needs to be examined with combined kavalactones or total extract to confirm its physiological relevance. However, it is interesting that kava is known for creating a relaxed but alert state (Cass and McNally 1998).

The functional significance of thromboxane A_2 inhibition by kava is not certain. More needs to be understood about the functions of prostaglandins in the CNS, but given the inhibition of $GABA_A$ by thromboxane A_2, kava's suppression of thromboxane A_2 synthesis could conceivably contribute to its anxiolytic and sedative effects. More research is needed to determine if this mechanism of action is physiologically significant at normal kavalactone concentrations.

Pharmacokinetics

Pharmacological effects of kavalactones are estimated to occur at plasma concentrations of 50–150 μM/L (Kretzschmar and Meyer 1968). Kavalactones peripherally administered quickly gain access to the CNS (Keledjian et al. 1988). Five minutes after a 100 mg/kg bolus injection (IP) in mice, the following brain concentrations of kavalactones were obtained (ng/mg): dihydrokavain (64.7 ± 13.1), kavain (29.3 ± 0.8), desmethoxyyangonin (10.4 ± 1.5), and yangonin (1.2 ± 0.3). These accumulate and are eliminated at different rates: whereas kavain and dihydrokavain accumulate and are eliminated quickly, yangonin and desmethoxyyangonin do so slowly. Metabolites of kavalactones are detectable in human urine (Duffield et al. 1989).

A pharmacokinetic synergy occurs with kavalactones. When a kava resin is administered (containing combined kavapyrones), levels of kavain and yangonin in the brain are multiplied 2 and 20 times, respectively, as compared to individual administration (Keledjian et al. 1988). Although the mechanism of this synergy is uncertain, it may be due to competition for plasma binding sites. Some report that these synergistic effects occur with yangonin and desmethoxyyangonin and other kavalactones, implying an influence on intestinal absorption. Thus, results from studies using individual kavalactones must be generalized cautiously, because they do not account for the magnified effects of the naturalistic combined administration of kavalactones.

The preparation of kava used may greatly affect its effectiveness. A comparison was made between aqueous and lipid-soluble extracts of kava in mice (Jamieson et al. 1989). The lipid-soluble extract produced sedation, analgesia, and local anesthesia, while the aqueous extract was ineffective orally.

There is evidence to suggest that limited tolerance to kava develops (Duffield and Jamieson 1991). A kava extract parenterally administered daily for three days produced little physiological or behavioral tolerance in mice. However, kava extract and ethanol were found to interact, potentiating each other's sedative effects and increasing the toxicity of kava (Jamieson and Duffield 1990). Similarly, synergistic interactions occur between kavalactones and barbiturates (Jussofie et al. 1994).

Physiological Effects

Physiological studies of kava constituents have focused on several of their effects: muscle relaxant, sedative, analgesic, antiseizure, and neuroprotective.

Neuromuscular effects The muscle relaxant effect of kava was studied in mouse and frog muscles. It produced direct neuromuscular effects, reducing the amplitude of end-plate potentials and miniature end-plate potentials, and depressed muscle action potentials. This effect was not reversed by application of Ca^{2+}. It was concluded that the mechanism of neuromuscular relaxation in kava was similar to that of local anesthetics: by a direct blocking effect on ion channels of the muscle.

Analgesia Analgesic effects of kava components have been investigated in mice (Jamieson and Duffield 1990). Kava extract and kavalactones were both found to effectively produce analgesia that was not mediated by opioid mechanisms, because it was not reversed by naloxone. Although speculative, the GABAergic and monoamine actions of kava could account for its analgesic effects.

Neuroprotective effect At last, kavain has been examined for its neuroprotective effect. The neuroprotective effect is probably mediated by its blocking of voltage-gated Na^{+} and Ca^{2+} channels. Similar to other neuroprotective Na^{+} channel blockers (i.e., tetrodotoxin), kavain inhibits the metabolic consequences of anoxia in neurons (Gleitz et al. 1996b). Kava was found to diminish the volume and area of infarcted tissue in mice, which was probably mediated by methysticin and dihydromethysticin (Backhauss and Krieglstein 1992).

Electrophysiological and cognitive effects The effects of kava on brain electrophysiology were investigated in cats (Holm et al. 1991). Kavain produces high-amplitude delta activity, spindlelike formations, and continuous alpha or beta activity in the amygdala. Similar to barbiturates, kavain prolongs synchronized sleep.

The effects of kavain on human electrophysiology was examined in a double-blind, placebo-controlled study (Frey 1991). Dose-dependent increases were seen in delta, theta, and alpha 1 power, and decreases ocurred in alpha 2 and beta power. These changes were suggestive of a sedative effect of kavain, and were maximal in frontal areas. Interestingly, an initial activating effect was seen at the lowest dose (200 mg) but not at the largest dose (600 mg).

Event-related potentials (ERPs) were used to study the cognitive effects of kava, as compared to oxazepam (Münte et al. 1993). In a double-blind crossover study, subjects were given a verbal memory task (word recognition). While oxazepam impaired performance, kava actually improved performance. Whereas oxazepam caused a poorer recognition rate and reduced the electrophysiological difference between old and new words, kava increased the new/old difference and led to a slightly improved recognition rate. Another double-blind study used ERPs to examine the effects of a kava root extract on visual search (Heinze et al. 1994). Again, whereas oxazepam reduced task-associated potentials in frontal, parietal, and occipital areas, kava was associated with increases.

A study of the cognitive effects of kava on psychometric tests was undertaken by Foo and Lemon (1997). They employed a number of measures to assess attention, reaction time, visuomotor tracking, and short-term memory. Of several measures given, kava only produced minor effects on the digit symbol task, but no other tests of attention or concentration. Unlike ethanol, kava produced no effects on subjective measures of impairment given to the subjects. However, when given together, kava and ethanol potentiated each other's effects on subjective and objective cognitive measures.

Antiseizure effects Kavalactones have been investigated for their antiseizure effects in animals (Kretzschmar et al. 1969; Jamieson et al. 1989; Gleitz et al. 1995, 1996a). This action appears to be mediated by suppression of voltage-gated ion channels, although a contribution from their GABAergic or noradrenergic activity could contribute. Inhibition of ion channels and facilitating of GABA activity are mechanisms shared by many antiseizure medications. Kavain was found to reduce excitatory activity in hippocampal slices, but not to affect long-term potentiation or synaptic plasticity (Langosch et al. 1998). However, kava extracts were found to only have a weak effect on strychnine-induced seizures (Jamieson et al. 1989). Concentrations of 10–100 µM/L of methysticin had antiseizure effects in slices of hippocampus and entorhinal cortex.

Although there is some evidence for an antiseizure effect of kava, it is not clear whether these effects extend to humans. There have not been any studies that have demonstrated its effectiveness in clinically controlling seizures. Individuals who are being treated for epilepsy are urged not to attempt to replace their current medications with kava, and especially not without the direction of a physician.

Anxiolytic effects Several methodologically controlled studies have been performed to assess the anti-anxiety effects of kava. The studies employed standardized doses of kavalactones ranging from 60 to 240 mg per day, and were 4 to 24 weeks in duration (Pittler and Ernst 2000). Subjects presented with anxiety symptoms that were diagnosed with criteria from the DSM-III-R, and/or several psychometric measures of anxiety (Hamilton Anxiety Scale and Adjective Check List [of Janke and Debus], Anxiety Status Inventory and Zung's Self-Rating Anxiety Scale, and State-Trait Anxiety Inventory). A review and meta-analysis of methodologically controlled studies of kava for treating anxiety was undertaken by Pittler and Ernst (2000). They found kava to be superior to placebo across all seven controlled studies. A meta-analysis of three studies that used the Hamilton Anxiety Scale found a significant reduction in anxiety.

Some studies found kava to be effective using only 2 acute doses (preoperatively), while others found benefit after chronic doses (Bhate et al. 1989; Lehmann et al. 1989; Volz and Kieser 1997). Another interesting study found kavain to be equivalent in efficacy to the benzodiazepine oxazepam on standard measures of anxiety (Anxiety Status Inventory and Zung's Self-Rating Anxiety Scale) (Lindenberg and Pitule-Schodel 1990). There were no serious side effects reported in the clinical studies reviewed by Pittler and Ernst (2000).

Toxicity

No health hazards are known with the proper use of kava (Gruenwald et al. 1998). Kava has been approved by the German Commission E for treatment of anxiety and insomnia. In clinical studies of kava for anxiety, adverse effects were uncommon and did not differ across placebo and kava groups.

There do not appear to be any studies published on the effects of acute overdosage with kava. Given its CNS depressant effects, it should not be taken with other similar drugs, including benzodiazepines, barbiturates, ethanol, or antiseizure medications. Animal research shows an interaction between kava and ethanol, increasing the toxicity of kava (Jamieson and Duffield 1990). There is one clinical report of combined administration of kava and the benzodiazepine alprazolam (Almeida and Grimsley 1996). A 54-year-old man taking the two presented in a disoriented and lethargic state that resolved after several hours. The use of kava during pregnancy has not been formally studied.

Kava dermopathy A scaly skin eruption called kava dermopathy is reported to occur from kava use (Norton and Ruze 1994). It is reversible, and appears to only occur with heavy chronic use. A suspected contribution of niacin deficiency to kava dermopathy was ruled out (Ruze 1990).

Parksinsonism Four cases were reported of dyskinesia presenting with kava use in individuals (Schelosky et al. 1995). These consisted of dystonia, tonic head rotation, twisting of the trunk, oculogyric crises, and increased duration of "off" periods in a parkinsonian patient. These symptoms subsided with discontinuation of kava and treatment with a cholinergic muscarinic antagonist (biperiden). The authors suggest that this represents a dopamine antagonist action of kava, and raise caution about its use in the elderly.

Summary

Kava is an herbal drug known for centuries through the South Pacific islands, with therapeutic, social, and cultural uses. Its chemical constituents, the kavalactones, create psychoactive effects by altering central GABA transmission, blocking voltage-gated ion channels (Na^+ and Ca^{2+}), monoamine mechanisms, and possibly eicosanoid systems. Although kavalactones create significant effects individually, they exhibit pharmacokinetic synergy, reaching higher brain concentrations when administered collectively. Kava's long-reputed effect for creating relaxation is supported pharmacologically, and a few controlled studies have confirmed its usefulness in treating anxiety. Formal studies on improving sleep have not been conducted, but are warranted. There appears to be little toxicity with proper use of kava. Perhaps one of the most useful

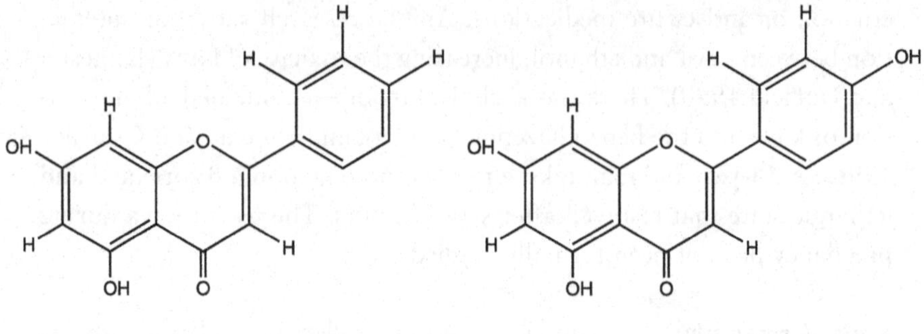

Chrysin

Apigenin

Figure 6.6
Chemical structure of chrysin and apigenin.

properties is that it produces a relaxed but alert state in lower doses, with minimal effects on cognition.

Passionflower

History and Botany

There are a few members of the passionflower family (Passifloraceae) that have psychotropic effects. The one most studied is *Passiflora incarnata*, although some work has been done on *Passiflora coerulea* and *Passiflora edulis. P. incarnata* is a colorful, flowering plant with five white or lavender petals, a purple or pink corona, and five brightly colored stamen (Gruenwald et al. 1998). The parts of the plants used for medicinal effect are the whole plant or aerial parts. It is native to the mid- to southeastern United States. Passionflower has a history with Native Americans as a poultice to treat bruises, and as a tea for sedative/anxiolytic effects (Kowalchick and Hylton 1987). It is one of the most common herbs commercially available in Britain (Tyler 1994).

Chemical Constituents

There are three categories of constituents in passionflower: flavonoids, maltol, and indole alkaloids. Among flavonoids are chrysin (5,7-dihydroxyflavone), vitexin, coumerin, and umbelliferone (figure 6.6). The greatest accumulation of flavonoids occurs in the leaves (Menghini and

Mancini 1988). Flavonoids vary across the ontogenic cycle, with the highest concentration of isovitexin occurring between preflowering and flowering stages. The indole alkaloids are small amounts (up to 0.01%), including harman, harmine, harmaline, and harmalol (Tyler 1994).

Mechanisms of Action

Perhaps the most studied constituent of passionflower is the flavonoid chrysin. Chrysin was isolated from *P. coerulea*, a species closely related to *P. incarnata*. It binds to benzodiazepine receptors with micromolar affinity ($K_i = 3$ μM) and competes for binding with the benzodiazepine flunitrazepam (Medina et al. 1990). Behavioral assays (see below) suggest that chrysin acts as a partial agonist at central benzodiazepine receptors (Wolfman et al. 1994).

Other flavones in passionflower (vitexin, coumerin, umbelliferone) have not been well characterized for their neuropharmacological action. Vitexin (derived from millet in one study) was found to have antithyroid properties. The remaining constituents, maltol and harman alkaloids, are present in small quantities and not presumed to contribute to the psychotropic effects (Meier 1995). Harman alkaloids in greater quantities are hallucinogenic and presumed to work through 5-HT receptors (Grella et al. 1998).

Physiological Effects

Sedative and anxiolytic effects A number of flavonoids have been shown to bind to benzodiazepine receptors and have anxiolytic effects (Medina et al. 1997). The anxiolytic effects of chrysin were examined in mice (Wolfman et al. 1994). Chrysin (1 mg/kg IP) reduces behavioral measures of anxiety (elevated-plus maze) in a manner similar to diazepam (0.3–0.6 mg/kg), which was reversed by pretreatment with a benzodiazepine antagonist, Ro 15-1788. The anxiolytic effect is not likely due to sedation because there is no concurrent reduction in motor activity at the doses used. Unlike diazepam, chrysin does not produce muscle relaxation at higher doses.

The sedative and anxiolytic effects of passionflower were examined in two other animal behavioral assays (staircase test, light/dark box choice test). Both anxiolytic and sedative effects occur, as well as potentiation of pentobarbital sedation, at 400 mg/kg of hydroalcoholic extract in mice (Soulimani et al. 1997). The anxiolytic and sedative activity occur in a dose-dependent continuum (Della Logia et al. 1981). *Passiflora edulis* has sedative effects as well (Maluf et al. 1991).

Despite neuropharmacolgical and animal data to support sedative and anxiolytic effects of passionflower, there have not been any such controlled studies in humans. Two studies have been published that examined the effects of combined herbal extracts on anxiety, including passionflower (Bourin et al. 1997). Although there were significant and experimentally controlled effects, a combined herbal treatment confounds the ability to selectively identify the effects of passionflower. A second controlled study was similarly confounded by the use of a three-herb combination (Gerhard et al. 1991).

General physiological effects Physiological and electrophysiological changes in response to chronic passionflower treatment were studied in the rat (Sopranzi et al. 1990). There was no change in body weight, core body temperature, motor coordination, or analgesia (as measured by the tail-flick test). There was some general reduction of activity (in the one-arm radial maze), but the EEG appeared normal.

Cognitive effects A study of the effects of chrysin on memory was performed in the rat (Salgueiro et al. 1997). Chrysin does not have any amnestic effects on either acquisition or retention in three tests of memory (inhibitory avoidance, shuttle avoidance, and habituation to an open field), even at higher doses than required to produce anxiolytic effects. The cognitive effects of passionflower have not been examined in humans.

Analgesic effects Although pharmaceutical benzodiazepine drugs and certain flavones have analgesic effects, chrysin and vitexin do not (Salgueiro et al. 1997; Rylski et al. 1979). However, an extract of *Passiflora incarnata*, administered orally or IP did raise nociceptive thresholds, raising the possibility of nonchrysin analgesic flavones present in *P. incarnata* (Speroni and Minghetti 1988). Chrysin was shown to reduce morphine withdrawal in a physiological assay (guinea pig ileum contraction) in a dose-dependent manner (Capasso et al. 1998).

Antiseizure effects One study examined antiseizure effects of chrysin on chemically induced (pentylenetetrazol) seizures in mice (Medina et al. 1997). Peripheral (IP) administration produced inconsistent effects, but central (intracerebroventricular) injection (40 μg) had a significant anticonvulsant effect. Further, this effect was abolished by prior injection of the benzodiazepine antagonist, Ro 15-1788 (3 mg/kg IP).

Toxicity

There have been no formal studies of the toxicity of passionflower, but adverse effects have not been reported. There is one report of a case of inflammatory vasculitis associated with a preparation of passionflower (Smith et al. 1993). Like other herbs in this category, its putative benzodiazepine action contraindicates its combined use with other CNS depressants.

Chamomile

History and Botany

Chamomile refers to two similar species of plants: German chamomile *(Matricaria recutita)* and Roman Chamomile *(Chamaemelum nobile)*, both of which are members of the Asteraceae family (figure 6.7). *C. nobile* is a low-growing perennial herb, while *M. recutita* is a tall, annual plant (Kowalchick and Hylton 1987). Chamomile has been used throughout history, including ancient Egyptian, Roman, and Greek cultures. The two species look very much like daisies, with white petals and a yellow central disc. They are both native to Europe, Africa, and Asia and have been naturalized in North America. The most common form of ingestion is to dry the flowering tops and brew them in a tea. Although there are many reported uses of chamomile, it is best known for its antispasmodic, anti-inflammatory, and mild calming effects (Leyel 1994; Gruenwald et al. 1998).

Chemical Constituents

Chamomile contains the terpenoids (−)-alpha-bisabolol, (−)-alpha-bisabololoxides A and B, and a gauianolide lactone called matricin. Also contained are the flavonoids apigenin and apigenin-7-glucoside (see figure 6.6) (Tyler 1994; Robbers et al. 1996). Apigenin was found

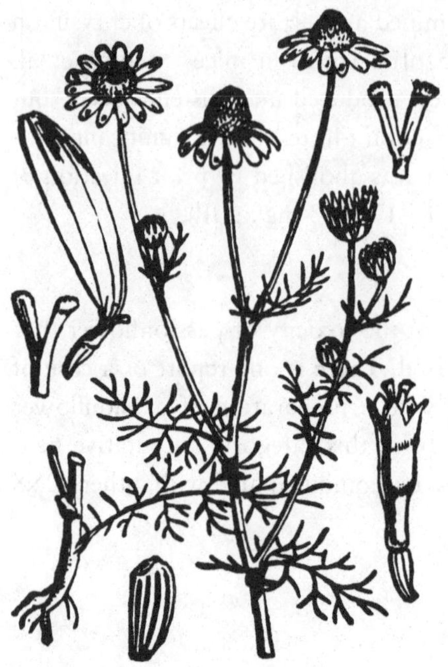

Figure 6.7
Chamomile *(Matricaria recutita)*. Reprinted from Culbreth DMR. (1927). *Materia Medica and Pharmacognosy*, 7th ed. Philadelphia: Lea & Febiger.

to have low solubility in hydrophilic or nonpolar solvents (Li et al. 1997). Thus, nonaqueous extracts would contain far more than a tea preparation.

Mechanisms of Action and Physiological Effects
The sedative and anxiolytic effects of chamomile are likely mediated by the ability of apigenin to bind to benzodiazepine receptors (Viola et al. 1995). It binds with micromolar affinity at benzodiazepine receptors (4 μM), but has no effect at muscarinic, α_1 adrenergic receptors, or the GABA binding site of the $GABA_A$ channel. Apigenin has anxiolytic effects in mice in a behavioral assay (the elevated plus maze), but no anti-seizure effects occur (Viola et al. 1995). At doses ten times greater than required for anxiolytic effects, apigenin showed mild sedative effects (in ambulatory locomotor activity and the hole-board test). No myorelaxant effects were noticed.

A study of the effects of apigenin on memory was performed in the rat (Salgueiro et al. 1997). It does not show any amnestic effects on either acquisition or retention in three tests of memory (inhibitory avoidance, shuttle avoidance, and habituation to an open field), even at doses higher than those required to produce anxiolytic effects.

Studies of apigenin on the rat thoracic aorta have found apigenin to have vasodilatory effects (Ko et al. 1991). This effect was probably mediated by an inhibition of voltage- and ligand-gated Ca^{2+} channels. It would be interesting to see if this effect also occurs in the CNS.

There is some evidence for apigenin actions on the monoamine systems. Apigenin was found to stimulate uptake of tyrosine into adrenal chromaffin cells in a concentration-dependent manner, resulting in increased monoamine production (Morita et al. 1990). Apigenin was also found to be a competitive inhibitor of a protein-tyrosine kinase (p40) (Kellis and Vickery 1984). Finally, apigenin was found to inhibit MAO, and to inhibit uptake of norepinephrine in the rat atria (Lorenzo et al. 1996). Again, it would be interesting to see if these effects extend to the CNS and chamomile's psychotropic effects, especially when administered peripherally, and if they have behaviorally significant actions in the amounts derived from common over-the-counter preparations.

There is some literature that examines flavonoids such as apigenin as ligands for the estrogen beta receptor, and as an inhibitor of the enzyme estrogen synthetase (aromatase) (Kuiper et al. 1998; Kellis and Vickery 1984). These compounds do so potently, but the behavioral significance of amounts observed in common preparations needs to be further investigated.

Apigenin has been found to inhibit release of histamine (Middleton and Drzewiecki 1984). Although inhibition of histamine by apigenin could potentially have psychotropic effects, it would need to be demonstrated that this effect occurs in the CNS (Loring and Meador 1989; Kim et al. 1996). This may not be the case, because apigenin's effect on histamine release is dependent on immunoglobulin antigens (Middleton and Drzewiecki 1984).

Thus, the best candidate for chamomile's psychotropic effects is the activity of apigenin at benzodiazepine receptors. There are other potential mechanisms that may contribute to its effects, but they need to be further investigated for the magnitude of their contribution.

Toxicity
Chamomile appears very low in toxicity. It has been listed as Generally Regarded as Safe (GRAS) by the Food and Drug Administration (Tyler 1994). Adverse reactions may include allergic reactions to the pollen in the flowers (Kowalchick and Hylton 1987; Subiza et al. 1990).

Remaining Sedative and Anxioltyic Herbs

There are several remaining herbs that are reputed to have sedative effects: skullcap, geranium, hops, and catnip. However, the neuropharmacological mechanisms have not been well characterized, and behavioral data in animals and humans are lacking. The existing knowledge on these plants is presented here.

Catnip

Catnip *(Nepeta cataria)* is a coarse green-grey leaved perennial plant with spotted white tubular flowers (Kowalchick and Hylton 1987). It has a long recorded history of use, extending back to ancient Roman civilization. Among its many reported uses, catnip is noted for sedative properties. The active agent for this effect is uncertain, but catnip has in it several terpenes, including nepetalactone. One terpene, *cis-trans*-nepetalactone was hypothesized to be responsible for the sedative effect based on its structural similarity to valepotriates, the depressant principles from valerian.

Paradoxically, catnip fed to mice had stimulant effects, with increased rearing, locomotion, and stereotypical behavior, increased susceptibility to chemically induced (picrotoxin and strychnine) seizures, and decreased sleeping time after barbiturate administration (Massoco et al. 1995). The LD_{50} for nepetalactone in mice was reported to be quite high at 1300 mg/kg (Harney et al. 1978). In chicks, an alcohol extract of catnip had biphasic effects, where low to moderate doses (25–1800 mg/kg) produced sedative effects, while higher doses (>2 g/kg) had less sedative and perhaps stimulant effects (Sherry and Hunter 1979). Humans have reported sedative effects of catnip, and one accidental ingestion by a young child reportedly produced sedative effects (Osterhoudt et al. 1997).

The inconsistencies in the effects of catnip could be attributed to a few possible causes. As Sherry and Hunter illustrated (1979), the effects could be biphasic and thus dose dependent. Another possibility is interspecies differences. A more dramatic illustration of this is in the reaction that cats have to catnip (Siegel 1989). Cats will sniff, lick, and chew the leaves of the plant, followed by short periods of blank staring into space and shaking the head from side to side. Next they will rub their body against the plant and some fall over and roll in it. When introduced to catnip, cats will later return to the site where they encountered it. These behaviors indicate a pleasurable state, and both male and females may adopt mating postures with erections occurring in the males. Nepetalactones are believed to mimic a scent in cat urine that triggers sexual behaviors. The sexual nature of the feline response to catnip is suggestive of pheromonal activity at the vomeronasal organ (VNO). The VNO is a chemical sense organ found in the nasal sinuses that is involved in sexual behaviors and hormonal effects, and not the sense of smell (Halpern 1987). Counterintuitively though, the effects of catnip on felines is mediated by the main olfactory system, and not the VNO (Hart and Leedy 1985).

There was some association of hallucinogenic effects with catnip in humans, particularly through administration by smoking. This was reported in a 1969 paper, but apparently resulted from confusion with cannabis (Tyler 1994). Any reports of hallucinogenic or sedative effects of catnip in humans, at this point, are purely anecdotal.

Hops

Hop *(Humulus lupulus)* is a flowering vine that grows in Europe, Western Asia, and North America, and is reported to have anxiolytic/sedative effects (figure 6.8) (Kowalchik and Hylton 1987). It is an ingredient of beer, but is also consumed as a tea. The female flowers are placed in a pillow to treat insomnia by their fragrance. It has not been well studied, but the responsible agent is believed to be 2-methyl-3-butene-2-ol, because it produces sedation when injected intraperitoneally in mice (Hänsel et al. 1980). In humans, one study found no CNS depressant effects when administered orally (Hänsel and Wagener 1967). However, the effects produced by inhalation (thus avoiding digestion and absorption issues), have not been studied.

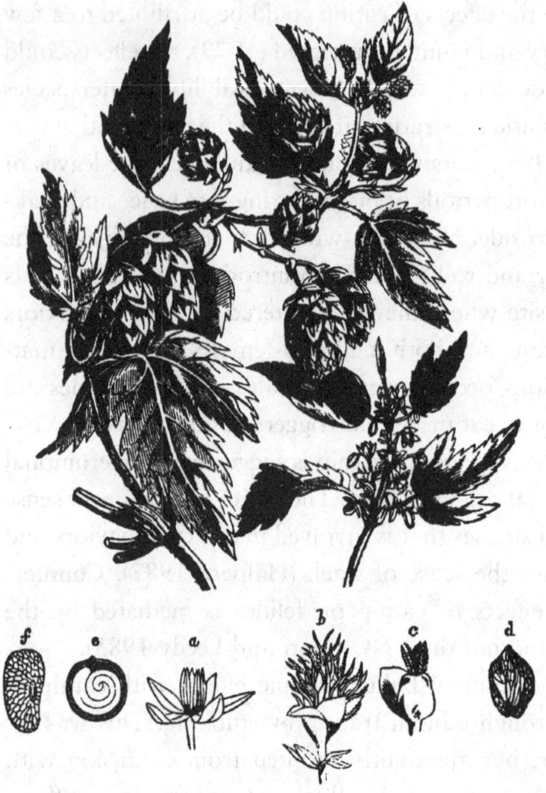

Figure 6.8
Hops *(Humulus lupus)*. Reprinted from Culbreth DMR. (1927). *Materia Medica and Pharmacognosy*, 7th ed. Philadelphia: Lea & Febiger.

Skullcap

Skullcap *(Scutellaria lateriflora)* is an herb that has been used in Chinese and Western medicine for sedative and antiseizure effects (Wong et al. 1998). Its pharmacological and behavioral effects have not been established in animals or humans.

Lemon Balm

Lemon balm *(Melissa officinalis)* is an upright flowering perennial, and a member of the mint family (Kowalchick and Hylton 1987). It is reputed to have anxiolytic effects in humans, but no formal studies have been done. In mice, lemon balm has sedative effects in familiar (staircase test) and unfamiliar (two-compartment test) environments, and to have analgesic activity (writhing test) (Soulimani et al. 1991). It also increased the sedative activity of a barbiturate (pentobarbital). Although these effects are promising, further work would be needed to identify active constituents and confirm whether effects occur in humans.

Geranium

There are several members of the Geranium family (Geraniaceae), some of which have been anecdotally reported to have anxiolytic or sedative effects. However, there is a paucity of research to support the use of this herb as a CNS depressant (Manolov et al. 1977; Tasev et al. 1969).

Summary and Conclusions

There are several herbs with CNS depressant effects that have been used mostly for anxiolytic and sedative effects historically. This has been supported by neuropharmacological, animal, and human studies (table 6.1). In some cases, the herbs meet Class I criteria for therapeutic treatment (table 6.4). Much work remains to be done in further testing the efficacy of these drugs and more firmly delineating their biochemical mechanisms.

Several other herbs have weaker evidence for CNS depressant effects, but hold potential for further research and evaluation. Certain herbs have also had historical use for treating epilepsy, before the invention of several modern, very effective synthetic antiseizure medications. There is, at present, absolutely no evidence that the CNS depressant herbs will be effective or sufficient in the treatment of epilepsy. Much further research would be needed to support this contention. Further, withdrawal of current antiseizure medications would put an individual at high risk for recurrence or worsening of seizures.

7

Psychotherapeutic Herbs

Long before the advent of modern pharmaceutical drugs, several herbal medications were employed for the alleviation of mental disorders. Some of these are considered impractical by today's standards for treatment of psychopathology. For a short time, Freud advocated the use of cocaine to alleviate depression. Cannabis and opium were used to treat agitation. Other herbal medications are being supported by scientific research and seriously considered by the medical community. Some are offered here more for historical interest, and yet others have only recently added psychotherapeutic value to their list of potential benefits.

As will be discussed in detail here, these herbs may create several effects, due to multiple neuropharmacological actions or even due to a single action. For the sake of convenience, the herbs have been broadly classified here into antidepressant/anxiolytic and antipsychotic categories due to their frequently overlapping effects.

The Psychopharmacological Era

The twentieth century has witnessed a revolution in the discovery of drugs for the treatment of mental illness (Baldessarini 1996; Lickey and Gordon 1991). Formerly, many drug treatments were either ineffective or nonspecific. The first modern psychopharmacological treatment came from the Australian psychiatrist John F. J. Cade, who proposed the use of lithium salts to treat bipolar disorder. Although slow to gain acceptance, lithium has become a standard treatment. In 1950, chlorpromazine was synthesized in France and successfully tested for treatment of psychotic agitation. The first antidepressant drug, iproniazid, was originally developed to treat tuberculosis and serendipitously found to have antidepressant effects in the late 1950s. Meprobamate was introduced as an anxiolytic in the mid-1950s. Although it has fallen into disuse, it heralded the discovery of a series of modern sedative and anxiolytic drugs.

The discovery of psychopharmacological medications was revolutionary because they provided a means of treating illnesses that were otherwise intractable. With the exception of electroconvulsive treatments for severe depression, there were no medical treatments for disorders that did not respond to psychotherapy. Once established, the drugs led to an ongoing search for more effective and safer medications. A second reason for their revolutionary status is that they furthered understanding of mental illnesses and normal brain function. Investigations of their therapeutic mechanisms led to theories of the neurochemical bases of mental illnesses.

The advent of clincal psychopharmacology had an enormous socioeconomic impact as well. The number of patients residing in psychiatric hospitals had been steadily increasing in the United States to a peak of 550,000 following World War II (Lickey and Gordon 1991). Since the introduction of psychotherapeutic medications, there has been a steady decline to 111,000 by 1986. Drug treatments allowed for briefer hospital stays. Unfortunately, there was a gap in social services for some time, when adequate follow-up care was not provided to the mentally ill who were released from hospitals but still not functionally independent. Nonetheless, the discovery of psychotherapeutic drugs has alleviated unquantifiable amounts of human suffering. With careful research, some herbal medications may add to this effort.

Depression and Anxiety

Major depression is one of the most common mental disorders. It has a lifetime prevalence of 17% in the general population, and a current prevalence of 4.9%, constituting a significant public health problem (Blazer et al. 1994). It is characterized by intense sadness and cognitive impairments most notable in concentration, worry, pessimism, and lowered self-esteem (American Psychiatric Association 1994). Interpersonal relationships may suffer and social withdrawal occurs. Physiological changes are common in homeostatic functions such as appetite, sleep, sex drive, and hormonal levels. Although sadness and grief are normal emotions, major depression is a pathological condition that is distinguished by its duration and severity. Unike normal emotions, major depression lacks the adaptive benefits that normal emotions provide, and causes a resulting impairment in social and occupational functioning.

Anxiety disorders are a collection of heterogeneous disorders including panic disorder, phobias, obsessive-compulsive disorder, posttraumatic stress disorder, and generalized anxiety disorder (APA 1994). What they all share is anxiety as a principal symptom—in greater frequency or degree than normal experience and leading to behavioral maladjustment. Anxiety includes a subjective component with feelings of dread, emotional tension, and worry. Behavioral manifestations include avoidace of anxiety-producing situations, motor impairment, and cognitive impairment (e.g., inability to concentrate). Physiological manifestations of anxiety include muscle tension and sympathetic autonomic reactions such as increased heart rate and blood pressure, sweating, dry mouth, nausea, dizziness, and diarrhea. Although low levels of anxiety are adaptive, their severity, frequency, and duration make them maladaptive in anxiety disorders.

Pharmaceutical Antidepressants and Anxiolytics

There are numerous antidepressant medications on the market (table 7.1). Following development of monoamine oxidase (MAO) inhibitors were tricyclic antidepressants, selective serotonin reuptake inhibitors (SSRIs), and several atypical antidepressants (Baldessarini 1996). Successive generations of antidepressants have not necessarily become more effective in treating depression, but rather offer more favorable side-effect profiles—a crucial factor in effective clinical pharmacotherapy. An effective medication is not useful if its side effects are intolerable.

The variety of antidepressant agents developed all seem to share one commonality: alteration of monoamine systems (Bolden-Watson and Richelson 1993; Bonhomme and Esposito 1998). Only very recently have drugs that work outside of monoamine systems been shown to have reliable antidepressant effects.

Table 7.1
Examples of pharmaceutical antidepressant drugs

Class	Generic name	Trade name	Mechanism
MAOI	Phenelzine	Nardil	MAO inhibition
	Tranylcypromine	Parnate	MAO inhibition
	Moclobemide	Aurorex	MAO_A inhibition
Tricyclic	Imipramine	Tofranil	Reuptake inhibition (NE > 5-HT)
	Amitriptyline	Elavil	Reuptake inhibition (5-HT > NE)
	Clomipramine	Anafranil	Reuptake inhibition (5-HT > NE)
	Nortriptyline	Pamelor	Reuptake inhibition (5-HT > NE)
	Desipramine	Norpramin	Reuptake inhibition (NE ≫ 5-HT)
SSRI	Fluoxetine	Prozac	Reuptake inhibition (5-HT)
	Sertraline	Zoloft	Reuptake inhibition (5-HT)
	Paroxetine	Paxil	Reuptake inhibition (5-HT)
	Fluvoxamine	Luvox	Reuptake inhibition (5-HT)
	Citalopram	Celexa	Reuptake inhibition (5-HT)
Atypical	Nefazodone	Serzone	Reuptake inh. (5-HT), 5-HT_2 antagonist
	Mirtazapine	Remeron	α_2 antagonist, 5-HT_2 & 5-HT_3 antagonist
	Bupropion	Wellbutrin	Reuptake inhibition (NE, DA)
	Venlafaxine	Effexor	Reuptake inhibition (5-HT, NE)
Antagonists	Ondansetron	Zofran	5-HT_3 antagonist
	Mianserin	—	5-HT_2 antagonist

Source: Adapted from Baldessarini 1996; Julien 1997; Cooper et al. 1996; Stahl 1998.

The MAO inhibitors irreversibly bind to mitochondrial MAO, preventing oxidative deamination of the monoamines dopamine, norepinephrine, and serotonin. These bind to both forms of MAO (MAO_A and MAO_B) and include the drugs phenelzine, tranylcypromine, and isocarboxazid (Baldessarini 1996). These drugs also prevent hepatic breakdown of tyramine (a substance found in many foods such as aged cheese, red wine, and figs) by MAO_B, which can precipitate a hypertensive crisis. A newer class of reversible, short-acting MAO inhibitors (e.g., moclobemide) are being investigated that are selective to MAO_A, and thus do not have the same tyramine toxicity problems. Thus, the antidepressant effect of MAO inhibitors is believed to lie in their ability to increase available monoamines.

Tricyclic drugs have, as the name implies, a three-ring structure, and interfere with reuptake of norepinephrine and/or serotonin into axon terminals. Tricyclic drugs include imipramine (Tofranil), amitriptyline (Elavil), clomipramine (Anafranil), and nortriptyline (Pamelor, Aventil). Tricyclics have the occasional but unfortunate cardiovascular side effects of arrhythmia and postural hypotension. Newer, nontricyclic antidepressants have been developed that are collectively referred to as SSRIs. These have a potent and selective action on serotonin, and lack the cardiovascular side effects of the tricyclics. These include fluoxetine (Prozac), paroxetine (Paxil), sertraline (Zoloft), and fluvoxamine (Luvox). A fifth SSRI, citalopram (Celexa) has been used in Europe and has recently been approved in the United States. Venlafaxine (Effexor) blocks reuptake of norepinephrine and serotonin, while bupropion (Wellbutrin) acts on both dopamine and norepinephrine.

Mirtazapine (Remeron) is a newer antidepressant that also blocks 5-HT reuptake, but additionally has antagonistic effects at adrenergic α_2, 5-HT_2, and 5-HT_3 receptors (Stahl 1998). Mirtazapine appears to have indirect agonistic effects on 5-HT_{1A} receptors, which may contribute to its antidepressant effect (Berendsen and Broekkamp 1997). Nefazodone, as well, has SSRI and 5-HT_2 antagonist effects. The 5-HT_2 antagonist effects of these antidepressants is believed to be responsible for their lower incidence of sexual side effects (Nutt 1997).

In addition to acute effects, chronic use of antidepressants causes chronic receptor adaptations. For example, venlafaxine blocks reuptake of serotonin and norepinephrine and chronically causes a reduction of β_1 adrenergic receptors in frontal cortex (McGrath and Norman 1998). Imipramine causes alterations in serotonin release in both raphe nuclei and frontal cortex (Maione et al. 1997). Both imipramine and fluoxetine alter the expression of dopamine receptors (Dziedzicka-Wasylewska et al. 1997). Chronic administration of SSRIs and MAO inhibitors desensitizes 5-HT_{1A} and 5-$HT_{1B/1D}$ receptors (Bonhomme and Esposito 1998; Le Poul et al. 1997). Others have shown a tonic activation of 5-HT_{1A} receptors after chronic treatment with antidepressant drugs (Maione et al. 1997; Haddjeri et al. 1998). Although there does not appear to be a single unifying hypothesis that accounts for all of the effects created by the diverse mechanisms of antidepressant drugs, increased function in monoamine systems and receptor modulation are consistent findings (Bonhomme and Esposito 1998; Maione et al. 1997).

In summary, the antidepressant drugs discussed here all have a common effect on monoamine systems, either by preventing enzyme degradation, blocking reuptake, or direct receptor effects. Also common to all of these drugs is the lag of 2–3 weeks for therapeutic effects to begin after treatment is started. It is likely that the actual antidepressant mechanism of these medications is the receptor alterations. Reuptake occurs immediately after taking the drug, but the therapeutic effects correlate well with chronic receptor adaptations.

There is a high comorbidity of depression and anxiety, suggestive of common neurobiological substrates (Rodney et al. 1997; Flint 1994; Gorman 1996–97; Enns et al. 1998; Eison MS 1990; Montgomery 1983; Paul 1988). Therefore, it is not surprising that pharmacological treatments that address one disorder may have ameliorative effects on the other. Indeed, some antidepressants have been tested for effectiveness in treating generalized anxiety disorder and were found to be as effective (trazodone) or better (imipramine) than diazepam (Rickels et al. 1993; Schweizer et al. 1998).

Other serotonergic drugs that are direct receptor agonists or antagonists have been found to have anxiolytic effects (Stahl 1998; Bonhomme and Esposito 1998). A novel class of anxiolytic drugs called azapirones act as partial agonists at 5-HT_{1A} receptors (Yocca 1990). Clinically, they are represented by BuSpar, which was approved for use in 1986 (Eison

AS 1990). Several 5-HT_{1A} agonists have been found to produce anxiolytic effects in animal models and in human clinical trials (File et al. 1996; Krummel and Kathol 1987; Goldberg and Finnerty 1979). Furthermore, they have antidepressant effects; they augment the antidepressant effects of serotonin reuptake inhibitors, and they decrease the therapeutic latency (Bouwer and Stein 1997; Artigas et al. 1996; Sussman 1998; Rickels et al. 1991; Wieland and Lucki 1990; Jenkins et al. 1990; Fabre 1990). However, results have not been uniformly positive, such as in refractory severe depression (Sussman 1998; Fischer et al. 1998)

Drugs acting as antagonists at 5-HT_2 receptors have been found to have antidepressant and anxiolytic effects, including the antidepressant nefazodone (Deakin 1988; Martin and Lemonnier 1994; Graeff et al. 1996). Mianserin is a more selective 5-HT_2 antagonist, which is undergoing the FDA drug approval process. It has been shown to have antidepressant and anxiolytic effects (Granier et al. 1985; Brogden et al. 1978; Murphy 1978). 5-HT_3 antagonists, such as ondansetron, have been developed as antiemetic drugs, primarily due to the role of 5-HT_3 receptors in emesis (Costall and Naylor 1992). 5-HT_3 receptors involved in this effect are found in the human brain stem (area postrema, dorsal vagal complex) and enteric nervous system. However, 5-HT_3 receptors are also located in the hippocampus, amygdala, nucleus accumbens and basal ganglia (Parker et al. 1996; Abi-Dargham et al. 1993). 5-HT_3 antagonists have shown some antidepressant and nonsedating anxiolytic effects in animal models, and hold potential for application to humans (Martin et al. 1992; Costall et al. 1990; Bloom and Morales 1998). There is also some physiological and anecdotal evidence to suggest that 5-HT_3 antagonists might serve as adjuncts to pharmacotherapy of schizophrenia (Gerlach 1991; Greenshaw and Silverstone 1997; Greenshaw 1993).

One final mechanism that has recently shown promise for antidepressant effects appears distinct from all of the monoamine systems. A study published in 1998 demonstrated that a substance P antagonist (MK-869) had antidepressant effects in humans (Kramer et al. 1998). Substance P is localized to many areas of the brain that are involved in emotional processing, including the amygdala, dentate gyrus, subiculum, nucleus accumbens, striatum, locus coeruleus and periaqueductal grey (Kramer et al. 1998; Quirion et al. 1983). Substance P antagonists have shown antidepressant effects in animal models, and levels of substance P are reduced in forebrain areas after chronic treatment with antidepressants (Kramer et al. 1998, Shirayama et al. 1996). Conversely, withdrawal of chronic antidepressant treatment increases sensitivity to substance P in the cingulate gyrus (Jones and Olpe 1984).

Although several putative anxiolytic herbs are discussed in chapter 6, a select few are discussed here because of their similarity to antidepressant medications in terms of neuropharmacological activity, and because of the close relationship between depression, anxiety, and their pharmacological treatment in general. Whereas the anxiolytic herbs discussed previously have anxiolytic effects through more-general CNS depressant actions, the ones discussed here seem to have more-specific actions, particularly on serotonin.

Psychotic Disorders

Schizophrenia is a group of psychotic disorders characterized by several key disturbances: cognitive, emotional, and behavioral (American Psychiatric Association 1994; Goodwin and Guze 1996). Symptoms have been traditionally divided into positive and negative. Positive symptoms are excesses, which include hallucinations and delusions. Negative symtoms consist of deficits in psychological function. Among these are such cognitive disturbances as difficulties in logical and abstract thinking, attention, thought organization, lack of volition, affective flattening, and social withdrawal.

The duration and nature of the psychotic disorder present determines which diagnosis is given: schizophrenia, schizophreniform, or brief psychotic disorder. Schizoaffective disorder is diagnosed when there is a significant concurrent mood disturbance such as major depression, mania, or bipolar disorder. Delusional disorder is a condition where nonbizarre delusions persist for at least one month, but other symptoms of schizophrenia are not present. Subtypes of schizophrenia are recognized, which are defined by their predominant symptoms. These include paranoid, disorganized, and catatonic types. Catatonic schizophrenia is characterized by maintaining unusual postures for long periods of time.

Table 7.2
Pharmaceutical antipsychotic drugs

Class	Generic name	Trade name
Phenothiazines	Chlorpromazine	Thorazine
	Thioridazine	Mellaril
	Mesoridazine	Serentil
	Trifluoperazine	Stelazine
	Fluphenazine	Prolixin
	Prochlorperazine	Compazine
Thioxanthenes	Chlorprohixine	Taractan
	Thiothixene	Navane
Butyrophenone	Haloperidol	Haldol
Dibenzoxapine	Loxapine	Loxitane
Dihydroindolone	Molindone	Moban
New generation	Clozapine	Clozaril
	Risperidone	Risperidal
	Olanzepine	Zyprexa
	Sertindole	Serlect

Pharmaceutical Antipsychotics

Despite the existence of several available antipsychotic (neuroleptic) medications, they are uniformly potent antagonists of dopamine receptors (table 7.2). The potency of the medications' antagonism at D2 receptors correlates linearly with their antipsychotic efficacy. These facts, combined with knowledge that dopamine-activating drugs (cocaine, amphetamines) can create a paranoia-like and a schizophrenia-like psychosis have led to the dopamine-hypothesis of schizophrenia. Although consistent, this does not explain all aspects of schizophrenia, like negative symptoms of cognitive and affective deficits. Other theories have proposed neurodevelopmental underpinnings of schizophrenia and amino acid neurotransmitter bases (Akbarian et al. 1996; Weinberger 1996). Whereas prefrontal abnormalities have been associated with negative symptoms, temporolimbic abnormalities are associated with positive symptoms. (Casanova 1997; Bogerts 1997; Mattson et al. 1997). These theories are not mutually exclusive. To summarize, it seems that genetic predispositions and prenatal insults result in aberrant brain development involving prefrontal and temporolimbic areas. The functional activity of these regions and neurotransmitter systems are altered, resulting in the symptomatology of schizophrenia.

Whatever the underlying causes may be, neuroleptic medications are the most effective treatment for schizophrenia. All antipsychotic medications have some form of dopamine receptor antagonism and they are distinguished by their chemical class. The phenothiazines include chlorpromazine (Thorazine), thioridazine (Mellaril), mesoridazine (Serentil), trifluoperazine (Stelazine), fluphenazine (Prolixin), and prochlorperazine (Compazine). The thioxanthenes include chlorprohixine (Taractan) and thiothixene (Navane). Butyrophenones are represented by haloperidol (Haldol). Loxapine (Loxitane) is a dibenzoxapine, and molindone (Moban) is a dihydroindolone.

A newer generation of antipsychotics have been introduced in the 1990s that have the dual advantages of reduced extrapyramidal effects and amelioration of negative symptoms. These drugs include clozapine (Clozaril), risperidone (Risperidal), and olanzepine (Zyprexa). Pharmacologically, they antagonize 5-HT_{2A} receptors as well as dopamine receptors. Sertindole (Serlect) is yet another new generation antipsychotic that has a variety of dopamine and serotonin antagonist effects. With the discovery of dopamine receptors beyond the D_1/D_2 dichotomy, many antipsychotics were found to have effects there too. For example, clozapine has less efficacy at the D_2 receptor, but stronger effects at D_4 receptors. Haloperidol is an antagonist at D_3 as well as D_2 receptors.

Side Effects

Antipsychotic drugs vary according to their side-effect profiles regarding sedation, autonomic effects, and extrapyramidal motor symptoms. Sedation and autonomic effects are mediated, in part, by the muscarinic cholinergic and alpha adrenergic effects of the drugs. While the binding to D_2 receptors predicts dosage and efficacy for antipsychotic drugs, it also predicts extrapyramidal motor symptoms (Seeman 1987). These include akathisia (or motor restlessness), dystonic postures, and parkinsonism (resting tremor, bradykinesia, and limb rigidity). Due to the functional relationship between dopamine and acetylcholine in the basal ganglia, anticholinergic effects of antipsychotic drugs may actually reduce the parkinsonism they produce. Unfortunately, anticholinergic drugs tend to impair such cognitive processes as attention and memory—an effect that schizophrenics do not need. Agranulocytosis is an occasional (occuring in 1–2%) and reversible side effect of clozapine, for which patients taking the medication must be monitored.

Tardive dyskinesia is a condition that sometimes results from chronic neuroleptic treatment lasting from months to years (Baldessarini 1996; Stahl et al. 1982). It occurs in 15–25% of treated chronic psychotic patients and is characterized by repetitive, athetoid writhing and stereotyped choreiform movements of the face, eyes, mouth, extremities, and trunk. Discontinuation of neuroleptic medication allows the symptoms to gradually decline, but sometimes they can persist indefinitely. The pathophysiology of tardive dyskinesia is poorly understood, but it appears to involve supersensitive postsynaptic dopamine receptors in the basal ganglia.

Neuroleptic malignant syndrome is an acute iatrogenic condition caused by neuroleptics, characterized by tremor, catatonia, fluctuating consciousness, hyperthermia, and cardiovascular instability. It is relatively uncommon, occuring in 1–1.5% of patients but is fatal in 11–38%, most often due to cardiovascular collapse (Jahan et al. 1992). The pathogenesis of neuroleptic malignant syndrome is poorly understood, but it is believed to result from altered dopamine and serotonin transmission in the hypothalamus, spinal cord, and striatum. Treatment includes discontinuation of neuroleptics and administration of drugs that increase dopamine transmission: bromocriptine or L-dopa (Jahan et al. 1992; Baldessarini 1996).

Herbal Antidepressants and Anxiolytics

Saint-John's-Wort

History and Botany

Saint-John's-wort *(Hypericum perforatum)* is a perennial herb with round stems having two distinct lengthwise ridges (Kowalchik and Hylton 1987; Leyel 1994). It produces bright yellow flowers with five

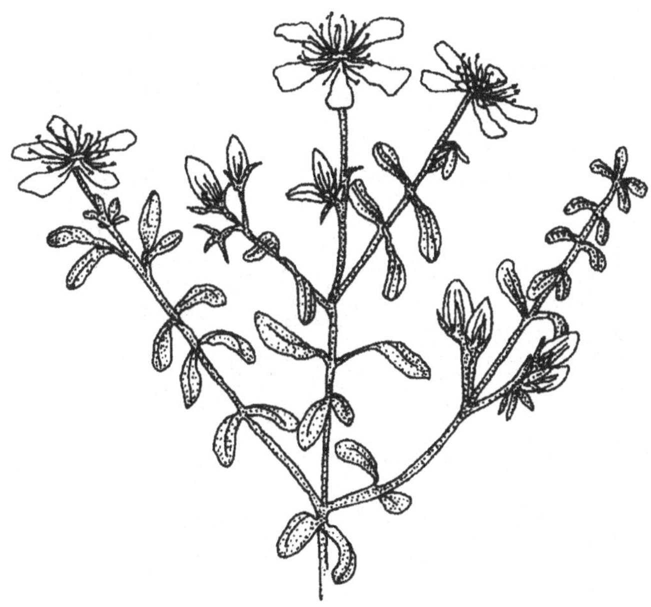

Figure 7.1
Saint-John's-wort *(Hypericum perforatum)*. Reprinted with permission from Sturdivant and Blakely. (1999). *Medicinal Herbs in the Garden, Field, and Marketplace.* Friday Harbor, WA: San Juan Naturals. Illustration by Peggy Sue McRae.

petals and sepals, and three stamen bundles (figure 7.1). The leaves are light green, oblong, and grow in pairs on opposing sides of the stems. There are several species of hypericum, but for the sake of convenience, the name hypericum will be used here to refer to *H. perforatum* throughout this work, unless otherwise specified.

Saint-John's-wort was used in ancient Greece and medieval Europe, where it was believed to ward off evil spirits. Its name derives from *wort*, the Old English word for herb, and the fact that it was harvested in Europe on the eve of St. John's day (June 24th) and burned to purify the air (Heiligenstein and Guenther 1998). Traditional uses include treatment of depression, insomnia, enuresis, and anxiety. Modern use has focused on its antidepressant effects and possible antiviral effects for treatment of the human immunodeficiency virus (HIV) (Heiligenstein et al. 1998) (table 7.3). There has been some interest in its antiglioma effects as well (Couldwell et al. 1993).

Table 7.3
Psychotherapeutic herbs

Herb	Proposed use	Active principles	Mechanisms
Saint-John's-wort	Antidepressant	Hypericin	Monoamine reuptake inhibition*
		Pseudohypericin	MAO inhibition
		Hyperforin	COMT inhibition
		Procyanidins	$GABA_A$, $GABA_B$, benzo., reuptake
		Flavonoids	Opioid μ and κ binding
		Sigma receptor binding	
		PKC inhibitor	
		PTKinase inhibitor	
		IL-6 inhibitor	
Ginger	Antidepressant	Shogaols	5-HT_3 antagonist
	Anxiolytic	Gingerols	Eicosanoid inhibition
		Galanolactone	Ca^{2+}/ATPase
		Zingiberene	Substance P release
		Zingiberol	
Ginkgo biloba	Antidepressant	Flavonoid glycosides	Monoamine (5-HT_{1A}, α_2), MAO?
	Anxiolytic	Terpene lactones	Vasodilator (NO, PAF)
		Ginkgolic acids	Decreased glucocorticoid release
Rauwolfia	Antipsychotic	Reserpine	Monoamine depletion via vesicular reuptake inhibition
		Rescinnamine	
		Deserpidine	
		Tetrahydroserpentine	
		Raubasine	
		Ajmalicine	

See text for references.

Table 7.4
Hypericum constituents

Naphthodianthrones	Hypericin Pseudohypericin
Flavonoids	Amentoflavone Catechin Epicatechin Hyperoside Kaemferol Luteolin Myricetin Quercetin Iso-quercetin Rutin
Phloroglucinols	Hyperforin Adhyperforin
Phenolic acids	Caffeic acid Chlorogenic acid Gentisic acid Ferulic acid
Terpenes	Monoterpenes Sesquiterpenes
Xanthones	1,5-dihydroxyxanthone 5-hydroxy-1methoxyxanthone 6-deoxyjacareubin

See text for references.

Not all species of Saint-John's-wort have antidepressant effects. While *H. calycinum* has been found to have antidepressant-like effects in animal models equal to *H. perforatum*, others *(H. hyssopifolium ssp. elongatum)* do not (Ozturk 1997).

Constituents

Extract of hypericum contains at least ten constituents that may contribute to its pharmacological effect (see table 7.4) (Heiligenstein and Guenther 1998). They are categorized into six classes: naphthodianthrones, flavonoids, phloroglucinols, phenolic acids, xanthones, and terpenes (Nahrstedt and Butterweck 1997; Erdelmeier 1998). The naph-

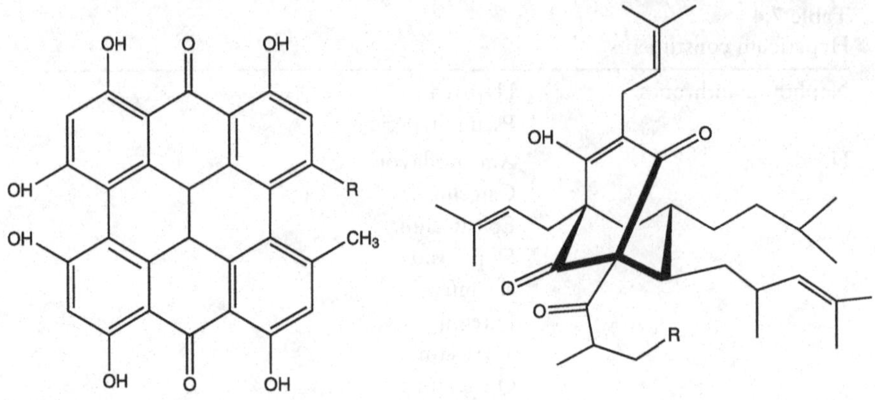

Napthodianthrones
Hypericin R = CH_3
Pseudohypericin R = CH_2OH

Phloroglucinols
Hyperforin R = H
Adhyperforin R = CH_3

Figure 7.2
Chemical structure of Saint-John's-wort constituents.

thodianthrones, hypericin and pseudohypericin, are probably the best known constituents due to their MAO-inhibiting properties (figure 7.2). Flavonoids include amentoflavone, catechin, epicatechin, hyperoside, kaemferol, luteolin, myricetin, quercetin, isoquercetin, and rutin. The phloroglucinols are hyperforin and adhyperforin. The phenolic acids identified are caffeic acid, chlorgenic acid, gentisic acid, and ferulic acid. The terpenes in hypericum are monoterpenes and sesquiterpenes. Some xanthones identified are 1,5-dihydroxyxanthone, 5-hydroxy-1methoxyxanthone, and 6-deoxyjacareubin (Rocha et al. 1994).

Pharmacokinetics

Extracts of hypericum may vary considerably in terms of the quantity and ratio of their constituents based on the extraction process used. Maximum extraction of hypericin and pseudohypericin is obtained with an 80% methanol solvent at 80 °C (Wagner and Bladt 1994). Hyperforin is a lipophilic constituent of hypericum that is present in the oil extract (Chatterjee et al. 1998a). It is not very stable, but its presence is sustained by hot maceration of the flowers and storage in the absence of air (Maisenbacher and Kovar 1992).

The pharmacokinetics of hyperforin have been studied in rats and humans (Biber et al. 1998). In rats, after a 300 mg/kg oral dose of hypericum extract (WS 5572, containing 5% hyperforin), maximum plasma levels of 370 ng/ml (690 nM) are achieved at 3 hours. The half-life of hyperforin is 6 hours. Humans given a 300 mg tablet of hypericum (containing 14.8 mg hyperforin) showed maximum plasma levels of 150 ng/ml (280 nM) at 3.5 hours. The half-life is 9 hours, and mean residence time is 12 hours. Pharmacokinetics of hyperforin are linear up to 600 mg, and no accumulation occurs after repeated doses. By comparison, effective and safe plasma levels of paroxetine and fluoxetine vary between 40 and 200 ng/ml (Preskorn 1997). The effective plasma concentration of hyperforin predicted from computer-fit data is approximately 97 ng/ml (180 nM), which could be easily monitored (Biber et al. 1998). There is a linear correlation between oral dose of hyperforin and plasma levels, and steady-state concentrations of 100 ng/ml (180 nM) could be achieved with three-times-daily dosing.

The pharmacokinetics of hypericin and pseudohypericin plasma have been studied as well (Brockmöller et al. 1997). Human subjects receiving placebo, or 900, 1800, or 3600 mg of a standardized hypericum extract (LI 160), which contained 0, 2.81, 5.62, and 11.25 mg of total hypericin and pseudohypericin, achieved maximum total plasma concentrations at 4 hours (0.028, 0.061, and 0.159 mg/L, respectively). The half-lives of absorption, distribution, and elimination were 0.6, 6.0, and 43.1 hours, respectively, using 750 μg of hypericin, and are slightly different for 1578 μg of pseudohypericin (1.3, 1.4, and 24.8 hours, respectively) (Kerb et al. 1996). The systemic availability of the hypericum extract LI 160 is between 14 and 21%. Comparable results are found in another study using LI 160 (Staffeldt et al. 1994). Long-term dosing of 3 × 300 mg per day showed that steady-state levels of hypericin are reached after 4 days.

The oral bioavailability of hypericum may be altered and improved by a combination of its constituents. A hypericum extract containing naphthodianthrones is inactive in a water suspension, but very effective when another constituent, procyanidin, is present. Procyanidin had the effect of increasing the water solubility of naphthodianthrones, and thus increasing their pharmacokinetic availability (Butterweck et al. 1997). Further, the facilitative effect of procyanidin exhibited an inverted U curve.

This is a prime example of how plant constituents can act cooperatively, and isolation of a single constituent may reduce its effectiveness.

Reported clinical doses of hypericum extract range from 300 to 1200 mg per day. (Heiligenstein and Guenther 1998; Linde et al. 1996)

Mechanisms of Action

Monoamine The constituents of *Hypericum perforatum* and a few other species of hypericum have several pharmacological mechanisms that could account for its antidepressant effects. Much attention had been given to the ability of hypericin to inhibit MAO. Hypericum extract (LI 160) does inhibit both MAO_A and MAO_B, but does so weakly, occuring only in the millimolar range (Muller et al. 1997; Thiede and Walper 1994). MAO inhibition is attributed to both hypericin and flavonol content (Bladt and Wagner 1994). Thus, inhibition of MAO alone is insufficient to explain the antidepressant effect of hypericum. Inihibition of 35% of COMT activity occured at the millimolar range as well, for which flavonols are chiefly responsible. Although these actions may contribute to the antidepressant effect, they are inadequate by themselves to account for it. MAO inhibition has been found by xanthones extracted from other hypericum species such as *H. brasiliense* (Rocha et al. 1994).

Although the individual inhibition of either MAO or COMT may be comparatively minor in isolation, their combined inhibition along with other monoamine or nonmonoamine actions could have additive if not synergistic effects. For example, a fraction with combined hypericin and flavonoids had antidepressant effects in an animal model (Butterweck et al. 1997). Hypericum is a particular case wherein a single isolated principle may be sufficient for the desired effect, but less effective than the entire plant extract.

Another action of hypericum constituents that is particularly relevant to antidepressant effects is the ability to inhibit neuronal reuptake of monoamines. The half-maximal inhibition for monoamine uptake is 100 times lower than for the inhibition of MAO_A or MAO_B (Chatterjee et al. 1998a). Hyperforin is the major contributor to this action, blocking reuptake of 5-HT, norepinephrine, and dopamine (Muller et al. 1998). Half-maximal inhibition occurs at nanomolar concentrations (80 to

200 nM). Affinity for inhibition of reuptake was equal (2 μg/ml) for all three monoamines studied (Muller et al. 1997). The antidepressant effects are accompanied by increases in urinary metabolites of dopamine and norepinephrine (Muldner and Zollner 1984). Not only is hyperforin more potent than hypericin, but also present in higher concentrations in hypericum (>2.5% vs. <0.4%, respectively). Thus, the plasma concentrations of hyperforin used in a pharmacokinetic study are very close to those used in in vitro experiments that demonstrate synaptosomal reuptake inhibition of serotonin, norepinephrine, and dopamine (Biber et al. 1998). Radiolabeled hyperforin does cross the blood-brain barrier and penetrates brain tissue (Ostrowski 1988). Hypericin itself has minor reuptake inhibition effects on DA (22% inhibition in the low micromolar range), but not on NE or 5-HT.

In addition to reuptake effects, subchronic treatment with hyperforin down-regulates β adrenergic receptors and up-regulates 5-HT_2 receptors in frontal cortex of the rat (Muller and Rossol 1994, 1997, 1998). Chronic (26-week) daily treatment with 2700 mg/kg of a hypericum extract (LI 160) up-regulates the affinity and density of both 5-HT_{1A} and 5-HT_2 receptors by 50%. This appears selective to hyperforin, because other hypericum constituents (hypericin and kaemferol) fail to show the same effect. There may be a direct effect on 5-HT receptors, because activity in the guinea pig ileum and Bezold-Jarisch reflex assays indicate 5-HT_3 and/or 5-HT_4-like effects (Chatterjee et al. 1998a, 1998b). However, hypericin inhibits 5-HT_{1A} receptors (30% inhibition) in the low micromolar range (Raffa 1998) The monoamine activity of hypericum is differentially influenced by the extract used (Bhattacharya et al. 1998). The ethanol extract (containing 4.5% hyperforins) showed more dopaminergic activity, whereas the CO_2 extract (containing 38.8% hyperforins) showed more serotonergic activity, but no dopaminergic activity.

Amino acid neurotransmitter Constituents of hypericum also appear to have effects on amino acid neurotransmission, particularly GABA. Hypericin and a crude extract bind to $GABA_A$ and $GABA_B$ receptors (Cott 1997). Hyperforin also inhibits synaptosomal GABA reuptake in the low micromolar range (IC_{50} values of 0.05–0.10 μg/ml). Activity at $GABA_A$ benzodiazepine receptors was noted in extracts of four hypericum species *(H. perforatum, H. hirsutum, H. patulum,* and *H. olympicum).* Amentoflavone is the responsible constituent, displacing flumazenil from benzodiazepine receptors in the nanomolar range (IC_{50} 14.9+/–1.9 nM). Again, no such effect is observed for hypericin. Amentoflavone acts as a partial agonist at GABA benzodiazepine receptors. However, it remains in question whether this constituent crosses the blood-brain barrer because it does not inhibit central flunitrazepam binding when administered peripherally (Nielsen et al. 1988). In addition to GABA activity, hyperforin inhibits reuptake of glutamate at 0.05–0.10 μg/ml (Baureithel et al. 1997). Activity on GABA transmission is consistent with anxiolytic or even antidepressant effects of hypericum.

Opioid A recent study has shown activity of hypericum extracts at opioid receptors (Simmen et al. 1998). Extracts displace naloxone from μ and κ opioid receptors in the micromolar range (IC_{50} 25 and 90 μg/ml, respectively). In contrast, extracts of the sedative herb *Valeriana officinalis* do not have this effect. This effect is due to unidentified constituents and not by the flavonoids quercetin or kaemferol. Opioids are known to have effects on emotion, so it is conceivable that activity of hypericum at μ and κ receptors contributes to its therapeutic effects (Gerra et al. 1998; Tejedor-Real et al. 1995; Walker and Zacny 1998). Although they are not conventional treatment for depression, opioids such as buprenorphine have been effective in treatment of refractory depression (Bodkin et al. 1995). However, for any further conclusions to be drawn, it would be necessary to further elucidate the opioid effects of hypericum to determine what functional effect, if any, hypericum has on the receptors.

Sigma receptor Several other mechanisms of action have been identified in hypericum and its extracts. Hypericin inhibits greater than 40% of binding at muscarinic and σ (sigma) receptors in the low micromolar (1.0 μM) range (Raffa et al. 1998). The σ receptor was originally classified as an opioid receptor, but was later identified to be nonopioid in nature (Martin et al. 1976; Johnson and Jones 1990). Along with the NMDA receptor, the σ receptor was found to be a major target of the dissociative anesthetic drug phencyclidine (PCP, angel dust). The physiological roles and endogenous ligand of the σ receptor are not yet fully understood. Certain neurosteroids (dehydroepiandrosterone and pregnenolone) have antidepressant effects in an animal model (Porsolt forced-swim test), which are mediated in part by the σ receptor (Reddy et al. 1998).

Protein kinases Hypericin also inhibits protein tyrosine kinase activity in the nanomolar range, and protein kinase C (PKC) in the micromolar range (Agostinis et al. 1995; Takahashi et al. 1989; Harris et al. 1996), which has led to its consideration as an antiglioma treatment (Zhang et al. 1997; Couldwell et al. 1994). The psychotherapeutic ramifications of this finding are not readily apparent, but PKC is integral to many intracellular communication mechanisms in the brain. Relatively little attention has been paid to this effect of hypericin, but the activity of protein kinases is intimately related with the function of monoamine systems, decreased in the brains of depressed suicide victims, and increased by antidepressant drugs (Hrdina et al. 1998; Blakely et al. 1998; Tadokoro et al. 1998). Specific mechanisms of monoamine-protein kinase interactions are beginning to be elucidated. For example, activators of PKC decrease the expression of the norepinephrine transporter, and thus the rate of norepinephrine reuptake from the synapse (Apparsundaram 1998). Further, these antidepressant-protein kinase interactions have some anatomical specificity to areas such as the frontal cortex (Tadokoro et al. 1998).

Other mechanisms A few other effects of hypericin, and a crude hypericum extract have been found, including affinity for NMDA, inositol triphosphate, and adenosine receptors. However, these are not likely to be significant to its therapeutic effects because concentrations required for these interactions are not likely to be achieved by oral administration (Cott 1997). Vasoactive effects are possible because hypericum extracts blocked the vasoconstricting effects of histamine and prostaglandin $F_{2\alpha}$ in porcine coronary arteries, and some vasorelaxation occurs in one particular fraction. These effects are hypothesized to be mediated by inhibition of phosphodiesterase (Melzer et al. 1991).

Hypericum also has effects on cytokine levels (Thiele et al. 1994). A hypericum extract (LI 160) given to people with depression and healthy volunteers almost completely suppressed interleukin-6 (IL-6), interleukin-1β (IL-1β), and tumor necrosis factor-α. IL-6 and IL-1β are both known to reduce the release of corticotrophin-releasing hormone, which is implicated in depression (Arborelius et al. 1999).

Finally, a thorough receptor binding study by Raffa and colleagues (1998) showed that hypericin extracts had no effect at adrenergic (alpha or beta), adenosine, angiotensin, benzodiazepine, dopamine, bradykinin, neuropeptide Y, PCP, NMDA, opioid, cholecystokinin A, histamine H_1, or nicotinic ACh receptors. Although comprehensive, this study did not look at the binding of any other hypericum constituents.

Mechanisms: summary Thus, although much attention has been focused initially on MAO inhibition, there are several pharmacological mechanisms possessed by hypericum that could account for its reputed antidepressant effects. These include increased monoamine activity through inhibition of degrading enzymes and blocking reuptake, GABA receptor activity and blocking reuptake, inhibition of protein kinase C, binding to opioid and σ receptors, and suppression of interleukins. Whereas some of these effects (e.g., blocking monoamine reuptake) may be sufficient to explain the antidepressant effect, a combined additive or synergistic effect of the collective actions is .feasible (Bennett et al. 1998). Furthermore, different constituents of hypericum have been demonstrated to have different effects, so that a single isolated constituent may be less effective than the whole plant extract.

Physiological Effects

Electrophysiological effects Extracts of hypericum were examined for their electrophysiological effects in animals. The onset of effects occurred 3–4 hours after administration. Frequencies affected first were in the alpha range and were maximal in the frontal cortex (Dimpfel and Hofmann 1995). Another study examined the EEG effects for two hypericum extracts in rats: one extract high in hyperforin and lacking naphthodianthrones (CO_2), and another extract (LI 160) low in hyperforin. Both extracts showed similar early alpha effects, but only LI 160 had a late effect of increased delta frequencies. The alpha effects are comparable to those found in pharmaceutical serotonin reuptake inhibitors, and the delta effects are comparable to those found with NMDA antagonists such as MK-801 (Dimpfel et al. 1998).

To date, four methodologically controlled studies have been published that examined the electrophysiological effects of hypericum. One study used 18 subjects taking 900 mg per day for 8 days, with quantitative EEG performed on days 1 and 8 (Schellenberg et al. 1998). Effects peaked between 4 and 8 hours after administration. This study also attended to extracts that differed in hyperforin content (0.5% and 5.0%), while keeping the hypericin content constant. The higher dose of hyperforin (5.0%) produced increases in delta (1.25–4.5 Hz) and beta-1 (12.75–18.5) frequencies. Theta (4.75–6.75) and alpha-1 (7.0–9.5 Hz) effects were more pronounced on day 8 than day 1. A second study compared hypericum to the tricyclic antidepressant maprotiline on EEG and evoked potentials (Johnson et al. 1994). Opposing effects occurred in the theta band for the two drugs, but similar effects ocurred on alpha and beta. The third study examined the effect of the extract LI 160 on sleep EEG. Increases in slow-wave sleep (stages 3 and 4) were seen throughout the total sleep period. No effects were seen on sleep continuity, onset, duration, or wake-up phases (Schulz and Jobert 1994). The effects of hypericum extract on sleep EEG were examined (Sharpley et al. 1998). Two doses (0.9 and 1.8 mg of "Kira," Lichtwer Pharma) increased the latency to enter REM in nondepressed volunteers. This effect is consistent with pharmaceutical antidepressants, which increase REM latency and/or reduce total REM duration.

Cognitive effects The effects of LI 160 on cognitive performance of subjects being treated for depression were examined. A significant antidepressant effect was seen and with low incidence of side effects, but no adverse cognitive effects were found on measures of attention, concentration, or reaction time (Schmidt and Sommer 1993).

Antidepressant effects Hypericum has been shown to have antidepressant effects in several animal models. An extract fraction high in naphthodianthrones showed antidepressant effects in the forced-swim test, and was attenuated by a dopamine antagonist (sulpiride) (Butterweck et al. 1997). A commercially available extract of hypericum, LI 160, is rich in flavonoids and naphthodianthrones and has antidepressant effects in the forced-swim and tail suspension tests. These antidepressant effects occurred in an inverted U shape and were reduced by dopamine antagonists (Butterweck et al. 1997). Preparations high in hyperforin but devoid of hypericin have antidepressant effects in the behavioral despair and learned helplessness paradigms (Chatterjee et al. 1998a, 1998b). These latter studies suggested that hyperforin is sufficient to produce an antidepressant effect, although it is not necessarily the only constituent with that effect.

Studies in mice have shown a hypericum extract to increase exploration in an unfamiliar environment, prolong sedative sleep time, and antagonize the effects of reserpine. Other antidepressant-like effects are found on the water-wheel test, and chronic administration decreased aggression in socially isolated male mice (Okpanyi and Weischer 1987).

Several human clinical studies have been performed on the effectiveness of hypericum in depression (Linde et al. 1996; Volz 1997). There has been a wide variety in the methodology used with respect to experimental controls, doses, preparations used (extracts, whole herb), hypericin contents, and sample size. Most studies ranged from 4 to 12 weeks in duration, and employed doses of 350–1000 mg of extract. Diagnoses were made using DSM or ICD criteria, and subjects were typically rated in the mild to moderate range in severity of depression. Many studies employed quantitative psychometric instruments such as the Hamilton Depression Rating Scale, Clinical Global Impression Scale, and the Depression Self-Rating Scale. Improvements were noted in mood, as well as in somatic symptoms of depression such as fatigue, disturbed sleep, and inactivity (Hubner et al. 1994). One study suggested that hypericum may be effective in treatment of seasonal affective disorder as well (Kasper 1997).

Methodological controls. Some published studies on the effectiveness of hypericum have experimental design flaws, but there are several that are methodologically controlled, employing double-blind, randomization, and placebo controls. Randomized, placebo-controlled studies were summarized and evaluated in a meta-analysis by Linde and colleagues (1996). The combined subject pool was 1,757 outpatients with mild to moderate depression. In total, 23 randomized studies were found, of which 15 were placebo controlled. Hypericum was superior to placebo across studies. One study used a second phase where the placebo group was crossed over to active treatment (LI 160) producing significant improvement (Hansgen et al. 1994). A more stringent meta-analysis, which also used double-blind as an inclusion criteria, found Saint-John's-wort to be superior to placebo and equivalent to tricyclics in efficacy (Kim et al. 1999).

Responsible Constituents. The contribution of the different constituents of hypericum was examined by one methodologically controlled study (Laakmann et al. 1998). A large sample ($n = 174$) of subjects diagnosed by DSM-IV criteria were tried on 300 mg of either of two extracts (WS 5572 and WS 5573), relative to a placebo group. These two extracts differ in their hyperforin content (5.0% and 0.5%, respectively). The high-hyperforin group showed the greatest improvement, suggesting that it is very relevant to the antidepressant response. Further, a dose-response relationship was shown between the hyperforin content of hypericum extracts and its antidepressant effect. A sizable reduction in ratings of depression (Hamilton rating scale for depression, 10.3 ± 4.6) was found with WS 5572. Because these two extracts differ primarily by their hyperforin, it appears that hyperforin content may be the most salient chemical constituent for standardization in the future, rather than hypericin.

Pharmaceutical Comparison. At least 8 studies to date have examined the effectiveness of hypericum compared to the pharmaceutical antidepressants imipramine, amitriptyline, and maprotiline. Preliminary results indicate that hypericum is equivalent to standard antidepressants in effectiveness (Linde et al. 1996; Vorbach 1997). Similar to the pharmaceutical antidepressants, there is a 10–14 day lag for therapeutic effects of hypericum (Harrer et al. 1994). Indeed, the differences seen between hypericum and placebo groups becomes apparent between 2 and 4 weeks (Sommer and Harrer 1994). Hypericum has been reported to have a more favorable side-effect profile than several pharmaceutical antidepressants as well (Vorbach et al. 1994; Harrer et al. 1994). In double-blind studies, subjects have reported fewer and less-severe side effects. Although these initial results are promising, Linde and colleagues (1996) have concluded that the present evidence is inadequate to establish whether hypericum is as effective as other antidepressants and whether it has fewer side effects.

Toxicity

Although used extensively, there have not been any published reports of serious drug interactions or toxicity for hypericum (Heiligenstein and Guenther 1998). The long-term safety of hypericum has not been evaluated.

Side effects In an open study with 3,250 subjects, the most common side effects reported were gastrointestinal irritation (0.6%), allergic reactions (0.5%), fatigue (0.4%), and restlessness (0.3%). A review of case reports, clinical trials, post-marketing surveillance, and drug monitoring studies concurrently showed that the most common side effects were gastrointestinal, dizziness/confusion, and sedation (Ernst et al. 1998). Importantly, the side effects of hypericum in this study were comparable to placebo levels. A pharmacokinetic study showed that plasma levels of up to 300 ng/ml were well tolerated. Headache occured in one subject who was taking 1200 mg extract (59 mg hyperforin, plasma conc. >400 ng/ml) (Biber et al. 1998).

The meta-analysis by Linde and colleagues (1996) found greater incidence of side effects reported by taking pharmaceutical antidepressants (52.8%) than those taking hypericum (19.8%). The meta-analysis by Kim and colleagues (1999) found that subjects were more likely to discontinue treatment with tricyclics than Saint-John's-wort, and tricylics were twice as likely to cause side effects.

Phototoxicity Hypericum has been noted to cause a phototoxicity in cell cultures and a dermatitis and inflammation of nasal mucosa in grazing animals that consume the plant (Brockmöller et al. 1997). There have been no reported cases in humans, but perhaps caution is advised to individuals receiving significant sun exposure or who are particularly photosensitive (Tyler 1994). The responsible element for this photosensitivity is believed to be hypericin. One methodologically-controlled study quantified the response of subjects taking hypericum (LI 160) to ultraviolet radiation (UVA and UVB) (Brockmöller et al. 1997). In a single-dose phase, a comparison of light sensitivity did not differ between hypericum extract and placebo groups, and there was no dose relation in light sensitivity. Sensitivity to selective UVA light was increased only after the highest dose (3600 mg of extract) with marginal statistical significance. In the multiple-dose phase (1800 mg/day, 15 days), there was a slight increase in light and UVA sensitivity. However, the photosensitivity occurred at doses much higher than those used for antidepressant effects.

Pharmacokinetic interactions Preliminary evidence suggests that Saint-John's-wort induces the cytochrome oxidase enzyme isoform CYP3A4 (Ernst 1999). This raises the potential for pharmacokinetic interactions with drugs metabolized by the same enzyme. A few cases have been reported of reduced warfarin levels (Yue et al. 2000). Similar interactions have also been reported for concurrent use with digoxin, theophylline, and cyclosporin (Nebel et al. 1999; Ruschitzka et al. 2000; Johne et al. 1999). As with any other medication, potential interactions should be considered when taking a combination of drugs.

Cytotoxicity There has been some concern raised over cytotoxic and mutagenic in-vitro effects of hypericum, which have been ascribed to the constituent quercetin (Tyler 1994). However, quercetin is a flavonoid that is present in many plants and vegetables, and it is estimated that the average person consumes 50 mg per day. Consumption of hypericum would not significantly add to this (1 mg in commonly used amounts). The German Commission E has concluded that this is not of great concern.

Hypomania and use with other antidepressants One case has been reported of concurrent use of hypericum with an SSRI. Gordon (1998) reported a case of a 50-year-old woman taking 600 mg/day of hypericum for chronic depression. She had discontinued taking Paxil 10 days prior to hypericum and experienced no ill effects at that time. However, she added 20 mg of paroxetine to her regimen of hypericum to improve her sleep. She presented with lethargy, nausea, and weakness, but vital signs and mental status were normal. Following discontinuation of medications, she returned to normal status the next day.

Two cases of hypomania resulting from hypericum have been reported (O'Breasail and Argouarch 1998). One case involved post-stroke depression with a history of unsuccessful treatment with other antidepressant treatments: paroxetine, fluoxetine, and ECT, but not concurrent with the hypericum. After 6 weeks with hypericum (dosage unspecified), he developed increased drive, pressured speech, irritability, grandiosity, and alterations of concentration and sleep. His behavioral problems persisted after discontinuation of hypericum, but were controlled by valproate. The second case reported was of a patient presenting with manic features: irritability, increased drive, anger, mood lability, grandiosity, flight of ideas, and sleep disturbance. A year prior to this he witnessed a fatal accident and began experiencing anxiety, depression, and some post-traumatic stress symptoms. His manic symptoms began following 3 months of treatment with hypericum. He was treated with lithium carbonate and his mood symptoms stabilized over 2 weeks.

Given the wide availability and usage of hypericum, manic reactions such as the ones described appear to be uncommon. As expected, concomittant use of hypericum with pharmaceutical antidepressant medication appears to be contraindicated. Although some antidepressant medications can be given in combination, this must be done with caution and with dosage considerations to account for additive or synergistic effects.

Sexual function One of the potential benefits of hypericum is the apparent reduced or lack of adverse effects upon sexual function, compared to pharmaceutical antidepressants. The SSRIs are particularly notorious for inhibition of sexual function, whereas antidepressants with dopaminergic actions (e.g., bupropion) do not, and may actually enhance sexual function (Rosen et al. 1999; Piazza et al. 1997). Anecdotal reports and the fact that there are no clinical reports of sexual dysfunction with hypericum is encouraging, but it remains to be tested empirically.

Conclusions

Thus, the long tradition of hypericum as a treatment for depression has been well supported by modern scientific research. Several active constituents have been identified, including naphthodianthrones (e.g., hypericin), phloroglucinols (e.g., hyperforin) and flavonoids (amentoflavone). Research has delineated its pharmacokinetic properties, and many of its neurochemical mechanisms have been identified: enhancing monoamine transmission (MAO, COMT, reuptake inhibiton, and chronic receptor alterations), enhancing GABA transmission, and affecting transmission in opioid, sigma, protein kinase, and interleukin systems. Antidepressant effects of hypericum are consistent across animal and human studies.

Future directions for research on hypericum may continue the work done in clinical efficacy. More specifically, studies may be of interest that examine its effects in treatment of more severe depression and different subtypes of depression. The comparative efficacy of different hypericum preparations could be further investigated, and optimum dosages need to be established (Linde et al. 1996). Further work is needed to compare hypericum's efficacy and side effects with those of the SSRIs or atypical antidepressants, because published studies to date have only compared it with tricyclics.

Other directions hypericum research might take would be to examine analgesic effects of hypericum. Numerous antidepressants have been found to have analgesic effects, or to potentiate the effects of opioid analgesia, due to the role of monoamine systems in analgesia (Clifford 1985). Further, the opioid and σ effects of hypericum could create analgesic effects, but the nature of hypericum's action at opioid receptors needs to be elucidated. Given that clomipramine and selected SSRIs have been found to be effective in treating obsessive-compulsive disorder, the possibility of whether hypericum would have a similar effect may be investigated (Pigott and Seay 1999). Finally, given that antidepressants are effective in treating anxiety, controlled trials may be attempted for hypericum as well (Rickels et al. 1993).

Ginger

History and Botany

Ginger is a rhizome, or underground stem, of the plant *Zingiber officinale* from the Zingiberaceae family (figure 7.3). It is a tropical perennial that grows 6–12-inch stalks and dense, cone-like flowers at the end. Its leaves are long and grasslike, typically 6–12 inches in length and 0.75 inch wide (Kowalchik and Hylton 1987).

Ginger's use was well known among the ancient Greeks and Romans, and was a common import from Asia during the eleventh and thirteenth

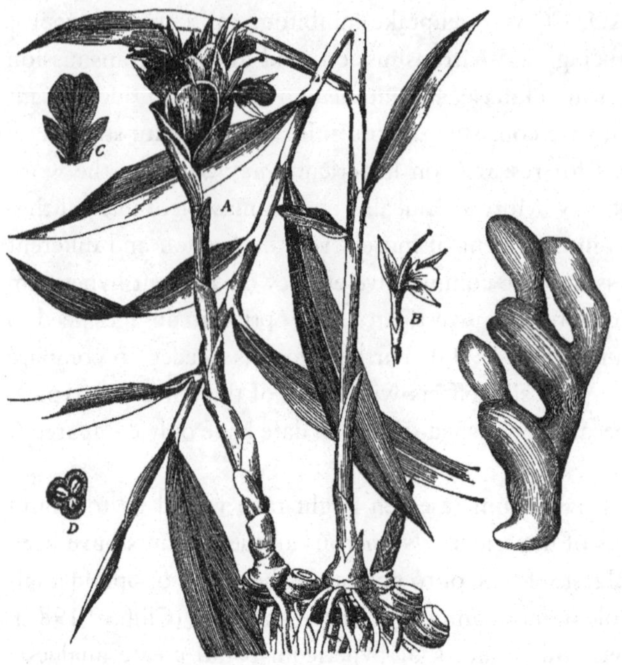

Figure 7.3
Ginger *(Zingiber officinale)*. Reprinted from Culbreth DMR. (1927). *Materia Medica and Pharmacognosy*, 7th ed. Philadelphia: Lea & Febiger.

centuries A.D. (Kowalchik and Hylton 1987). It was known in China as early as the fourteenth century B.C. It is mentioned in the Koran as part of a divine drink (Mustafa et al. 1993). The name *zingiber* derives from the Arabic word *Zinschebil* meaning root of *Zindschi*, or India (Robbers et al. 1996). In the Unani-Tibb and and Ayurvedic herbal traditions, it is given to treat rhinitis, gingivitis, toothache, painful menstruation, asthma, stroke, constipation, and diabetes (Mustafa et al. 1993). The Spanish had been using it as early as the sixteenth century, and introduced it to Jamaica and the West Indies, where it is now widely cultivated. Ginger is generally used for therapeutic effects on digestion and gastrointestinal function, and is widely known as a cooking spice.

Preparation Ginger is most commonly used as a food spice. It is harvested 8–9 months after planting to make dried ginger poweder, or after

Table 7.5
Ginger constituents

Aromatic ketones	Shogaols
	Zingerone
	Gingerols
	Paradol
Terpenoids	Zingiberene
	Zingiberol
	Bisabolene
	Galanolactone

See text for references.

5–6 months for fresh use (Govindarajan 1982a) . Sliced and ground fresh ginger is often used in cooking. Ginger is also crystallized and candied and made into syrups. Perhaps one of the most common forms of consumption of ginger is the beverage ginger ale, which is made from carbonated water and ginger syrup. "Ginger beer" as it is now commonly sold, is merely ginger ale with an increased amount of ginger content. It was traditionally made by fermenting ginger with other spices (e.g., licorice, clove, hops, and gentian) into an alcoholic beer. "Ginger Jake" was an alcoholic beverage made during the American Prohibtion era. Tragically, it was laced with a toxin that caused irreversible paralysis.

A ginger oil is produced from the steam distillation of dried root, and used in beverages, candies, and perfumes. Ginger oleoresin, or solvent extract, is now used as a flavoring agent as well.

Chemical Constituents

Several factors may affect the chemical composition of ginger, including maturity at harvest, agricultural climate, and geographic origin (Mustafa et al. 1993). Ginger has a lipid content of approximately 7%. The oil extract has a high proportion of sesquiterpenes, most notably zingiberene, as well as monoterpenes and oxygenated compounds. The primary pungent chemical in ginger is an aromatic ketone called gingerol, with homologues varying by carbon atoms in the side chain and designated as (6)-, (8)-, and (10)-gingerol (table 7.5). Gingerols are chemically converted to shogaol, zingerone, and alkanals (hexanal, octanal, and decanal). Shogaol may be further converted to paradol by hydrogenation. It is the commercial preparation that is responsible for some of these reactions, because zingerone and shogaol are found in small amounts in fresh ginger, but in large amounts in stored ginger (Mustafa et al. 1993; Ye et al. 1989). Thus, the composition of fresh and stored ginger may vary, potentially altering its pharmacological effects. The primary terpenoid in ginger is zingiberene. Other terpenes include zingiberol, bisabolene, and galanolactone (figure 7.4). Lesser components of ginger include curcuminoids (cassumunin A and B), and homologues of gingediol and gingediacetate (Mustafa et al. 1993; Nagano et al. 1997).

Pharmacokinetics

Few studies have looked at the pharmacokinetic properties of ginger constituents. One pharmacokinetic study in rats showed a rapid clearance of (6)-gingerol, with a terminal half-life of 7.23 minutes and a total body clearance of 16.8 ml/min/kg (Ding et al. 1991). There was also a high degree of serum binding for (6)-gingerol (92.4%). Further, the disappearance of [6]-gingerol from plasma is mediated by the liver, in part, but not the kidneys (Naora et al. 1992). Shogaol has been shown to be metabolized to paradol and dehydroparadol by liver fractions (Surh and Lee 1992).

Mechanisms of Action

Four prinicpal mechanisms have been cited to explain the diverse physiological mechanisms of ginger. Broadly, these are (1) eicosanoid inhibition, (2) serotonin antagonism, (3) substance P release, and (4) Ca^{2+}/ATPase activity.

Eicosanoid activity Eicosanoids are cellular messengers involved in numerous physiological processes and pathological conditions and are active in the central nervous system (Cooper et al. 1996). They are synthesized from phospholipids into arachidonic acid by the enzymes phospholipase A_2 and phospholipase C (see figure 7.5). Arachidonic acid is further converted by cyclooxygenases into prostaglandins and thromboxanes. Various lipoxygenases convert arachidonic acid into HPETEs (hydroperoxyeicosatetraenoic acid), which are then converted

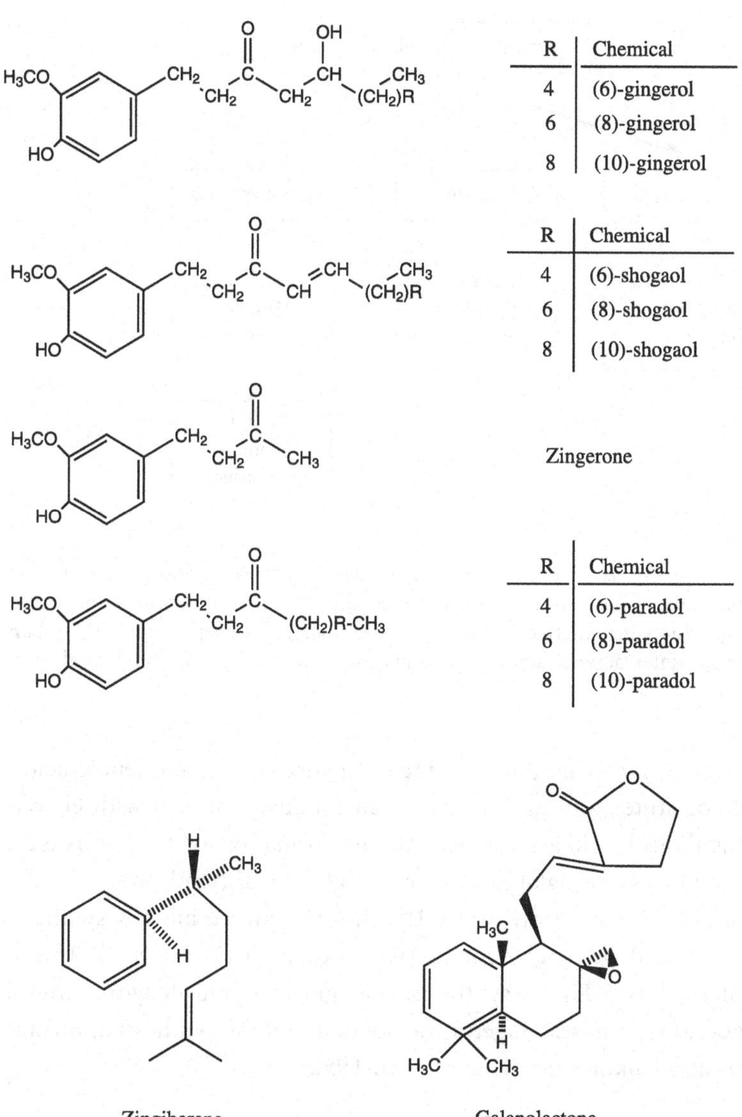

R	Chemical
4	(6)-gingerol
6	(8)-gingerol
8	(10)-gingerol

R	Chemical
4	(6)-shogaol
6	(8)-shogaol
8	(10)-shogaol

R	Chemical
4	(6)-paradol
6	(8)-paradol
8	(10)-paradol

Figure 7.4
Chemical structure of ginger constituents.

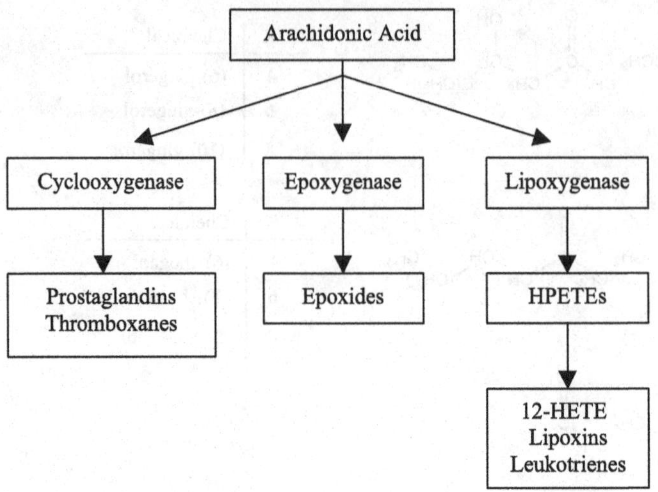

Figure 7.5
Eicosanoid synthesis. Arachidonic acid is converted by cyclooxygenases into prostaglandins, and thromboxanes. Lipoxygenases convert arachidonic acid into HPETEs, which are then converted to lipoxins, leukotrienes, and 12-HETE (hydroxyeicosatetraenoic acid). Epoxygenases convert arachidonic acid into epoxides.

to lipoxins, leukotrienes, and 12-HETE (hydroxyeicosatetraenoic acid). Several consitutents of ginger have been found to interact with eicosanoid metabolism. Ginger extract inhibits formation of thromboxanes, prostaglandins (prostaglandin $F_{2\alpha}$, prostaglandin E_2, and prostaglandin D_2), and leukotrienes (Srivastava 1986). Gingerdione inhibits synthesis of 5-HETE and prostaglandin E_2 ($IC_{50} = 18$ μM) (Flynn et al. 1986). Shogaol inhibits 5-HETE synthesis, and gingerol and dehydroparadol inhibit cyclooxygenase. Gingerol was found to inhibit synthesis of prostaglandins and leukotrienes (Kiuchi et al. 1992).

Serotonergic activity Several physiological functions of the 5-HT_3 receptor have been demonstrated in the central and peripheral nervous system. It has been implicated in cognitive, emotional, and physiological processes as a consequence of its neuroanatomical distribution and neurophysiological effects (Greenshaw 1993; Greenshaw and Silverstone 1997). The acetone extract of ginger was found to have serotonin antagonist effects (Huang et al. 1991). Galanolactone, a diterpenoid found in ginger, was responsible for this action in the guinea pig ileum assay and effective in the micromolar range (Huang et al. 1991). This effect was much more pronounced in the guinea pig ileum (predominantly a 5-HT_3 effect), but not in the rat fundis and rabbit aorta strips, which are respectively mediated by 5-HT_1 and 5-HT_2 receptors. Further, galanolactone had a much greater effect in response to a selective 5-HT_3 agonist (2-methyl-5-HT). Gingerol has also been shown to have 5-HT antagonist effects (Yamahara et al. 1989). Other physiological assays (5-HT-induced hypothermia and diarrhea) have shown serotonin antagonist activity from oral doses of ginger (Huang et al. 1990). Among the constituents from the effective fractions, (6)-shogaol was more effective than (6)-dehydrogingerdione and (8)- and (10)-gingerol in inhibiting 5-HT-induced diarrhea. The ability of the responsible constituents to cross the blood-brain barrier, however, has not yet been explicitly demonstrated.

Substance P Ginger has been shown to release substance P. Substance P is a peptide neurotransmitter present in the brain and spinal cord, and which has modulatory effects on several neural processes, including pain transmission. (6)-shogaol has been shown to dose-dependently cause a Ca^{2+}-dependent release of substance P from spinal dorsal horn, in a similar manner to capsaicin from chili peppers (Onogi et al. 1992). This action relates closely to the analgesic effects of ginger and will be discussed at greater length in chapter 8.

Ca^{2+}-ATPase A fourth mechanism of action of ginger involves activity on Ca^{2+}-related processes. Gingerol was found to enhance Ca^{2+}-pumping ATPase in the sarcoplasmic reticulum in cardiac and skeletal muscles (Kobayashi et al. 1987). It inhibits the enzyme in lower concentrations (0.24 μM), but activates it at higher concentrations (3–30 μM), suggesting that it increases the rate constant for the enzyme-substrate complex breakdown and decreases the affinity of the enzyme for Ca^{2+}. Gingerol had an inotropic effect in guinea pig atrial muscle, but there was no effect on Na^+-K^+-ATPase activity, suggesting that this was not due to cellular cAMP levels or an influx of extracellular Ca^{2+}.

Cytosolic calcium homeostasis is tightly regulated in neurons as well as in muscle cells. It is sequestered in intracellular pools, which is accomplished by three components: (1) a calcium-activated pump (Ca^{2+}-ATPase), (2) a calcium channel (such as the inositol trisphosphate receptor or ryanodine receptor), and (3) a calcium-binding protein such as calsequestrin or calreticulin (Johnson et al. 1993). Ca^{2+}/ATPase is present in organelles of neural tissues although neurons lack a sarcoplasmic reticulum. Neuronal Ca^{2+}/ATPase pumps exist in organelles and in plasma membranes as well (Johnson et al. 1993, Panfoli et al. 1997). In cerebellar neurons, Ca^{2+}/ATPase was found in cisternae of the endoplasmic reticulum and in intracellular compartments for storage of Ca^{2+}, called calciosomes (Villa et al. 1991). The Ca^{2+}/ATPase pump in muscle and neuronal tissue derive from the same gene, but appear to be alternately spliced in a tissue-specific manner (Baba-Aïssa et al. 1998).

The regulation of intracellular neuronal Ca^{2+} is of high functional significance. Ca^{2+}-dependent neurotransmitter release is reduced by the Ca^{2+}/ATPase pump (Fossier et al. 1993). Although immediate Ca^{2+} currents are mediated by ionotropic glutamate receptors (i.e., NMDA) in hippocampal neurons, a sizable portion of neurons show delayed Ca^{2+} increases from intracellular pools (Miller et al. 1996). These delayed changes were synaptically mediated and dependent upon endosomal Ca^{2+}/ATPase.

Whether ginger exerts psychotropic effects through this mechanism is highly dependent on a few factors. It still needs to be established that ginger constituents penetrate the blood-brain barrier in sufficient concentrations to cause this effect. Further, there are alternate splices of neuronal and muscle Ca^{2+}/ATPase, so it cannot be assumed a priori that ginger constituents that affect muscular Ca^{2+}/ATPase will bind to neuronal Ca^{2+}/ATPase or have the same degree of effect. The behavioral and large-scale neural consequences of Ca^{2+}/ATPase modulation in general also need to be further elucidated.

Physiological Effects

Ginger has numerous physiological effects, including increasing bile emptying, increasing gastric motility, antiulcer, anti-inflammatory, antipyretic, vascular pressor, cardiotonic, analgesic, and antiemetic effects (Mustafa et al. 1993; Yamahara et al. 1989). Pressor effects are centrally mediated and produced by shogaol (Suekawa et al. 1986). However, the pressor effects are dose dependent, because low doses of (6)-shogaol and (6)-gingerol had depressor effects (Suekawa et al. 1984). Other effects of ginger are increased bile secretion, antipyretic, and anti-inflammatory effects. (6)-shogaol was found to mediate the antipyretic effect, to a degree comparable with aspirin (Mascolo et al. 1989). The effects that will be concentrated on in this chapter are the antiemetic and anxiolytic/antidepressant ones, and those mediated by eicosanoid pathways.

Platelet inhibition Ginger extract has been found to inhibit platelet aggregation induced by arachidonic acid, epinephrine, ADP, and collagen (Srivastava 1984). The extract's ability to inhibit cyclooxygenase activity and thromboxane levels correlated well with inhibition of platelet aggregation (Srivastava 1984; Mustafa et al. 1993). The type of preparation used also affects platelet inhibition, because roasted and charcoal of ginger were effective, while ether extracts of raw and dried ginger were not (Wu et al. 1993).

Ginger's platelet inhibition effect was demonstrated with oral doses in humans (Srivastava 1989). Although this was not confirmed in a later study, it highlights the importance of dosage and preparation (Janssen et al. 1996). The effect is dose dependent, and while fresh ginger is effective, dried ginger is not (Lumb 1994).

Gastrointestinal effects: animal studies Ginger enhances gastric motility with an oral administration of acetone extract, involving (6)-shogaol and several gingerols (Mustafa et al. 1993). However, gastric motility was inhibited by intravenous gingerol and shogaol, suggesting that dosage and route of administration are critical. In one study using intravenous (6)-shogaol, gastric transit was inhibited at 3.5 mg/kg but facilitated at 35 mg/kg, indicating that a U-shaped dose-response curve may be in effect (Suekawa et al. 1984).

Ginger extracts (acetone, 50% ethanolic and aqueous) were investigated for antiemetic activity in dogs (Sharma et al. 1997). Emesis was induced by 3 mg/kg cisplatin (a 100% emetic dose IV) in healthy mongrel

Table 7.6
Clinical studies of the antiemetic/nausea efficacy of ginger

Type of nausea	Efficacy	Comparison	Ginger dose	Reference
GA	−	Droperidol (ineffective)	2 g	1
GA	−	Placebo	0.5, 1.0 g	2
GA	+	Metoclopramide	0.5 g	3
GA	+	Metoclopramide	1 g	4
SS	+	Placebo	1 g	5
HG	+	Placebo	0.25 g/day	6

Key: − Ineffective, + Effective, CD Crossover design, DB Double blind, GA General anesthesia (postoperative nausea), HG Hyperemesis gravidarum, PC Placebo control, RA Randomized assignment, SS Seasickness.
References: 1. Visalyaputra et al. 1998; 2. Arfeen et al. 1995; 3. Phillips et al. 1993; 4. Bone et al. 1990; 5. Grontved et al. 1988; 6. Fischer-Rasmussen et al. 1991.

dogs. Across a range of oral doses (25–200 mg/kg) the aqueous extract was ineffective. The acetone extract was more effective than ethanolic extract, and both were less effective than the 5-HT_3 antagonist granisetron. In contrast, neither of the ginger extracts was effective against apomorphine-induced emesis. In addition to nausea and vomiting, the cancer chemotherapeutic agent cisplatin causes inhibition of gastric emptying. The acetone and ethanolic extracts of ginger were found to reverse this effect of cisplatin in rats (Sharma et al. 1998). Ginger juice and acetone extracts were more effective than the ethanolic extract. This reversal was comparable to that produced by the 5-HT_3 receptor antagonist ondansetron. In fact, ginger juice was more efficacious than ondansetron.

Gastrointestinal effects: human studies To date, six methodologically controlled studies have been undertaken to evaluate the antinausea and antiemetic efficacy of ginger in humans (table 7.6). Despite overwhelming anecdotal evidence, the results of clinical studies have been variable. These differences in results may be accounted for, at least in part, by differences in methodology across studies. One paradigm in which ginger had mixed efficacy is postoperative nausea from general anesthesia. Of the four such studies conducted, two failed to support, while the other two supported this role of ginger (Visalyaputra et al. 1998; Arfeen et al. 1995; Phillips et al. 1993; Bone et al. 1990). However, one study, which failed to show an effect with ginger, also failed to show a benefit from droperidol, an antiemetic drug that has proven effective in several studies of postanesthetic nausea and emesis (Visalyaputra et al. 1998; Koivuranta et al. 1997; Fortney et al. 1998). In the studies that supported ginger's effects, its efficacy was comparable to the drug metoclopramide. Ginger has been shown to be effective for treatment of motion sickness and hyperemesis gravidarum (Grontved et al. 1988; Fischer-Rasmussen et al. 1991). For the prevention of seasickness, ginger reduced cold sweating and the incidence of vomiting. There was also a trend toward reduced nausea and vertigo. Further study showed ginger to reduce vertigo but not nystagmus in response to caloric stimulation of the vestibular system (Grontved and Hentzer 1986). Thus, there is emprical evidence to support the antinausea/emetic efficacy of ginger. The degree of this efficacy may vary depending on the intensity and/or source of the nausea (e.g., general anesthetic, pregnancy, motion sickness). It would be interesting to see ginger's efficacy in nausea of other etiologies such as viral, ethanol hangover, and chemotherapy.

Behavioral Effects and Electrophsyiology

Pharmacological studies of oral and intravenously administered ginger constituents produce behavioral effects (Suekawa et al. 1984). Intravenous (1.75–3.5 mg/kg) and oral (70–140 mg/kg) doses of (6)-shogaol inhibit spontaneous motor actvity and prolong hexabarbital-induced sleeping time. (6)-shogaol was more potent than (6)-gingerol. In an EEG study, intravenous (6)-shogaol shifted a low-amplitude fast-wave pattern to a high-amplitude slow-wave pattern after 5 minutes, which persisited for 60 minutes (Qian and Liu 1992; Suekawa et al. 1984).

Two studies have been done to date that address ginger's anxiolytic effects in an animal model (Hassenohrl et al. 1996, 1998). Unfortunately, both of these employ a combined treatment of ginger and *Ginkgo biloba* so they do not allow for differentiation of effects. The combination had diazepam-like effects in an animal model of anxiety (elevated-plus maze) (Hassenohrl et al. 1996). These effects were dose dependent and triphasic: low doses (0.5 mg/kg intragastrically) had anxiolytic effects, intermediate doses (1 and 10 mg/kg) had no effect, and higher doses (100 mg/kg) had anxiogenic effects. Unlike diazepam, the ginger/ginkgo combination did not have memory-imparing effects on spatial navigation memory (water maze) or inhibitory avoidance learning (Hassenohrl et al. 1998). The ratio of ginger to ginkgo affected the anxiolytic efficacy in the elevated-plus maze. The standard preparation with a ratio of ginger to ginkgo of 2.5 : 1 had anxiolytic efficacy, whereas other ratios, (1 : 1 or 1 : 2.5) were ineffective across all doses tested.

If ginger alone exerts anxiolytic effects, one potential mechanism is by 5-HT_3 antagonism by galanolactone, because pharmaceutical 5-HT_3 antagonists show antidepressant and anxiolytic effects (Huang et al. 1991; Martin et al. 1992; Costall and Naylor 1992; Costall et al. 1990; Menard and Treit 1999; Alvarez-Guerra et al. 2000). Another potential mechanism of anxiolytic effects of ginger is the eicosanoid inhibition (Kiuchi et al 1992; Srivastava 1984; Mustafa et al. 1993; Cooper et al. 1996). Apart from direct neuronal effects of eicosanoids, arachidonic acid and its metabolites inhibit $GABA_A$ transmission (Schwartz and Yu 1992). For example, thromboxane A_2 inhibits GABA receptor function, independent of its actions on cerebrovasculature and glial cells (Schwartz-Bloom et al. 1996). The interactions between eicosanoids and GABA are complex, but arachidonic acid levels increase along with increases in intracellular Ca^{2+} and GABA efflux, suggesting that it may be acting as an intrinsic feedback modulator in GABAergic neurons (Asakura and Matsuda 1984). Ginger constituents could hypothetically create an anxiolytic effect by facilitating GABA conductance through inhibition of arachidonic acid metabolites. Whether or not this occurs to a significant degree could be verified by in vitro and in vivo experiments with ginger constituents and assessing their effect on GABA transmission.

The antithromboxane effect of ginger is of potential significance in stress and depression. Hypercortisolism is found in approximately 50% of patients with major depression. Plasma thromboxane B levels correlated in a group of depressed patients with high levels of cortisol, but not with depressed individuals with low cortisol or with normal controls

(Piccirillo et al. 1994). The effects of thromboxane A_2 were examined in nondepressed, normal individuals. Thromboxane A_2 was found to have direct CNS effects on hemodynamic, ACTH, and cortisol responses (Cudd 1998). Whether ginger has a significant effect on these processes and whether it has an antistress or antidepressant effect is speculative, but the eicosanoid activites of ginger and relationship to depression warrant further investigation.

Toxicity

There is little known toxicity of ginger. The LD_{50} of oral ginger is very high (170 to 250 g/kg depending on the preparation) (Wu et al. 1990). It is listed by the Food and Drug Administration as Generally Regarded As Safe. No adverse reactions are noted in the normal doses of 2–4 g. It has been recommended not to take ginger in the presence of morning sickness or gallstones (Gruenwald et al. 1998).

Ginger Jake was rendered toxic only because of an adulterant organophosphate, triorthocresyl phosphate (TOCP), and not any constituent of ginger itself (Woolf 1995; Morgan and Tulloss 1976, Morgan and Penovich 1978). About 50,000 people ingested TOCP and experienced muscle pain, weakness, and minimal sensory impairment. TOCP causes irreversible central and peripheral neuronal damage, consisting of axonal dying-back neuropathy and upper motor neuron syndrome with spasticity and abnormal reflexes.

Summary and Conclusions

Four pharmacological mechanisms of ginger constituents have been investigated that could putatively mediate a central behavioral effect: (1) eicosanoid inhibition, (2) serotonin antagonism, (3) substance P release, and (4) Ca^{2+}/ATPase activity. Whether any of these occur is entirely contingent upon the passing of ginger constituents through the blood-brain barrier. Although there have been no studies that explicitly address this, electrophysiological and behavioral changes from peripheral administration provide indirect support.

Pharmacological data and experimental data indicate two potential uses of ginger: antiemetic and anxiolytic/antidepressant. Studies of antiemetic effects have brought generally positive results, although further research would allow stronger conclusions. Animal research and pharmacological mechanisms suggest an anxiolytic role of ginger, but there are no human studies to date that examine this. It is unlikely that ginger by itself will be sufficient as an antidepressant or anxiolytic for cases of clinical severity. However, ginger has few negative effects when used in reasonable quantities, and could augment other medications and/or counteract negative side effects.

Ginkgo

Although primarily recognized for its nootropic effects, ginkgo has been studied somewhat for psychotherapeutic effects. Because ginkgo has been discussed at length in chapter 5, this section will focus primarily on the studies of its anxiolytic and/or antidepressant effects.

Anxiolytic Effects

Two studies by Hassenohrl and colleagues (1996, 1998), which are described above, showed anxiolytic effects of a combined ginger and ginkgo preparation in an animal model. Again, the primary problem with these investigations is that they did not evaluate each herb in isolation. It is possible that each has anxiolytic effects and that combined they have synergistic effects. On the other hand, it is also possible that either of the two is ineffective and that a single herb is accounting for all of the effects. It is interesting to note, however, that in those studies, the ratio of ginger to ginkgo had significant effects on the anxiolytic potency.

A few other studies have been done that show anxiolytic effects of ginkgo in animal models. Ginkgo extract was found to reduce learning impairment induced by an auditory stressor on a discrimination task (Rapin et al. 1994). Young and old rats were given 20 days of oral treatment with EGb 761 (50 or 100 mg/kg/day). Although effective in both groups, EGb 761 was more effective in older than younger rats. Chronic administration of EGB 761 (50 and 100 mg/kg/day for 5 days) reduced avoidance deficits in the learned helplessness paradigm in rats, but was less effective when given afterward (Porsolt et al. 1990). Anxiolytic-like effects were also seen in an emotional hypophagia paradigm in mice.

Antidepressant Effects
Ginkgo has been tested in one study for treatment of seasonal affective disorder (Lingjaerde et al. 1999). This methodologically controlled study used a standardized extract, containing 48 mg flavone glycosides and 12 mg terpene lactones per day, for 10 weeks. Subjects were evaluated using the Mongomery-Åsberg Depression Rating Scale and an atypical symptom scale directed at symptoms of seasonal affective disorder (hypersomnia, hyperphagia, and carbohydrate craving). The results were negative, and failed to show an effect of ginkgo on any of the measures used. The authors cite a small number of subjects as a disadvantage of the study, potentially raising the probability of a false negative error. Other potential influences on the outcome may have been the dose used and the latency between symptom onset and treatment initiation.

Putative Mechanisms and Constituents
Ginkgolic acid conjugates (6-alkylsalicylates) were tested for anxiolytic effects in several animal paradigms (Satyan et al. 1998). Single oral doses (0.3 and 0.6 mg/kg) of ginkgolic acid conjugates showed dose-related anxiolytic effects in elevated-plus maze, the open field, and novelty-induced feeding tests. Diazepam had similar effects in the models used. The anxiolytic effects of ginkgo may be dependent on the extract used. The standardized ginkgo extract EGb 761, which lacks ginkgolic acid conjugates, showed lesser anxiolytic effects in some of the measures. The doses of ginkgolic acids were equivalent to what would be found in a 50 or 100 mg dose of extract, respectively. Further, given that the anxiolytic effects were obtained by oral administration, it indirectly suggests penetration of the blood-brain barrier. Paradoxically, acute and chronic administration of EGb 761 (8–16 mg/kg, IP) was found to reduce social contact in rats, which was reversed by diazepam, suggesting anxiogenic effects (Chermat et al. 1997). It should be noted that Satyan and colleagues (1998) showed anxiolytic effects of ginkgo in several measures but not in the social interaction test.

Monoamine There are several mechanisms that, alone or in combination, could account for ginkgo's potentially mood-altering effects. These are broadly categorized into monoamine and GABAergic effects. Ginkgo extract (EGb 761) increases uptake of 5-HT, but not dopamine, into synaptosomes, which is prevented by the 5-HT reuptake inhibitor clomipramine (Ramassamy et al. 1992). Hypothetically, increasing 5-HT reuptake could create anxiolytic effects by reducing 5-HT stimulation of 5-HT_2 receptors that have anxiogenic effects (Jenck et al. 1998). However, this action is contrary to the action of SSRIs, so reconciling an antidepressant action of ginkgo would likely necessitate other mechanisms. Aqueous and ethanolic ginkgo extracts as well as commercial preparations inhibit MAO_A and MAO_B in vitro (White et al. 1996). It remains to be shown that this occurs in the brain and at normal oral doses. But the authors also reported preliminary evidence that an oral dose of ginkgo could produce 30–50% inhibition of MAO_B in platelets in humans. However, a PET study of ginkgo extract in humans showed that it does not produce significant changes in the activity of brain MAO_A and MAO_B.

Although the monoamine mechanism of ginkgo is uncertain, treatment does alter monoamine receptors in animals. Chronic ginkgo extract reversed an age-related reduction in the maximal number of binding sites of 5-HT_{1A} receptors in aged (24-month-old) but not young (4-month-old) rats (Huguet et al. 1994). Chronic oral administration of ginkgo extract (EGb 761) also prevents the stress-induced desensitization of 5-HT_{1A} receptors, without altering their density or affinity (Bolanos-Jimenez et al. 1995). Drug discrimination paradigms also support that ginkgo extracts have effects on 5-HT_{1A}, but not 5-HT_2 receptors (Winter and Timineri 1999). Ginkgo chronically administered also reverses the decline in binding density of α_2-adrenergic receptors in aged rats (Huguet and Tarrade 1992).

GABA Another potential mechanism of ginkgo's psychotropic effects is amentoflavone. Amentoflavone is a flavonoid with benzodiazepine activity in the nanomolar range (Lobstein-Guth, et al. 1988; Baureithel et al. 1997). Amentoflavone seems to act as a partial agonist at GABA benzodiazepine receptors. However, it remains in question whether this constituent crosses the blood-brain barrer because it does not inhibit central flunitrazepam binding when administered peripherally (Nielsen et al. 1988). Still, there is some behavioral pharmacology evidence that supports a direct or indirect GABAergic action of ginkgo (Chermat et al. 1997).

Neuroendocrine Chronic treatment with oral ginkgo extract reduces stress-induced impairments in learning and elevation of stress hormones, in both young and old rats (Rapin et al. 1994). Ginkgolide B is one of the constituents responsible for this effect, which acts by reducing the binding and expression of peripheral-type benzodiazepine receptors in the adrenal cortex (Amri et al. 1996, 1997; Papadopoulos et al. 1998). In this way, it reduces production glucocorticoids, and may also act at the hypothalamic level to inhibit the hypothalamic-pituitary-adrenal (HPA) axis (Marcilhac et al. 1998).

Overactivation of HPA axis is associated with anxiety and depression. Elevated levels of cortisol occur during situational anxiety (Armario et al. 1996; Salmon et al. 1986). Dysregulation of the HPA axis occurs in such anxiety disorders as generalized anxiety and panic disorder (Avery et al. 1985). Concordantly, disruption of the glucocorticoid receptor gene is associated with reduced anxiety in mice (Tronche et al. 1999). Major depression is associated with disruption of the HPA axis due to impaired feedback mechanisms, resulting in elevation of cortisol levels (Carroll et al. 1981; Young et al. 1991). Chronic elevation of glucocorticoids is neurotoxic, and recurring depression is associated with neuropathological changes in the hippocampus (Sheline et al. 1996). Remission of depression is associated with a return of cortisol to normal levels (Steiger et al. 1989).

Thus, ginkgo's actions on the HPA axis may afford it anxiolytic and antidepressant-like effects, particularly when stress is a causal factor. Considering its neuroendocrine effects, investigation of ginkgo in depression may still be warranted, particularly where stress and anxiety play causal roles.

Summary and Conclusions

Ginkgo is most commonly known for its cognitive effects, but there is evidence to suggest it may have psychotherapeutic effects as well. As with its cognitive effects, the mechanisms responsible for its anxiolytic or antidepressant effects are uncertain, but likely involve monoamine and/or

GABAergic mechanisms. Animal studies suggest that ginkgo has anxiolytic effects that increase with advancing age. Despite evidence in several animal studies, there are few, if any, human studies that address its psychotherapeutic effects. Ginkgo remains to be tested in controlled clinical trials to determine in which disorders and at what doses it is effective.

There have been few, if any, studies on ginkgo and depression. Although it holds potential for psychotherapeutic effects, it does not seem that ginkgo could be used alone to treat anxiety or depression. More likely, it could serve as adjunctive treatment for anxiety or depression, and have positive side effects on those using it for nootropic effects.

Antipsychotic Herbs

Rauwolfia

History and Botany

Rauwolfia serpentina (serpentwood), of the Apocynaceae family, was reputed for thousands of years in India as a tranquilizer. In Sanskrit, it was referred to as *sarpagandha*, and in Hindi as *chandrika* (Robbers et al. 1996). Western medical interest in the plant began in the 1950s, when the constituent reserpine was identified. Rauwolfia is a small tree or shrub with numerous small pink and white flowers, deciduous leaves, and a fleshy ovoid fruit (Kowalchik and Hylton 1987). The medicinal part of the plant is the dried root (Gruenwald et al. 1998). Its name derives from Leonhard Rauwolf, a sixteenth century German botanist. Three primary species are recognized with distinct geographical distributions: *Rauwolfia serpentina* (India, Sri Lanka, Thailand, Indonesia, Burma), *R. tetraphylla* (southern Mexico to Colombia and the West Indies), and *R. vomitoria* (Africa, from Senegal to Mozambique).

Mechanism of Action

The psychoactive constituents of rauwolfia are alkaloids classified in three groups: (1) weakly basic indole alkaloids, (2) intermediate basic indoline alkaloids, and (3) strong anhydronium bases. Approximately 50 alkaloids have been identified, but the principal indole alkaloids

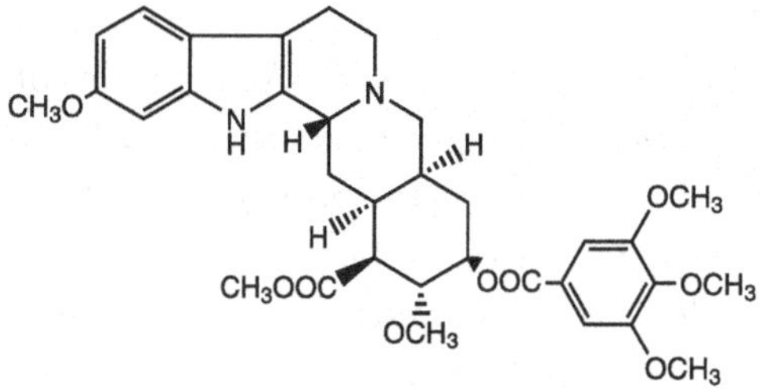

Reserpine

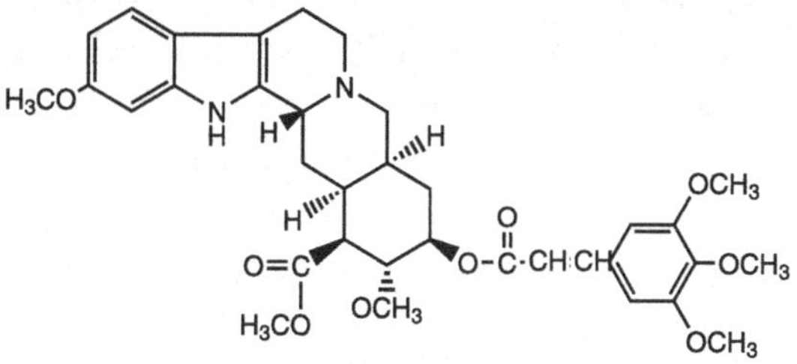

Rescinnamine

Figure 7.6
Chemical structure of rauwolfia alkaloids.

are reserpine, rescinnamine, and deserpidine (figure 7.6). Other indole alkloids are tetrahydroserpentine, raubasine, and ajmalicine. Ajmaline, isoajmaline, and rauwolfinine are also tertiary indoles, which have no therapeutic effects.

Reserpine blocks vesicular storage of monoamines, prolonging their presence in cytoplasm. There they are degraded by MAO, leading to a depletion of monoamines in synaptic terminals of central and peripheral neurons, so that little or no neurotransmitter is released when the neuron depolarizes (Oates 1996). Reversal of this process requires synthesis of new vesicles, which occurs over a period of days to weeks after discontinuation of the drug.

Therapeutic Uses

The primary medical uses of rauwolfia are antihypertensive and antipsychotic. However, it has drawbacks and its use has been supplanted with the invention of more modern antipsychotics such as piperazine, phenothiazines, butyrophenones, and thioxanthenes. Antagonism of dopamine receptors is a primary action of antipsychotic drugs (Carlsson 1978; Seeman 1987). Thus, reserpine may create antipsychotic effects by reducing the availability of dopamine or other monoamines. Despite the drawbacks, there is a place for the use of reserpine as an adjunct treatment for psychosis (Solon 1996; Wolkowitz et al. 1993). Schizophrenic patients on long-term neuroleptic treatment who were given adjunct reserpine showed a decrease in thought disturbance, agitation and hostility, and suspiciousness (Bagdy et al. 1988). However, these changes did not correlate with CSF changes in monoamine levels. In fact, although norepinephrine levels changed, other monoamine markers (CSF dopamine metabolites, platelet MAO, and serum dopamine-beta-hydroxylase) did not.

Rauwolfia derivatives became available in the 1950s in western medicine for the treatment of hypertension. The antihypertensive effects of rauwolfia alkaloids occur from their depletion of monoamines in adrenal chromaffin cells and sympathetic ganglia, and perhaps central neurons as well (Oates 1996).

Toxicity

The primary limiting effect of reserpine is depression. Depletion of central monoamines is believed to be the mechanism for this effect (Heninger et al. 1996; Charney 1998). The depression may occur in a gradual and insidious manner, and the causal association between the drug and depression may be missed (Oates 1996). Rauwolfia alkaloids are contraindicated in anyone with a history of depression, and careful vigilance is required to ensure that they do not induce depression in otherwise normal individuals. Additional side effects are sedation and difficulty with concentration and performing complex mental tasks.

Psychotherapeutic Herbs: Conclusions

The discovery of pharmaceutical medications for the treatment of mental illnesses has revolutionized treatment and our understanding of the brain. Several herbal medications have been employed historically for the treatment of mental illness, many of which are ineffective or impractical. However, a few hold promise. Rauwolfia has long been used as a tranquilizer and antipsychotic medication, which is likely related to its depletion of monoamine neurotransmitters. Although this has an antipsychotic effect, it also has the unfortunate side effects of depression and cognitive impairment. Although it may have some use as an adjunctive treatment for schizophrenia, the advent of neuroleptics and newer atypical antipsychotic drugs are likely to render it obsolete.

Hypericum not only has a long tradition of use as an antidepressant, but also a considerable amount of scientific research to support it. More research is needed, but it certainly works better than placebo and may be as efficacious as pharmaceutical antidepressants. The mechanism of this effect is not certain although monoamine reuptake mechanisms are most likely involved. Various other mechanisms may contribute additive or synergistic effects.

Ginger is most commonly used as a spice, but has significant antiemetic effects and may have anxiolytic or antidepressant effects. It may not likely be sufficient by itself, but it could augment other medications and/or counteract negative side effects. At least four mechanisms have been found that may mediate ginger's central effects. Although known for its cognitive effects, ginkgo may also have anxiolytic or antidepressant effects. Ginger and ginkgo have potential as psychotherapeutic herbal medications, but far more research is needed to establish their basic efficacy.

It is not likely that herbal psychotherapeutic medications will replace the use of pharmaceutical treatments. Herbal treatments are too few, and those known at present need more research to establish their use. By far, hypericum has the best potential of this class.

8
Analgesic and Anesthetic Plants

Pain is a basic sensory, emotional, and cognitive phenomenon that signals some type of harm to the organism. It is practically universal to human experience, and although it is initially adaptive, it frequently outlives its usefulness and impedes one's ability to function. Accordingly, plants that alleviate pain have become essential to human civilization.

The plant drugs discussed here for their analgesic and anesthetic effects are diverse in form as well as pharmacology, reflecting the diverse neurochemistry of the sensory and analgesic branches of the nervous system. They are grouped here by their pharmacological mechanism, including: opioid (poppy, myrrh), cholinergic (tobacco, lobelia, areca), eicosanoid (willow, feverfew), neurokinin (chili, ginger), purinergic (coffee, tea, chocolate, guarana, maté, kola), cannabinoid, monoamine (coca, khat), and uncertain mechanisms (ginseng). Plants discussed here for their local anesthetic effects are coca and clove.

Definition of Terms

Whereas *pain* is used to refer to the total subjective phenomena associated with injury and suffering, *nociception* more specifically refers to the aspect of sensory transmission. Nociception is the more correct term for the experimental study of pain, because it is objectively measured through a behavior in animals and humans alike (e.g., withdrawal reflexes, verbal ratings). The actual subjective experiences are private and known to each subject alone. However, for the sake of convenience, the word *pain* will be used here to address both aspects. Similarly, the word *analgesia*, meaning the relief from pain, will be used in place of the more objective term *antinociception*.

Another distinction must be made between *analgesia* and *anesthesia.* While *anesthesia* refers to blocking of all sensations, *analgesia* refers to the specific blocking of pain, leaving other cutaneous senses (e.g., touch, pressure, temperature) intact. Among anesthetics, local and general anesthetics are distinguished. *Local anesthesia* refers to local blockade of nerve conduction, whereas *general anesthesia* involves inducing deep unconsciousness with a depressant drug. The anesthetic plant medications discussed here are solely local anesthetics. Although they effectively block all sensation, local anesthetics are ultimately applied to prevent painful sensations (e.g., dental procedures).

Pain and Analgesia Systems

Sensory Transmission of Pain

In order to accurately appreciate drugs that block pain, it is necessary to have at least a cursory understanding of pain and analgesia in the nervous system. Pain typically begins with injury to bodily tissue and stimulation of primary afferent neurons (Price 1988; Kandel et al. 1991). Although many types of axons participate in different aspects of pain, the primary types are Aδ and C fibers. Thermal and mechanical pain is mediated by the small-diameter Aδ fibers, conducting signals at 5 to 30 m/sec, while C fibers are polymodal, and thus activated by several high-threshold stimuli. They also conduct at a slower rate (0.5–2 m/sec). Aδ and C fibers are distributed throughout the skin and deeper tissues. The cell bodies of primary afferents are in the dorsal root ganglion, and they project to the dorsal horn of the spinal cord.

In addition to mechanical and thermal stimulation, there are a number of endogenous chemicals that activate or sensitize primary afferents. These include K^+, serotonin, bradykinin, histamine, prostaglandins, leukotrienes, and neurokinins such as substance P.

Aδ and C primarily project to lamina II and V of the dorsal horn, where they synapse onto local interneurons or directly onto upward-projecting neurons (figure 8.1). These primary afferents release a number of neurotransmitters to relay pain, including glutamate, aspartate, substance P, neurokinin A and B, and calcitonin gene-related peptide (table 8.1). NMDA, non-NMDA and neurokinin receptors are involved in re-

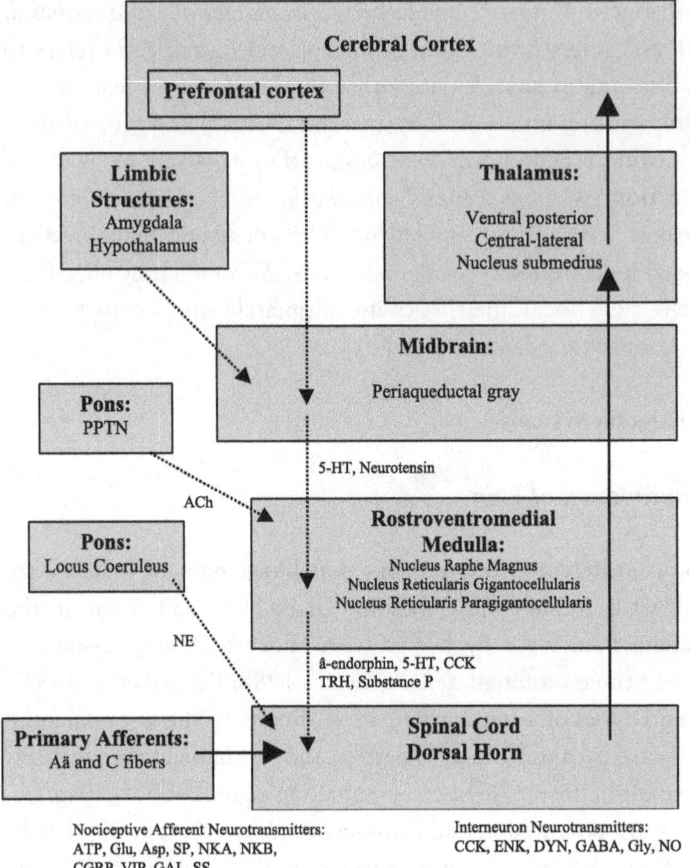

Figure 8.1
Central pain and analgesia systems. Abbreviations: 5-HT, serotonin; ACh, acetylcholine; ATP, adenosine triphosphate; Asp, aspartate; CCK, cholecystokinin; CGRP, calcitonin gene-related peptide; DYN, dynorphin; ENK, enkephalin; GABA, gamma-aminobutyric acid; GAL, galanin; Glu, glutamate; Gly, glycine; NE, norepinephrine; NK, neurokinin; NO, nitric oxide; SS, somatostatin; SP, substance P; TRH, thyrotropin-releasing hormone; VIP, vasoactive intestinal peptide.

Table 8.1
Neurotransmitters released by nociceptive afferents in the dorsal horn

Adenosine triphosphate (ATP)
Glutamate
Aspartate
Substance P
Neurokinin A
Neurokinin B
Calcitonin gene-related peptide
Vasoactive intestinal peptide
Galanin
Somatostatin

Table 8.2
Neurotransmitters released by interneurons in the dorsal horn

Cholecystokinin
Enkephalin
Dynorphin
GABA
Glycine
Nitric oxide

ceiving the signal and exciting projection neurons. Dorsal horn interneurons release a number of neurotransmitters, including opioids and GABA (table 8.2). Afferents from cutaneous and visceral sources may converge in the spinal cord. This sometimes causes *referred pain*, where pain originating in one part of the body may be experienced in another part. Thus, a heart attack is sometimes experienced as chest and left-sided ulnar pain.

Projection neurons in the dorsal horn send ascending axons through anterolateral pathways in the spinal white matter. These reach the thalamus, but send collaterals to brain stem sites along the way. Among the ascending tracts are the spinothalamic tract and spinoreticular tract. Thalamic nuclei receiving nociceptive afferents are the central lateral nucleus and ventroposterolateral nuclei. The central-lateral nuclei have widespread projections and a diffuse influence on the cortex. In contrast, the ventroposterolateral nuclei convey fine-scale epicritic information, and project to specific sensory areas such as primary and secondary somatosensory cortex (SI, SII) in the parietal lobe. Pain activates several other cerebral areas, including limbic structures, the insula, anterior cingulate, and orbitofrontal cortex.

Neural Inhibition of Pain

The nervous system has its own mechanisms for controlling pain. Endogenous control of pain is accomplished through a descending set of projections involving multiple structures from supraspinal to spinal levels. Findings from anatomical studies combined with pharmacological and electrophysiological studies have yielded an approximate working model of analgesia (Basbaum and Fields 1984). In general, the system receives input from multiple brain areas and incoming sensory information. When sufficient pain is encountered, it activates a descending system in the brain stem that projects down to the spinal cord and dampens or blocks the pain transmission at the level of the dorsal horn. The rest of this section will consider the relevant neuroanatomical areas in more detail.

Running through the center of the midbrain is the cerebral aqueduct, which conducts cerebrospinal fluid, and surrounding it is the periaqueductal grey (PAG) (Bandler and Shipley 1994). The role of the PAG is perhaps best summarized as receiving sensory input to integrate analgesic, defensive/aggressive, sexual, and autonomic responses (Mayer and Price 1976; Bandler and Shipley 1994). The ventrolateral section of the PAG is of particular interest for analgesia. The PAG connects reciprocally multiple brain areas, including the forebrain (e.g., frontal cortex, cingulate, amygdala, hypothalamus) (Van Bockstaele et al. 1991; Bandler and Shipley 1994). It also connects with brain stem regions such as raphe and reticular nuclei (Van Bockstaele et al. 1991). Both electrical and neurochemical stimulation of the PAG produces analgesia.

The nucleus locus coeruleus (LC) in the pons is an important source of noradrenergic projections in the central nervous system, with extensive forebrain, brain stem, and spinal projections (Lindvall and Björklund 1974). Particularly relevant to analgesia are projections from the LC to nuclei in the rostral ventromedial medulla (RVM) (see review: Moore and Bloom 1979). Stimulation of the LC faciltates analgesia produced by both electrical stimulation and morphine microinjection (Bodnar et al. 1988, 1991; Segal and Sandberg 1977). Projections from the RVM to LC and then to the spinal cord are important in mediating analgesia (Clark and Proudfit 1991). Analgesia elicited through the vlPAG and LC depends in part on α_2 receptors in the dorsal horn (Peng et al. 1996).

Another pontine area of interest regarding analgesia is the pedunculopontine tegmental nucleus (PPTN), which is a major brain stem source of cholinergic cells. The PPTN has projections to the RVM and spinal cord (Iwamoto and Marion 1993). The RVM receives input from many brain areas relevant to analgesia, and has projections to the spinal cord (Fields et al. 1991; Zagon 1995).

Thus, the primary descending circuit that mediates analgesia involves projections from the PAG to the RVM, and from the RVM to the spinal cord, with various forebrain and brain stem areas modulating the circuit (Basbaum and Fields 1984). A number of neurotransmitters are used in this system, including serotonin, norepinephrine, GABA, neurotensin, excitatory amino acids, and opioids. (Clements et al. 1985; Moore and Bloom 1979; Clements et al. 1987; Beitz 1982). Serotonergic neurons in this circuit corelease Substance P and thyrotropin-releasing hormone or enkephalin (Hokfelt et al. 1977). So, administering various receptor antagonists, including serotonin, excitatory amino acid, and acetylcholine, into the RVM blocks the descending transmission of signals that inhibit pain (Kiefel et al. 1992a, 1992b, 1993; Spinella and Bodnar 1996; Spinella et al. 1997, 1999).

Opioid Neurotransmitters and Analgesia

The classic endogenous opioid peptides are derived from one of three families of precursors: pro-opiomelanocortin (POMC), pro-dynorphin, and pro-enkephalin. Many active opioid peptides are derived from these three, but the best known are β-endorphin, enkephalin, and dynorphin. POMC is produced by nuclei in the hypothalamus and medulla (Khachaturian et al. 1985; Watson et al. 1978; Bloom et al. 1978). Enkephalin and dynorphin neurons are distributed to all levels of the central nervous system (Hokfelt et al. 1977; Khachaturian et al. 1983; Sar et al. 1978; Khachaturian et al. 1985).

Table 8.3
Opioid subtypes and ligands

Receptor	Agonist	Antagonist	Endogenous ligands
μ	Morphine, DAMGO	β-FNA	EM, ENK, β-END
μ_1	—	Naloxonazine	
μ_2	—	—	
δ	DSLET, DADLE	Naltrindole	ENK
δ_1	DPDPE	DALCE	
δ_2	Deltorphin	NTII	
κ	U50,488H	nor-BNI	DYN

Key: DAMGO—D-Ala^2, met-Phe^4, Gly(ol)^5-enkephalin; DADLE—D-Ala^2, D-Leu^5-enkephalin; DALCE—D-Ala^2, Leu^5, Cys^6-enkephalin; DPDPE—D-Pen^2, D-Pen^5-enkephalin; DSLET—D-Ser^2, Leu^5-enkephalin, Thr^6; DYN—Dynorphin; EM—endomorphin; ENK—enkephalin; β-FNA—β-funaltrexamine, NTII—naltrindole 5′-isothiocyanate; nor-BNI—Nor-binaltorphimine.

Recently, a few new opioid peptides have been identified (Taylor and Dickenson 1998). In 1995 a peptide called orphanin FQ (alternately referred to as nociceptin) was identified, which binds to an *opioid-like receptor*, entitled ORL1 (Reinscheid et al. 1995). Similar to other opioid receptors, ORL1 is a g-protein-coupled metabotropic receptor. Unlike other opioids, orphanin FQ/nociceptin can create analgesic or hyperalgesic effects, depending on the dose used and site of injection (Yamamoto et al. 1999; Rossi et al. 1998). Two other novel opioid neuropeptides have been discovered, entitled endomorphin$_1$ and endomorphin$_2$ (Zadina et al. 1997). Both show a high affinity and selectivity for the μ receptor. Endomorphins appear to localize to many areas of the brain, but not necessarily to all areas in which mu receptors are found. Physiological actions of endomorphins are similar or identical to those produced by μ-selective agonists.

Opioids create their effects by acting at opioid receptors (table 8.3). These are, namely, μ, κ, and δ. Each is further divided into subtypes, which are differentially distributed throughout the nervous system: μ_1, μ_2, δ_1, δ_2, κ_1, and κ_3. A κ_2 receptor was defined pharmacologically, but no one to date has cloned a receptor that resembles it (Zukin et al. 1998). Selective agonists have been developed for the receptor subtypes (see table 8.3). Naloxone is a general antagonist for all classical opioid receptors. All opioid receptors create cellular effects through G-protein-

Table 8.4
Classification of analgesic and anesthetic plants

Mechanism	Plants
Analgesic Plants	
Opioid	Opium poppy, myrrh
Cholinergic	Tobacco, lobelia, areca
Eicosanoid	Willow, feverfew
Neurokinin	Chili, ginger
Purinergic	Coffee, tea, cocoa, guarana, maté, kola
Cannabinoid	Cannabis
Monoamine	Khat, coca
Uncertain	Ginseng
Local Anesthetic Plants	
Block of Na^+ channels	Coca, clove

coupled mechanisms. They inhibit adenylate cyclase activity, activate receptor-gated K^+ currents, and inhibit voltage-gated Ca^{2+} currents (Reisine and Pasternak 1996).

Many opioid receptors have now been cloned and their amino acid sequences determined (Evans et al. 1992; Kieffer et al. 1992).

Analgesic Drugs

Thus, there are numerous neurochemical systems that participate in pain transmission and analgesia systems in the brain. Potentially, any drug that interferes with any of these systems could have analgesic effects. As will be demonstrated in this chapter, there are many plants with analgesic and anesthetic effects, working through a variety of pharmacological mechanisms (table 8.4).

Analgesic Plants

Opium Poppy

History and Botany

The opium poppy *(Papaver somniferum)* is a blue-grey annual plant growing 30 to 150 cm in height (Robbers et al. 1996; Gruenwald et al.

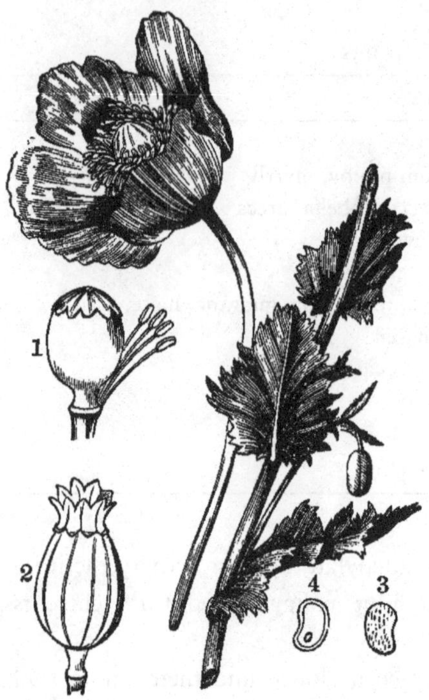

Figure 8.2
The opium poppy *(Papaver somniferum)*. Reprinted from Culbreth DMR. (1927). *Materia Medica and Pharmacognosy*, 7th ed. Philadelphia: Lea & Febiger.

1998). It has a single erect stem with a round seed pod at the top. Its seeds are small, reniform, and black or blue in color (figures 8.2, 8.3). After being sterilized, the seeds are commonly used for baking. The flowers are violet-white or red in color. *Papaver* is the Latin name for the opium poppy, and *somniferum* is also from Latin, meaning "sleep-producing." *Opium* comes from the Greek word *opion*, meaning poppy juice (Robbers et al. 1996). Whereas the word *opiate* refers to drugs derived from the poppy, *opioid* encompasses both natural and synthetic drugs in this class, as well as endogenous neurotransmitters. *Narcotic* is an archaic term for opioids, and its usage has been confused with other illicit drugs.

The opium poppy is one of several plants that have profoundly affected human history. It has provided an unmatched medicine for

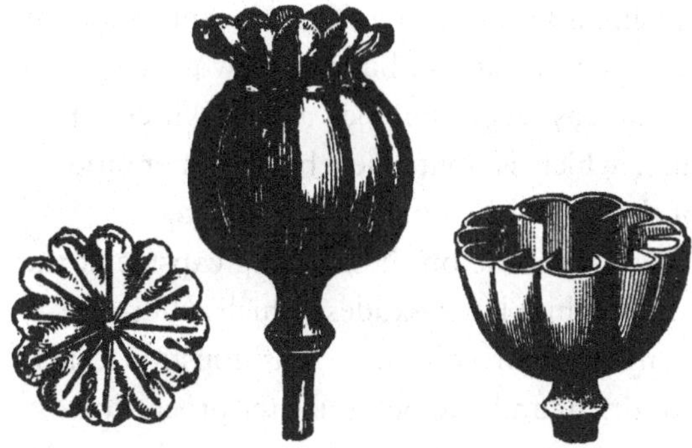

Figure 8.3
Seed pod of the opium poppy *(Papaver somniferum)*. Reprinted from Culbreth DMR. (1927). *Materia Medica and Pharmacognosy*, 7th ed. Philadelphia: Lea & Febiger.

relieving pain and suffering. On the other hand, opioids' powerful emotional and reinforcing effects have made addiction to them a persistent and prevalent dilemma. The opium poppy has probably been used throughout much of human history. Poppy seeds were discovered in lake villages in Switzerland dating back to the Neolithic period and Bronze Age (Rudgley 1993). Its use was known among the ancient Romans, Greeks, and Egyptians, and the first known writings come from Theophrastus in the third century B.C.E. The Arabs used opium as a medical treatment and introduced it to East Asia, where it was used to treat dysentery. During the eighteenth century, smoking of opium became popular in East Asia. Use of opioids in the United States was legally unrestricted until the twentieth century, when addiction gained prominence (Musto 1991).

Some major alkaloids were isolated from opium during the nineteenth century, which led to the use of pure alkaloids rather than the crude preparation. A series of synthetic opioids have been developed in the twentieth century, including meperidine and methadone, as well as the opioid antagonists naloxone and naltrexone. Understanding of opioids has continued in this century with the identification of opioid receptors and the isolation of endogenous opioid neuropeptides. Although many neurotransmitters are involved in analgesia, it was the research into the powerful mechanisms of opium alkaloids that began the understanding of analgesia.

Cultivation of the plant in India began in the fifteenth century C.E. It was probably originally cultivated in Europe, but it is now grown in an area between Turkey and Southeast Asia. Poppies are grown commercially for pharmaceutical use, which is controlled by the International Narcotics Control Board of the United Nations.

To extract opium, razor cuts are made on the ripening capsule at the proper stage of development. A white latex exudes, which oxidizes to a red-brown color overnight and is later collected. This constitutes raw opium, which is compressed, dried, and shipped for later processing.

Chemical Constituents

More than 30 alkaloids have been identified in opium (Robbers et al. 1996). The most relevant are morphine (4–21%), codeine (0.8–2.5%), noscapine (4–8%), papaverine (0.5–2.5%), and thebaine (0.5–2%) (figure 8.4). Other opium alkaloids include narceine, protopine, laudanine, codamine, cytopine, lanthopine, and meconidine. Numerous other opioids have been synthesized from opium alkaloids. Among them is heroin, or diacetylmorphine.

Mechanisms of Action

As discussed in greater detail above, endogenous and exogenous opioids alike create their effects by binding to μ, κ, and/or δ opioid receptors. The physiological actions of opioids depend also on their neuroanatomical distribution. Concerning analgesia, presynaptic opioid receptors are present on the terminals of sensory neurons in the spinal cord. Stimulation of those receptors causes decreased release of substance P. Postsynaptic effects of morphine also occur on interneurons and ascending spinothalamic neurons. Agonists of δ and κ receptors act similarly in the spinal cord. In addition to spinal mechanisms, several supraspinal sites mediate opioid analgesia. Administration of opioids in combinations of supraspinal and/or spinal sites produces supra-additive or synergistic effects (Yeung and Rudy 1980; Bodnar et al. 1991; Rossi et al. 1993, 1994).

Indirect Mechanisms

Opioids dose-dependently reduce the release of acetylcholine in several brain areas, including the hippocampus, striatum, and cerebral cortex

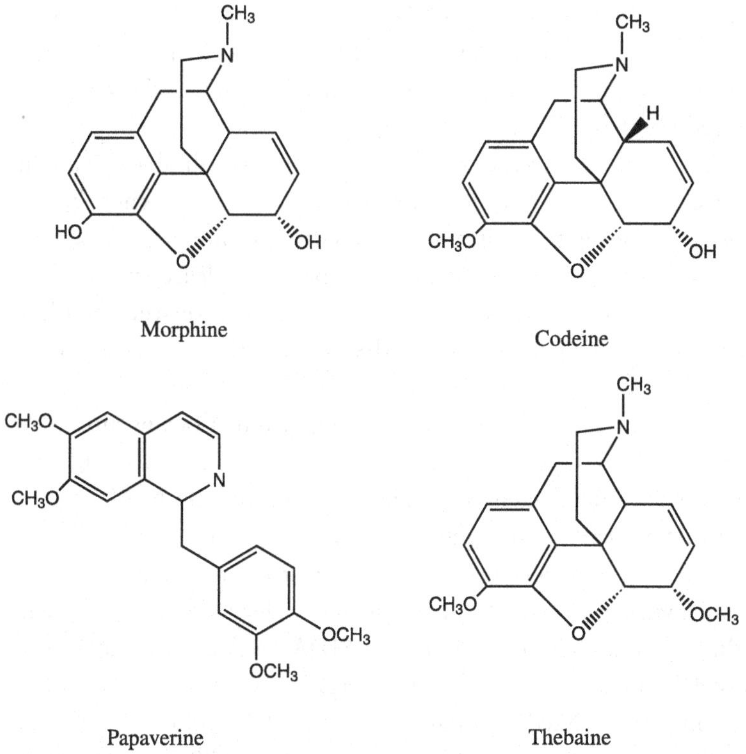
CH3
N
HO
OH
O
Morphine
CH3
N
H
CH3O
OH
O
Codeine
CH3O
CH3O
N
OCH3
OCH3
Papaverine
CH3
N
CH3O
OCH3
O
Thebaine

Figure 8.4
Chemical structure of opium alkaloids.

(Lapchak et al. 1989). Interspecies differences are found, however, where κ agonists reduce acetylcholine release in the guinea pig hippocampus, while μ receptors have this effect in the rat. Although species differences exist, inhibition of acetylcholine release by opioids commonly involves Ca^{2+} mechanisms and do not appear to involve GABAergic mechanisms (Feuerstein et al. 1996). However, they may be mediated by interneurons releasing somatostatin (Feuerstein et al. 1998).

Central monoamine release is influenced by opioids. Indeed, opioid analgesic mechanisms are known to depend on descending monoamine projections (Basbaum and Fields 1984). However, opioids and monoamines also interact at other levels of the neuraxis. Opioid agonists of μ, κ, and δ receptors inhibit release of norepinephrine in the cortex and hypothalamus (Werling et al. 1987; Diez-Guerra et al. 1987). This effect is mediated by μ receptors located on noradrenergic neurons. Cortical serotonin projections, in contrast, are relatively unaffected by opioids (Hagan and Hughes 1984).

Overall, μ agonists increase transmission in the mesolimbic dopamine system (Devine et al. 1993; Johnson and North 1992). They inhibit GABAergic neurons in the ventral tegmental area, disinhibiting dopamine activity. In contrast, κ agonists inhibit dopamine release in the same system. As with other drugs of abuse, an influence on the mesolimbic dopamine is believed to mediate the positive reinforcing effects of opioids.

Opioids also interact with excitatory amino acid neurotransmitters. At lower micromolar concentrations, μ agonists (e.g., DAMGO) enhance NMDA activity in the nucleus accumbens, but inhibit non-NMDA activity (Martin et al. 1997). At higher concentrations (5 µM), NMDA currents are reduced. Conversely, central administration of glutamate can precipitate a withdrawal syndrome in morphine-dependent animals, similar to the opioid antagonist naloxone. NMDA mechanisms also appear to be involved in the development of morphine tolerance. Competitive and noncompetitive NMDA antagonists and inhibitors of nitric oxide synthase reduce or eliminate tolerance to morphine (Elliott et al. 1995; Bilsky et al. 1996). However, this does not occur for tolerance to κ opioids.

Pharmacokinetics

Opioids are administered in several ways. Opium was most commonly taken recreationally by smoking, but intravenous administration has become most common since the isolation of opium alkaloids and invention of the hypodermic needle. The development of heroin from morphine at the turn of the twentieth century led to more intense euphoric effects and greater risk for addiction. Heroin may also be snorted, or it can be smoked when added to a medium such as tobacco. Medically, opioids are commonly given through oral, subcutaneous, intravenous, transdermal, or rectal routes.

The presence of alkaloids in poppy seeds has led to arguments that they may result in positive drug screens, even when no illicit drugs have been taken. This concern was common enough to be satirized in an episode of the American television show *Seinfeld.* Morphine concentrations found in poppy seeds are approximately 167 μg/g, and codeine concentrations are around 44 μg/g (Paul et al. 1996). While the amount of alkaloid is not sufficient to cause significant psychoactive effects, they may be detectable on drug screen tests, leading to false positive results. In an attempt to avoid this confusion, a cutoff concentration of 300 ng/ml is used to distinguish between opioid levels obtained from drug use and poppy seed ingestion. Consumption of bread rolls sprinkled with poppy seeds will most likely (but not always) yield negative results, but ingestion of poppy seed cakes or streusels can easily exceed cutoff levels (Meadway et al. 1998). In one study, positive screens occurred for 24 hours after consuming cakes that contained an average of 4.69 g of seed (dose equivalent to 0.07 g poppy seed/kg). One proposed way to discriminate between poppy seed ingestion and illicit drug use in forensic screenings involves thebaine, because it is only found in poppy seeds (Cassella et al. 1997). However, the elimination of thebaine varies between individuals, so the absence of thebaine does not necessarily mean use of illicit drugs (Meadway et al. 1998). A better discriminant is 6-monoacetylmorphine, which is present in urine after heroin use, but not after poppy seed consumption (Mulé and Casella 1988).

Opioids are generally well absorbed enterally (Reisine and Pasternak 1996). However, blood levels of morphine only reach half of those reached by injection. The more lipid soluble opioids are absorbed through the nasal mucosa or transdermally (e.g., fentanyl). Transdermal adminstration is much slower and more prolonged, avoiding the fluctuating levels produced by injection.

Opioid levels in the brain are significant within seconds to minutes after injection. As mentioned before, heroin is more lipid soluble than morphine, so a greater amount penetrates the brain. Lipid solubility and ionization are the predominant factors that determine the distribution of opioids (Mather 1987). At therapeutic concentrations, about one-third of morphine is bound to protein in the blood.

When heroin is administered, it is rapidly converted to 6-monoacetylmorphine and then to morphine in the brain. Heroin is also more lipid soluble, suggesting that its increased potency is due to increased distribution into the brain. The major metabolic pathway for morphine is conjugation with glucuronic acid to form morphine-6-glucuronide (M6G). While morphine itself is active, M6G may account for the majority of morphine's effects. Glucuronidation of the 6-hydroxyl group of morphine and codeine does not affect their μ affinity, but slightly increases their affinity for δ receptors and reduces their κ affinity (Mignat et al. 1995). Morphine is eliminated in urine, mostly as morphine-3-glucuronide.

General Effects

Analgesia Opioid analgesics, namely morphine and codeine, are potent analgesics. In addition to reducing the sensory aspect of pain, opioids alter the emotional aspect, where the pain may still be present but less troubling. However, even intrathecal morphine alone will reduce pain, so emotional changes are not solely responsible. Generally, continuous, dull pain is more responsive to opioids than sharp, intermittent pain, but sufficient doses can reduce both types. Although pain from tissue damage responds to opioids, pain due to nerve injury (neuropathic pain) does not. While actions in spinal and brainstem areas may be sufficient to explain the block of the sensory aspects of pain, involvement in cortical, limbic, and thalamic structures may dull the emotional response to pain.

Cardiovascular Morphine has no significant cardiovascular effects on a person laying supine, but orthostatic hypotension may occur due to peripheral vasodilation and inhibited baroreceptor reflexes. Myocardial effects are not significant in normal individuals, but may be more variable during myocardial infarction.

Miosis Morphine causes constriction of the pupil by a direct action on the parasympathetic nerve. Miosis is pathognomonic of opioid (specifically μ agonist) overdose, but mydriasis occurs with respiratory suppression and asphyxiation.

Respiratory μ and δ ligands participate in the regulation of respiration (Su et al. 1998). Respiratory suppression is a regular feature of morphine, which suppresses all phases of respiration. Respiratory arrest is the most frequent cause of death from morphine or heroin overdose. In normal therapeutic doses, however, respiratory effects are not problematic in people without pulmonary disease. Respiratory depression results from altering the response of brainstem areas to carbon dioxide levels.

Digestive system μ agonists decrease secretion of stomach acid, reduce gastric motility, and prolong gastric emptying. Pancreatic, biliary, and intestinal secretions are reduced. Intestinal transit is also slowed. Peristaltic movements are reduced, but tone is increased, sometimes causing spasm. As a result, constipation is a frequent problem with opioid use. Bile duct pressure is also increased by opioids.

Morphine also causes nausea and vomiting by stimulation of the area postrema. Nausea is a common reaction to intravenous injection, but tolerance develops to this effect over repeated use.

Cough Opioids are effective cough suppressants, through direct effects on a cough center in the medulla. This was a prominent use of opioids, but effective nonopioid agents have been developed for this purpose that are nonaddicting and do not suppress respiration. Ironically, heroin was developed as a cough medicine in the hopes that it would have less toxic and addicting effects.

Neuroendocrine Through hypothalamic actions, morphine inhibits the release of gonadotropin-releasing hormone and corticotrophin-releasing hormone (Desjardins et al. 1990; Grossman 1983; Reisine and Pasternak 1996). Consequently, there is a decrease in circulating levels of luteinizing hormone, follicle-stimulating hormone, adrenocorticotrohpic hormone, β-endorphin, testosterone and cortisol. Increased prolactin levels occur, possibly through interactions with dopaminergic systems. However, tolerance to these neuroendocrine effects develops with chronic administration.

Behavioral effects Opioids produce sedation, but not as profoundly as CNS depressants like barbiturates or general anesthetics. A person administered an opioid is generally lethargic but arousable.

Opioids have noted effects on ingestive behavior and appetite (Bodnar 1996). Morphine increases food intake, and μ antagonists conversely decrease food intake. Similarly, δ agonists increase spontaneous food intake, but κ agonists have marginal effects.

Morphine generally has sedative effects, reducing overall activity. But local injections into dopaminergic systems can increase locomotor activity, and daily administration can also sensitize one to the locomotor effect (Kalivas and Duffy 1987). High doses of opioids create muscle rigidity and catalepsy.

Emotional effects Morphine creates a pleasant, euphoric state, which is an aspect of the behaviorally reinforcing effect. The subjective state produced by opioids is often described as ecstatic and is compared to a sexual experience. These effects are most likely mediated by μ and possibly δ receptors, and interactions with the mesolimbic dopamine system (Shippenberg et al. 1993; Di Chiara and North 1992; Wise 1989). In contrast, κ opioids have dysphoric and psychotomimetic effects (Kumor et al. 1986).

Morphine has anxiolytic effects in humans. Users typically experience a sense of contentment and complacency. This effect is most likely mediated by opioid receptors in limbic structures such as the amygdala (File and Rodgers 1979).

Cerebral blood flow The differential mood-altering effects of μ and κ opioid agonists is reflected in neuroimaging studies. Hydromorphone, a μ agonist, increases CBF in the anterior cingulate cortex, bilateral amygdala, and the thalamus, as measured by single photon emission computed tomography (SPECT) (Schlaepfer et al. 1998). In contrast, butorphanol (which has kappa activity) produces a less-distinct pattern of activation, with increases primarily in the temporal lobes. Cerebral blood flow differences in opioid-dependent subjects tend to normalize within 2 weeks after discontinuation (Rose et al. 1996).

Neuroimaging of people with opioid dependence shows differences in this population compared to controls (Gerra et al. 1998). However, these differences may be more related to concurrent psychiatric disturbances than the opioid effects (Gerra et al. 1998). Chronic opioid dependence with comorbid depression is associated with decreased perfusion in the right frontal and left temporal lobes. A negative correlation exists between left temporal cerebral blood flow and the Depression subscale scores on the Minnesota Multiphasic Personality Inventory. A decrease in right frontal perfusion is also seen in opioid-dependent subjects who have antisocial tendencies.

Cognitive Opioids affect cognition through receptors located in many parts of the cerebrum and brain stem. Clinical doses of opioids generally have modest or mixed effects on cognition in humans, depending on the drug and cognitive paradigm used. To further complicate the picture, many studies are done on people suffering from a severe illness and significant levels of pain, which themselves affect cognitive function and may confound experimental results. Thus, results of such studies must be interpreted with caution. However, studies of opioids in nonclinical populations confirm their cognitive effects.

Opioids are sedating and cause a reduction in processing speed in clinical populations (e.g., Digit Symbol Substitution Test) (Wood et al. 1998). However, a study in healthy subjects did not confirm these effects on digit substitution (Walker and Zacny 1998). Improvements are seen in choice reaction time after morphine administration (Hanks et al. 1995). Deficits have been reported in early-stage visual processing (O'Neill et al. 1995; Hanks et al. 1995). By comparison, morphine's cognitive effects are lesser than those of lorazepam, but milder than hydromorphone (Rapp et al. 1996; Hanks et al. 1995).

Opioid effects on memory are consistent in humans and animal models (Braida et al. 1994; Saha et al. 1991). Verbal and visual memory are impaired by morphine one hour after oral administration (Hanks et al. 1995; Kerr et al. 1991). These could be due to direct neuronal effects of opioids, or perhaps through indirect effects on cholinergic transmission. However, in some animal paradigms morphine can enhance memory consolidation through indirect dopaminergic mechanisms (Castellano et al. 1994).

Addiction and Dependence

Tolerance and dependence are characteristic of repeated administration of opioid drugs, which limits their use in treatment. It has been proposed that tolerance results from desensitization of opioid receptors and altered intracellular G-protein/adenylate cyclase interactions (Reisine and Bell 1993). As mentioned above, NMDA and nitric oxide mechanisms have also been implicated.

Dependence is evident with chronic use of opioids, and discontinuation precipitates a withdrawal syndrome. A withdrawal syndrome can also be rapidly precipitated by an antagonist. The opioid withdrawal syndrome is characteristic and aversive (Farrell 1994; Milhorn 1992). Within 8 hours after discontinuation, one experiences tearing, yawning, sweating, and runny nose. By 12–14 hours, tossing, restless sleep occurs. The peak occurs at 48–72 hours, with pupil dilations, inability to eat, gooseflesh, restlessness, tachycardia, motor tremors, muscle cramps, nausea, diarrhea, intestinal spasms, and alternating chills and flushing. During this time, the person is understandably irritable, anxious, and dysphoric.

Treatment of acute opioid withdrawal is largely pharmacological. Most commonly, a replacement strategy is used where the person is switched to a longer-acting, oral opioid such as methadone. This maintains the person in a steadier state and avoids the fluctuations that occur with injecting a shorter-acting opioid (e.g., heroin). While some treatment programs seek to maintain users on methadone indefinitely, others slowly taper the dose down. Tapering avoids the severe acute withdrawal symptoms, but prolongs the discomfort over a longer period of time. A second opioid has been approved for this purpose, L-α-acetylmethadol (LAAM), which has the advantage of a longer duration of action than methadone (Houtsmuller et al. 1998).

Another pharmacological approach is to reduce the intensity of the symptoms with the α_2 adrenergic antagonist clonidine, which is normally used to treat hypertension. Overactivity of the locus coeruleus is associated with opioid withdrawal signs such as tachycardia, nausea, vomiting, and sweating. Thus, clonidine attenuates these symptoms by reducing firing of the locus coeruleus.

A protracted opioid withdrawal syndrome is recognized, consisting of mood disturbance and drug craving and may last months or longer after discontinuation. Accordingly, release from treatment after acute withdrawal and without any further treatment is associated with a high relapse rate. Follow-up treatment is essential to address longer-term aspects of opioid addiction. Relapse is treatable with methadone, and due to methadone/heroin cross-tolerance, people taking methadone who inject heroin report that the effects are not as intense. For those completely withdrawn from opioids and with high motivation and cooperation, maintenance on the opioid antagonist naltrexone (Trexan) will reduce or prevent the reinforcing effects of heroin. Thus, it helps reduce the short-term temptation to relapse.

Toxicity

Acute toxicity results from intentional or accidental overdoses of opioids (Reisine and Pasternak 1996). After an overdose, consciousness is impaired and arousal is difficult, sometimes to the point of coma. The respiratory rate lowers and may stop entirely. Cyanosis and a fall in blood pressure occur subsequent to hypoxia. The skin becomes cold and clammy, and skeletal muscles become flaccid. Seizures may occur, but respiratory arrest is the primary cause of death in opioid overdose. Fortunately, opioid antagonists such as naltrexone (Trexan) are very fast and effective in reversing an acute overdose, when applied in time. However, antagonists can precipitate an acute withdrawal syndrome in people who are dependent, and rebound sympathetic effects must be monitored.

Neonatal toxicity Opioid use during pregnancy causes dependence in the neonate, who undergoes withdrawal symptoms after birth (Franck and Vilardi 1995). Opioid abuse is associated with lower birth weight and increased risk of neonatal mortality (Hulse et al. 1997, 1998). Preliminary evidence suggests that the μ partial agonist buprenorphine may be a more attractive treatment than methadone for opioid-dependent pregnant women (Fischer et al. 1998).

Myrrh

History and Botany

Myrrh *(Commiphora molmol)* is a shrub that grows in eastern Mediterranean regions and Somalia (Gruenwald, 1998). It grows irregular, knotted branches, trifoliate leaves, and yellow-red flowers (figure 8.5). The part used is a resin that exudes from the bark. It was made into an oint-

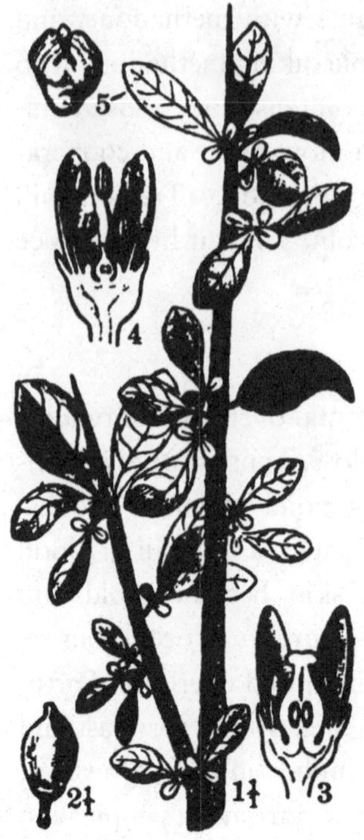

Figure 8.5
Myrrh *(Commiphora molmol)*. Reprinted from Culbreth DMR. (1927). *Materia Medica and Pharmacognosy*, 7th ed. Philadelphia: Lea & Febiger.

ment and used topically. Its use was known to the ancient Egyptians, Jews, Romans, and Greeks (Dolara et al. 1996). Hippocrates recommended it to treat sores. In the Bible, "vinum murratum," a wine containing myrrh, was offered to Christ before his crucifixion.

Chemical Constituents
Myrrh contains many sesquiterpenes such as delta-elemene, β-eudesmol, α-copaene, and several furosesquiterpenes (Gruenwald 1998). Also contained are the triterpenes 3-epi-α-amyrin and α-amyrenone.

Analgesic Effects
When given enterically (via gavage) to mice, the constituent furanoedesma-1,3-diene (FED) (figure 8.6) produced analgesic effects in the

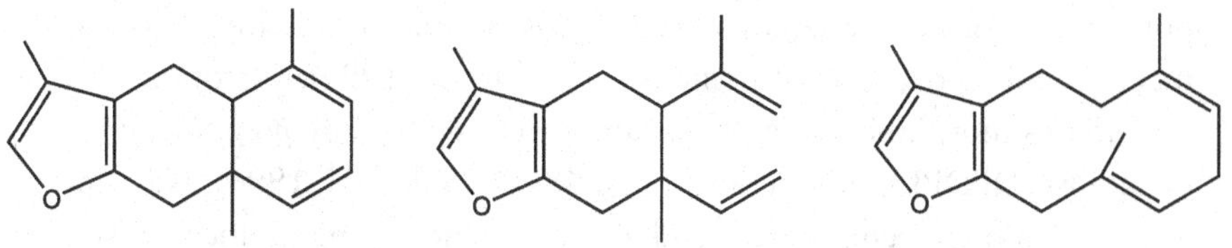

Furanoeudesma-1,3-diene Curzarene Furanodiene

Figure 8.6
Chemical structure of analgesic myrrh constituents.

acetic acid writhing test and hot-plate test (Dolara et al. 1996). A dose of 1.25 mg/kg of FED was comparable to 5 mg/kg PO of morphine. Further, the FED analgesia was reversible by naloxone, indicating the involvement of opioid receptors. FED also displaced [^{3}H]diprenorphine from central opioid receptors, but with a high inhibition constant.

It is unlikely that myrrh will be used clinically for analgesic purposes, given the presence of other superior analgesics. However, it is mentioned here for the historical and ethnopharmacological aspects.

Cholinergic Analgesics

Given the role of acetylcholine receptors in analgesic circuits, it is not surprising that a number of plants with cholinergic mechanisms have analgesic effects. The RVM has muscarinic and nicotinic receptors (Cortés and Palacios 1986; London et al. 1985). The PAG has nicotinic receptors as well (Segal et al. 1978).

The stimulant aspects of nicotine, the primary alkaloid from tobacco, are discussed in greater detail in chapter 4. But nicotine also has significant analgesic effects. Nicotine produces analgesia when injected into the midbrain ventrolateral PAG (Llewelyn et al. 1981). Nicotine injected into the PPTN or RVM increases hot-plate and tail-flick latencies in rats, which is blocked by muscarinic drugs in both sites (Iwamoto 1989, 1991). Recently, a high-potency nicotinic agonist has been developed, ABT-594, that has analgesic efficacy comparable to morphine in a number of measures (Bannon et al. 1998). Cholinergic analgesic mechanisms also interact with opioid mechanisms. Subanalgesic doses of nicotine potentiate morphine analgesia, and a cross-tolerance develops between nicotine and morphine (Zarrindast et al. 1996, 1999). Nicotine only potentiates morphine analgesia, and not that induced by β-endorphin, a δ_1 agonist (DPDPE), or κ agonist (U50,488H) (Suh et al. 1996). Nicotine analgesia alone seems to depend on endogenous opioid mechanisms (Zarrindast et al. 1997).

Similar to tobacco, lobelia may also have analgesic effects. However, it depends on the mode of administration (Damaj et al. 1997). Intrathecal lobeline produces analgesia on the tail-flick test, but subcutaneous administration is ineffective. On the other hand, subcutaneous lobeline dose-dependently enhances nicotine analgesia. Tolerance develops to this effect of lobeline after 10 days. Lobeline can also produce hyperalgesic effects when administered into the dorsal posterior mesencephalic tegmentum (Hamann and Martin 1994). However, the relevance of this to peripheral administration of lobelia is questionable because chronic injections (IP) of lobeline in rats induced no changes in tail-flick latencies (Sopranzi et al. 1991).

Areca is another stimulant plant with cholinergic mechanisms and analgesic effects. Its chemical constituents (arecoline, arecaidine, guvacoline, and guvacine) have muscarinic agonist effects as well as GABAergic mechanisms. However, the muscarinic actions are sufficient to explain arecoline's analgesic effect in rats on the tail-flick test, because they are prevented by cholinergic antagonists (Gower 1987).

Eicosanoid Analgesics

Willow

History and Botany

Willows are several species of the *Salix* genus. *Salix nigra* is the American willow. It is a tree growing 6 to 18 meters in height with gray bark. The leaves are small and lanceolate. Its flowers are yellow or green, depending on the sex of the tree. The medicinal part of the tree used is its bark.

Willow bark has been used throughout recorded history to treat pain, fevers, and inflammation. Its uses have been independently discovered in cultures as diverse as the ancient Greeks, Hottentots, and American

Indians. The active principle, salicin, was isolated in 1829. It is chemically converted to the active principle, salicylic acid, in the intestine and liver. The chemically modified acetylsalicylic acid was first marketed in 1899 as *aspirin.* Salicin is also found in meadowsweet *(Filipendula ulmaria*, then referred to as *Spireaea ulmaria)*, from which the name *aspirin* derives (*a*cetyl *spiric* acid). The sodium salt of salicylic acid has the drawback of producing gastrointestinal irritation, but acetylsalicylic acid is well tolerated.

Eventually the drug was synthesized rather than extracted from willow. Until the invention of acetaminophen, ibuprofen, and other related drugs, aspirin was the most widely used analgesic drug. Between 10,000 and 20,000 tons of aspirin are consumed annually in the United States (Insel 1996).

Chemical Constituents

Salix species contain several glycosides and esters yielding salicylic acid, including salicin (0.1–2%), salicortin (0.01–11%), and other salicylin derivatives (Gruenwald et al. 1998). Also contained in Salix species are tannins and flavonoids.

Pharmacokinetics

Salicin occurs in small amounts in willow, making raw preparations impractical for treatment (Tyler 1994). Between 3 and 20 cups of willow bark tea, depending on salicin content, would be necessary to get an effect. At such high doses, the presence of tannins in the bark would also cause aversive effects. Thus, aspirin is needed to reach therapeutic effects.

Orally ingested aspirin is rapidly absorbed and significant blood levels occur within 30 minutes, peaking at 2 hours. Rectal absorption is slower and less reliable, but absorption through the skin is fairly rapid. Salicylates are distributed to most body tissues, and 80 to 90% is bound to plasma proteins such as albumin. Aspirin competes for several plasma binding sites, including those shared by certain thyroid hormones (thyroxine, triiodothyronine), phenytoin, bilirubin, penicillin, and other NSAIDs. The plasma half-life of aspirin is 15 minutes, but salicylate has a half life of 2 to 3 hours. The major metabolic products are salicyluric acid, and glucuronide conjugates. Some salicylic acid is exrcreted in urine unchanged.

Mechanisms of Action

The therapeutic effects of aspirin and other nonsteroidal anti-inflammatory drugs (NSAIDs) derive from their ability to inhibit prostaglandin synthesis. Prostaglandins are a subgroup of eicosanoids, synthesized from phospholipids into arachidonic acid, which may then be converted into prostaglandins by cyclooxygenases. Specifically, aspirin inhibits cyclooxygenase, preventing conversion from arachidonic acid to prostaglandins (Insel 1996).

General Effects

Several characteristic effects are known of aspirin, which are present to varying degrees in other NSAIDs. These include analgesic, antipyretic, anti-inflammatory, and anticoagulant effects.

Prostaglandins released during tissue injury sensitize the endings of peripheral sensory nerves to other pain transmitters such as histamine and bradykinin. Thus, inhibition of prostaglandins inhibits the initiation of pain signals in the periphery, creating analgesia. However, there may also be some central analgesic effects of aspirin, through monoamine mechanisms (Shyu and Lin 1985; Taiwo and Levine 1988). Aspirin is an effective analgesic for low- to medium-intensity pain, but is not effective for high-intensity pain. Aspirin's effectiveness also varies with the type of pain: it is effective for headache and musculoskeletal pain, less effective for toothaches and sore throat, and ineffective for visceral and traumatic pain (Insel 1996).

In addition to analgesic effects, aspirin has antipyretic effects, reducing fevers caused by infection. Normal body temperature is not lowered by aspirin and it has no effect on hyperthermia induced by exercise. Fevers from infections are initiated by cytokines in the blood stream that enter the brain through circumventricular organs and cause production of PGE_2 in the hypothalamus (Saper and Breder 1994). Thus, salicylates reduce fever by inhibiting PGE_2 production.

Toxicity

Aspirin is generally low in toxicity and produces comparatively little tolerance and no addiction. However, its effects are not entirely benign, especially in certain medical conditions. Acute overdose of aspirin is fatal in doses of 10 to 30 mg, although some high doses have been reported without lethality (Insel 1996). Mild intoxication manifests as headache, dizziness, tinnitus, dimmed vision, hearing difficulty, confusion, sweating, nausea, hyperventilation, and diarrhea. Higher doses create skin eruptions, acid-base balance disturbances, and more pronounced disturbance of the central nervous system, including seizures and coma. The anticoagulant effects of aspirin increase bleeding time and hemorrhage is occasionally seen. Treatment is directed at cardiovascular and respiratory support, and correction of acid-base imbalances.

Reye's syndome is a rare but serious sequela of aspirin use, occuring primarily in people under age 20 who were given aspirin during a viral infection, especially influenza or chicken pox. It manifests as continuous vomiting, disorientation, behavior changes, and lethargy. Encephalopathy and death are occasional consequences, with the mortality rate around 31% (Belay 1999). Since it was reported in 1980, there has been a steep decrease in the number of cases. A rediagnosis of many cases also found a high percentage (69%) to have an underlying metabolic disorder that mimicked the clinical symptoms of Reye's syndrome.

Feverfew

History and Botany

Feverfew *(Tanacetum parthenium)* has a traditional reputation for treating pain and anxiety. It is a strongly aromatic flowering plant growing 15 to 60 cm in height, with daisylike flowers (figure 8.7) (Gruenwald 1998). Feverfew originated in southeast Europe, but now grows in most parts of Europe, as well as Australia and North America. It may be consumed by chewing fresh or freeze-dried leaves, but extracts are now also commercially available. Its modern uses include treatment of arthritis, rheumatic illnesses, migraine, and, as the name suggests, fevers.

Chemical Constituents and Mechanisms

The primary active chemical constituent in feverfew is parthenolide, a sesquiterpenoid lactone (figure 8.8) (Robbers et al. 1996). Levels of sesquiterpene lactones vary across different types of extracts: ethanol extracts contain about 0.5%, whereas aqueous ones contain 0.3% (Gromek et al. 1991). The sesquiterpene lactones in feverfew inhibit the

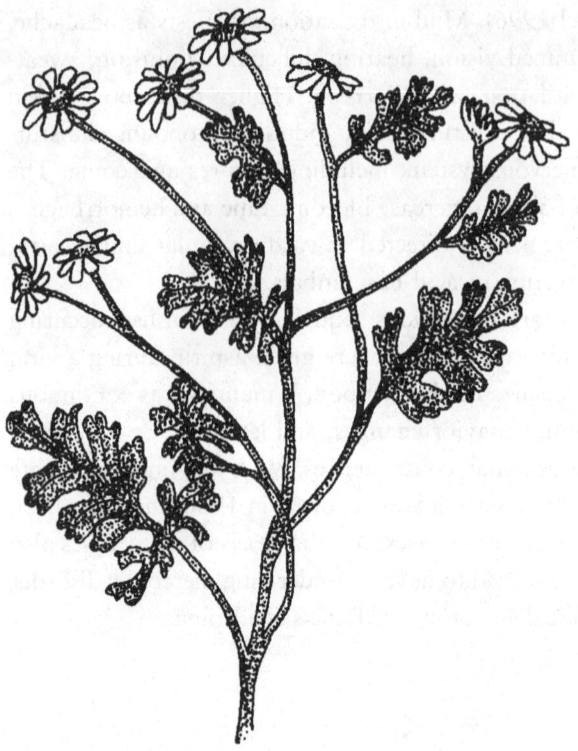

Figure 8.7
Feverfew *(Tanacetum parthenium)*. Reprinted with permission from Sturdivant and Blakely. (1999). *Medicinal Herbs in the Garden, Field, and Marketplace.* Friday Harbor, WA: San Juan Naturals. Illustration by Peggy Sue McRae.

synthesis of the eicosanoids thromboxane B_2 and leukotriene B_4 in rat and human leukocytes, with IC_{50} values in the 5–50 µg/mL range (Sumner et al. 1992). These effects were irreversible but not time dependent.

Feverfew may create analgesic and/or anti-inflammatory effects through inhibtion of eicosanoids. Feverfew extract inhibits cyclooxygenase and lipoxygenase in rat leukocytes (Capasso 1986). More specifically, parthenolide inhibits the expression of cyclooxygenase and proinflammatory cytokines (tumor necrosis factor-α and interleukin-1) (Hwang et al. 1996). Parthenolide was specifically found to inhibit production of PGE_2 from arachidonic acid in the micromolar range (IC_{50} 11–14 µM), a mechanism shared by aspirin and other NSAIDs (Pugh and

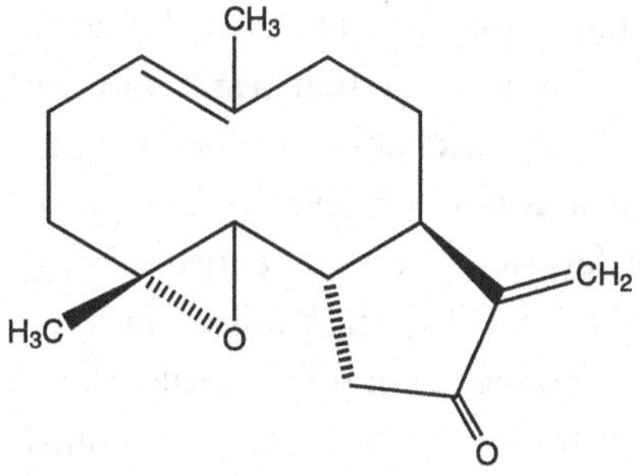

Figure 8.8
Chemical structure of parthenolide.

Sambo 1988). Nonsesquiterpene lactones in feverfew were also found to inhibit eicosanoid synthesis with high potency (Sumner et al. 1992).

Parthenolide acts as a low-affinity antagonist at 5-HT_{2A} receptors (Weber et al. 1997b). Feverfew also inhibits the release of serotonin from platelets, which correlates with its sesquiterpene content (Marles et al. 1992). In contrast, parthenolide does not appear to bind to 5-HT_{1A} receptors (Weber et al. 1997a). Whereas a parthenolide-containing extract of feverfew inhibited contraction of smooth muscle, a chloroform extract (not containing parthenolide) elicited potent and sustained contractions (Barsby 1993). Furthermore, this contraction by the chloroform extract was not mediated through 5-HT_2 receptors.

Analgesic Effects

One animal study showed analgesic and anti-inflammatory effects of feverfew in rats and mice (Jain and Kulkarni 1999). Dose-dependent analgesic effects were seen on the acetic acid-induced writhing test and carrageenan-induced paw edema using either feverfew extract or isolated parthenolide. These appear to be due to analgesic effects and not nonspecific behavioral effects, because higher doses failed to alter other aspects of behavior including locomotor activity or pentobarbital-induced sleep. The analgesic/anti-inflammatory effects of feverfew have yet to be thoroughly investigated in humans. One methodologically controlled study of feverfew was undertaken for treatment of rheumatoid arthritis (Pattrick et al. 1989). However, chronic (6-week) doses of chopped feverfew (70–86 mg/day) showed no benefit over placebo.

The analgesic effects of ferverfew have not been tested in humans. Feverfew's inhibitory effects on the eicosanoid system, especially on cyclooxygenase and PGE_2, is the most likely mechanism of its analgesic effects. Inhibition of PGE_2 could also account for feverfew's reputed antipyretic effects. Analgesic effects of feverfew through central $5\text{-}HT_{2A}$ receptors are another possibility. Central $5\text{-}HT_{2A}$ mechanisms may be partly responsible for the analgesic effects of acetaminophen (Srikiatkhachorn et al. 1999). Peripheral administration of a $5\text{-}HT_2$ antagonist (ketanserin) has analgesic effects, perhaps through removal of inhibition of descending serotonergic projections (Alhaider 1991). On the other hand, administration of ketanserin also inhibits the analgesic effects of morphine, as well as opioid and nonopioid forms of stress-induced analgesia (Paul et al. 1988; Kellstein et al. 1988; Kiefel et al. 1989). Thus, the analgesic effects of feverfew through central serotonergic mechanisms is a possiblity, but is not a necessary conclusion. Of course, this is also contingent on whether feverfew constituents penetrate the blood-brain barrier, which has not yet been specifically investigated.

Feverfew appears to treat migraines through vascular serotonin receptors. Some clinical studies of feverfew support its use in the prevention of migraine (Murphy et al. 1998; Johnson et al. 1985). This includes a reduction in the number and severity of attacks, and in the degree of vomiting caused by the attacks. A systematic review of clinical trials of feverfew for migraine identified five methodologically controlled studies (Vogler et al. 1998). Although the majority of studies support feverfew in this respect, its effectiveness has not yet been established beyond doubt.

Toxicity

No significant adverse effects are known to result from typical doses of feverfew (Gruenwald 1998). A contact dermatitis occurs infrequently. Because feverfew also inhibits human blood platelet aggregation, interactions are possible with antithrombotic medications such as aspirin or warfarin (Groenewegen and Heptinstall 1990). Abrupt discontinuation of feverfew by people taking it chronically for treatment of migraine can produce rebound withdrawal symptoms. These consist of migraines, anxiety, poor sleep patterns, and stiffness of the muscles and joints.

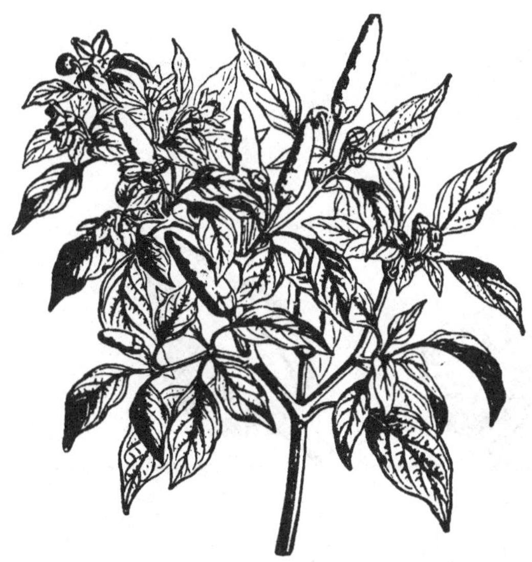

Figure 8.9
Chili pepper *(Capsicum frutescens)*. Reprinted from Culbreth DMR. (1927). *Materia Medica and Pharmacognosy*, 7th ed. Philadelphia: Lea & Febiger.

Neurokinin Analgesics

Chili Peppers

History and Botany

Chili or Cayenne peppers *(Capsicum annum, C. frutescens)* are members of the Solanaceae family and are characteristically known for the burning sensation they produce on contact (figure 8.9) (Gruenwald 1998; Robbers et al. 1996). It is estimated that they are eaten on a daily basis by one-quarter of the world's population. Numerous varieties are available, including the ultrahot *habanero*. *C. annum* is an annual plant cultivated in temperate to semitropical climates. It grows 20–100 cm in height with solitary leaves. The fruit produced (or peppers) are hollow and boxlike (hence the name derivation from the Latin *capsa*, or box). The wall of the fruit is tough and may be red, yellow-green, or brownish. Its seeds are numerous, small, and disc shaped (figure 8.10). Although indigenous to Central America, the plant was later introduced

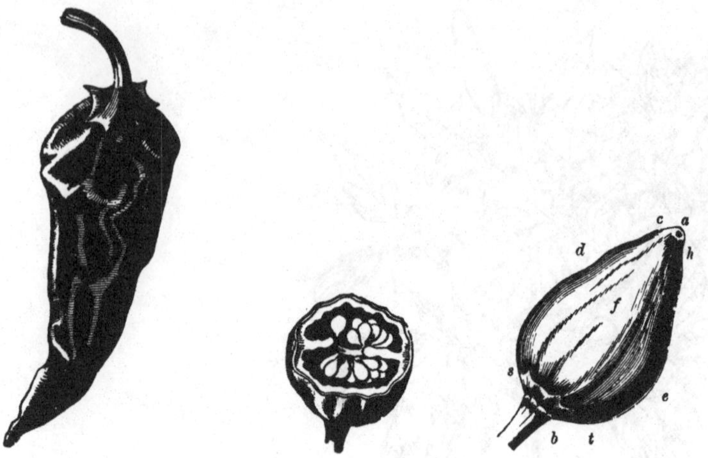

Figure 8.10
Fruit of *Capsicum annuum*. Reprinted from Culbreth DMR. (1927). *Materia Medica and Pharmacognosy*, 7th ed. Philadelphia: Lea & Febiger.

to Asia and Africa by the Portugese. It is now cultivated in many areas with warmer climates.

The first known written record of chilies dates to 1494, by the physician Chauca, who accompanied Columbus to the West Indies. *Chili* is the Nahuatl word for the plant (Szallasi and Blumberg 1999).

It is interesting to note that most of our modern uses of chili peppers are preceded by ancient Mesoamericans. Capsaicin, the active chemical constituent, is used today as an irritant in self-defense sprays, and dried chilis were burned by the Inca to blind the invading Spaniards. Just as we apply capsaicin for analgesia, native Americans used to rub chili on the gums to relieve the pain of a toothache. Eunuchs serving Chinese Emperors were castrated after hot pepper extracts were chronically applied to their scrotums.

Capsaicin was extracted and named by Thomas Thresh in 1846, and its chemical structure was determined in 1919. The Scoville Unit was also developed in 1912 as a measurement of the hotness of chili peppers (Scoville 1912). A pepper with 1000 Scoville Units means that an alcoholic extract must be diluted 1:1000 before it ceases to be hot. The Mexican *habanero* pepper has an astonishing 350,000 Scoville Units.

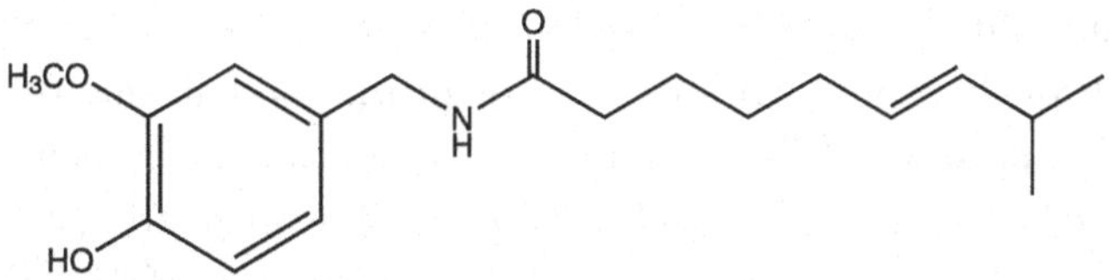

Figure 8.11
Chemical structure of capsaicin.

Chemical Constituents
The primary chemicals of interest in chilies are capsaicinoids, namely capsaicin (0.02%) and dihydrocapsaicin (figure 8.11). Also found are flavonoids, carotenoids (capsanthin), steroid saponins (capsicidin), and ascorbic acid or vitamin C (0.2%). Capsaicin has a vanilloid chemical structure.

Mechanisms of Action
Capsaicin is an agonist at the vanilloid receptor (Szallasi and Blumberg 1999). A vanilloid receptor has been cloned (termed VR1), which is a chemically and thermally gated cation channel. It is nonselective for cations and composed of six transmembrane segments and one partial segment. While heat opens the channel, capsaicin and acids lower its activation threshold. Through these receptors, capsaicin selectively activates $A\delta$ and C fibers, which transmit nociceptive information to the spinal cord. Immunoreactivity for the vanilloid receptor in the spinal cord was found in lamina I (zone of Lissauer) and the inner layer of lamina II (substantia gelatinosa) (Guo et al. 1999). There is speculation about an endogenous vanilloid, although a specific one has not been identified to date (Szallasi and Blumberg 1999).

Activation of vanilloid receptors by capsaicin results in a release of several neuropeptides, among which is the neurokinin substance P. Substance P normally signals pain in nociceptive afferents, so capsaicin creates a false pain/burning sensation even though no actual tissue damage occurs.

General Effects
Capsaicin may treat pain through a few mechanisms. In muscle soreness due to exercise, capsaicin effects are attributed to improved local circu-

lation (Szallasi and Blumberg 1999). Acutely, capsaicin may affect other forms of pain through counterirritation, although the mechanisms of this are not well understood. When administered chronically, capsaicin depletes substance P, by continuously releasing it and downregulating its expression. There is also a desensitization of vanilloid receptors after the initial stimulation.

Therapeutic use of capsaicin is primarily through a topical cream containing 0.025–0.075% of the chemical. The cream is applied locally to treat various forms of pain, including those associated with rheumatoid arthritis, osteoarthritis, postherpetic neuralgia, diabetic neuropathy, postmastectomy and postamputation neuroma (or phantom limb pain). When the cream is applied acutely, a mild burning sensation occurs. But when applied 4 to 5 times daily for several days to weeks, the painful sensation may subside. Unfortunately, it is not possible to do double-blind studies of capsaicin due to the burning sensation it produces.

Toxicity

The predominant adverse effect of clinical use of capsaicin is the burning sensation it produces. Many find it intolerable, and withdrawal rates from clinical studies have been reported as 30% or higher (Szallasi and Blumberg 1999). Excessive ingestion of chili peppers can cause visceral pain, increased peristalsis and diarrhea (Gruenwald 1998). Excessive external application can cause blister and ulcer formation. Very high doses can cause a serious hypothermia.

An occasional common side effect of capsaicin exposure is bronchoconstriction, in asthmatic people, caused by inhaled airborne particles. In nonasthmatic people, this induces a cough. This is prevented by washing the skin surface where capsaicin was applied after 30–40 minutes of exposure. Chronic overdosage can cause chronic gastritis, kidney and liver toxicity, and neurotoxic effects.

Ginger

Ginger is a rhizome, or underground stem, of the plant *Zingiber officinale*. It is discussed in greater detail in chapter 7, but will be mentioned briefly here for its analgesic effects. Micromolar doses of (6)-shogaol have been shown to dose-dependently cause a release of substance P from spinal dorsal horn in a Ca^{2+}-dependent manner, similar to capsaicin from chili peppers (Onogi et al. 1992). However, this effect is 1/50 as potent as capsaicin, where 100 μM of shogaol produces half the effect of 10 μM of capsaicin.

The clincal usefulness of this effect of ginger is not established. Ginger does have analgesic effects in animals (Suekawa et al. 1984). Systemically administered (6)-shogaol at 160 mg/kg in rats produces an analgesic effect, peaking between 15 and 30 minutes. However, a smaller dose of 80 mg/kg is ineffective. Ginger extract was ineffective in supressing writhing induced by intraperitoneal acetic acid. Ginger's analgesic effects have not been formally tested in humans, but one study examined the postsurgical antiemetic effects of oral ginger and failed to observe any differences in the need for postoperative analgesics between placebo and ginger groups (Philips et al. 1993). A more specific study would be needed to confirm or rule out clinically relevant analgesic effects of ginger in humans.

Purinergic Analgesics

There are several herbal medicines that contain the methylxanthines caffeine, theobromine, and theophylline. These are stimulant drugs, which are discussed in greater detail in chapter 4. Namely, they are coffee *(Coffea arabica)*, tea *(Camellia sinensis)*, cocoa *(Theobroma cacao)*, guarana *(Paullinia cupana)*, maté *(Ilex paraguariensis)*, and kola *(Cola nitida* and *C. acuminata)*. The primary pharmacodynamic mechanism of the methylxanthines is antagonism of presynaptic adenosine receptors. This prevents the synaptic negative feedback of adenosine and increases neurotransmitter release. The methylxanthines are mentioned here briefly for their analgesic effects. Adenosine and adenosine triphosphate (ATP) are involved in pain transmission at peripheral and spinal sites (Sawynok 1998).

Caffeine alone may produce analgesic effects in some forms of pain, but clinically it is most often used as an adjuvant medication (Laska et al. 1983; Ghelardini et al. 1997; Kraetsch et al. 1996; Forbes et al. 1991). It enhances the analgesic effects of nonsteroidal anti-inflammatory drugs such as acetaminophen and also speeds the onset of analgesia. It is effective in different types of clinical pain, including uterine cramping, episiotomy, and molar extraction.

Caffeine and theophylline potentiate morphine analgesia in rats (Malec and Michalska 1988; Misra et al. 1985). Chronic caffeine lowers the ED_{50} for morphine analgesia (Ahlijanian and Takemori 1986). Conversely, peripheral administration of adenosine agonists (2-chloroadenosine and L-N^6-phenylisopropyladenosine) reduce morphine analgesia in rats on the tail-flick tests (Mantegazza et al. 1984). Caffeine prevents the reduction of morphine analgesia by adenosine agonists. The interaction of purinergic drugs and morphine analgesia is believed to be mediated by actions on adenylate cyclase.

There is also evidence for cholinergic involvement in caffeine analgesia (Ghelardini et al. 1997). The muscarinic antagonists atropine and pirenzepine, and the choline uptake inhibitor hemicholinium-3 prevent caffeine analgesia. In contrast, it was unaffected by an opioid antagonist (naloxone) or a tyrosine hydroxylase inhibitor (α-methyl-*p*-tyrosine).

The role of caffeine in migraine headaches is due to its vasoconstrictor effects. Caffeine is used in combination with ergotamine for migraine (Sawynok 1995; Sargent et al. 1988). However, discontinuation or missing a dose of caffeine after chronic use can precipitate headaches (Fennelly et al. 1991; Couturier et al. 1992).

Cannabinoid Analgesia

Cannabinoids are known to reduce pain. THC, the prinicpal active constituent of *Cannabis* species, is effective in models of both phasic and tonic pain (Moss and Johnson 1980). Several other cannabinoids also have analgesic effects at the level of the spinal cord, including 11-hydroxy-delta 9-THC, delta 9-THC, and delta 8-THC, although they each have different ED_{50} values (Welch and Stevens 1992). The analgesia produced by different cannabinoids is differentially blocked by a CB_1 antagonist (SR141716A), with 15-fold differences in some cases (Welch et al. 1998). On the other hand, some cannabinoids antagonize the analgesia produced by others. For example, cannabidiol dose-dependently antagonizes the analgesia produced by THC and cannabinol (Welburn et al. 1976).

The analgesic effects are mediated through CB_1 receptors, and reversed by cannabinoid antagonists (Lichtman and Martin 1997; Vivian et al. 1998). THC produces analgesic effects at both spinal and supraspinal levels (Reche et al. 1996). THC activates structures in the descending pain inhibiting system, involving the RVM (Basbaum and Fields 1978, 1984; Meng et al. 1998). Cannabinoid agonists injected into the RVM elevate tail-flick latencies by more than 50%, which is reduced by a CB_1 antagonist (Martin et al. 1998). Actions of THC in the RVM are similar to morphine but pharmacologically distinct (Meng et al. 1998). Cannabinoid antagonists reverse THC analgesia at supraspinal sites more effectively than at spinal sites (Welch et al. 1998). Still, THC produces analgesia in mice with spinal transections, suggesting independent spinal mechanisms (Smith and Martin 1992).

The cellular mechanism of cannabinoid analgesia is uncertain. Although cAMP and adenylate cyclase mediate other effects of cannabinoids, they do not appear to be involved in cannabinoid-induced analgesia (Cook et al. 1995). Instead, other mechanisms such as cannabinoid receptor-coupled calcium or potassium channels may be responsible.

THC and Opioid Analgesia

There are several lines of evidence that suggest opioid and cannabinoid systems interact in analgesia. Inhibition of opioid peptidases potentiates THC analgesia, which is blocked by supraspinal μ and spinal κ opioid receptors (Reche et al. 1998). An intrathecally administered κ antagonist (nor-binaltorphimine) blocks THC cannabinoid analgesia, but not other physiological effects of cannabinoids (e.g., hypothermia, hypoactivity, and catalepsy) (Smith et al. 1994). Cross-tolerance occurs between morphine and THC for analgesic and hypothermic effects (Bloom and Dewey 1978).

Cross-tolerance occurs at the spinal level between THC and κ agonists (U-50,488H and CI-977) on analgesic tests, but not between THC and agonists of μ (DAMGO) or δ (DPDPE) receptors. Convergently, antisense studies suggest that cannabinoid analgesia is related to spinal κ_1, but not μ or δ receptors (Pugh et al. 1995).

Synergistic effects are produced by co-administration of morphine and cannabinoids (Pugh et al. 1996; Welch and Stevens 1992). THC enhances morphine analgesia when with either central (intracerebroventricular or intrathecal) or peripheral (PO or SC) administration (Smith et al. 1998). The ED_{50} of THC is reduced by morphine, and vice versa, on several measures of nociceptive threshold (the tail-flick test, hot-plate test, jump test, and paw-lick responses) (Reche et al. 1996; Welch and Stevens 1992; Hine 1985). THC enhancement of morphine analgesia is mediated by the CB_1 receptor and reduced with a selective CB_1 antagonist. Supraspinal synergy between morphine and THC also involves μ and spinal κ opioid receptors (Reche et al. 1996; Pugh et al. 1996).

Nonopioid Mechanisms of THC Analgesia

Although cannabinoids interact with opioids in analgesia, there also appear to be opioid-independent mechanisms (Hamann and di Vadi 1999). The analgesia produced by cannabinoids alone is not abolished by pretreatment with the general opioid antagonist naloxone (Gilbert 1981; Welch and Stevens 1992; Ferri et al. 1986).

There is evidence to suggest that cannabinoids create analgesia by activating descending noradrenergic neurons. The catecholamine neurotoxin, 6-hydroxydopamine, reduces THC analgesia (Ferri et al. 1986). Further, THC analgesia is blocked by an intrathecal α_2-noradrenergic antagonist (yohimbine), but not by a nonspecific serotonin antagonist (methysergide) (Lichtman and Martin 1991). Yohimbine blocks THC analgesia at lumbar but not thoracic regions.

Some cannabinoids may create analgesia though eicosanoid systems. Delta 1-THC-7-oic acid, a metabolite of delta 1-THC, creates analgesia through inhibition of eicosanoid synthesis (Burstein et al. 1988). In contrast, delta 1-THC creates hyperalgesic effects by elevating levels of prostaglandins.

Endocannabinoids in Analgesia

Similar to exogenous cannabinoids, anandamide has analgesic effects (Fride and Mechoulam 1993). Peripheral anandamide (10 mg/kg IM) produces antinociception in primates. However, centrally administered anandamide does not alter pain perceptive thresholds (Murillo-

Rodriguez 1998). THC- and anandamide-induced analgesia also have different durations (90 min and 15 min, respectively) (Smith et al. 1998).

Similarities in receptor binding are observed between cannabinoids and anandamide. Binding to CB receptors by anandamide, a selective CB_1 antagonist (SR 141716A), and CB agonist (CP 55,940) shows that all three ligands compete for the same cannabinoid receptor (Adams et al. 1998). Still, THC and anandamide may create analgesia through different mechanisms. CB_1 antagonists block THC analgesia but have no effect on anandamide analgesia, strongly suggesting different sites of action for THC and anandamide in some processes (Smith et al. 1998; Adams et al. 1998). Anandamide also has pharmacological effects distinct from CB receptors: anandamide, but not THC, has direct effects on the NMDA receptor (Hampson et al. 1998). The cross-tolerance between anandamide and THC in analgesic paradigms was differentially cross-tolerant to opioids. While THC produced cross tolerance to κ opioids, anandamide did not (Welch 1997).

Anandamide may reduce pain by a peripheral action, by acting on CB_1-like receptors located outside the CNS (Calignano et al. 1998). Palmitylethanolamide (PEA) is an endocannabinoid that is coreleased with anandamide and activates peripheral CB_2 receptors. When the two are administered together, they show a 100-fold synergistic effect on analgesic measures. Measurements of anandamide and PEA levels in the skin show that there are sufficient amounts to create tonic activation of local cannabinoid receptors. Thus, endocannabinoids may tonically inhibit cutaneous pain.

Analgesic Effects of THC in Humans

The clinical analgesic efficacy of THC is prominent. In a study of cancer patients, 10 mg of THC was equivalent to 60 mg of codeine (Noyes et al. 1975). This dose produced sedative but no other psychoactive effects. A dose of 20 mg was more effective, but produced additional dizziness, ataxia, blurred vision, and psychoactive effects.

The analgesic response to THC may be variable and appears to depend on personality characteristics of the subject (Raft et al. 1977).

Objective measures of personality found those with the characterstics of submissiveness, rigidity, low introspection, and high-state anxiety to be poor responders to the analgesic effects of THC. Unfortunately, although there is ample evidence to support the analgesic efficacy of cannabinoids, there is little clinical research to match it.

Monoamine Analgesics

Khat

Khat alkaloids are monoamine stimulants, causing a release of neurotransmitters in a manner similar to amphetamine (see chapter 4). The major alkaloid cathinone has analgesic effects on the tail-flick test in rats (Nencini et al. 1984). It also enhances the analgesia induced by brief electric foot shock (Nencini et al. 1988). The analgesia produced by cathinone is long lasting, with effects seen at both 30 minutes and 24 hours. Cathinone-induced analgesia depends on α adrenergic receptors, followed by release of opioid peptides and by activation of serotonergic pathways (Della Bella et al. 1985). It is prevented by monoamine depletion with reserpine or *p*-chlorophenylalanine. Cathinone potentiates morphine analgesia, and cathinone analgesia is blocked by naloxone (Della Bella et al. 1985; Nencini et al. 1984). The cathinone metabolite norpseudoephedrine does not have intrinsic analgesic effects on the hotplate test, but it potentiates the analgesic effects of morphine (Nencini et al. 1998). In contrast, there is no apparent contribution from adrenohypophyseal hormones to cathinone analgesia (Nencini et al. 1984).

Coca

Cocaine, from the coca plant, is one of the few drugs with dual analgesic and local anesthetic effects. These are distinct actions, which occur through different pharmacological mechanisms. (The local anesthetic effects are discussed below.) Given the role of monoamines in analgesia, it is not surprising that cocaine has analgesic effects in the central nervous system. This is likely to involve dopaminergic mechanisms at both supraspinal and spinal levels (Lin et al. 1989; Pertovaara and Tukeva 1990; Kiritsy-Roy et al. 1994). Cocaine alone produces analgesia in the hot-plate, but not the paw-pressure test (Waddell and Holtzman 1999).

Interactions are seen between cocaine and the opioid system in analgesia. A synergistic effect occurs when cocaine is combined with a μ agonist (morphine) in the hot-plate test and a κ agonist (U69,593) in the hot-plate test (Waddell and Holtzman 1999). Cocaine enhances morphine analgesia in several analgesic paradigms (e.g., formalin test, hot-plate test, and thermal tail-flick test) (Kauppila et al. 1992). The synergistic interaction between cocaine and opioid analgesia likely involves noradrenergic mechanisms, supraspinal μ and δ receptors, and spinal μ receptors (Misra et al. 1987; Sierra et al. 1992).

Interestingly, one study has shown that cocaine may be a direct antagonist at nicotinic receptors (Damaj et al. 1999). Cocaine blocks several of nicotine's effects, including analgesia on the tail-flick test, independent of its monoamine activity or local anesthetic effects.

Uncertain Analgesic Mechanisms

Ginseng

Ginseng species are discussed at length in chapter 5, but mentioned briefly here for their analgesic properties. Ginsenosides produce dose-dependent analgesic effects in the formalin test when administered intrathecally in microgram doses (Yoon et al. 1998). They also dose-dependently inhibit pain behaviors induced by intrathecal injection of substance P. Ginsenoside Rf has dose-dependent analgesic effects when administered systemically with effects in two measures of pain: acetic acid abdominal constriction test and biphasic formalin test (Mogil et al. 1998). Analgesic effects in the acetic acid abdominal constriction test were comparable at concentrations similar to those reported for aspirin and acetaminophen. Ginsenoside Rf is effective in the tonic phase of the formalin test, but ineffective in the acute phase. It is also ineffective in the thermal tail-flick and hot-plate tests. A possible (but not necessary) conclusion is that ginsenoside Rf is effective in tonic but not acute forms of pain. Opioid analgesia is mediated through Ca^{2+} channels in sensory neurons, so it is possible that the block of Ca^{2+} channels by ginsenoside Rf is a responsible mechanism. However, it inhibits large, but not small, nociceptors, which is inconsistent with tonic pain. So, mechanisms other than Ca^{2+} block are likely involved.

Systemic (IP) administration of ginseng extract produces analgesia and hypothermia in rats, which is not reversed by the opioid antagonist naltrexone (Ramarao and Bhargava 1990). However, ginseng reduces the analgesia, hyperthermia, and catalepsy induced by morphine. This effect shows an inverted-U dose-respone curve, where morphine analgesia is blocked by ginseng at 25 and 50 mg/kg doses, but not by 12.5, 100, and 200 mg/kg doses. Spinal ginsenosides reduce the analgesic effect of supraspinal morphine (intracerebroventricular, 2 μg) in the tail-flick test for at least 6 hours (Suh et al. 1997). Individual ginsenosides having this effect are Rb2, Rc, Rd, and Rg1, but not Rb1. While individual ginsensosides have this effect, total extract of ginseng may not. Ginseng's antagonistic effects on opioid analgesia may rely on serotonergic mechanisms (Kim et al. 1992). Ginsenoside reduction of κ opioid-induced (U50,488H) analgesia was prevented by treatment with the serotonin precursor, 5-hydroxytryptophan (5-HTP). The dopamine precursor L-dopa did not have the same effect.

Constituents of Vietnamese ginseng *(Panax vietnamensis)* also show analgesic effects and antagonism of opioid analgesia. Majonoside-R2, a saponin from Vietnamese ginseng, dose-dependently reduces analgesia induced by subcutaneous mu (morphine) or kappa (U-50,488H) opioid agonists in the tail-pinch test (Huong et al. 1997). This effect was produced when majonoside-R2 is administered peripherally (IP) or supraspinally (intracerebroventricular). Also, majonoside-R2 also antagonizes the opioid analgesia when they are co-administered intracerebroventricular or intrathecal. Diazepam had similar effects, and both were reversed by the benzodiazepine antagonist flumazenil and the GABA channel blocker picrotoxin. Thus, majonoside-R2 antagonizes opioid analgesia at spinal and supraspinal levels, at least partly by acting through $GABA_A$ receptors. Systemic and central majonoside-R2 also antagonizes analgesia induced by the alpha-2 agonist clonidine in the tail-pinch test (Nguyen et al. 1996, 1997). Again, this antagonistic effect was reversed by flumazenil and picrotoxin, suggesting $GABA_A$ mediation.

Similar to naloxone, majonoside-R2 also reduces stress-induced analgesia measured by the tail-pinch test (Nguyen et al. 1995).

In summary, species of ginseng have analgesic effects in several animal models. *Panax ginseng* creates analgesia through nonopioid mechanisms and is antagonistic to opioid and adrenergic analgesia. Antagonism of opioid analgesia occurs at spinal and supraspinal levels and is mediated by serotonergic mechanisms. Other putative mechanisms are antagonism of substance P receptors and Ca^{2+} channels. *Panax vietnamensis* shows similar analgesic effects and antagonism of opioid analgesia and involves $GABA_A$ mechanisms. Despite notable evidence for an analgesic effect of ginseng, there have not been any controlled studies carried out in humans to date. Although it has not been examined in the context of analgesia, nonginsenoside constituents of ginseng have nicotinic activity, which could contribute to analgesic effects.

Local Anesthetics

Local anesthesia involves the blockade of nerve conduction in order to stop sensation. Because local anesthetics act on all nerve fibers they may also temporarily create motor paralysis. The usefulness of local anesthetics is their ability to completely block axonal transduction, which is reversible and without any apparent lasting effects.

Coca

Cocaine was probably the first drug with recognized local anesthetic effects (Catterall and Mackie 1996). Natives of Peru have long known that chewing coca leaves produces oral numbness (Young and MacKenzie 1992). When cocaine was first isolated from the coca plant by Albert Nieman in 1860, he noticed that it had a numbing effect on his tongue when he tasted it. Carl Koller introduced cocaine as a local anesthetic for ophthalmologic surgery in 1884. Given that the euphoric and autonomic effects of cocaine are unwanted during clinical anesthesia, Einhorn and colleagues began searching for a more tolerable synthetic substitute in 1892, and synthesized procaine (Novocain) in 1905. Since then, many related synthetic local anesthetics have been developed,

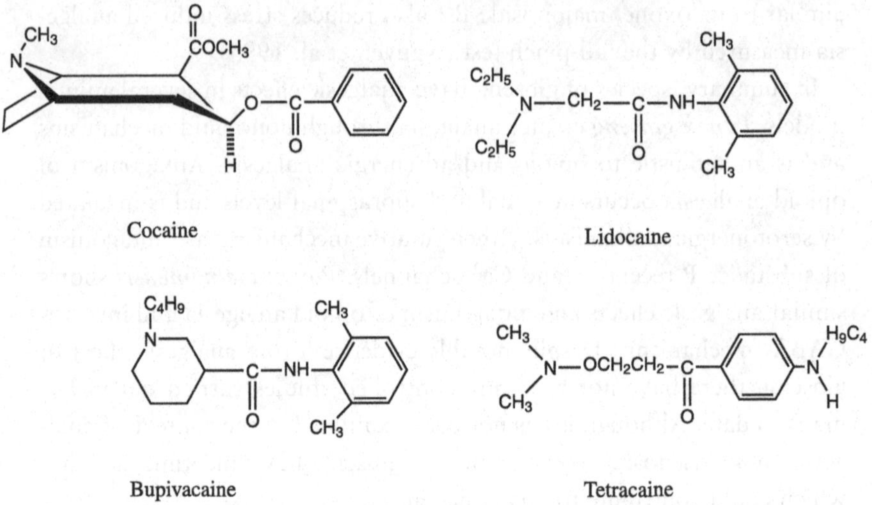

Cocaine

Lidocaine

Bupivacaine

Tetracaine

Figure 8.12
Chemical structure of cocaine and synthetic local anesthetics.

including lidocaine (Xylocaine), bupivacaine (Marcaine), and tetracaine (Pontocaine) (figure 8.12). The use of cocaine for local anesthesia has been largely replaced by synthetic drugs that produce less psychoactive effects. However, cocaine is still used sometimes for topical anesthesia of the upper respiratory tract.

Mechanism of Action

The local anesthetic actions of cocaine are independent of its well-known actions on monoamines. Rather, the local anesthetic effects occur as a consequence of its interaction with voltage-gated Na^+ channels (Matthews and Collins 1983). Cocaine's cerebral vasoconstrictor effects occur through local anesthetic rather than sympathomimetic mechanisms (Albuquerque and Kurth 1993).

The site of action on the Na^+ channel for cocaine and its analogs appears to be on the intracellular side of the channel, so cocaine must evidently cross the cell membrane to be effective (Narahashi and Frazier 1971). The Na^+ channel is composed of a large protein divided into α, β_1, and β_2 subunits. The α subunit is further divided into four domains, each of which contains four transmembrane segments (designated I–IV).

This protein is fixed in the cell membrane, and is sensitive to voltage. When the cell is sufficiently depolarized, a conformational change occurs in the protein, allowing flow of Na^+ across the membrane. After several milliseconds, an inactivation gate closes, ceasing the flux of Na^+. The inactivation gate is likely located on an intracellular loop between domains III and IV.

The inhibition produced by local anesthetics is both frequency- and voltage-dependent, and also referred to as "use-dependent block." Nerves that are more stimulated encounter a greater degree of inhibition, while resting axons are relatively less sensitive (Butterworth et al. 1987). The duration of action is prolonged by vasoconstrictors because they keep the drug in contact with the nerve longer rather than it being carried away in the blood stream. Different size nerve fibers also have varying sensitivity to local anesthetics. Smaller C and $A\delta$ fibers are more sensitive than the larger $A\gamma$, $A\beta$, and $A\alpha$ fibers. Thus, sensory and autonomic nerves are more susceptible than motor and proprioceptive nerves.

Clove Oil

Clove oil is used as a local anesthetic. Clove comes from the tree *Syzygium aromaticum* (formerly referred to as *Eugenia caryophyllus* or *Caryophyllus aromaticus*) (Gruenwald et al. 1998; Tyler 1994; Robbers et al. 1996). It is an evergreen tree that grows up to 20 meters in height. The spice derives from the characteristic nail-shape cloves of the tree (figure 8.13). Clove oil, which is the preparation used for local anesthesia, is steam-distilled from the flowers. A large proportion of clove produced is ground and added to tobacco. These are referred to as *kretek* in Indonesia, or as simply as *clove cigarettes* in the West. They contain approximately 60% tobacco and 40% clove (Clark 1989). Although more popular in Indonesia, they have made their way to the West.

Clove was known to the Chinese as early as 266 B.C.E. The Dutch wished to monopolize the trade of clove in the seventeenth century, and so destroyed all of the trees except those on Ambon and Ternate. However, the tree has since been introduced to many other regions. Indigenous to the to the Molucca Islands, it is also grown on several islands of

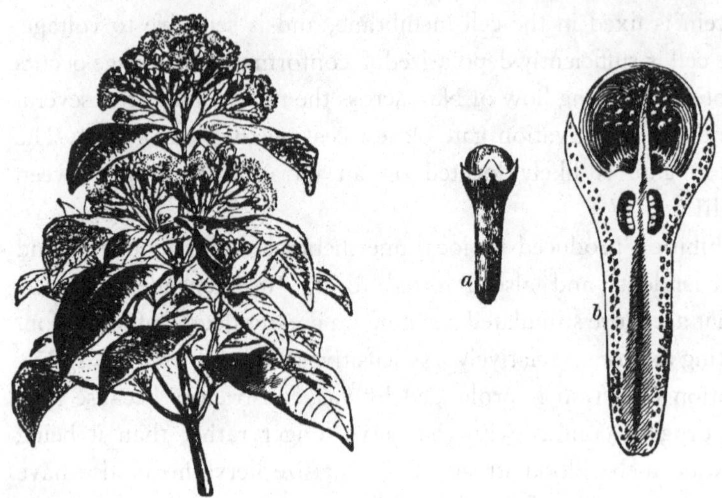

Figure 8.13
Clove *(Syzygium aromaticum)*. Reprinted from Culbreth DMR. (1927). *Materia Medica and Pharmacognosy*, 7th ed. Philadelphia: Lea & Febiger.

Africa, Asia, and the West Indies. The majority of the world's supply comes from Tanzania and Zanzibar.

Chemical Constituents
There are several related phenolic compounds found in the volatile oil of clove. The primary one is eugenol, accounting for 85% of the total (figure 8.14) (Tyler 1994; Robbers et al. 1996).

Mechanism of Action
The anesthetic action of clove is attributable to eugenol and its natural analogs. Little is really known about the local anesthetic mechanism of eugenol. As mentioned above, eugenol is a phenolic compound, and phenol itself acts as a local anesthetic (Kizelshteyn et al. 1992). Phenol acts synergistically with bupivacaine, and most likely blocks Na^+ channels. Eugenol has not been specifically shown to block Na^+ channels, but its phenolic structure suggests that it does.

Low millimolar concentrations of eugenol activate a Ca^{2+} channel (Ohkubo and Kitamura 1997). Further, a Cl^- channel may indirectly activate in response to the Ca^{2+} influx. Eugenol acts on Ca^{2+} channels

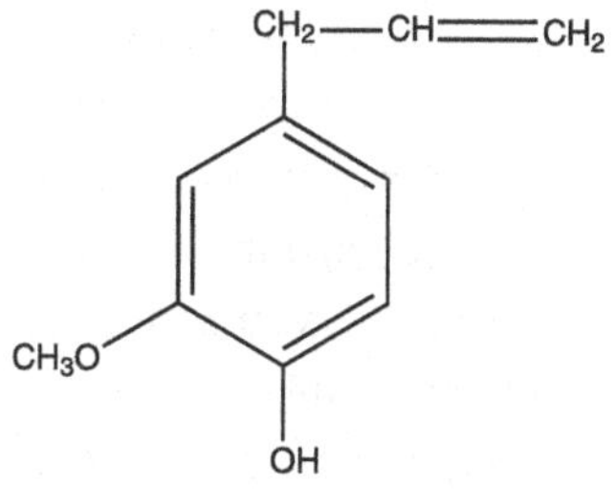

Figure 8.14
Chemical structure of eugenol.

through at least two mechanisms, one involving the capsaicin receptor and the other independent of it. While blockade of Na^+ channels is suspect for any drug that reduces action potentials and sevres as a local anesthetic, no such studies have specifically addressed this with eugenol.

Another mechanism that potentially contributes to clove oil's effects is inhibition of prostaglandin synthesis through both cyclooxygenase and lipoxygenase pathways (Tyler 1994). Accordingly, local injections of clove oil supressed joint swelling in arthritic rats (Sharma et al. 1994).

General Effects

In addition to eugenol's phenolic structure, it displays several properties of a local anesthetic drug (Brodin and Røed 1984). Submillimolar concentrations of eugenol reversibly inhibit action potentials and increase the threshold for nerve stimulation. At concentrations above 2.44 mM, the nerve block is irreversible. At the neuromuscular junction, eugenol has both pre- and postsynaptic effects on end-plate potentials and miniature end-plate potentials. Consistent with use-dependent block, little effect is seen on the resting membrane potential of muscle. A synergistic effect occurs with eugenol and d-tubocurarine, suggesting a possible common mode of action for the two drugs.

Eugenol may be mixed with zinc oxide as a temporary tooth filling, where the eugenol seeps into the pulp of the tooth and has anesthetic effects (Markowitz et al. 1992).

Intraperitoneal injections of eugenol and its natural analogs produce unconsciousness in rats, accompanied by slow-wave activity on the EEG (Sell and Carlini 1976). Cerebral levels of dopamine, norepinephrine, and serotonin are not apparently altered.

The central effects of eugenol in humans are uncertain, and what perpetuates clove's addition to cigarettes is also uncertain. However, other local anesthetics have profound effects on the CNS. For example, in animals, intravenous procaine activates electrical activity in limbic structures and suppresses activity in neocortical structures (Servan-Schreiber et al. 1998; Ketter et al. 1996). In humans, procaine similarly induces limbic activation, including the anterior cingulate, insula, and amygdala/parahippocampal gyrii. Decreases in activity occur in the left inferior parietal lobule, right thalamus, and bilateral cerebellum. Reported subjective phenomena include a variety of emotional experiences, ranging from euphoria to depression and anxiety. In some instances, the anxiety reaches the intensity of panic, and it correlates with left amygdala activation. Subjects who do not experience panic have greater activation in the anterior cingulate bilaterally and in the left inferior frontal cortex. Thus, local anesthetics produce emotional effects by activation of central limbic structures. Whether eugenol replicates this pattern remains to be seen.

Toxicity

Clove is listed as Generally Regarded as Safe (GRAS) by the U.S. Food and Drug Administration, and is approved by the German Commission E for use as a local anesthetic.

Because clove cigarettes also contain tobacco, they carry all of the hazards of regular tobacco smoking (Council on Scientific Affairs 1988). Several cases of serious medical illness have been associated with clove cigarettes in the United States (Guidotti et al. 1989). These include cases of hemorrhagic pulmonary edema, pneumonia, bronchitis, and hemoptysis. Because eugenol anesthetizes the respiratory tract, it inhibits the normal gag reflex and has led to aspiration pneumonia in at least one case. Accidental overdoses in children have led to CNS depression, urinary abnormalities, and anion-gap acidosis. These cases were treated successfully with supportive measures (Lane et al. 1991).

Conclusion

As is evident in this chapter, a wide variety of plants have been found to have analgesic and/or anesthetic effects. Their pharmacological diversity reflects the diverse neurochemistry and neurophysiology of pain and analgesia systems in the nervous system.

Some of the plants and drugs discussed here are widely known for their analgesic/anesthetic effects. They have become an integral part of our medical treatment, advanced our understanding of pain and analgesia, and led to the development of similar drugs with better clinical properties. Namely, these are the opioids from poppy, salicylates from *Salix* species, and cocaine from coca. Together, these drugs and their synthetic relatives account for the vast majority of clinical pain relief.

The other plants and drugs are discussed for the purpose of elucidating the mechanisms behind their long-known clinical effects (e.g., clove). It is also interesting to note that many stimulant drugs (tobacco, areca, lobelia, khat, coca) have incidental but significant analgesic effects. Few people smoke tobacco for the purpose of relieving pain, but it is effective in that regard. It remains to be studied empirically, but perhaps people smoke tobacco more when in pain without explicitly knowing it.

9

Hallucinogenic Plants

Hallucinogenic plants constitute a wide variety of species, all of which profoundly distort perception, cognition, and mood. Although some synthetic hallucinogenic drugs have been produced, the majority of this class are derived from plants. Both traditional shamans and modern scientists are equally captivated by the effects of these drugs, whether for unlocking secrets of the spirit world or for unlocking secrets of the human mind and brain.

The use of hallucinogens is fairly prevalent in western cultures. A 1990 national survey estimated that 7.6% of the U.S. population over age 12 had tried a hallucinogenic drug once in their lives, and 1.1% had done so within the last 12 months (National Institute on Drug Abuse, 1990). After marijuana, hallucinogens were the most commonly tried illicit drugs. Use of hallucinogens is most common among people between the ages of 18 and 25.

Terminology

Considerable thought has been given to which term most appropriately labels this class of drugs, and how they are best defined to differentiate them from other drugs with overlapping effects. The toxicologist Louis Lewin termed them *phantasticants* in 1924. Although appropriate, the term is rarely used today. *Psychedelic* translates from Greek as "mind manifesting" or "mind-expanding," but its implications are uncertain. William James suggested, "Our normal waking consciousness, rational consciousness as we call it, is but one special type of consciousness, whilst all about it, parted from it by the flimsiest of screens, there lie potential forms of consciousness entirely different" (James 1902). In this framework, hallucinogens demonstrate subjectively how much "external reality" is really an internal construction by the brain. Although this may apply well to the monoamine hallucinogens, the cholinergic hallucinogens can cloud consciousness. They create a state more accurately described as an amnestic delirium than an expansion of consciousness.

The term *psychotomimetic* was coined to compare the effects of hallucinogens to the symptoms of schizophrenia and other psychotic conditions. However, the effects produced by hallucinogens and mental illness are qualitatively different. While drug-induced hallucinations tend to be more visual, auditory hallucinations are most common in schizophrenia. The hallucinogenic drugs discussed here may induce positive symptoms (e.g., hallucinations), but do not induce the negative symptoms (e.g., cognitive deficits, social withdrawal) of schizophrenia.

The term *hallucinogen* derives from the Latin word *alucinari*, meaning to "wander in mind" (Abraham et al. 1996). However, hallucinogens are not the only drugs capable of creating hallucinations. If given in high enough doses, other drugs such as cocaine, opioids, and cannabis can do the same. Instead, the term is used to label drugs for which hallucinations are their most prominent effect, even at low doses. Thus, a hallucinogen may be defined as "any agent that causes alterations in perception, cognition, and mood as its primary psychobiological actions in the presence of an otherwise clear sensorium" (Abraham et al. 1996). This definition, however, excludes the cholinergic hallucinogens because they certainly cloud consciousness.

Perhaps there is no completely satisfactory term for this class of drugs, but the term *hallucinogen* will be used to collectively refer to them throughout this chapter.

Historical Uses of Hallucinogenic Plants

Given the powerful ability of these plants to alter perceptions, it is not surprising that humans have ascribed magical powers to them. The modern interpretation of the effects of these drugs is rooted in their effects on the brain, altering the apparatus through which we construct reality. But that explanation arose in the context of knowledge about the brain, and the neural basis of thought and perception. For generations of people in nonindustrial cultures with traditional beliefs, the supernatural explanation is the most sensible one. Many cultures, such as those of the Aztec and ancient Greeks, incorporated them into religious rituals (Grinspoon and Bakalar 1997; Schultes and Hofman 1980, 1992).

Modern interest in hallucinogenic drugs increased in the West after the synthesis of LSD by Albert Hofman in 1949. Aldous Huxley wrote perhaps the most famous account of hallucinogens, describing his experiences with mescaline in his book, *The Doors of Perception* (Huxley 1954). In the 1960s, some experimented with hallucinogens in an attempt to expand consciousness, while others proposed that they could create a temporary model of schizophrenia in humans. Hallucinogenic drugs were classified under Schedule I of the Controlled Substances Act of 1970. This restricted their use, asserting that they have a high potential for abuse and lack any therapeutic value. However, the use of peyote by the Native American Church was protected by the Religious Freedom Restoration Act in 1993.

Classification of Hallucinogens

There are many ways to potentially classify hallucinogenic drugs. They are organized here by their primary mechanism of action: monoamine, cholinergic, and amino acid. The monoamine hallucinogens are further subclassified as indole (indolealkylamine) or catechol (phenethylamine) in structure, although actions at serotonin receptors are likely to underlie all of their hallucinogenic effects (Rech and Commissaris 1982).

Monoamine Hallucinogens

The monoamine hallucinogens are a diverse group of plants, consisting of fungi (ergot and psilocybe), cacti (peyote, San Pedro, cawe), vines (yage, morning glory, Hawaiian rosewood), and trees (nutmeg) (table 9.1). They have convergently evolved biochemical constituents that interfere with monoamine activity.

Table 9.1
Monoamine hallucinogens

Common	Botanical	Type	Active principles
Ergot	*Claviceps purpurea*	Fungus	*d*-isolysergic acid *d*-lysergic acid
Psilocybe	*Conocybe silineoides* *Panaeolus sphinctrinus* *Psilocybe aztecorum* *P. caerulescans* *P. mexicana* *Stropharia cubensis*	Fungus	Psilocin, psilocybin
Peyote	*Lophophora williamsii* *Trichocereus pachanoi*	Cactus Cactus	Mescaline, etc. Mescaline 3,4-dimethoxyphenyl-ethylamine 3-methoxy-tyramine
Cawe	*Pachycereus pecten-aboriginum*	Cactus	4-hydroxy-3-ethoxy-phenylethylamine
Yage	*Banisteriopsis caapi*	Woody vine	Harmala alkaloids Dimethyltryptamine
Morning Glory			
Ololiuqui Badoh Negroh	*Turbina corymbosa* *Ipomoea violacea*	Flower-ing vine	Lysergic acid amide Lysergic acid hydroxy-ethylamide
Hawaiian Baby Rosewood	*Argyreia nervosa*		Lysergic acid amide
Iboga	*Tabernanthe iboga*	Shrub	Ibogaine Ibogamine Tabernanthine Coronaridine
Nutmeg	*Myristica fragrans*	Tree	Myristicin Elemicin

See text for references.

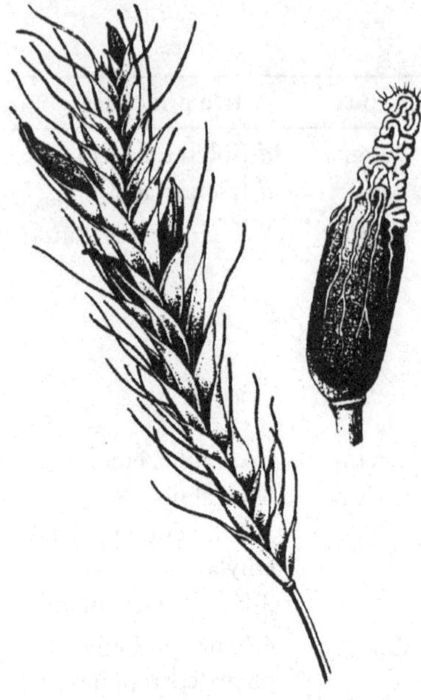

Figure 9.1
Ergot *(Claviceps purpurea)*. Reprinted from Barron et al., "The Hallucinogenic Drugs." *Scientific American*. April 1964. Illustration by Alex Semenoick.

Ergot

History and Botany

Ergot *(Claviceps purpurea)* is a parasitic fungus that grows on rye *(Secale cereale)* and other grains, particularly during wet seasons (Gruenwald et al. 1998). It is black and hard, and protrudes from the grains. Insects carry and deposit the spores, which grow hyphae down into the ovary of the rye to access its nutrients. When the ovary is destroyed, a mycelium grows. A long black sclerotium grows to a length of 8 cm, which eventually falls to the ground. In the following spring, pink fruiting bodies grow from it, releasing thread-like acospores (figure 9.1).

The ergot fungus and its noxious effects were known to the Mesopotamian cultures of Assyria and Babylonia (van Dongen and de Groot 1995). The earliest known written mention of ergot is an Assyrian cuneiform tablet dating circa 600 B.C.E., referring to it as a "noxious pustule in the ear of grain." Ironically, it was not until 1676 C.E. that the symptoms of ergot poisoning (or ergotism) were associated with ingestion of ergot. The Romans referred to ergotism as *Ignis sacer*, or Holy Fire. This name was carried through to the European Middle Ages, and refers to the burning sensation it causes in the extremities. Casualties from ergotism were significant: one epidemic in Europe during 944 C.E. was responsible for the deaths of 40,000 people (Abraham et al. 1996).

Saint Anthony was a monk who lived in the third and fourth centuries C.E. A shrine was named after him in the south of France in 1039 C.E., where an outbreak of ergotism occurred. The shrine became a popular pilgrimage for those suffering from ergotism. Thus, ergotism became known as *Saint Anthony's fire*. It is speculated that increased peripheral circulation from walking and change in diet accounted for the healing properties of such a journey.

There are still occasional modern outbreaks of ergotism, such as in Ukrania and Ireland in 1929, and in Belgium in 1953. It has been suggested that the Salem witch trials of 1692 may have been sparked by ergotism, although others favor a social psychological explanation for the events (Matossian 1982; Spanos 1983).

Chemical Constituents

Ergot possesses two general classes of alkaloids: amine and amino acid (Peroutka 1996). The amine alkaloids have antagonist effects on serotonin receptors, while the amino acid alkaloids are less selective and act upon other monoamine receptors. While some amine alkaloids are of interest for cognition-enhancing effects (e.g., Hydergine), certain amino acid alkaloids are known for their hallucinogenic effects. Namely, these are *d*-isolysergic acid and *d*-lysergic acid (figure 9.2). LSD (*d*-lysergic acid diethylamide) is a synthetic compound derived from ergoloids, but it serves as a model for plant-derived psychedelics. Both likely work through similar or identical mechanisms and differ only in efficacy or potency. The majority of research in this area has focused on LSD, rather than on naturally occuring hallucinogenic ergoloids.

Pharmacology

LSD is odorless and tasteless and is effective in microgram doses. Doses of 25–50 µg produce an intensification of perceptions, while larger doses are needed for full hallucinations. The total duration of the drug effect

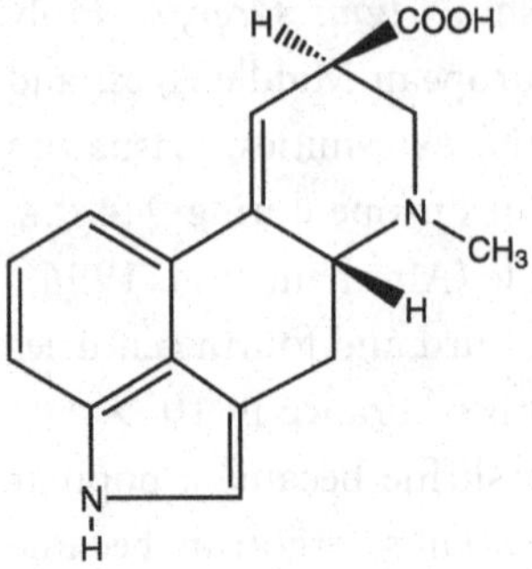

Lysergic Acid
(*Claviceps purpurea*)

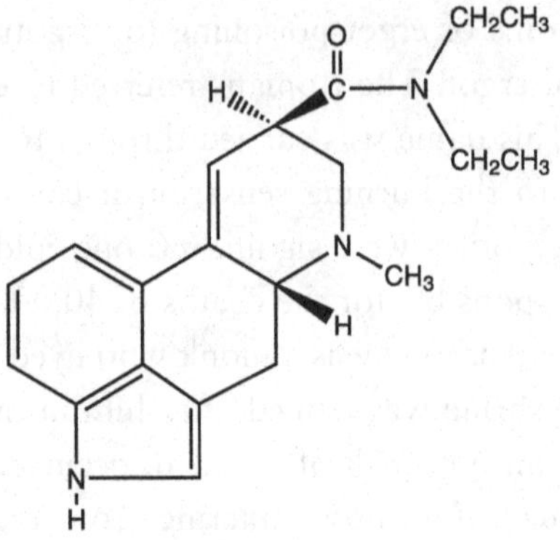

Lysergic Acid Diethylamide
(*synthetic*)

Figure 9.2
Chemical structure of LSD and lysergic acid diethylamide.

is 6–12 hours. Tolerance develops to the behavioral effects after daily administration for 4–7 days, and lasts for 3 days. LSD develops cross-tolerance to other monoamine hallucinogens, such as mescaline and psilocybin. The authenticity of illicit LSD is questionable; many seized samples do not contain the actual drug.

Mechanisms of Action

Serotonin LSD is an agonist at 5-HT_{1A}, 5-HT_{2A}, and 5-HT_{2C} receptors (Welsh et al. 1998; Krebs-Thomson et al. 1998; Burris et al. 1991). However, actions at 5-HT_2 receptors may best account for the hallucinogenic effects of LSD and other monoamine hallucinogens because a high correlation exists between their 5-HT_2 binding affinity and their efficacy (Titeler et al. 1988; Marek and Aghajanian 1996). LSD creates half-maximal effects at 5-HT_{2A} and 5-HT_{2C} receptors in the nanomolar range (7.2 nM and 27 nM, respectively) (Egan et al. 1998; Burris and Sanders-Bush 1992). In contrast, drugs that act solely at 5-HT_{1A} receptors are not hallucinogenic. More recently, LSD has been shown to bind to 5-HT_5, 5-HT_6, and 5-HT_7 receptor subtypes.

Debates have arisen over whether LSD is an agonist or antagonist, but its effects are probably best characterized as partial agonist (Glennon

1990; Marek and Aghajanian 1996; Pierce and Peroutka 1990a; Zhang and Dyer 1993). LSD has inhibitory effects on raphe neurons, but this is dissociable from its behavioral effects, suggesting a postsynaptic site of action (Trulson 1986; Vandermaelen and Aghajanian 1983; Blier et al. 1989). However, LSD shows a preferential activation of phospholipase A_2-arachidonic acid pathways. Still, LSD stimulates phosphoinositide hydrolysis at 25% of that maximally achieved by serotonin, consistent with a partial agonist effect (Sanders-Bush et al. 1988; Berg et al. 1998). LSD also decreases spontaneous activity in the locus coeruleus, but increases its response to stimulation (Rasmussen and Aghajanian 1986).

Significant tolerance develops to the effects of LSD. Daily repeated administration of LSD downregulates 5-HT_2 receptors, but not 5-HT_{1A}, 5-HT_{1B}, adrenergic, or dopaminergic receptors (Buckholtz et al. 1990, 1988). Further, down-regulation of 5-HT_2 receptors closely parallels the development of behavioral tolerance to LSD. In contrast to cortical 5-HT_2 receptors, there is no reduction in 5-HT_{1A}, 5-HT_{1B}, β-adrenergic, α_1 or α_2 adrenergic, D_2 receptors, or a serotonin reuptake site (Buckholtz et al. 1990).

Dopamine A few studies have examined the dopaminergic effects of LSD. The affinity of LSD for D_2 receptors is similar to its affinity for 5-HT_2 sites, and it has a slightly lower affininty for D_1 receptors (Watts et al. 1995). LSD has partial agonist effects at D_2 receptors as seen in the inhibition of prolactin release (Giacomelli et al. 1998). Neuroleptic drugs are also used clinically to terminate an LSD experience. Thus, the effects of LSD on dopaminergic function may contribute to its hallucinogeinc effects.

General Effects

Autonomic LSD produces sympathomimetic effects, including pupil dilation, tachycardia, increased blood pressure, piloerection, hyperreflexia, nausea, and fever.

Behavioral LSD typically suppresses locomotor and exploratory behaviors (Mittman and Geyer 1991). It reduces attention and response to external stimuli, presumably reflecting greater attention to internal stimuli (e.g., illusions, hallucinations). LSD does induce a conditioned place preference in rats (Meehan and Schechter 1998).

Electrophysiology LSD hyperpolarizes pyramidal neurons in somatosensory cortex, whereas serotonin initially depolarizes and then causes a long-lasting hyperpolarization (Pierce and Peroutka 1990b). In cats, the EEG effects of LSD indicate increased arousal and wakefulness (Kay and Martin 1978). During sleep, LSD decreases REM sleep and sleep spindles. Chronic treatment with selective serotonin reuptake inhibitors (SSRIs) decreases the electrophysiological responsiveness to LSD (de Montigny et al. 1990). Through 5-HT_2-mediated mechanisms, LSD enhances nonsynchronous glutamatergic EPSPs in cortical pyramidal cells (Aghajanian and Marek 1999).

The effect of LSD on cerebral blood flow was studied in the rat (Goldman et al. 1975). An intravenous injection of LSD increased blood flow to frontal and parietal cortex within 10 minutes, and to the cerebellum within 20 minutes. Increases (significant or nonsignificant) were evidenced in all brain areas assessed, except for the hippocampus, where a minor, nonsignificant reduction was noted.

Neuroimaging An LSD analog [N1-([^{11}C]-Methyl)-2-Br-LSD ([^{11}C]-MBL)]was used to assess 5-HT2 binding in the human brain with positron emission tomography (PET) (Wong et al. 1987). A distinctly serotonergic pattern of binding is seen with highest levels of labeling in frontal, temporal, and parietal cortex. Lower levels of binding are observed in caudate and putamen. There are no studies that address the hallucinatory effects of LSD with functional neuroimaging, but one exists for mescaline (see below).

Cognitive and subjective effects The effects of LSD on attention have been examined in animal paradigms. LSD reduces accuracy on a multiple-choice reaction time task, which is reversed by a 5-HT_2 antagonist (Carli and Samanin 1992). LSD produces gross alterations in time perception, which holds true in animal models as well as human reports (Frederick et al. 1997).

The hallmark effects of LSD are profound perceptual distortions and hallucinations. It produces a heightened awareness of sensations, where mundane sensations become vivid and intense. Lower doses produce illusions and alterations of perception, including intensification of colors and distortions of shade, movement, and form. One may experience macropsia or micropsia, which are the perceptions that visual objects are getting larger or smaller, respectively. Visual afterimages may be prolonged and visual percepts may overlap. Emotional meaning is intensified and experience may take on a magical or epiphanic intensity (Abraham et al. 1996). Higher doses may produce geometric visual patterns or fully formed hallucinatory experiences. Hallucinations are most typically visual in nature, and begin 2–3 hours after drug administration. Auditory hallucinations are rare, but distortions of body image are not uncommon. LSD enhances classical conditioning, through actions at 5-HT_{2A} and 5-HT_{2C} receptors (Welsh et al. 1998). Memory is generally unimpaired, and past memories may be vividly reexperienced.

Another effect of LSD is an altered sense of self. Many experience a derealization or a "spectator ego," where one feels like a passive observer of one's own experiences. Many also experience a lessened sense of interpersonal boundaries. In a positive social context, this can result in a sense of union with others. However, if it becomes frightening it can result in anxiety and fears of depersonalization.

The effects of LSD are highly variable between and within individuals, and are highly influenced by one's mental state and environmental setting (Abraham et al. 1996). Those taking the drug alone are more likely to experience anxiety, speech disruption, and reduced motility, while those taking it in a group setting are more likely to experience euphoria. More adverse experiences are reported by those who are unaware that they are receiving it.

Addiction and Dependence

LSD produces a rapid and complete tolerance, but it is not powerfully reinforcing the way drugs of abuse like cocaine and heroin are. LSD does not produce any known withdrawal syndrome (Abraham et al. 1996). It does not produce positive reinforcement in animal self-administration models. Concurrently in humans, it does not lead to patterns of repetitive, compulsive use. Regular LSD users typically show a pattern of usage consisting of periodic use spaced several weeks or more apart.

Toxicity

Massive overdoses of LSD are required to have lethal effects. Many of the symptoms of ergotism, excluding hallucinations, are not caused by lysergic acid, but by other ergoloids. A high safety margin exists with LSD, with fatal doses in the range of 150,000 mg/kg in rodents. No human fatalities have ever been reported from an overdose of LSD. The cases of eight people were reported, who snorted pure LSD, mistaking it for cocaine (Klock et al. 1975). The estimated doses taken were between 10,000 and 100,000 μg. They experienced confusion, hallucinations, and hemorrhaging (through inhibition of platelet formation), but all recovered.

Ergotism Ergotism is a constellation of symptoms that occurs as a result of eating the ergot fungus. The effects of ergotism were apparent to ancient writers on the subject (Schultes and Hofman 1980, 1992). Two general forms are distinguished: a neurological form consisting of seizures and hallucinations, and a vascular form consisting of gangrene and loss of extremities (noses, ear lobes, fingers, toes, and feet). The vascular symptoms of ergotism are due to the vasoconstricting effect of ergoloids, and the neurological form seems to result from ergot occurring primarily in wild grasses. Another effect of ergot is uterine contractions, frequently causing spontaneous abortions. This effect was taken advantage of by European midwives, who employed ergot to assist contractions during difficult births. Although it is not a drug of choice due to unpredictable side effects, the ergoloid ergotmetrine is still available for treatment of postpartum hemorrhage (van Dongen and de Groot 1995).

Bad trips A commonly known outcome of hallucinogenic experience is colloquially known as a bad trip. This essentially consists of a panic episode, sometimes brought on by a dislike of the hallucinogenic effects and fear that the experience will not end. Given that LSD prolongs one's perception of time, it may seem as if the experience will never end and it is easy to understand how such fears may rapidly escalate into panic. This reaction responds to supportiveness and a familiar environment, although some contend that reassurance may worsen the condition (Abraham et al. 1996). Anecdotal clinical experience indicates that benzodiazepines and neuroleptics may be useful as acute pharmacological treatments.

Hallucinogen-persisting perception disorder Hallucinogen-persisting perception disorder (HPPD), commonly called flashbacks, are phenomena where the person reexperiences aspects of the hallucinogenic trip long after it has ended. This is reported by approximately 15% of LSD users. Some precipitants of HPPD are cannabis use, anxiety, fatigue, and sudden movement into a dark environment. This may be a normal function of memory that becomes exaggerated due to the intense nature of the hallucinogenic experience. Alternately, it may also be a direct pharmacological effect.

In LSD users who presented with visual disturbances, the disorder remained after 5 years in half of the sample (Abraham 1983). Common visual disturbances reported were geometric percepts, false fleeting perceptions in the peripheral visual field, flashes of color, and afterimages. Diagnosis of HPPD may seem relatively simple on the surface because hallucinogenic drugs are known to have these effects in a subset of the population. However, one must rule out other potential diagnoses that could mimic HPPD, such as toxic exposures, stroke, brain tumors, central infections, and brain trauma.

HPPD has been studied with quantitative EEG. Compared to controls, people with HPPD show a faster alpha frequency and shorter visual-evoked-response latency, consistent with LSD-induced cortical disinhibition (Abraham and Duffy 1996). Conversely, the auditory-evoked-response latency is increased. Analyses indicate that these differences are predominant in temporal and left parietal regions.

A few cases have been reported of exacerbation of HPPD by risperidone (Risperdal) (Abraham and Mamen 1996). The exact reason for this is uncertain, but the fact that risperidone and LSD both act at 5-HT_2 receptors is probably causative. Also, two cases have been reported of an exacerbation of HPPD by selective serotonin reuptake inhibitors (Markel et al. 1994).

Other adverse effects LSD is not teratogenic, but it can increase spontaneous abortions due to uterotonic effects. Use during pregnancy is unnecessary and clearly contraindicated. LSD appears to have weak, if any, mutagenic effects (Cohen and Shiloh 1977–78). Claims of chromosomal damage have showed conflicting results, and have not been supported in humans.

Psilocybe

History and Botany

There are several related species of mushrooms that have hallucinogenic effects. Many are in the psilocybe genus, including *Psilocybe aztecorum*, *P. caerulescans*, and *P. mexicana* (Schultes and Hofman 1980, 1992). Other related species include *Stropharia cubensis*, *Panaeolus sphinctrinus*, and *P. foenisecii* (see table 9.1 and figure 9.3).

Use of these mushrooms was well known to Native American civilizations in Central America. The Aztec referred to them as *Teonanacatl*, meaning "divine flesh," or "god flesh" and reserved them for use in religious ceremonies. Religious use of hallucinogenic mushrooms is also known to the Mazatec, Chinantec, Mije, Zapotec, and Mixtec of Oaxaca. The Mazatec still actively employ mushrooms in religious ceremonies, referring to them as *Nti-si-tho*. There is evidence that mushrooms were also used by the Maya.

Chemical Constituents

The two principal hallucinogenic constituents of psilocybe mushrooms (and related genera) are psilocybin and psilocin (Schultes and Hofman 1980, 1992) (figure 9.4). They are very similar, having a dimethyltryptamine structure and differing only by a phosphoric acid molecule. Psilocybin may be called 4-phosphoryl-DMT and psilocin may be called 4-hydroxy DMT. They are both approximately 1/200 as potent as LSD. Absorption is adequate through the oral route, making this a common form of consumption.

The levels of psilocybin are generally twice that of psilocin, and levels may vary greatly across different samples of mushroom (Bigwood and Beug 1982). Psilocybin is generally absent from the first or second fruiting of the mushroom grown from culture, and maximizes in the fourth

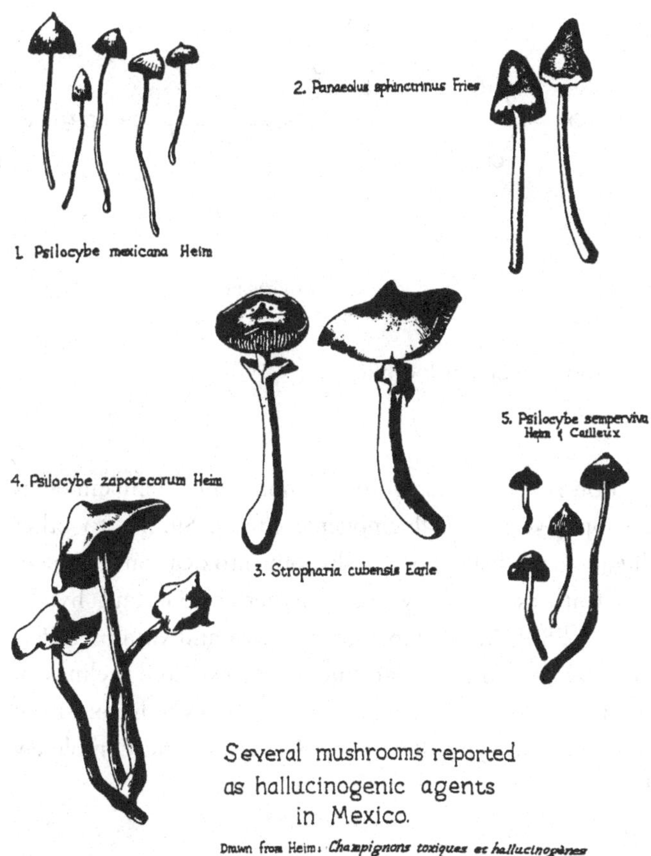

Figure 9.3
Psilocybe and related species. Reprinted with permission from Schultes RE, Hofman A. (1980). *The Botany and Chemistry of Hallucinogens*, 2nd ed. Springfield, Ill.: Charles C. Thomas Publishers.

fruting. Psilocybin levels vary by a factor of four in controlled cultures, and by a factor of seven in wild samples (Beug and Bigwood 1982).

Mechanisms of Action

Psilocybin and psilocin are believed to work through mechanisms similar to LSD and other indole hallucinogens. Similar to LSD, chronic psilocybin in take also down-regulates 5-HT_2 receptors, which parallels the development of behavioral tolerance (Buckholtz et al. 1990).

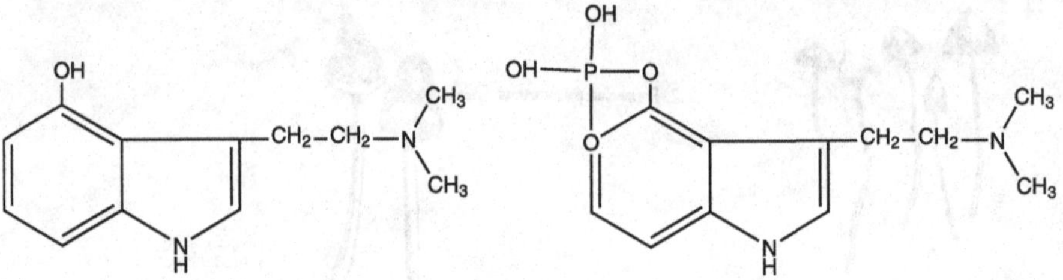

Figure 9.4
Chemical structure of psilocin and psilocybin.

General Effects
Psilocybe intoxication is very similar to other monoamine hallucinogens in terms of the subjective and hallucinogenic effects. Similar to other monoamine hallucinogens, psilocybe mushroom intoxication produces sympathomimetic features of tachycardia, hypertension, and hyperreflexia (Peden et al. 1982). Many experience nausea and vomiting. Perceptual distortions are primarily visual, but paresthesia and feelings of depersonalization also occur. The acute effects of psilocybe intoxication are shorter-lived than LSD, typically lasting 4–6 hours and completely clearing by 12 hours.

Peyote

History and Botany
Peyote *(Lophophora williamsii)* is a small, spineless cactus that grows in the deserts of northern Mexico and the Rio Grande valley (Anderson 1996; Schultes and Hofman 1980) (figure 9.5). It was originally classified as *Anhalonium williamsii,* until reassigned to the *Lophophora* genus. Another related species is *Lophophora diffusa.*

The peyote cactus is prepared for use by cutting the crown and drying it into buttons, which retain potency for a long time. They are then eaten or made into a tea for drinking. Purified mescaline crystals are dissolved and taken orally or injected. Doses vary considerably, ranging from 4 to more than 30 buttons.

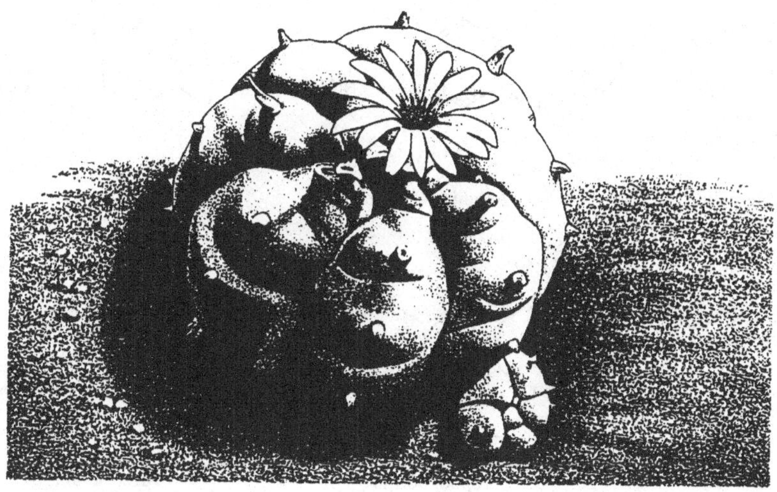

Figure 9.5
Peyote *(Lophophora williamsii)*. Reprinted from Barron et al., "The Hallucinogenic Drugs." *Scientific American.* April 1964, p. 210. Illustration by Alex Semenoick.

The word peyote derives from the Nahuatl word for the cactus, *peyotl.* Religious use of peyote was well established at the time of European arrival. Early European reports date peyote use back at least as far as 300 B.C.E. among the Chichimecas and Toltecs (depending on the accuracy of interpretation of native calendars), but samples found in caves have been carbon dated to 8,000 years ago. The Spanish tried to eradicate the use of peyote, but only succeded in driving its use into secrecy. Peyote use was known in Texas in 1760, but began to spread among tribes by 1880. The Native American Church was founded in 1918 by several groups practicing ceremonial peyote use and currently has over 250,000 members.

Mescal Bean

Due to similarities in their names, the mescal bean is often confused with mescaline (Schultes and Hofman 1980, 1992). These derive from entirely different plants: whereas mescaline derives from peyote cactus, the mescal bean grows on the shrub *Sophora secundiflora.* The mescal bean itself has psychoactive effects, and was used since prehistoric times by Indians in the Rio Grande basin. Samples have been found dating back

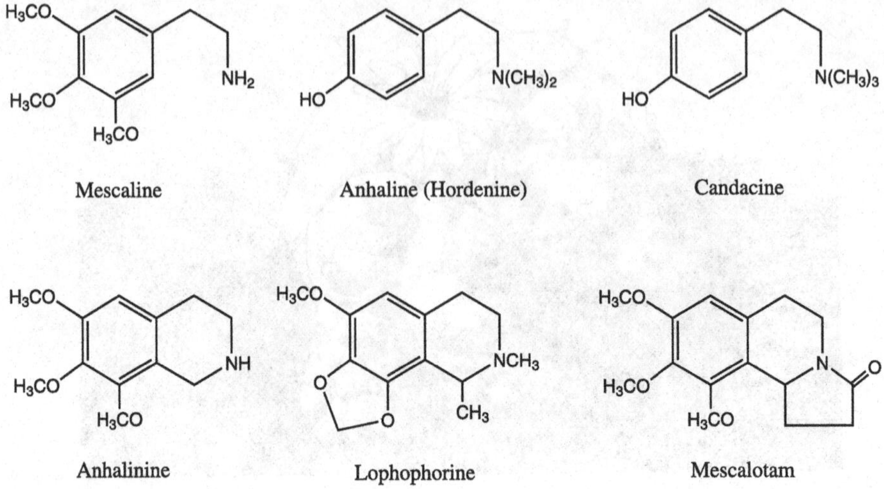

Figure 9.6
Chemical structure of peyote alkaloids.

to 1500 B.C.E. Use by the Arapaho and Iowa tribes in North America is recent, dating back to 1820 C.E. However, with the advent of peyote and formation of the Native American Church, many have abandoned use of the mescal bean. The beans contain the alkaloid cytisine, which has nicotinic cholinergic effects. Although nicotine itself is not hallucinogenic, sufficient doses of mescal will create a hallucinogenic delirium. High doses can cause death by respiratory failure.

Chemical Constituents
More than 55 alkaloids have been isolated from peyote. Mescaline (3,4,5-trimethoxy-β-phenethylamine) is the primary psychoactive alkaloid of the peyote cactus, and by far the one that has been most studied (figure 9.6). These may be categorized into phenethylamines (including mescaline), isoquinolones, and Krebs acid conjugates. See table 9.2 for a partial list of peyote alkaloids.

Pharmacology
It was estimated that the mescaline content of peyote is approximately 3%, and that 1% is available when one chews and swallows the dried

Table 9.2
A partial list of peyote alkaloids

Phenethylamines
N-acetylmescaline
Anhaline (or hordenine)
Candicine
Mescaline (3,4,5-trimethoxy-β-phenethylamine)
N-methylmescaline
Tetrahydroisoquinolones
Anhalamine
Anhalonine
Anhalidine
Anhalotine
Anhalonidine
Lophophorine
Lophotine
Peyophorine
O-methylanhalonidine
Pellotine
Peyotine
Krebs Acid Conjugates
Mescalotam
Peyoglutam
Peyonine
Peyoglunal

Adapted from Anderson 1996; Schultes and Hofman 1980.

buttons. After oral intake of mescaline, peak plasma concentrations occur at 90–120 minutes (Demisch and Neubauer 1979). Mescaline poorly passes the blood-brain barrier because of its low lipid solubility, so high amounts are needed to produce an effect (Ray and Ksir 1990). The half-life of the drug is 6 hours, and psychoactive effects may last for 10 hours. It is not metabolized, but excreted unchanged in urine (Julien 1998).

Mechanisms

Monoamine Mescaline has monoamine mechanisms similar to that of LSD and other monoamine hallucinogens. Mescaline has many neurochemical effects in common with LSD, but with a few differences as well. It binds to 5-HT_2 receptors with high nanomolar affinity (302 nM), and activates phosphoinositide hydrolysis at 5-HT_{2A} receptors (Newton et al. 1996; Titeler et al. 1988). But chronic mescaline use does not alter binding to 5-HT_2 receptors as LSD does (Buckholtz et al. 1990). Mescaline increases the acoustic startle, which is prevented by 5-HT_2 antagonists (Davis 1987). Also similar to LSD, mescaline decreases the spontaneous activity of the locus coeruleus, but increases its activation in response to stimulation (Rasmussen and Aghajanian 1986; Aghajanian 1980). There is evidence that mescaline's effects are mediated by dopaminergic as well as serotonergic mechanisms (Trulson et al. 1983; Ahn and Makman 1979). Drug discrimination studies in rats indicate that mescaline generalizes to LSD and psilocybin (Appel and Callahan 1989).

Unlike LSD, dorsal raphe neurons are insensitive to mescaline, and unlike LSD and psilocybin, mescaline does not down-regulate 5-HT_2 receptors (Penington and Reiffenstein 1986; Buckholz et al. 1990). Mescaline also fails to directly inhibit 5-HT neurons (McCall 1982). Some tolerance develops with repeated administration of mescaline, which also shows cross-tolerance with LSD, but not amphetamine (Colasanti and Khazan 1975).

Acetylcholine Mescaline, in micromolar concentrations, decreases the release of acetylcholine at the neuromuscular junction, with subsequent effects on end-plate potentials and motor function (Ghansah et al. 1993). Whether or not any similar effect occurs on central cholinergic systems has not been investigated.

General Effects

Little is known specifically about the effects of mescaline compared to LSD. Much information about it relies upon its similarities with other monoamine hallucinogens. The majority of attention is given here to mescaline, but some brief mention of the diverse effects of other peyote alkaloids (of which little is known) is deserved. Often, their effects are very different from mescaline. Many alkaloids are present in sufficent concentrations to alter human physiology after oral consumption of peyote. Lophophorine in humans causes a "sickening feeling in the back of the head," a decrease in pulse, and a blushing in the face (Anderson 1996). Anhalodine has CNS stimulant properties. Pellotine has sedative effects, causing drowsiness and reduced motivation for activity, bradycardia, and reduced blood pressure.

Behavioral and motor effects Mescaline and its analogs inhibit cholinergic neuromuscular transmission by blocking release of acetylcholine and reducing end-plate potentials in the micromolar range (Ghansah et al. 1993). This effect has not been investigated in humans, but it could reduce the force of muscle contractions and motor control.

Similar to LSD and other monoamine hallucinogens, mescaline suppresses locomotor and exploratory behavior in novel environments (Wing et al. 1990). Also similar to LSD, tolerance develops to the behavioral effects of chronic doses of mescaline (Murray et al. 1977). Mescaline increases aggression in rat models (Sbordone et al. 1978); however, this is an elicited aggression (by electric shock) and does not necessarily generalize to human behavior. Increased aggression is not characteristic of humans using mescaline.

Neuroendocrine Mescaline increases release of prolactin to levels four times greater than baseline, and also stimulates secretion of growth hormone (Demisch and Neubauer 1979).

Electrophysiology and neuroimaging Similar to LSD, peripheral injections of mescaline produce desynchronization of the EEG and increase arousal in the rat (Colasanti and Khazan 1975). This period lasts for 2–3 hours, and is followed by a period of slow-wave and REM sleep with normal sleep cycles.

A SPECT imaging study of mescaline showed a hyperfrontal pattern in cerebral blood flow, with greater increases on the right side (Hermle et al. 1992). Increases are also seen in inferior temporal cortex and the hippocampus. Decreases in cerebral blood flow occur in occipital and parietal cortical regions.

Subjective effects The subjective effects of equipotent doses of mescaline and LSD are said to be indistinguishable (Schwartz 1988). Behavioral evidence also concurs temporally with the neuropharmacological effects of mescaline. This is supported by drug discrimination paradigms in rats (Appel and Callahan 1989).

Toxicity

There is no clear evidence for genetic toxicity of mescaline. Chromosomal damage in lymphocytes was not evident in Huichol Indians, who have a 1,600-year cultural tradition of religious peyote use (Dorrance et al. 1975).

However, mescaline is teratogenic and has adverse effects when given during pregnancy, with decreased reproductive success evident in hamsters (Hirsch and Fritz 1981). One effect is a delay in ossification of the skull, sternum, and metatarsals. Given the serotonergic mechanisms of mescaline, it may also affect uterine contractions. Mescaline, like any other hallucinogenic drug, is probably best avoided during pregnancy. Its developmental effects are uncertain and the risks far outweigh any potential benefit from religious, psychotherapeutic, or recreational use.

Other Hallucinogenic Cacti

There are other species of cactus with hallucinogenic effects. One is the San Pedro cactus *(Trichocereus pachanoi)*, which grows in the Andes region of Peru, Ecuador, and Bolivia. It is a branched, spineless, and columnar cactus, growing to a height of 9–20 feet. San Pedro is also noteworthy in that it contains mescaline and other related phenethylamines such as 3,4-dimethoxyphenylethylamine and 3-methoxytyramine (Pardanani et al. 1977; Schultes and Hofman 1980, 1992). Mescaline levels in dried samples reach 2%. Use of San Pedro dates back to 1300 B.C.E. in Peru. Similar to other hallucinogenic plants, it has been used in religious ceremonies.

Cawe *(Pachycereus pecten-aboriginum)* is yet another species of hallucinogenic cactus, which grows in Mexico. It is also a columnar cactus, growing up to 35 feet in height. It is known as *Cawe* or *Wichowaka* to the Tarahumara. Studies have identfied 4-hydroxy-3-methoxyphenylethylamine and 4-tetrahydroisoquinoline alkaloids as the probable psychoactive constituents.

Yage

History and Botany

Yage (also known as *yaje, hoasca, ayahuasca, caapi, pinde,* or *natema*) consists of one or more hallucinogenic plants combined, but most importantly *Banisteriopsis caapi* or *B. inebrians* (Schultes and Hofman 1980, 1992) (figure 9.7). Other plants commonly added are *Psychotria viridis, P. carthagenensis,* or *B. rusbyana. Banisteriopsis* are lianas (thick woody vines) with dark ovate leaves and grow in Brazil, Bolivia, Columbia, Ecuador, Peru, and Venezuela. The combination of plants is reported to prolong and intensify the hallucinogenic effects of yage due to pharmacological interactions.

The bark of *Banisteriopsis* is prepared in cold or boiling water. It may also be chewed or administered as a snuff. Liquid preparations are bitter and may induce dizziness, nausea, and vomiting.

Chemical Constituents

Banisteriopsis caapi The primary hallucinogenic constituents of *B. caapi* are the *β*-carbolines. These include harmaline, tetrahydroharmine, harmol, harmic acid methyl ester, harmic amide, acetyl norharmine, harmine *N*-oxide, harmalinic acid, and ketotetrahydronorharmine (figure 9.8). *B. rusbyana* also contains DMT, as well as *N*-methyltryptamine, 5-methoxy-N,*N*-dimethyltryptamine, and 5-hydroxy-N,*N*-dimethyltryptamine (bufotenin). *N*-methyltetrahydro-*β*-carboline is found in trace amounts.

Psychotria viridis and P. carthagenensis *Psychotria* species contain DMT, *N*-methyltryptamine, and *N*-methyltetrahydro-*β*-carboline. However, a more recent study of *P. carthagenensis* showed the plant to be devoid of psychoactive alkaloids (Leal and Elisabetsky 1996).

Mechanisms of Action

There are two major types of hallucinogenic alkaloids in yage. These are DMT and the harmala alkaloids (or *β*-carbolines).

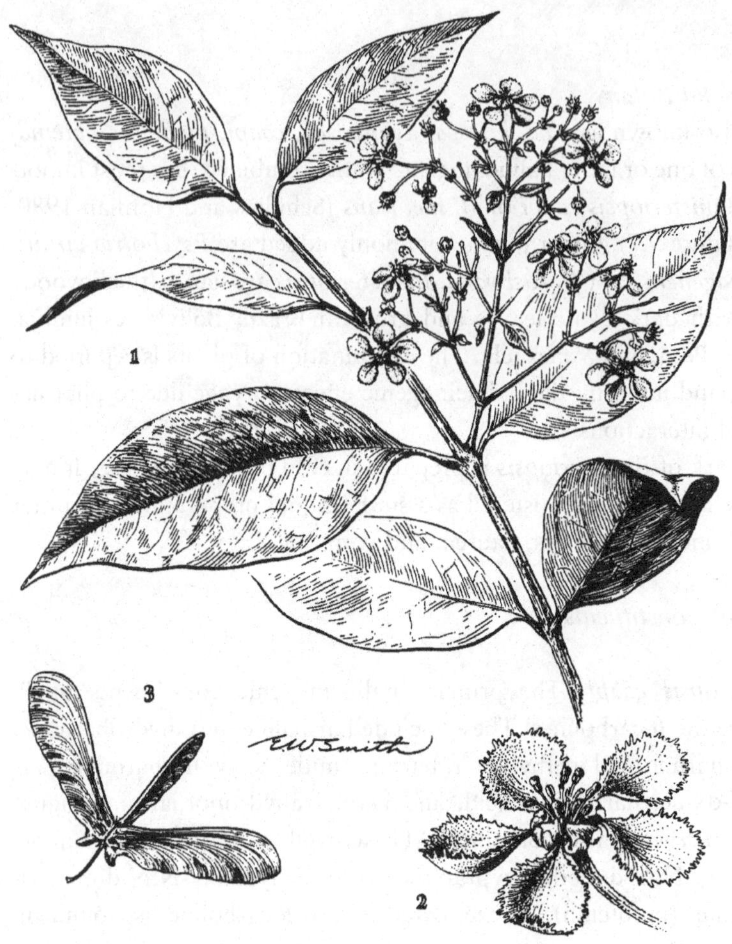

Figure 9.7
Banisteriopsis caapi. Reprinted with permission from Harner, MJ. (1973). The role of hallucinogenic plants in European witchcraft, in *Hallucinogens and Shamanism*. Harner MJ, ed. London: Oxford University Press.

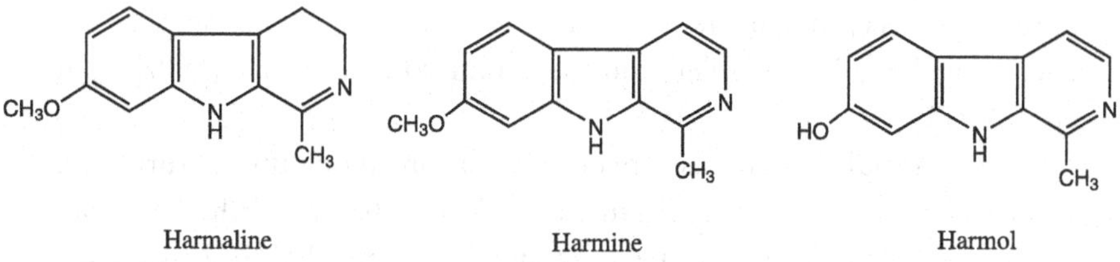

Harmaline Harmine Harmol

Figure 9.8
Chemical structure of banisteriopsis alkaloids.

Dimethyltryptamine DMT acts as an agonist at 5-HT_{2A} and 5-HT_{2C} receptors, stimulating phosphoinositide hydrolysis to a degree comparable to serotonin (Smith et al. 1998). Drug discrimination paradigms similarly show DMT to generalize with the 5-HT_{2A} agonist DOI [1-(2,5-dimethoxy-4-iodophenyl)-2-aminopropane]. In choroid plexus, DMT acts as a partial agonist at 5-HT_{2C} receptors. The 5-HT_{2C} receptor, but not 5-HT_{2A}, shows desensitization with repeated exposure to DMT over time. Because psychoactive effects of DMT are reported to be fairly resistant to tolerance, it suggests that the 5-HT_{2C} may play a minor, if any, role in this effect. Similar to LSD, DMT inhibits firing of raphe neurons (McCall 1982).

DMT behaves as an agonist at 5-HT_{1A} receptors (Deliganis et al. 1991). A 5-HT_{1A} agonist increases the subjective effects of DMT, suggesting a buffering effect of 5-HT_{1A} on the hallucinogenic effects of 5-HT_2 receptors (Strassman 1996). In vivo binding studies of radiolabeled DMT show greatest accumulation in the cerebral cortex, caudate, putamen, and amygdala (Yanai et al. 1986).

β-carboline Mechanisms

Monoamines Harmala alkaloids have direct actions on monoamine receptors. β-carbolines, including norharmane, harmaline, and harmane inhibit binding of tryptamine in the nanomolar range, and 5-HT_1 and 5-HT_2 in the micromolar range (Airaksinen et al. 1987). Some β-carbolines bind to 5-HT_2 receptors with affinity in the high nanomolar range (Grella et al. 1998). Like other classical hallucinogens, β-carbolines probably act as partial agonists at 5-HT_2 receptors (Grella et al. 1998). Actions at α_2

adrenergic receptors by harman and 3-methylharman are implied by effects on the guinea pig ileum in the submicromolar range (Dolzhenko et al. 1983).

Also, harmala alkaloids create effects on monoamine turnover. Postnatal rats administered harmaline (shortly before birth) have elevations in brain levels of the norepinephrine metabolite 3-methoxy-4-hydroxy-phenylglycol (MHPG), but decreases in the dopamine and serotonin metabolites 3,4-dihydroxyphenylacetic acid (DOPAC) and 5-hydroxyindole acetic acid (5-HIAA) (Okonmah et al. 1988). Harmine pretreatment increases brain levels of L-dopa with concurrent increases in striatal dopamine (Meneguz et al. 1994). However, this effect is species-specific, occurring in the rabbit but not in the rat.

Harmala alkaloids are inhibitors of brain MAO. Harmane inhibits MAO_A in the submicromolar range (5×10^{-7} M) and MAO_B in the micromolar range (5×10^{-6} M) (Glover et al. 1982). Harmine inhibits MAO_A, but also has additional unspecified monoamine modulatory effects (Meneguz et al. 1994; Fernández de Arriba et al. 1994). Harmaline or its metabolites may also stimulate aldehyde reductase or catechol O-methyltransferase (COMT) (Okonmah et al. 1988).

Excitatory amino acids Harmaline competitively displaces MK-801 binding in the micromolar range, suggesting that it binds to the channel site of the NMDA receptor-channel (Du et al. 1997). However, unlike MK-801 or PCP, which block the channel, it has been proposed that harmaline acts as an inverse agonist at this site, opening the cation channel and increasing Ca^{2+} flux. The effects of harmaline at NMDA receptors is blocked by MK-801 (Du and Harvey 1997).

$GABA_A$ benzodiazepine β-carbolines act as inverse agonists of the $GABA_A$ benzodiazepine receptor (Mehta and Ticku 1989). Whereas benzodiazepines such as diazepam stimulate Cl^- influx, β-carbolines inhibit it. Harmine, harmaline, harmane, and harmalol inhibit flunitrazepam binding in the micromolar range (half-maximal inhibition between 28 and 130 µM) (Mousah et al. 1986).

Endogenous β-carbolines, such as harmane, have also been found in the human brain, but their endogenous functions are uncertain (Tse et al.

1991; Rommelspacher et al. 1980). Harmaline tremor is reversed by the benzodiazepine agonist diazepam (Valium) (Robertson 1980).

Pharmacology

Ingestion of yage in healthy volunteers yields plasma concentrations of 10 to 250 ng/mL for harmine and 1.0 to 25.0 ng/mL of harmaline (Callaway et al. 1996). The dose-concentration relationships are linear in this range. DMT shows linear dose-concentration relationships for plasma concentrations between 5 and 1000 ng/mL. Systemically administered β-carbolines penetrate brain tissue, with relatively even distribution (Moncrieff 1989). DMT taken alone is not absorbed well orally. It may be taken as a snuff or smoked, or mixed with other plants to improve absorption.

Harmine and harmol are metabolized by three liver microsomes to 6-hydroxy-7-methoxyharman and 3- or 4-hydroxy-7-methoxyharman, which are further metabolized to unidentified metabolites (Tweedy and Burke 1987). Protein binding of harmine and harmol occurs, and is dependent on metabolism alkalinity.

Unlike most hallucinogens, tolerance to subjective effects is not observed with DMT, even over several closely spaced doses (Strassman 1996). In contrast, tolerance was evident to hormonal and heart-rate responses.

General Effects

Autonomic effects Harmala alkaloids, as well as isolated harmine and harmaline, produce a dose-dependent hypothermia (Abdel-Fattah et al. 1995). This effect is serotonin-dependent, and partly mediated by 5-HT_{1A} receptors.

On the other hand, DMT produces a dose-dependent hyperthermia (Strassman and Qualls 1994). Although statistically significant, these effects are small. DMT produces mydriasis, which is probably mediated by 5-HT_2 receptors.

Neuroendocrine effects DMT causes a transient increase in release of several hormones. In humans intravenously administered DMT (0.4 mg/kg), increases are seen in β-endorphin, corticotrophin, prolactin, cortisol, and growth hormone, but not melatonin (Strassman and Qualls 1994).

Cardiovascular effects Harmala alkaloids have cardiovascular effects (Aarons et al. 1977). Harmine, harmaline, and harmalol decrease heart rate, but increase pulse pressure, peak aortic flow, and myocardial contractile force in dogs. Harmine reduces systemic arterial blood pressure and peripheral vascular resistance. Vascular resistance effects are not mediated by β-adrenergic or histamine H_1 receptors.

DMT elevates pulse rate and blood pressure. In one study, heart rate elevated from around 70 beats per minute at baseline to 100 beats per minute at the highest dose (0.4 mg/kg, IV).

Neurophysiological effects Harmane produces excitation in the nucleus accumbens in nanomolar concentrations, but depression in micromolar concentrations (Ergene and Schoener 1993). Harmine and *B. caapi* extract decrease the acoustic startle, which is reversed to some degree by DMT (Freedland and Mansbach 1999). β-carbolines may have antioxidant effects through inhibiting oxidative enzymes in the microsomal system (Tse et al. 1991).

Motor effects Harmaline produces a motor tremor (8–14 Hz) through activation of cells in the inferior olive, which is blocked by noncompetitive NMDA antagonists (Du et al. 1997; Stanford and Fowler 1998). Harmaline tremor is also reversed by benzodiazepine agonists (Robertson 1980). The tremor is initiated by synchronous rhythms in the olivocerebellar system and red nucleus (Lorden et al. 1988; Gogolák et al. 1977; Batini et al. 1980). The tremor is associated with increased cGMP in the cerebellum, and tolerance with a relative normalization of cGMP (Lutes et al. 1988). Rapid tolerance develops to this effect with repeated doses.

Subjective effects The subjective effects of DMT are very much like those of the other monoamine hallucinogens. Animal drug discrimination paradigms indicate that DMT and related compounds produce similar effects to LSD (Helsley et al. 1998). However, β-carbolines do not substitute well for LSD in these paradigms. Maximal substitution occurs with harmane only at intermediate levels. Some have reported that unlike other hallucinogens, ecstatic feelings are not experienced with yage. Amazonian Indians ingesting yage often report seeing snakes and jaguars, likely due to their prominent role in that culture.

One feature that distinguishes DMT is the short duration of effect (Strassman et al. 1994). The onset of effect is very rapid, partially due to administration method, and subsides completely in 30 minutes. With intravenous doses, subjects commonly report a "rush," where the rapid onset of effects is acutely experienced. In some, this creates feelings of anxiety and being overwhelmed. Intravenous doses of DMT at 0.2 mg/kg was a threshold for halluinogenic effects, while 0.05 mg/kg was often not discriminated from placebo.

β-carbolines have anxiogenic effects, likely through inverse agonism of the $GABA_A$ benzodiazepine receptor (File et al. 1982). However, prominent anxiety has not been noted with yage in comparison to other monoamine hallucinogens. It is possible that the effects of harmala alkaloids are not sufficient to produce this effect, or that they may be offset by other pharmacological mechanisms.

Toxicity

Harmala alkaloids are potent inhibitors of monoamine oxidase (Callaway and Grob 1998). Thus, if combined with other antidepressants, such as selective serotonin reuptake inhibitors, there is potential for serious side effects. Harmaline or its metabolites also cross the placental barrier (Okonmah et al. 1988).

Harmaline has also been found to have neurotoxic effects on Purkinje neurons (O'Hearn and Molliver 1997). This likely results from excitotoxic consequences induced by prolonged stimulation of inferior olivary neurons. Whether this occurs in levels reached during human consumption has not been specifically addressed. Prolonged neurological symptoms have not been reported in those who consume the drug.

Morning Glory and Related Species

History and Botany

There are several species of flowering vines with hallucinogenic properties, commonly referred to as morning glory (Schultes and Hofman

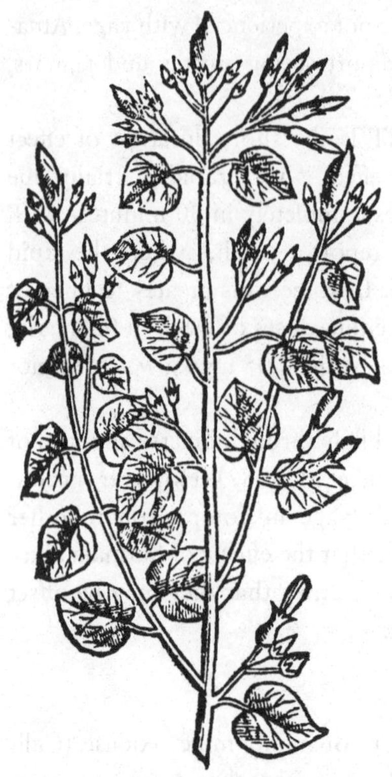

Figure 9.9
Ololiuqui *(Turbina corymbosa).* Reprinted with permission from Schultes RE, Hofman A. (1980). *The Botany and Chemistry of Hallucinogens*, 2nd ed. Springfield, Ill.: Charles C. Thomas Publishers.

1980, 1992; Shawcross 1983). Perhaps the most popular is ololiuqui *(Turbina corymbosa*, formerly *Rivea corymbosa).* It is a large vine with heart-shaped, green leaves and multiple bell-shaped flowers (figure 9.9). *Ololiuqui* is the Nahuatl word for the seed, literally meaning "round object." Its hallucinogenic effects were known to the Aztecs, who used it in religious ceremonies. Another related species is known as badoh negro *(Ipomoea violacea)* among the Zapotec, and among the Aztec as *tlililtzin.* Several varieties of this plant are commonly known as "heavenly blue," "pearly gates," and "flying saucers." The Hawaiian Baby Woodrose *(Argyreia nervosa)* is another related species that appears to have the highest concentration of hallucinogenic chemicals among these species.

Chemical Constituents

The identified psychoactive constituents of the morning glories are lysergic acid alkaloids, similar to those isolated from ergot. These include *d*-lysergic acid amide (or ergine), lysergol, lysergic acid hydroxyethylamide, and *d*-isolysergic acid amide. As the names imply, lysergic acid amide and lysergic acid diethylamide (LSD) only differ by the replacement of two hydrogen atoms with ethyl groups. As a result, LSD is about 100 times more potent.

Mechanisms and Effects

Based on structural similarities, the neuropharmacological mechanisms of morning glory alkaloids are likely similar or identical to those of LSD. The subjective effects are also similar, but the lower potency of the alkaloids requires larger doses for hallucinogenic effects. Somatic effects tend to be pronounced, with nausea and gastrointestinal symptoms being very common.

Nutmeg and Mace

Nutmeg and mace are spices derived from the tree *Myristica fragrans* (Schultes and Hofman 1980, 1992; Julien 1998). It is an evergreen tree, growing up to 15 meters in height, bearing flowers and a fleshy, round fruit (Gruenwald et al. 1998) (figure 9.10). Other species of the *Myristica* genus also yield nutmeg and mace, including *M. malabarica*. *Myristica fragrans* was native to the Molucca islands, but is now cultivated throughout tropical regions (Robbers et al. 1996). Islands of the Malay archipelago are the primary source. Their use in Europe began when it was introduced by Arabs in the first century C.E. However, their use was well known in ancient Egypt and India, where nutmeg is sometimes snuffed together with tobacco.

Nutmeg is prepared from the seed of the tree, while mace is prepared from the fleshy covering that surrounds it. Differing composition of the

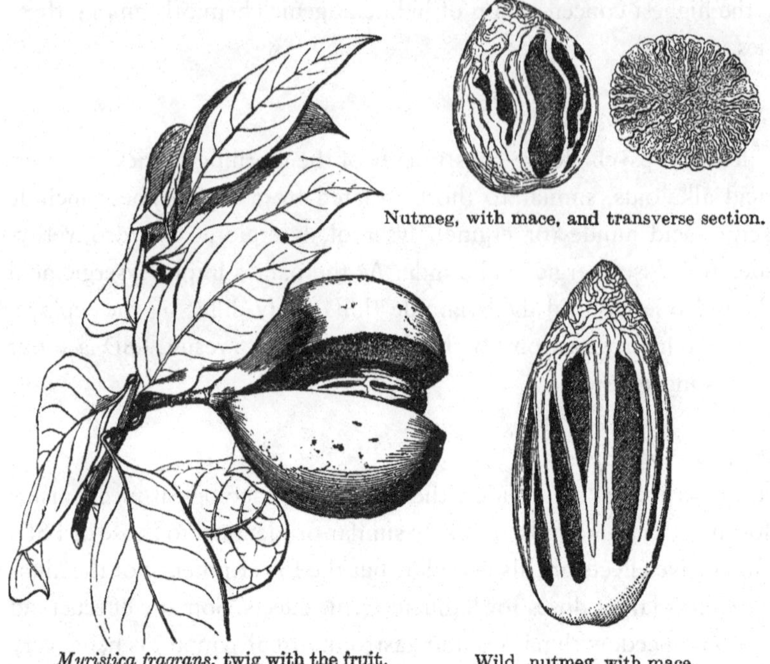

Figure 9.10
Nutmeg and mace *(Myristica fragrans)*. Reprinted from Culbreth DMR. (1927). *Materia Medica and Pharmacognosy*, 7th ed. Philadelphia: Lea & Febiger.

essential oils gives the two spices different tastes. The psychoactive chemicals in nutmeg and mace are the terpenoids *myristicin* and *elemicin*. Structurally, these bear resemblance to amphetamine and phenethylamine hallucinogens such as mescaline (figure 9.11).

A large amount of spice must be consumed (~15 g) to produce psychoactive effects. Somatic effects are prominent, and include tachycardia, dry mouth, and flushing of the skin. Subjective effects begin after 2–5 hours, and may involve euphoria, visual hallucinations, anxiety, depersonalization, and derealization. A hangover-like feeling is also reported to occur after the intoxication. Nutmeg and mace are reputed to be used recreationally in places where other psychoactive drugs are (supposedly) harder to obtain (e.g., prisons). However, the side effects are often aversive enough to usually discourage use.

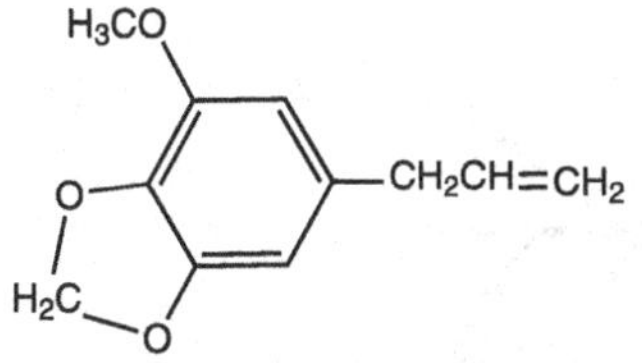

Myristicin

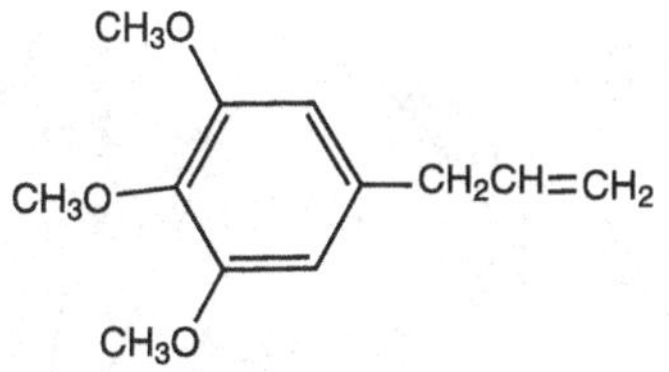

Elemicin

Figure 9.11
Chemical structure of myristicin and elemicin.

Iboga

History and Botany

Iboga *(Tabernanthe iboga)* is a shrub native to west-central Africa, and used in cultures of the Gabon and Congo (Schultes and Hofman 1980, 1992). It grows to a height of 4–6 feet in the undergrowth of tropical forests, but has also been cultivated. Its leaves are ovate, 3–4.5 inches in length and 1.25 inches wide, with a green color on top and yellowish-green underneath. Tiny flowers grow in groups of 5–12 with whitish, yellowish, or pinkish color. Its fruits are yellow-orange in color, ovoid, and grow as large as olives (figure 9.12).

The plant is used in elaborate religious ceremonies, which vary from area to area. Adherents use the plant to communicate spiritually with their ancestors. In lower doses, it is used to counteract fatigue and hunger. Warriors and hunters have used it to remain awake at night. Some Europeans have claimed that it has aphrodisiac effects as well. More recently, anecdotal reports have indicated possible antiaddictive effects of iboga, stimulating a rush of scientific research into the neurochemical effects of the plant (Mash et al. 1998).

Chemical Constituents

Several indole alkaloids have been isolated from the iboga plant, but the principal psychoactive agent is ibogaine. However, other alkaloids have physiological effects, and may also have psychoactive effects (figure 9.13). These include ibogamine, coronaridine, and tabernanthine. Some research has also focused on the effects of noribogaine (12-hydroxy-

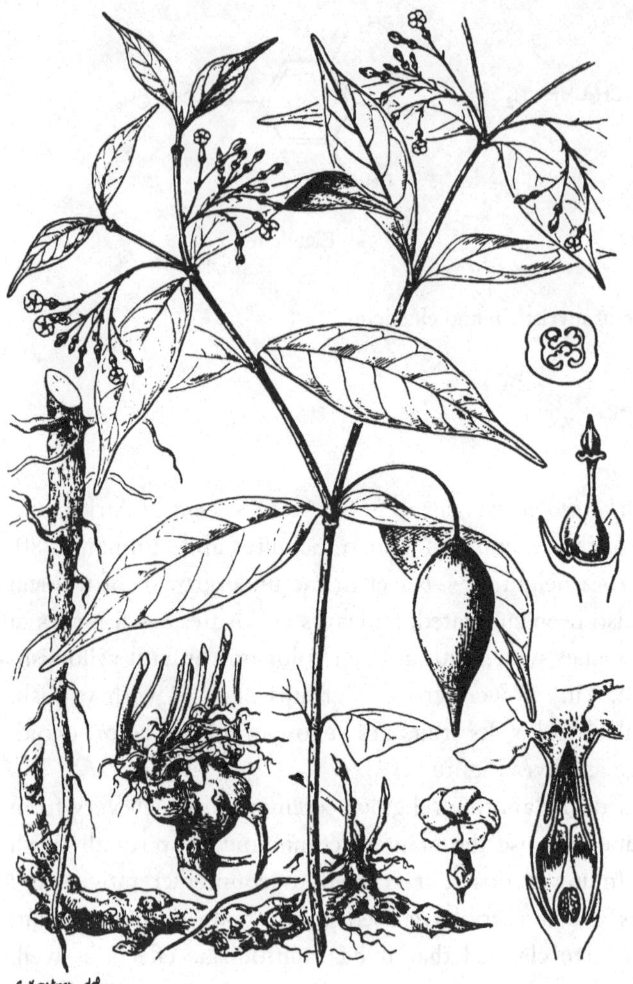

Figure 9.12
Iboga *(Tabernanthe iboga)*. Reprinted with permission from Schultes RE, Hofman A. (1992). *Plants of the Gods: Their Sacred, Healing, and Hallucinogenic Powers*. Rochester, VT: Healing Arts Press.

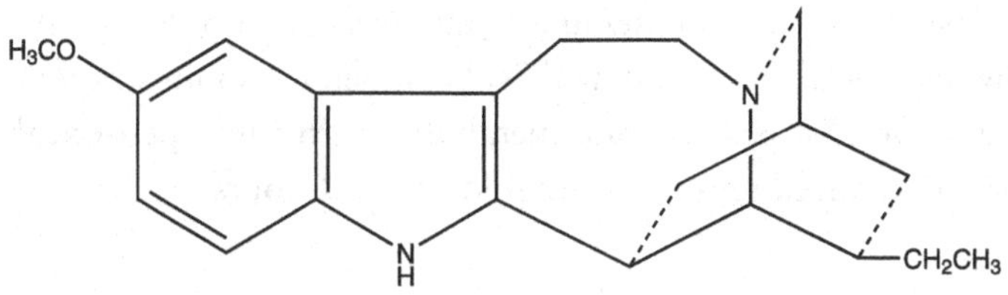

Figure 9.13
Chemical structure of ibogaine.

ibogamine), a metabolite of ibogaine. A congener of coronaridine has been synthesized, 18-methoxycoronaridine (18-MC), which may have a better clinical profile. For example, it is anticipated that 18-MC may not have hallucinogenic effects (Wei et al. 1998).

Pharmacology

The pharmacokinetics of ibogaine have not been fully elucidated (Popik and Glick 1996). Its absorption, distribution, metabolism, and excretion are not fully clear. The route of administration notably affects ibogaine's efficacy, with greater effects subcutaneously than intraperitoneally (Pearl et al. 1997). The half-life of ibogaine is approximately 1 hour in rodents, and it is not detectable in the brain after 12 hours, although the assays used may have lacked sensitivity (Dhahir 1971; Zetler et al. 1972; Popik and Glick 1996).

Ibogaine undergoes first pass metabolism and is O-demethylated to the primary metabolite 12-hydroxy-ibogamine, (O-demethylibogaine or noribogaine) (Mash et al. 1995). This transformation is accomplished by hepatic microsomal enzyme cytochrome $P\text{-}450_{2D6}$ (Obach et al. 1998). After several hours, brain and plasma levels of ibogaine and noribogaine are greater in female animals than male, even when both receive the same proportional dose (Pearl et al. 1997). These are likely to reflect sex differences in the bioavailability of ibogaine. Approximately 4–5% of ibogaine is excreted in urine unchanged (Dhahir 1971).

Long-term effects of ibogaine may be due, in part, to its slow release from fat tissue and conversion to noribogaine (Glick and Maisonneuve 1998). A significant accumulation of ibogaine occurs in adipose tissue (Hough et al. 1996). One hour after an intraperitoneal dose (40 mg/kg) of ibogaine, plasma levels of 106 ng/ml and fat levels of 11,308 ng/g are obtained. Higher levels are found with subcutaneous administration, suggesting extensive first-pass hepatic metabolism after intraperitoneal dosing. Levels are reduced ten- to twentyfold after 12 hours.

Mechanisms of Action

Acetylcholine Ibogaine functionally blocks nicotinic acetylcholine receptors in the low to intermediate micromolar range (Fryer and Lukas 1999). Ibogaine also blocks ion flux through ganglionic nicotinic channels in the nanomolar range (20 nM) (Badio et al. 1997). However, it was much weaker at neuromuscular nicotinic receptors, with half-maximal inhibition in the micromolar range (2 µM). Ibogaine inhibits the nicotine-mediated release of catecholamines at concentrations below 10 µM (Mah et al. 1998; Maisonneuve et al. 1997; Schneider et al. 1996).

Although ibogaine binds to muscarinic M_1 and M_2 receptors in the micromolar range, its action there is uncertain (Sweetnam et al. 1995). It fails to alter the adenylyl cyclase activity of a muscarinic agonist carbachol (Rabin and Winter 1996b).

Monoamine Ibogaine blocks uptake of both dopamine and serotonin, with half-maximal effects in the low- to mid-micromolar range (Wells et al. 1999). Noribogaine also blocks reuptake of serotonin in vivo (Wei et al. 1998). Both ibogaine and its metabolite noribogaine bind to the cocaine site of the serotonin transporter (Staley et al. 1996; Mash et al. 1995). However, ibogaine prevents cocaine-induced increases in serotonin levels in the brain (Sershen et al. 1997). Ibogaine also reduces release of dopamine induced by nicotine, cocaine, and morphine (Benwell et al. 1996; Sershen et al. 1997; Glick and Maisonneuve 1998). It causes a release of cytoplasmic dopamine in the striatum, which is reversed by dopamine uptake inhibitors (e.g., cocaine) (Harsing et al. 1994). However, the effects of ibogaine on dopamine release outlast the elimination time of the drug (Maisonneuve et al. 1991). The effects of a single dose of ibogaine on dopamine levels last up to a week, but are not seen at one month after injection (Maisonneuve et al. 1992).

The effects of ibogaine on monoamine turnover are complex. Acute intravenous ibogaine causes a short-lasting excitement of dopaminergic neurons in the ventral tegmental nucleus, but pretreatment fails to alter basal activity or activity stimulated by morphine and cocaine (French et al. 1996). It causes dramatic reductions in dopamine levels and increases in the metabolites DOPAC and HVA (Baumann et al. 1998; Binienda et al. 1998). These effects occur in the striatum and frontal cortex as soon as 30 minutes after intraperitoneal administration (Ali et al. 1996). It has been suggested that ibogaine's inhibitory effects on dopamine release in the accumbens and striatum are mediated by κ opioid receptors (Reid et al. 1996). It also blocks serotonin-induced release of dopamine in the striatum, which may be mediated by the 5-HT_{1B} receptor (Sershen et al. 1994a). Tabernanthine, as well, increases synthesis and elimination of catecholamines in many areas of the brain, but not the hypothalamus (Prioux-Guyonneau et al. 1984).

Ibogaine may release and block reuptake of serotonin (Wei et al. 1998). Reports exist of both increases and decreases of serotonin levels in frontal cortex (Ali et al. 1996; Binienda et al. 1998). However, increases in 5-HIAA occur in frontal cortex and decreases occur in the striatum and nucleus accumbens (Ali et al. 1996; Benwell et al. 1996). Like many other monoamine hallucinogens, ibogaine has affinity for 5-HT_{2A} receptors in the high micromolar range (92.5 μM) (Helsley et al. 1998). Animal drug discrimination studies support ibogaine agonist activity at 5-HT_{2A} and 5-HT_{2C} receptors, but not 5-HT_{1A} or 5-HT_3 antagonists (Helsley et al. 1998a, 1998b). Ibogaine and noribogaine increase the inhibition of adenylyl cyclase by morphine and serotonin, but do not alter basal levels (Rabin and Winter 1996b).

Amino acids Ibogaine is a competitive inhibitor of the NMDA receptor. It binds to the MK-801 receptor site within the NMDA channel in the submicromolar range, but not to the NMDA receptor itself (Itzhak and Ali 1998). Ibogaine's antagonism of the NMDA channel is also voltage-dependent (Popik et al. 1995; Chen et al. 1996). Noribogaine also has antagonistic effects at the MK-801 site, with potency 4–6 times greater than ibogaine (Mash et al. 1995; Ali et al. 1996). In contrast, ibogaine fails to affect kainate or GABA currents.

The NMDA antagonist effects of ibogaine are significant in light of the fact that MK-801 also reduces tolerance to opiates and alcohol, and reverses tolerance to stimulants (Trujillo and Akil 1991; Khanna et al. 1993; Karler et al. 1989).

Neurotensin Ibogaine treatment increases levels of neurotensin in the striatum, substantia nigra, and nucleus accumbens, but not frontal cortex (Alburges and Hanson 1999). This effect occurs 12 hours after administration and is blocked by a dopamine antagonist. Iboga also blocked release of neurotensin by cocaine. Neurotensin colocalizes with dopamine in neurons of the ventral tegmental area, and is altered by abused drugs (Cooper et al. 1996; Pilotte et al. 1991; Morley et al. 1980).

Opioids Iboga alkaloids have several effects at opioid receptors. Ibogaine has low micromolar affinity for κ opioid receptors (~3 μM), less for μ receptors (~11 μM), and no specific affinity for δ receptors (>100 μM) (Pearl et al. 1995). Noribogaine has even higher affinity for all three opioid receptors assayed: κ (~0.96 μM), μ (~2.66 μM), and δ (~24 μM). Thus, noribogaine may play a greater role than ibogaine in opioid actions. Others have found affinity for the μ opioid receptor to be in the nanomolar range (130 nM) (Codd 1995). Noribogaine is a full agonist at μ opioid receptors, stimulating G-protein activity at submicromolar concentrations (Pablo and Mash 1998). It also reduces tolerance to chronic morphine in mice (Bhargava and Cao 1997). Other iboga alkaloids have micromolar affinity for the μ receptor (coronaridine), δ receptor (coronaridine and tabernanthine), and κ receptor (ibogamine, coronaridine, and tabernanthine) (Deecher et al. 1992).

Both ibogaine and noribogaine enhance morphine analgesia in morphine-tolerant, but not morphine-naive rats (Sunder Sharma et al. 1998; Bhargava and Cao 1997). However, ibogaine does not alter tolerance to κ or δ opioid agonists (Cao and Bhargava 1997). Noribogaine does have affinity for the κ_1 opioid receptor (Ali et al. 1996).

Sigma receptors Ibogaine binds to both σ_1 and σ_2 receptors, with affinities in the range of 1.5–3 μM (Itzhak and Ali 1998). Some have reported that affinity is higher for σ_2 receptors (201 nM) than σ_1 receptors (8 μM) (Bowen et al. 1995). Activity at σ_2 receptors is believed to partly mediate ibogaine's neurotoxicity (Glick and Maisonneuve 1998).

Ion channels Ibogaine and other iboga alkaloids have micromolar affinity for voltage gated Na^+ channels (Deecher et al. 1992). Tabernanthine is also a Ca^{2+} channel blocker, producing half-maximal inhibition in the micromolar range (7–21 μM) (Miller and Godfraind 1983).

Intracellular messengers Noribogaine, but not ibogaine, stimulates phosphoinositide hydrolysis (Rabin and Winter 1996a). This effect was unaltered by tetrodotoxin or ω-conotoxin, indicating that it is not secondary to release of other neurotransmitters.

Physiological Effects

Cardiovascular A moderate rise (10–15%) in blood pressure occurs after administration of ibogaine, peaking at 1.5 to 2 hours and lasting up to 5 hours (Lotsoff 1995). On the other hand, tabernanthine alone produces bradycardia and hypotension, which is independent of autonomic innervation and muscarinic receptors (Hajo et al. 1981). In micromolar concentrations, it antagonizes arterial contractions induced by norepinephine and Ca^{2+} in the rat (Hajo-Tello et al. 1985). It also has a negative inotropic effect in heart muscle. The mechanisms of tabernanthine's cardiovascular effects are seemingly complex, but involve stimulation of vascular β_2 adrenergic receptors and cellular Ca^{2+} homeostasis (Miller and Godfraind 1983).

Neuroendocrine Preliminary research has been done on the hormonal effects of iboga. The findings consist of elevated levels of corticosterone and prolactin by ibogaine in rats (Baumann et al. 1998; Ali et al. 1996).

Behavioral and cognitive effects As might be expected, ibogaine has powerful sensory and motor effects. Rats administered ibogaine (20–60 mg/kg) show slower response times on sensory and sensory-motor tests (Kesner et al. 1995). Motor reflexes are impaired at 40–60 mg/kg, and there is an overall reduction in activity and emotionality. Ibogaine induces a tremor and ataxia (O'Hearn and Molliver 1997). Tabernanthine also induces tremor, which is mediated by $GABA_A$ benzodiazepine receptors (Trouvn et al. 1987).

Ibogaine itself stimulates locomotor activity in rats. However, it reduces the locomotor activity induced by morphine, with greater effects in female animals than males (Pearl et al. 1997). It also reduces locomotor activity induced by cocaine and amphetamine (Sershen et al. 1992a, 1992b; Blackburn and Szumlinski 1997). However, the interaction between ibogaine and cocaine is time-dependent, with motor activity inhibited at short delays, but potentiated at long delays (Maisonneuve et al. 1997).

Ibogaine has not shown any adverse effects on learning or memory retrieval in animals performing a maze task (Helsley et al. 1997a). In fact, pretreatment with ibogaine or O-demethylibogaine, but not t-butyl ibogaine, improves memory retrieval in the Morris water maze task (Popik 1996).

Electrophysiology Little work has been done to characterize the electrophysiological effects of iboga. Rats administered ibogaine showed decreases in power in delta, theta, alpha, and beta frequencies during the first 30 minutes (Binienda et al. 1998). However, this recovered after 15 minutes. Tabernanthine derivatives produce electrophysiological activation, increase wakefulness, reduce slow-wave activity, and block REM sleep in animals (Da Costa et al. 1980).

Subjective effects Ibogaine has psychoactive effects at doses of 200–300 mg and above (Sheppard 1994). Despite its short half-life, the effects of ibogaine are long lasting, typically in the range of 24–36 hours. Use of the plant is also associated with behavioral and motor effects. At certain doses and periods of the intoxication, people experience stimulation, whereas at other doses the subject typically stares into space and eventually collapses into a catatonic-like state. In African cultures, it is believed that the person's soul has left the body during this time and entered into the spirit world. Feelings of bodily levitation or floating have also been reported. A rainbowlike aura is seen around objects.

Time perception is altered, where short periods may seem extremely long. Users also report depersonalization or a sense of detachment, as if externally observing one's own actions. Another feature of ibogaine intoxication seems to be a panoramic recall of events from long-term memory, primarily in visual memory. The ability of iboga to allow one to commune with ancestors is most likely not a pharmacological property of the drug, but rather a result of set and setting influenced by culture.

Given ibogaine's monoamine and indole actions (particularly actions at 5-HT_2 receptors), it is likely that it produces hallucinations in a manner similar to those produced by other monoamine hallucinogens. However, the additional actions of iboga on other neurochemical systems, such as NMDA, may also modulate the quality of the hallucinogenic experience. Animal drug discrimination paradigms indicate generalization between LSD and ibogaine (Palumbo and Winter 1992). Intermediate degrees of generalization occur between ibogaine and noribogaine in animal drug discrimination tests (Helsley et al. 1997b, 1998b). However, almost complete (83.5%) generalization occurs between ibogaine and harmaline. Ibogaine generalizes to noribogaine in animal stimulus discrimination paradigms, but not to the NMDA antagonist MK-801 or κ opioid agonist U50,488 (Zubaran et al. 1999).

Antiaddictive Effects

The putative antiaddictive effects of ibogaine come from its reputed ability to reduce or eliminate withdrawal syndromes and cravings for long periods of time (Mash et al. 1998). Although these derived from anecdotal reports and were discovered serendipitously in humans, they have been supported by empirical research.

Several lines of research in animals support this contention. Ibogaine reduces cocaine intake in mice, which sustains for longer periods by repeated administration (Cappendijk and Dzoljic 1993; Sershen et al. 1994b). It also suppresses withdrawal symptoms in morphine-dependent rats precipitated by naltrexone, independent of tremor effects (Glick et al. 1992b). However, a reduction of opioid withdrawal symptoms is not evident in mice (Frances et al. 1992). While ibogaine pretreatment reduces acquisition of place preference with drugs of abuse such as morphine and amphetamine, it does not abolish previously established place preferences (Luxton et al. 1996; Moroz et al. 1997). Ibogaine binds to nicotinic receptors in the nanomolar range (IC_{50} 20 nM)(Badio et al. 1997; Glick and Maisonneuve 1998). It has been reported to curtail smoking and have antinicotinic effects, and may do so by reducing the dopaminergic response to nicotine (Maisonneuve et al. 1997).

Possible neurochemical mechanisms The interactions of ibogaine with various drugs of abuse may be mediated by different receptors, or combinations of receptors (Glick and Maisonneuve 1998). Combined treatment with a κ opioid antagonist and NMDA agonist partially block the effects of ibogaine, suggesting a role for these two receptors in ibogaine's antiaddictive effects (Glick et al. 1997). Ibogaine's effect on morphine dependence is related to it's NMDA antagonist activity (Layer et al. 1996). Effects on morphine-induced dopamine release may be dependent on prior exposure (Pearl et al. 1996). Serotonergic and dopaminergic actions of ibogaine also mediate its antiaddictive actions (Sershen et al. 1997). In particular, serotonergic actions may be more important for ibogaine's reduction of alcohol intake (Glick and Maisonneuve 1998). Similar to ibogaine, noribogaine decreases morphine and cocaine self-administration, the locomotor stimulant effect of morphine, and extracellular dopamine in the accumbens and striatum (Glick et al. 1996b).

Some, but not all of ibogaine's effects may involve pharmacokinetic actions. Although ibogaine does not alter brain morphine or alcohol levels, it does alter amphetamine levels, suggesting a possible hepatic interaction (Glick et al. 1992a; Rezvani et al. 1995).

Alternative iboga alkaloids Potential neurotoxic effects of ibogaine have raised concern over its clinical use. It is possible that the antiaddictive and neurotoxic actions of ibogaine are discrete, allowing for potential separation of clinical and toxic effects (Molinari et al. 1996). Some other iboga alkaloids may have these properties, such as 18-MC.

18-MC is a synthetic iboga alkaloid that may retain ibogaine's antiaddictive effects, but lack the effects of neurotoxicity and tremor (Glick et al. 1996). Acute administration of 18-MC decreases self-administration of morphine and cocaine in rats, for a period of days to weeks (Glick et al. 1996a). It also reduces alcohol consumption and preference in rats (Rezvani et al. 1997). On the other hand, 18-MC does not show any cerebellar toxicity, even after high doses (100 mg/kg) (Glick et al. 1996). 18-MC also has similar actions to ibogaine in reducing morphine withdrawal (Rho and Glick et al. 1998). Similar to ibogaine, it reduces nicotine-induced release of dopamine (Glick et al. 1998).

Other iboga alkaloids besides ibogaine (tabernanthine, R- and S-coronaridine, R- and S-ibogamine, and desethylcoronaridine) decrease morphine and cocaine intake in animals shortly after administration, and in some cases one day after administration (Glick et al. 1994). R-ibogamine was the most consistent in this effect, reducing intake for several days after a single injection.

Studies in humans An open trial of ibogaine was carried out in seven subjects with opioid dependence, who were administered 700–1800 mg. After a prolonged hallucinatory period (24–38 hours), none of the subjects showed significant withdrawal symptoms. However, one who had taken the lowest dose resumed opioid use in two days. Of the subjects taking 1000 mg or greater, half relapsed and half remained abstinent for at least 14 weeks (Sheppard 1994). There are other case studies in humans in the medical literature (Cantor 1990; Luciano 1998; Sisko 1993; Kovera et al. 1998; Mash et al. 1998). Commonly reported phenomena are reductions in drug craving and opiate withdrawal symptoms within 1 to 2 hours, followed by a total resolution of the withdrawal syndrome within 24 hours. A review of cases indicates a 10% success rate at two years following a single treatment (Lotsoff 1995).

In 1996, the National Institute of Drug abuse discontinued clinical trials of ibogaine. Research is currently undertaken by researchers outside of the United States. Far more empirical research is needed to establish the antiaddictive effects of ibogaine. The neuropharmacological mechanisms support possible antiaddictive effects, and results of case studies suggest further investigation. If successful, it would still be necessary to complement it with psychosocial support and counseling, as with other addiction therapies.

Toxicity

Ibogaine has demonstrated toxic effects, which could potentially limit its usefulness in treating addiction. However, the proper dosage of alternative iboga alkaloids may avert this problem. The median lethal dose of ibogaine is 82 mg/kg in the guinea pig and 327 mg/kg in the rat (Dhahir 1971; Delourme-Houde 1946). Use of ibogaine for addiction treatment has been associated with two deaths overseas.

Neurotoxicity In sufficient concentrations, ibogaine produces cerebellar neurotoxicity in rats, characterized by degeneration of Purkinje cells in the vermis, intermediate, and lateral cerebellum (Molinari et al. 1996; O'Hearn and Molliver 1997). Ibogaine's cerebellar toxicity is likely due to excitation of neurons in the inferior olive, causing release of glutamate from climbing fibers apposed to Purkinje cells. Congruently, ablation of the inferior olive prevents this toxicity. Ibogaine neurotoxicity is accompanied by a late induction of neuronal nitric oxide synthase adjacent to Purkinje cells, which is likely to contribute to the excitotoxic cascade (O'Hearn et al. 1995). Acute high doses of ibogaine are also accompanied by reactive gliosis in the vermis, hippocampus, olfactory bulbs, brain stem, and striatum (O'Callaghan et al. 1996).

One caveat to the neurotoxic effect of ibogaine is that the effect is dose-dependent (Molinari et al. 1996). Ibogaine does not show neurotoxic effects at doses that produce clinically related effects in rats (40 mg/kg IP).

Monoamine Hallucinogens: Collective Issues

Therapeutic Uses

Some have used hallucinogenic drugs to facilitate the psychotherapy process, soon after the discovery of LSD in 1949 (Abraham et al. 1996; Grinspoon and Bakalar 1986). This has sometimes been referred to as *psycholytic therapy*. However, the Drug Abuse Control amendments to the Harrison Narcotics Act in 1965 restricted such use. Studies at that time used widely varying methodology, but a meta-analysis incorporating over 1600 subjects showed "good/very good" outcome in 40–60% of cases (Mascher 1967). While this could be due to altered cognitive processing of emotions and experiences during the hallucinogenic state, there may also be a direct pharmacological action as well. An uncontrolled study of LSD in depression showed robust antidepressant effects (Savage 1952; Strassman 1995).

LSD has been examined for treatment of alcoholism. Some have reported that it was as effective as other treatments available at the time, but did not have any particular advantage (Ludwig et al. 1969; Abuzzahab and Anderson 1971). Peyote use in the Native American Church has been anecdotally reported to alleviate alcoholism, for which there is a possible pharmacological basis (Blum et al. 1977). However, it is also feasible that the therapeutic effect is due to intense experiences elicited by the ceremony and the context of increased social involvement.

During the early 1960s, Timothy Leary conducted the Concord Prison Experiment to study the psychotherapeutic use of hallucinogenic drugs in prison inmates. Treatment involved administration of psilocybin and group psychotherapy in 32 prisoners. A follow-up study of recidivism in these prisonsers concluded that there was no long-term treatment effect and emphasized the value of postrelease social support (Doblin 1998).

There is no formal consensus on this subject, but it seems that people do benefit from psychotherapy with hallucinogenic drugs. This benefit is not necessarily greater or worse than traditional psychotherapy; it has not clearly been demonstrated that hallucinogens give any clear advantage. At present, the variable methodology of many past studies prevent a firm conclusion. When one weighs the benefits against the elaborate safety precautions that would be needed for such therapy and potential liability, it becomes apparent why this form of therapy has not flourished as it might have. Empirical research on ibogaine for addiction treatment represents the most solid evidence for a therapeutic use of a hallucinogenic drug. Further research is needed to establish the safety and effectiveness of this drug in humans.

Monoamine Hallucinogens and Concurrent Psychotherapeutic Medications

Administration of certain therapeutic psychotropic medications has been shown to alter responsiveness to hallucinogenic drugs. This is not surprising, because they both have actions on monoamine systems, sometimes even the same receptor subtytpes. Tricyclic antidepressants and lithium enhance the effects of LSD, whereas MAO inhibitors and selective serotonin reuptake inhibitors (SSRIs) decrease the effects (Bonson and Murphy 1996; Bonson et al. 1996). Three-week administration of an SSRI abolished the effect of LSD in some cases.

Monoamine Hallucinogens and Chronic Psychosis

A few cases have been described where use of large amounts of LSD were thought to contribute to the development of a chronic psychosis (Boutros and Bowers 1996). Many cases involve polydrug use, and hallucinations occured spontaneously or with cannabis use. LSD psychosis may be multifactorial, involving family history, premorbid personality, and exposure to other drugs (Strassman 1984). Indeed, predictors of poor outcome following LSD psychosis are suggestive of neurological predispositions. Parental alcohol abuse also appears to be a predisposing factor. Epidemiologic studies show an increase in the admission diagnosis of schizophrenia and paranoid disorders to state hospitals during times when use of hallucinogenic drugs increased in the general population. People with psychoses are also more likely to abuse hallucinogenic drugs (Tsuang et al. 1982). The literature in this area suffers from methodological problems, limiting the confidence of conclusions that can be made (Boutros and Bowers 1996). However, it does seem reasonable to suggest that heavy use of hallucinogenic drugs can facilitate a psychotic disorder in those with risk factors.

A psychological assessment of long-term religious users of yage was undertaken using diagnostic interviews, personality testing, and neuropsychological evaluation was performed, using age-matched controls as reference group (Grob et al. 1996). Yage users had an overall high functional status. A few cases were reported with remission of psychopathology after initiation of yage use, with no apparent detrimental effects on personality or cognition. Although these data by no means constitute empirical proof, they suggest that it is possible for people to use monoamine hallucinogens over time without adverse effects.

Chronic Cognitive Effects of Monoamine Hallucinogens

It is difficult to assess chronic cognitive effects of LSD or other hallucinogens in humans. This research faces the problem of lacking premorbid data, uncertainty of the actual drug used, and concurrent use of other psychoactive drugs. Of particular interest is premorbid cognitive problems in this research. It may well be that people with cognitive impairments are more likely to use psychoactive drugs. Indeed, abnormalities were found in the prefrontal cortex of polysubstance users when compared to normal controls (Liu et al. 1998). In hallucinogen users, statistical decreases were found in the Halstead category test and trail-making test A, but scores were still well within the normal range (Culver and King 1974; McGlothlin et al. 1969). Further, scores were not different on numerous other measures of cognitive function.

Cholinergic Hallucinogens

History and Botany

There are several plants classified as cholinergic hallucinogens, all belonging to the family *Solanaceae.* Namely, these are belladonna *(Atropa belladonna)*, henbane *(Hyoscyamus niger)*, and mandrake *(Mandragora officinarum).* This family also includes datura genus, of which there are many species. The most commonly known is perhaps jimsonweed *(Datura stramonium)*, also known as Jamestown weed or thorn apple (figure 9.14). Another species in this category is scopolia *(Scopolia carniolica)* (table 9.3).

The monoamine and cholinergic hallucinogens not only differ by neurochemical actions, but also by the qualitative alteration in consciousness they produce. Unlike the monoamine hallucinogens, the cholinergic hallucinogens produce partial or complete amnesia for the duration of their effect. Although they both induce hallucinations, the cholinergic hallucinogens create a state better characterized as delirium and sedation.

Belladonna

Belladonna is a perennial herb growing 1 to 2 meters in height. It has a straight woody stem and ovate pointy leaves. The flowers are solitary and hang from the plant, yellow on the inside with crimson veins (Gruenwald 1998). It grows in Europe, Iran, and northern Africa. The name *belladonna* comes from the Italian words meaning "beautiful woman," because the plant causes a prominent pupil dilation thought to

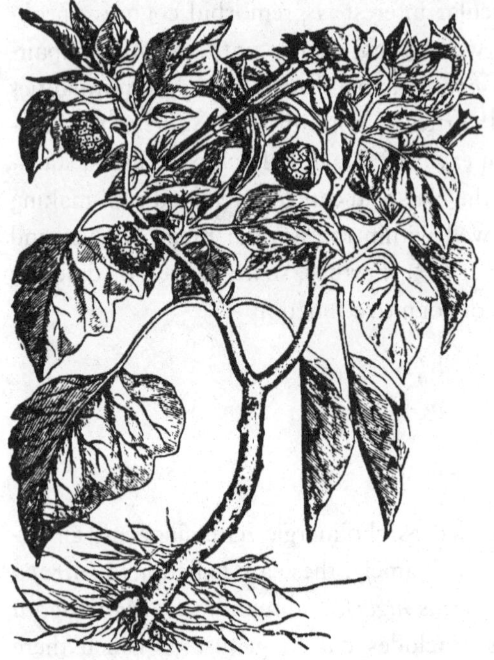

Figure 9.14
Thorn apple *(Datura stramonium)*. Reprinted with permission from Harner MJ. (1973). The role of hallucinogenic plants in European witchcraft, in *Hallucinogens and Shamanism*. Harner MJ, ed. London: Oxford University Press.

enhance attractiveness. The name *atropos* is from the eponymous Greek Fate who cuts the thread of life (Robbers et al. 1996).

Henbane
Henbane is a biennial herb growing wild in Europe, western Asia, and northern Africa, and cultivated in several other countries (Robbers et al. 1996). The ancient Egyptians mention its use in the Ebers Papyrus, written circa 1500 B.C.E. (Shultes and Hofman 1992). It was also mentioned in writings by the ancient Greek physician Pedanius Dioscorides for its medicinal uses. It has been suggested that the Oracle of Delphi inhaled smoke from henbane seeds to induce a prophetic trance. The plant is poisonous to livestock animals, as indicated by its common name *henbane*, and by its botanical name *hyoscyamus*, meaning "hog bean."

Table 9.3
Cholinergic and amino acid hallucinogens

Common Name	Botanical name
Cholinergic Hallucinogens	
Belladonna	*Atropa belladonna*
Datura	*Datura metel* *D. ferox*
Toloache	*Datura inoxia* *D. discolor* *D. kymatocarpa* *D. pruinosa* *D. quercifolia* *D. reburra* *D. stramonium* *D. wrightii*
Jimsonweed Thornapple	*Datura stramonium*
Henbane	*Hyoscyamus niger*
Mandrake	*Mandragora officinarum*
Scopolia	*Scopolia carniolica*
Amino Acid Hallucinogens	
Fly Agaric	*Amanita muscaria*

See text for references.

Mandrake

Mandrake was known to the ancient Egyptians, and has been found in several burial tombs (Rudgley 1993). The human-like form of the roots (sometimes resembling arms and legs), led early Europeans to believe that it could cure many human ailments (figure 9.15). Much superstition surrounds European lore regarding mandrake. It was believed to grow at the foot of gallows, springing from the semen of those who were hanged. Evil spirits were supposed to emit a shrieking sound when mandrake was uprooted.

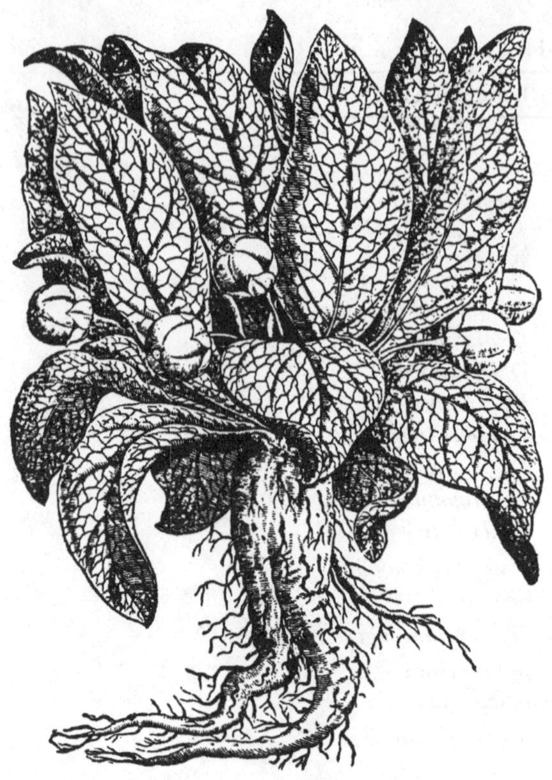

Figure 9.15
Mandrake *(Mandragora officinarum)*. Reprinted with permission from Harner MJ. (1973). The role of hallucinogenic plants in European witchcraft, in *Hallucinogens and Shamanism*. Harner MJ, ed. London: Oxford University Press.

Datura

There are many species of datura, the best known of which is probably jimsonweed *(Datura stramonium)*. It is an annual plant reaching a height of 1–2 meters, with large white solitary flowers (Gruenwald 1998) (figure 9.14). Datura is indigenous to many parts of the world, including Europe, Noth America, northern Africa, and eastern and southwestern Asia.

The word *datura* derives from its Sanskrit name, *dhattura*. *Stramonium* derives from the French word *stramoine*, meaning "stink weed," alluding to the unpleasant smell of the folium (Gruenwald 1998;

Robbers et al. 1996). It was grown in England by seeds imported from Constantinople, and known to settlers in Virginia (hence the name Jamestown weed or jimsonweed).

Historical Uses: Witchcraft, Lycanthropy, and Shamanism

Belladonna, henbane, and mandrake were used to induce hallucinatory states during witchcraft rituals in Europe. A salve was prepared using these plants, which was then applied to the skin (Harner 1973; Rudgley 1993). Absorption through the skin is questionable, but it was applied to the vaginal membranes, which are an effective site for drug absorption. Thus, an anointed broomstick was an effective way to apply the drug. The plants can create a sensation of flying, which is the source of the legend of witches flying on broomsticks. Use of such hallucinogenic herbs was also to induce a mental experience of lycanthropy, or changing into an animal form (such as a werewolf) (Harner 1973). Descriptions of lycanthropes in ancient Greece very closely resemble anticholinergic symptoms, including dry mouth, thirst, blurred vision, difficulty swallowing, and staggering gait.

Cholinergic hallucinogens were familiar to Native Americans long before the arrival of Europeans (Grinspoon and Bakalar 1997; Schultes and Hofman 1980, 1992). The Aztec used a plant called *toloache* or *toloatzin (Datura inoxia)* to prophesize, and it is still used among some Native American tribes for shamanic purposes. Carlos Castaneda wrote about the shamanic use of datura among the Yaqui in his book *The Teachings of Don Juan: A Yaqui Way of Knowledge* (Castaneda 1968).

Chemical Constituents

The cholinergic hallucinogens all have common chemical constituents that are responsible for their pharmacological effects (Robbers et al. 1996). These are the tropane alkaloids hyoscyamine, scopolamine (or hyoscine), and atropine (figure 9.16). It is scopolamine, and not atropine or hyoscyamine, which primarily produces the central and hallucinogenic effects because it is the only one that passes the blood-brain barrier sufficiently. However, all three have peripheral effects. *Datura stramonium* contains 0.1–0.65% tropane alkaloids, which is principally

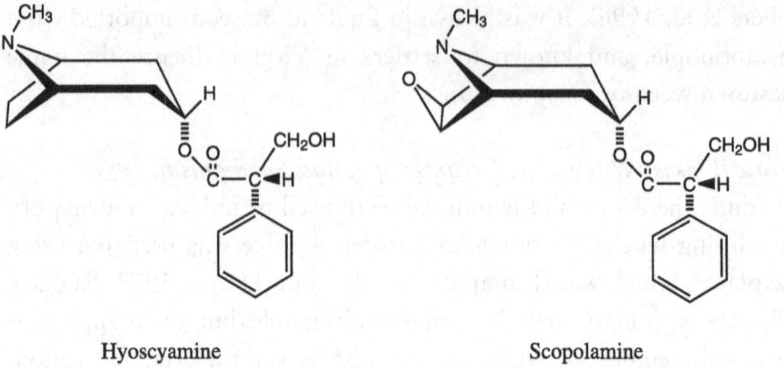

Figure 9.16
Chemical structure of the tropane alkaloids.

hyoscyamine, and scopolamine to a lesser extent. Belladonna contains 0.33–0.6% tropane alkaloids, primarily hyoscyamine. Henbane contains 0.05–0.28 tropane alkaloids, again primarily consisting of hyoscyamine. Scopolia contains 0.2–0.5% tropane alkaloids. The tropane akaloid content depends on the part of the plant used, with highest concentrations in the root (Gruenwald 1998). Drying the plant transforms some of the alkaloids, increasing the amount of atropine and scopolamine.

Mechanisms of Action

Acetylcholine

Tropane alkaloids are antagonists of muscarinic cholinergic receptors, competing with acetylcholine and other agonists (Brown and Taylor 1996). The antagonism is competitive, and can be overcome by larger concentrations of acetylcholine or other agonists. They are active at all known subtypes of the muscarinic receptor (Kebabian and Neumeyer 1994). Effects are seen at muscarinic receptors in all central and peripheral locations, including exocrine glands, smooth and cardiac muscle, and autonomic ganglia (Brown and Taylor 1996).

Monoamines

Cholinergic antagonists increase dopamine activity in the striatum, as measured in humans with PET (Dewey et al. 1993). The pedunculopontine and laterodorsal tegmental nuclei project to dopaminergic neurons of the substantia nigra pars compacta and ventral tegmental area (Yeomans 1995). Muscarinic antagonists like scopolamine disinhibit cholinergic neurons, which in turn excite dopaminergic neurons. Whereas cholinergic drugs for Parkinson's disease selectively block M_1 muscarinic receptors, the cholinergic hallucinogens are nonselective. This mechanism may explain the reinforcing effects of cholinergic hallucinogens. Reinforcement is associated with activity of the mesolimbic dopamine system originating in the ventral tegmental area, and scopolamine reduces the threshold for reinforcing brain stimulation (Yeomans et al. 1993). Ironically, anticholinergic hallucinogens are reinforcing even though the person may have little or no memory of the experience.

Other Neurotransmitters

Muscarinic receptors have modulatory effects on numerous other neurotransmitters in the brain (van der Zee and Luiten 1999). Of particular interest are interactions between glutamate and cholinergic systems in learning and memory (Aigner 1995).

Pharmacokinetics

Maximum serum concentrations of scopolamine occurred 10 to 30 minutes after subcutaneous administration (Ebert et al. 1998). The elimination half-life is approximately 220 minutes.

General Effects

Autonomic

Muscarinic receptors are present on ganglionic and postganglionic neurons, for both sympathetic and parasympathetic branches. Thus, the effect of systemic scopolamine is hard to predict and is often paradoxical (Brown and Taylor 1996).

Atropine and scopolamine have antispasmodic effects on the gastrointestinal tract. It partly inhibits vagal influence in the gut, reducing motility. However, the enteric nervous system also employs serotonin and dopamine, so parasympathetic innervation plays a modulatory role.

Nonetheless, a sufficient dose will reduce or temporarily halt peristalsis (Brown and Taylor 1996). Some effects on esophageal peristalsis may be mediated by central mechanisms (Bieger 1984).

Atropine reduces the tone and contractions of the ureter and bladder, and has antispasmodic effects on the gallbladder and bile duct. Negligible effects are produced on uterine contractions. Sweat glands are inhibited by atropine, and it can impair thermoregulation, especially in hot environments.

Cardiac Effects

Atropine generally increases heart rate, but it may briefly and mildly decrease it initially, due to M_1 receptors on postganglionic parasympathetic neurons. Larger doses of atropine produce greater tachycardia, due to M_2 receptors on the sinoatrial node pacemaker cells. There are no changes in blood pressure, but arrhythmias may occur. Scopolamine produces more bradycardia and decreases arterial pressure, whereas atropine has little effect on blood pressure (Vesalainen et al. 1997; Brown and Taylor 1996).

Respiratory Effects

Tropane alkaloids act as bronchodilators, but have been replaced clinically by methylxanthines and adrenergic drugs. They inhibit secretions from mucous membranes in the nose, mouth, pharynx, and bronchi.

Behavioral and Motor Effects

Central muscarinic antagonists reduce behavioral activity at higher doses by causing sedation. Scopolamine reduces locomotion and exploration in rats (Renner et al. 1992). However, they also produce some degree of euphoria, probably by indirect actions on dopaminergic systems (Yeomans et al. 1993). Muscarinic antagonists have long been used as antiparkinsonian agents, which is discussed in chapter 5.

Saccades are also affected by anticholinergic hallucinogens in humans (Oliva et al. 1993). Increases in saccade duration and latency occur along with decreases in velocity. Postsaccadic fixation is impaired as well, where the eye drifts after reaching the target.

Arousal and Sleep

Therapeutic doses of scopolamine produce CNS depression, characterized by drowsiness, amnesia, and dreamless sleep (Brown and Taylor 1996). It reduces arousal and increases the effort required to awaken (Parrott 1987). Higher therapeutic doses of atropine cause central excitation, characterized by restlessness, irritability, confusion, disorientation, hallucinations, and delirium. Larger doses produce central depression, paralysis, coma, and death by respiratory failure and cardiovascular collapse.

Tonic arousal and wakefulness are sustained by projections from the reticular formation to the thalamus, which affects thalamocortical processes (Young 1998). An important part of this ascending system is cholinergic projections from the pontine reticular formation, including the laterodorsal and pedunculopontine tegmental nuclei. Cholinergic reticular neurons also influence arousal through projections to the basal forebrain cholinergic nuclei, which in turn has widespread projections to the forebrain. Thus, scopolamine alters forebrain function through dual actions on brain stem and forebrain cholinergic nuclei.

Scopolamine supresses REM sleep in animals, and a rebound increase occurs during withdrawal from chronic treatment (Sutin et al. 1986; Zolotski et al. 1993). Similarly, scopolamine increases the latency for REM onset and decreases its total duration in humans (Sagalés et al. 1975). Decreases also occur in eye and body movements. This effect shows tolerance over chronic administration, and a rebound increase in REM occurs when scopolamine is replaced with saline placebo. Rapid eye movement (REM) sleep is driven by nuclei in the pontine reticular formation, namely the laterodorsal and pedunculopontine tegmental nuclei, and acetylcholine release is mediated by muscarinic autoreceptors (Shiromani and Fishbein 1986; Roth et al. 1996). Muscarinic receptors regulating REM are found throughout the brain stem, including dorsal raphe, locus coeruleus, and pontine reticular formation (Baghdoyan et al. 1994).

Electrophysiology

Scopolamine creates electrophysiological slowing in humans, with increases in absolute power in delta activity, and in relative power in delta and theta-1 activity over the central and parieto-occipital regions. Decreases occur in relative alpha-2 (9.2–12.8 Hz) over the frontal regions and in absolute alpha-2 over most recording sites. These EEG changes were congruent with changes on memory test (the Wechsler memory scale) (Kikuchi et al. 1999). Decreases also occur in fast alpha power (Ebert et al. 1998). In event-related-potential studies, scopolamine prolongs the latency of the P300 and reduces spectral power of long-latency-evoked potentials without altering earlier components (Meador et al. 1988). In contrast, the cholinesterase inhibitor physostigmine reverses these effects.

Functional Neuroimaging

Scopolamine increases cerebral blood flow to lateral occipital cortex bilaterally and to the left orbitofrontal region (Grasby et al. 1995). Decreases are seen in the right thalamus, precuneus, and lateral premotor areas bilaterally. When normal subjects are chronically administered scopolamine, there is a 12% increase in cerebral blood flow on single photon emission computed tomography (SPECT), but a decrease in cerebral muscarinic binding (Sunderland et al. 1995). On the other hand, acute administration dose-dependently reduces cortical blood flow, which is maximal in frontal cortex (Gitelman and Prohovnik 1992; Prohovnik et al. 1997).

In addition to altering cerebral blood flow, scopolamine alters cerebral glucose metabolism. In healthy older volunteers, absolute and normalized glucose metabolism are decreased in prefrontal and occipital regions and increased in parietal-occipital cortical regions and a left middle temporal region (Molchan et al. 1994). Metabolism is also reduced in the thalamus (Cohen et al. 1994).

Functional Activation in Cognitive Tasks

Some functional neuroimaging studies have examined the effects of scopolamine in cognitive tasks. Although scopolamine inhibits increases in cerebral blood flow to somatosensory stimulation, it does not inhibit the neural response (Ogawa et al. 1994). Thus, cholinergic systems may be involved in coordination of cerebral blood flow increases to neural activation. Subjects performing an attentional auditory discrimination task showed metabolic reduction in cingulate and increases in the basal ganglia (Cohen et al. 1994). The effects of scopolamine on memory have also been investigated using functional neuroimaging. Scopolamine reduces cerebral blood flow in left and right prefrontal cortex and the right anterior cingulate during performance of a verbal memory task (Grasby et al. 1995).

Collectively, these results indicate that scopolamine has profound effects on cerebral activity, both in resting and cognitive task-activation conditions. Of particular note are effects on frontal and striatal activity, which could well account for impairments on cognitive abilities such as working memory. Also of note is a decrease in thalamic activation, which could result from blocked activation from pontine tegmental cholinergic nuclei, and/or altered activity of fronto-striato-thalamic circuits. In either case, the functional imaging findings well account for the cognitive and subjective effects of central anticholinergic drugs.

Cognitive Effects: Animal Studies

Scopolamine impairs cognitive functions in a number of animal paradigms. Orientation of attention to a cued visual target (the Posner task) is reduced—in reaction time and accuracy (Davidson et al. 1999). It impairs working memory in both delayed match-to-sample and nonmatching-to-sample tasks in rats and primates (Granon et al. 1995; Rupniak et al. 1991; Bartus and Johnson 1976). Scopolamine produces memory deficits similar to lesions of basal forebrain cholinergic nuclei, characterized as impairments in visual discrimination learning, retention, and reversal (Harder et al. 1998).

Cognitive Effects: Human Studies

Scopolamine produces cognitive deficits in humans, which are more pronounced in the elderly (Zemishlany and Thorne 1991). Cognitive studies have focused on memory and attention, but some studies have shown impairments in a variety of cognitive functions.

Scopolamine produces dose-dependent impairments of attention and slows the speed of information processing (Ebert et al. 1998; Vitiello et al. 1997). It causes psychomotor slowing when it is administered to the elderly, and to young adults at higher doses (Flicker et al. 1992). Digit span is not affected by scopolamine in young volunteers, but more omissions are produced on letter cancellation tasks (Parrot 1987; Rusted 1988). Impairments are also seen in praxis and visual perception (Flicker et al. 1990). Deficits induced in problem solving and working memory are suggestive of effects on executive allocation of working memory (Rusted and Warburton 1988). Scopolamine impairs chess performance in trained players (Liljequist and Mattila 1979). On the other hand, no effects are observed in immediate and remote memory, language function, object sorting, or intrusion errors (Flicker et al. 1992, 1990; Zemishlany and Thorne 1991).

Scopolamine interferes with the encoding and consolidation of information into long-term memory. Reductions are seen in the overall score of the Wechsler memory scale after acute administration of scopolamine (Kikuchi et al. 1999). Impairments occur across both verbal and visual recall, and visual recognition as well (Flicker et al. 1990; Frumin et al. 1976; Rusted 1988). It significantly impairs delayed recognition of abstract shapes in humans when administered before the encoding stage (Rosier et al. 1998). However, the effect is only seen on delayed recognition: scopolamine does not affect immediate recognition or visuoperceptual discrimination. Impairments are seen in recall of paragraph information in humans, using the logical memory subtest of the Wechsler memory scale. Memory is also impaired on a verbal selective reminding test (Zemishlany and Thorne 1991; Rabey et al. 1996). Caffeine and nicotine partially reverse memory deficits induced by scopolamine in humans (Riedel et al. 1995).

Scopolamine produces greater impairment in older than younger subjects on cognitive tasks (Molchan et al. 1992; Zemishlany and Thorne 1991). Given the cognitive impairments it produces and the cholinergic nature of many dementias such as Alzheimer's disease, scopolamine has been explored as a pharmacological model of dementia in numerous animal and human cognitive studies. Although scopolamine intoxication mimics dementia in some respects, scopolamine does not completely create all of the symptoms (Ebert and Kirch 1998). A scopolamine-challenge is also ineffective as a probe for Alzheimer's disease, because it does not distinguish it from Parkinson's disease or vascular dementia, or predict cognitive decline (Rabey et al. 1996; Barker et al. 1998). However, a combined blockade of muscarinic and nicotinic receptors may provide a better pharmacological model of dementia (Little et al. 1998).

Toxicity

Toxicity from tropane alkaloids often results from their effects on autonomic function. Several species of *Datura* are freely available, either growing in the wild or cultivated as ornamental plants, such as angel's trumpet *(Datura sauveolens)*. Periodic outbreaks of jimsonweed use occur, when adolescents learn about the psychoactive effects of the plant and intentionally ingest it.

Transdermal scopolamine is used for treatment of motion sickness, causing relatively infrequent cases of confusion and visual hallucinations (Ayub et al. 1997; Wilkinson 1987). A case of paranoid delusions and hallucinations was reported after a two-week period of transdermal scopolamine, which continued 11 days after discontinuation (Rubner et al. 1997). Children may be particularly sensitive to adverse effects of anticholinergic drugs (Holland 1992). Others more sensitive to psychoactive side effects are the elderly, people with preexisting psychiatric illness, and those taking other anticholinergic medications (Ziskind 1988). Treatment of anticholinergic syndromes involves drugs that enhance cholinergic transmission, such as physostigmine.

Amino Acid Hallucinogens

Fly Agaric

Fly agaric *(Amanita muscaria)* is a mushroom that grows in forests, often under birches, firs, and larches (Schultes and Hofman 1980, 1992). It has a reddish, flat, and ovate cap, with distinct white warts over the surface. Another variety has an orange or yellowish cap, with yellow warts. The stem is white, cylindrical, and hollow, with a bulbous shape at the bottom (figure 9.17).

The *Amanita* genus comprises about 50 or 60 species, with varying chemical constituents—a number of which are toxic (Schultes and Hofman 1980, 1992). Fly agaric *(Amanita muscaria)* grows in widespread northern temperate zones of Eurasia and North America. In North

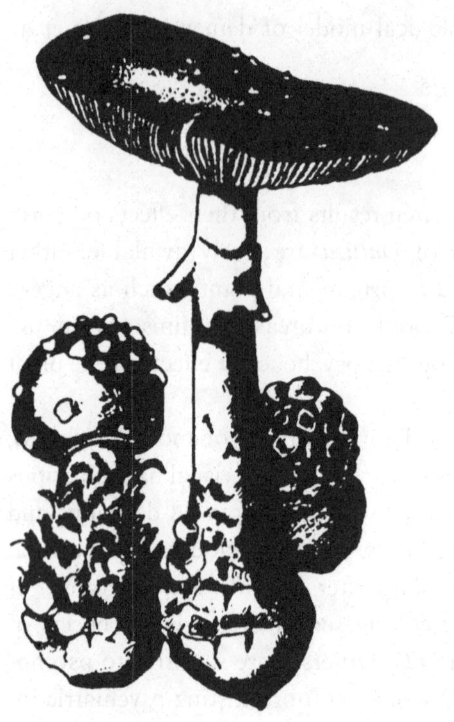

Figure 9.17
Fly Agaric *(Amanita muscaria)*. Schultes RE, Hofman A. (1980). *The Botany and Chemistry of Hallucinogens,* 2nd ed. Springfield, Ill.: Charles C. Thomas Publishers.

America, it was used by the Ojibway Indians of Michigan. In Eurasia, it has also been used by several tribes spanning Siberia. A related species, *Amanita pantherina*, is used in western Washington State.

Although less popular now, fly agaric may historically be the oldest and most widely used hallucinogen. Fly agaric was probably discovered in Siberia, through observation of its effect in intoxicated reindeer (Abraham et al. 1996). It is likely to be the drug known as *soma* in the ancient Indian Rig Veda.

Chemical Constituents
The psychoactive constituents of fly agaric are amino acid derivatives (Eugster et al. 1965; Schultes and Hofman 1980, 1992). These include ibotenic acid, muscimol, muscazone, muscarine, and (R)-4-hydroxy-

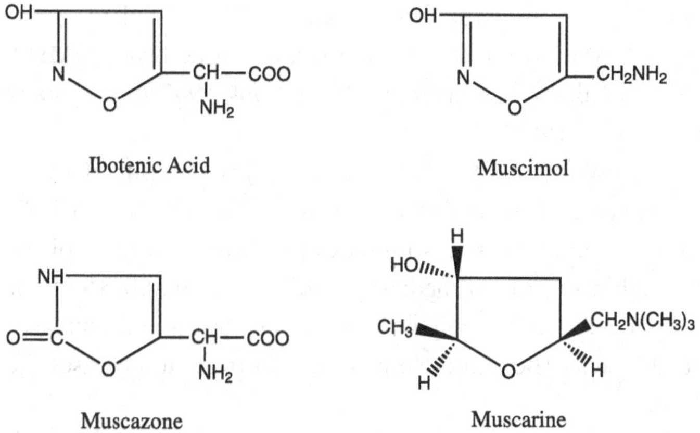

Ibotenic Acid

Muscimol

Muscazone

Muscarine

Figure 9.18
Chemical constituents of amanita muscaria.

pyrrolidone-(2) (figure 9.18 and see table 9.3). Ibotenic acid is present in amounts of 0.3–1 mg/kg of undried material. Muscimol is most likely formed by degradation of ibotenic acid. Muscazone is also formed from ibotenic acid but is less active pharmacologically.

Pharmacokinetics
Ingestion of one to four mushrooms is necessary for intoxication, and the onset of effects occurs about 15 minutes to 1 hour after ingestion. Little is known about the absorption and distribution of these chemicals. But muscimol does seem to pass the blood-brain barrier (Schultes and Hofman 1980, 1992).

The active constituents of amanita, and perhaps active metabolites as well, are excreted in urine. Because the mushrooms can be very expensive, many Siberian tribesmen drink their urine to prolong intoxication. Both ibotenic acid and muscimol are detected in urine. Up to 27% of muscimol injected into mice has been recovered from urine.

Mechanisms of Action

Acetylcholine Muscarine is an agonist at muscarinic acetylcholine receptors, for which the receptor was named. It is not certain what role this plays in the psychoactive effects of amanita.

Excitatory amino acids Ibotenic acid is structurally related to glutamate, the principal excitatory neurotransmitter, and it activates NMDA receptors (Madsen et al. 1990; Mayer and Westbrook 1987; Schwarcz et al. 1979; Honore et al. 1981).

Ibotenic acid is also a potent agonist at group I and group II metabotropic glutamate receptors (mGluRs) (Brauner-Osbourne et al. 1998). Similar to glutamate, ibotenic acid stimulates production of inositol triphosphates through a G-protein mediated mechanism (Scholz 1994). It stimulates phosphorylation of protein kinase C substrates and increases phospholipase D activity (Boss and Conn 1992). Further, it increases the release of glutamate.

Ibotenate creates neurotoxic and phosphoinositide effects through distinct receptors (Zinkand et al. 1992). The neurotoxic effects are prevented by MK-801 and enhanced by glycine, implying NMDA involvement. Phosphoinositide hydrolysis is mediated by metabotropic receptors, and is unaffected by NMDA agents.

GABA Muscimol is a $GABA_A$ agonist, creating effects in the low micromolar range (Bekar et al. 1999). Regional differences in the sensitivity of $GABA_A$ receptors to muscimol are seen across the cerebral cortex, hippocampus, and cerebellum (Ito et al. 1995). Muscimol induces long-term depression in the CA1 region of the hippocampus at concentrations of 10 μM (Akhondzadeh and Stone 1995, 1996). This occurs through actions at $GABA_A$, but not glutamate receptors.

General Effects

Although they apparently differ in their mechanisms of action, ibotenic acid and muscimol apparently produce a qualitatively similar subjective and behavioral state (Schultes and Hofman 1980, 1992). However, muscimol is approximately 5 times as potent as ibotenic acid. Vegetative functions do not appear to be grossly affected at usual doses.

Motor effects Amanita constituents cause a notable motor dysfunction in both animals and humans. A general inhibition of motor function occurs through supraspinal mechanisms. Other effects include twitching, trembling, or convulsive-like movements of the extremities.

Subjective effects A state of intoxication occurs with muscimol, characterized by confusion, disorientation, sensory disturbances (e.g., auditory, visual, numbness in the feet, etc.). Also common are fatigue and sedation, followed by sleep. Cognitive ability is diminished.

Animal drug discrimination paradigms suggest that muscimol generalizes well to other $GABA_A$ agonists such as THIP, but only partially to benzodiazepine agonists (diazepam), GABA uptake inhibitors (tiagabine), and not at all to GABA-transaminase inhibitors (valproate, vigabatrin) (Jones and Balster 1998). Thus, although they are all working through the GABAergic system, these drugs appear to create distinct subjective effects. Partial to full substitution occurs with the noncompetitive NMDA antagonist phencyclidine (PCP), depending on the dose and varying between individuals (Grech and Balster 1997).

Toxicity

Little is formally known about the toxicity of amanita use. Ibotenic acid is a potent neurotoxin, through excitatory amino acid mechanisms (Steiner et al. 1984; Schwarcz et al. 1984). It has been used extensively in animal research to create discrete neuroanatomical lesions. For example, it has been used to lesion the basal forebrain nuclei to create a putative animal model of Alzheimer's disease (Arbogast and Kozlowski 1988).

Intracerebral injections of ibotenic acid produce cell loss in several cerebral areas, including the striatum, the hippocampus, substantia nigra, and piriform cortex (Schwarcz et al. 1979). This degeneration is limited to the site of injection and does not affect axons, passage, or synaptic terminals originating in other areas.

Compared to other excitotoxic drugs, ibotenate has relatively lesser epileptogenic effects (Zaczek and Coyle 1982). However, intracerebroventricular infusion of ibotenic acid (6 nmol/min) induces clonic convulsions in mice (Laudrup and Klitgaard 1993).

10
Cannabis

History

Cannabis is one of civilization's oldest cultivated nonfood plants, and does not seem to exist anymore in its wild form (figure 10.1). In addition to its psychoactive effects, the cannabis plant has also been used for its fibers. Hemp fibers have been found in China dating from 4000 B.C.E., and hemp ropes were dated to 3000 B.C.E. in Turkestan, but it is not certain that cannabis was used for psychoactive purposes at those places and times (Schultes and Hofman 1992).

The psychoactive use of cannabis may be a relatively recent phenomenon, but it is also ancient. The earliest recorded psychoactive use of cannabis dates from 2000 B.C.E. in a Chinese pharmacopoeia by Emperor Shen Nung (Schultes and Hofman 1992). He recommended it for absent-mindedness and pain, as well as malaria, beri beri, constipation, and female disorders. Hoa-Glio, an ancient Chinese herbalist, recommended a combination of hemp resin and wine as an anesthetic for surgery. But its psychoactive use seems to have declined in China by the time of European contact. Assyrians used cannabis incense as early as 900 B.C.E. (Schultes and Hofman 1992). The Indian Vedas cite cannabis as a divine nectar: the favorite drink of the god Indra was made from it. Indian medical systems cited widespread uses for cannabis, including mania, leprosy, and dandruff. But they also recognized appetite-stimulant and digestive effects. *Bhang*, *charas*, and *ganja* are all Indian terms for preparations of the cannabis plant.

The Scythians are credited with spreading the use of cannabis to the Greeks from the steppes (Rudgley 1993). The ancient Greeks knew of the psychoactive effects of cannabis, although the prevalence of its use is

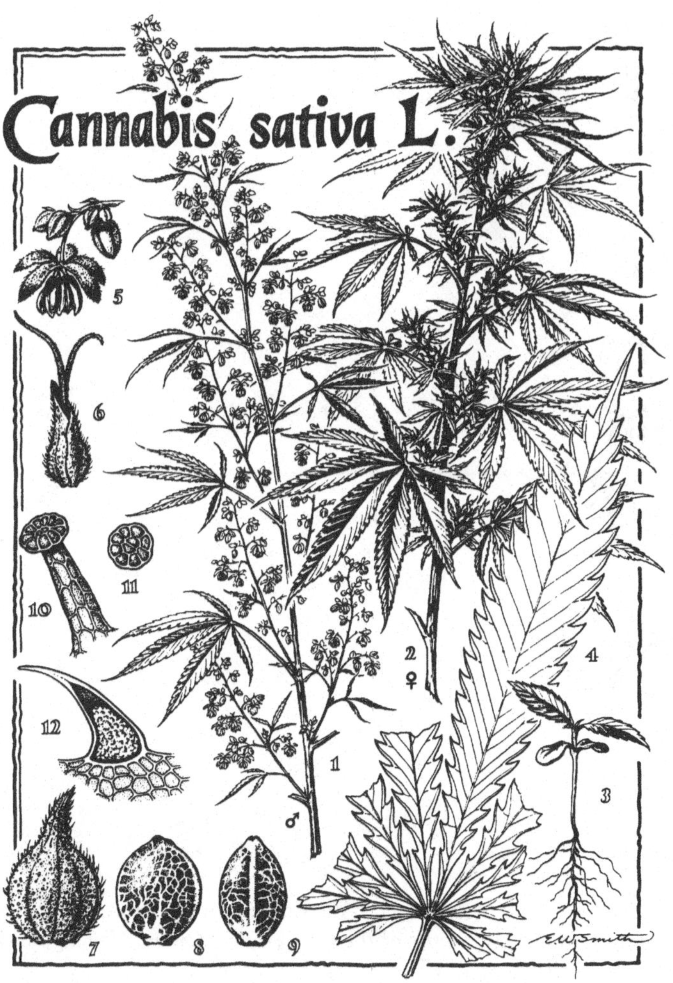

Figure 10.1
Cannabis (Cannabis sativa). Reprinted with permission from Schultes RE, Hofman A. (1992). *Plants of the Gods: Their Sacred, Healing, and Hallucinogenic Powers*. Rochester, VT: Healing Arts Press.

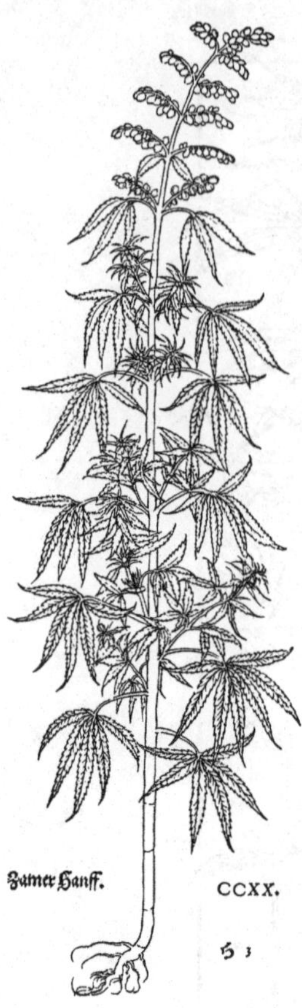

Figure 10.2
Woodcut of cannabis (Cannabis sativa). Reprinted with permission from Schultes RE, Hofman A. (1992). *Plants of the Gods: Their Sacred, Healing, and Hallucinogenic Powers*. Rochester, VT: Healing Arts Press.

not certain. Galen wrote that cakes made with hemp were intoxicating. Women of Thebes were said to use cannabis to dispel sorrow and bad humor (Bibra 1995). In medieval Europe, herbalists used cannabis for medicinal, but not psychoactive purposes. Cannabis was widely cultivated in Europe, and later in the American colonies (figure 10.2). Hemp fiber was a valuable commodity at the time, used to make rope and canvas. Although it is true that many farmers at the time grew hemp, including George Washington, there is nothing to indicate that they were aware of its psychoactive effects.

Cannabis was officially listed in the United States Pharmacopoeia until 1937, where it was recommended for a number of therapeutic uses, including sedation (Ray and Ksir 1990). The Marijuana Tax Act was passed in 1937 making it effectively illegal to grow, sell, buy, or distribute cannabis. From the early 1920s, cannabis use gained a public reputation as a menacing deviant drug, an attitude characterized in the movie *Reefer Madness*. By the 1950s and 1960s, cannabis use had gained popularity, particularly with American youths. Use peaked in the late 1970s, when 60% of high school seniors surveyed reported having used cannabis and 11% reported daily use (O'Brien 1996). By 1996, 35% of high school seniors had used cannabis at least once in the past year, but only 4.6% used it on a daily basis (Duffy and Milin 1996). In contrast, use of alcohol and cocaine had not changed across these time periods. In 1990, it was estimated that 6–10 million Americans smoke cannabis at least once per week.

The legal status of cannabis in the United States has varied greatly. The Controlled Substances Act of 1970 classified cannabis as a Schedule I drug, which implies that the drug has no currently accepted medical use and has a high potential for abuse. During the 1970s, however, a degree of tolerance grew. By 1977, most states considered possession to be a misdemeanor, and by 1980, eleven states had decriminalized possession (Grinspoon 1999). This atmosphere changed in the 1980s, when severe legal penalties were enacted and the toxic pesticide paraquat was sprayed on domestic cannabis crops.

The Dutch have depenalized and de facto legalized cannabis since 1976 (Engelsman 1989; MacCoun and Reuter 1997). Depenalization has not increased usage in the population since this time, but its commercial access has increased usage. However, parallel increases were also seen in the United States during this time period despite prohibition of cannabis use (Dutch cannabis use has remained equal or below that of the United States). How this example relates to the issue of American legalization or depenalization is a matter of debate.

Botany and Preparation

There was uncertainty in the early botanical classification of cannabis. It was originally designated a member of the Nettle family (Urticaceae),

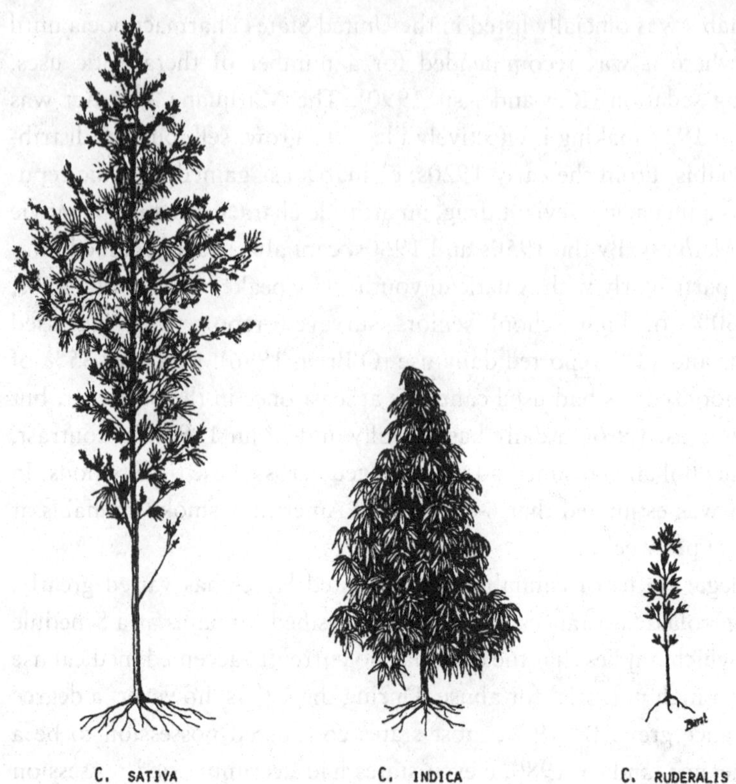

Figure 10.3
Three species of cannabis. Reprinted with permission from Schultes RE, Hofman A. (1980). *The Botany and Chemistry of Hallucinogens,* 2nd ed. Springfield, Ill.: Charles C Thomas Publishers.

but later assigned to the Fig family (Moraceae) (Schultes and Hofmann 1992). Today it is classified in its own family, Cannabaceae, of which the *Humulus* genus (Hops) is also a member. Three species of cannabis are recognized: *C. indica*, *C. ruderalis*, and *C. sativa* (figure 10.3).

Several products are derived from the cannabis plant (table 10.1). *Hashish* and *charas* are the dried resin exuded from the female flowers. These have the highest content of Δ^9-tetrahydrocannabinol (THC) at 10–20% and have the most potent psychoactive effects. *Ganja* and *sinsemilla* are the dried tops of the female plants, which averages 5–8%. *Marijuana* and *bhang* are derived from the rest of the plant and have the lowest THC concentration (2–5%).

Table 10.1
Cannabis preparations and THC content

Name	Preparation	THC Content
Hashish, charas	Dried resin exuded from female flowers	10–20%
Ganja, sinsemilla	Dried tops of female plants	5–8%
Marijuana, bhang	Remainder of the plant	2–5%

Throughout this chapter, the term *cannabis* is used to refer collectively to all of its products, unless otherwise specified.

Effects and Uses

Cannabis has been hard to characterize by its behavioral and psychological effects. It has mild sedative and anxiolytic properties. However, very high doses do not suppress respiration. But at higher doses it may produce euphoria, hallucinations, and heightened perceptual sensitivity, which makes it akin to psychedelic drugs. This is perhaps not surprising because there are many overlaps between behavioral classes of drugs. But more recently, since the characterization of endogenous receptors and ligands, cannabinoids have been viewed as their own unique class of drug.

Much debate has been waged over medicinal uses of cannabis. Several therapeutic uses have been proposed, including antiemetic, analgesic, appetite stimulant, and muscle relaxant. A synthetic cannabinoid, dronabinol (Marinol) has been marketed for clinical treatment of appetite loss, nausea, and vomiting. Although synthetic, it is identical to the main psychoactive chemical constituent of cannabis (Δ^9-THC).

Chemical Constituents

There are approximately 400 chemicals in the cannabis plant, 61 of which are unique and may be called cannabinoids. The most common psychoactive cannabinoid is Δ^9-tetrahydrocannabinol (Δ^9-THC) (Robbers et al. 1996) (figure 10.4). Other psychoactive cannabinoids include Δ^8-tetrahydrocannabinol (Δ^8-THC), 11-hydroxy-Δ^8-tetrahydrocannabinol (11-OH-Δ^9-THC), and 9-nor-9 β-hydroxyhexahydrocannabinol (β-

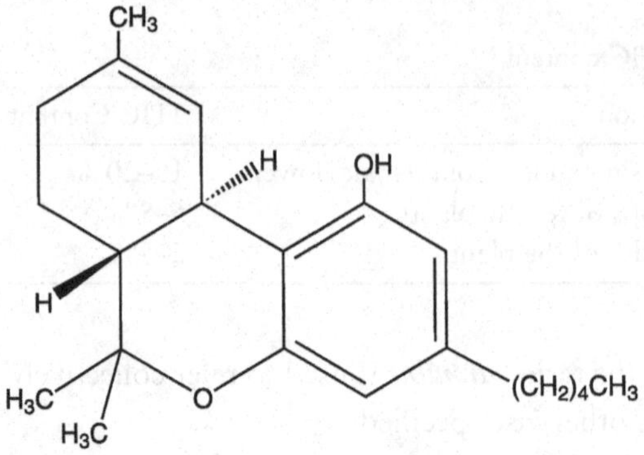

Figure 10.4
Chemical structure of delta-9-tetrahydrocannabinol (THC).

Table 10.2
Some identified endocannabinoids

Arachidonylethanolamide (anandamide)
sn-2-arachidonylglycerol (2-AG)
Docosatetraenoyl-ethanolamide
Di-homo-γ-linolenoyl-ethanolamide

See text for references.

HHC) (Tripathi 1987). Unless stated otherwise, THC will be used to refer to Δ^9-THC throughout the remainder of this chapter. Other cannabinoids that are not psychoactive include cannabinol and cannabidiol. More recently, endogenous substances have been identified that activate these receptors, and are referred to collectively as *endocannabinoids* (table 10.2).

Endocannabinoids

Several physiological roles of endocannabinoids have been identified, including memory, cognition, movement, and pain perception (Stella et al. 1997). Elucidation of the endocannabinoid systems is essential to the understanding of the effects of cannabis. There are both similarities and some pointed differences between the effects of exogenous and endogenous cannabinoids.

Table 10.3
Endocannabinoid synthesis and metabolism

Endocannabinoid	Anandamide	2-AG
Precursors	*N*-a-PEA	Diacylglycerol (DAG) 1-lyso-phosphatidylcholine
Synthesizing Enzymes	Phospholipase D	Phospholipase C Diacylglycerol lipase
Degrading Enzyme	FAAH	FAAH

See text for references.
Key: Fatty acid amide hydrolase (FAAH); *N*-a-PEA = *N*-arachidonoyl-phosphatidylethanolamine.

Identification and Synthesis

Anandamide (arachidonylethanolamide) was the first endocannabinoid to be identified (table 10.3) (Devane et al. 1992; Devane and Axelrod 1994). It was found to have THC-like effects and to produce cross-tolerance with THC (Di Marzo 1998; Fride 1995). A second endocannabinoid was later identified, *sn*-2-arachidonylglycerol (2-AG), which is present in the brain in concentrations 170 times greater than anandamide (DiMarzo 1998; Stella et al. 1997). 2-AG is produced in the hippocampus when Schaffer collaterals are stimulated. 2-AG acts as a full agonist at cannabinoid receptors, and prevents the induction of long-term potentiation at CA3-CA1 synapses. Other endocannabinoids identified are docosatetraenoyl-ethanolamide and di-homo-γ-linolenoyl-ethanolamide (Di Marzo et al. 1998) (figure 10.5).

Anandamide is believed to be synthesized from a phospholipid precursor, *N*-arachidonoyl-phosphatidylethanolamine, catalysed by phospholipase D (Di Marzo et al. 1998). The other proposed route of synthesis is from condensation of arachidonic acid and ethanolamine, although this has yet to be demonstrated in living cells. 2-AG is formed in a calcium-dependent manner, and mediated by the enzymes phospholipase C and diacylglycerol lipase (Kondo et al. 1998; Stella et al. 1997).

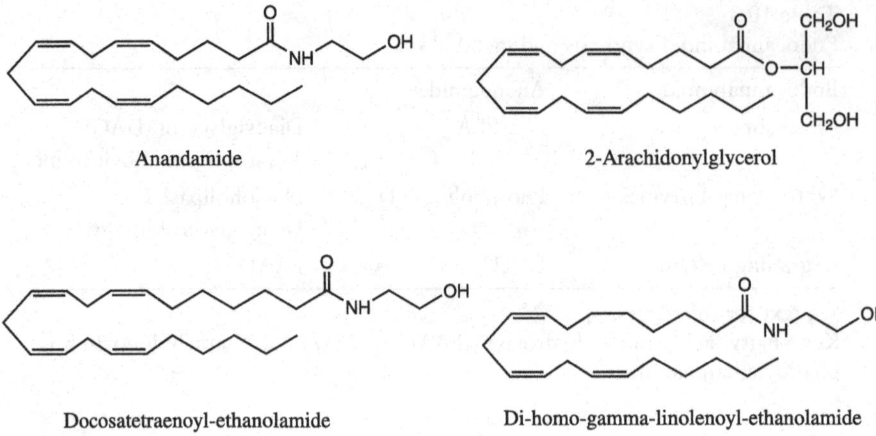

Figure 10.5
Chemical structure of the endocannabinoids.

Inactivation

Both anandamide and 2-AG are inactivated by enzymatic hydrolysis (Goparaju et al. 1998). Fatty acid amide hydrolase (FAAH) is an enzyme that catalyses their hydrolysis. High concentrations of FAAH were found in the cerebellum, hippocampus and neocortex of rat brain, which are also rich in cannabinoid receptors. Further, there is a complementary pattern of distribution of FAAH and the CB_1 receptor. For example, in the cerebellum, FAAH is found in the cell bodies of Purkinje cells and the CB_1 receptor is found in the axons of granule cells and basket cells, which are presynaptic to Purkinje cells. 2-AG may also be inactivated by direct esterification into membrane phospholipids.

Cannabinoid Receptors

Cannabinoid receptors were first suggested by the stereospecificity of THC enantiomers. The existence of the receptor was confirmed in 1984, which was followed by radioligand binding, receptor localization, and cloning of the cannabinoid CB_1 receptor (Howlett 1984; Childers and Breivogel 1998) (figure 10.6). There is a splice variant of the cannabinoid receptor, CB_{1A}, as well as a peripheral subtype, CB_2. It is the CB_1 recep-

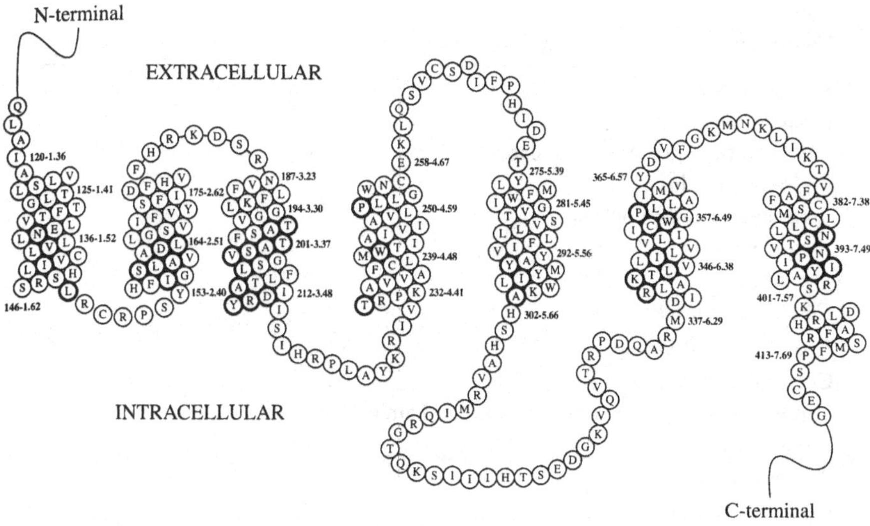

Figure 10.6
The cannabinoid receptor. Reprinted with permission from Julien, RM. (1997). *A Primer of Drug Action*, 8th ed. NY: W.H. Freeman.

tors in the brain that mediate the psychoactive effects of cannabis (Egertova 1998). The CB_2 receptor was identified in macrophages in the marginal zone of spleen (Munro et al. 1993). Both CB_1 and CB_2 belong to the 7 transmembrane domain, G-protein-coupled family of receptors (Childers and Breivogel 1998). CB_1 is longer by 72 amino acid residues, and there is 44% homology between the two subtypes. Through G proteins, cannabinoids inhibit adenylyl cyclase, decrease Ca^{2+} conductance, and increase inwardly rectifying K^+ conductance. They also induce release of arachidonic acid, stimulate formation of nitric oxide, and activate mitogen-activated protein (MAP) kinase (Childers and Breivogel 1998; Di Marzo 1998).

The cannabinoid receptors are distributed to many parts of the central nervous system (table 10.4) (Herkenham et al. 1991; Thomas et al. 1992). The highest density is seen in the basal ganglia (substantia nigra pars reticulata, globus pallidus, entopeduncular nucleus, caudate, and putamen) and cerebellum (molecular layer). Intermediate levels of binding were seen in the cortex (layers I and VI) and hippocampus (dentate gyrus and CA pyramidal cell regions). The cortical distribution of

Table 10.4
Central distribution of cannabinoid receptors

High Binding
Basal ganglia
substantia nigra pars reticulata
globus pallidus
entopeduncular nucleus
caudate
putamen
Cerebellum (molecular layer)
Intermediate Binding
Cerebral cortex (layers I and VI)
Hippocampus (dentate gyrus and CA pyramidal cells)
Frontal cortex
Amygdala
Cingulate gyrus
Low Binding
Spinal cord
Brain stem (medulla and pons)
Thalamic nuclei
Hypothalamus
Corpus callosum
Cerebellum (deep nuclear layer)

See text for references.

cannabinoid receptors is particularly high in the frontal cortex. Binding was also observed in limbic structures including the amygdala and cingulate gyrus. Low levels of binding were observed in the spinal cord and brain stem (medulla and pons), thalamic nuclei, hypothalamus, corpus callosum and the deep nuclear layer of the cerebellum. The neuroanatomical distribution of cannabinoid receptors well account for the cognitive, motor, and emotional effects of cannabis. In contrast, there are little or no cannabinoid receptors in the brain stem, which explains why cannabis has such a high fatal dose. Similarities in binding are observed between cannabinoids and anandamide. Binding to cannabinoid receptors by anandamide and a selective CB_1 antagonist (SR 141716A) and agonist (CP 55,940), showed that all three ligands compete for the same receptor (Adams et al. 1998).

Chronic exposure to THC causes a regulation of cannabinoid receptors, which appears to be region-specific (Zhuang et al. 1998). For example, while increases in cannabinoid receptor mRNA are seen in the cerebellum and hippocampus at 7 and 14 days of chronic treatment, decreases were seen in the striatum from days 2 to 14. However, levels returned to normal in all the regions by day 21, which coincides with reports of behavioral tolerance.

Physiological Effects of Endocannabinoids

Similar to exogenous cannabinoids, the endocannabinoids have roles in behavior, motor function, memory, thermoregulation and analgesia (Childers and Breivogel 1998; Adams et al. 1998). Endocannabinoids have a biphasic effect on locomotion, stimulating it at low doses and inhibiting it at higher doses, which has been attributed to cannabinoid receptors in the basal ganglia and cerebellum. Detrimental effects on memory are consistent with inhibitory effects of endocannabinoids in the hippocampus. Analgesic effects are produced at spinal and supraspinal levels, involving structures such as the dorsal horn and periaqueductal gray. Along with the similarities between endocannabinoids and cannabis constituents (referred to here as exocannabinoids), are significant differences. Although they have several common physiological effects, they are prevented by a CB_1 antagonist (SR 141716A) when induced by THC, but *not* when induced by anandamide (Adams et al. 1998).

Interaction with Other Neurochemical Systems

Amino Acids

Anandamide has dual effects on NMDA receptor function. It reduces NMDA Ca^{2+} currents, which is mediated by cannabinoid receptors and G-protein mechanisms (Hampson et al. 1998). However, anandamide *potentiates* NMDA currents due to a direct effect on the NMDA receptor itself. THC did *not* have the same effect. So anandamide appears to have at least one other CNS effect that is not through the cannabinoid receptors. THC also reduces AMPA/kainate activity, which is mediated by CB_1 receptors (Shen and Thayer 1999) (table 10.5). THC may in-

Table 10.5
Neuropharmacological effects of THC

Cannabinoid	Activation of cannabinoid (CB) receptors
Amino acids	reduces AMPA/kainate activity
Acetylcholine	Inhibition of ACh release (biphasic)
Monoamines	Activates mesolimbic DA Increases NE turnover
Opioids	Synergistic interaction with opioids
Neuroendocrine	Reduces testicular production of testosterone Enhances target responsivity to gonadotropins Reduces LH and prolactin secretion Increases adrenocorticotrophic hormone levels Increases corticosterone levels
Eicosanoids	Inhibition of PGE and PGF

See text for references.

teract indirectly with NMDA systems. THC-induced analgesia, but not hypothermia, is reduced by NMDA antagonists. These effects were not altered by nitric oxide manipulations (Thorat and Bhargava 1994).

There do not seem to be any direct GABA-mediated effects of THC (Pertwee et al. 1991). However, THC was found to enhance binding of ligands to the benzodiazepine receptor (Koe et al. 1985).

Acetylcholine

Cannabinoid agonists (e.g., THC) were found in vivo to produce a lasting inhibition of acetylcholine release in the medial-prefrontal cortex and hippocampus, in doses comparable to human use of cannabis (Gessa et al. 1998). This inhibition is dose dependent, mediated by the CB_1 receptor, and did not diminish after 7 days of chronic exposure (Carta et al. 1998). It is interesting to note that a higher dose of cannabinoid antagonist alone increased acetylcholine release, suggesting that acetylcholine release is under tonic inhibition by endogenous cannabinoids. High doses (30 mg/kg) of cannabinoids *increase* acetylcholine levels in several brain areas (Tripathi et al. 1987). The cataleptic effect of THC in higher doses (10 mg/kg IP in rats) was found to be mediated by central cholinergic pathways (Pertwee and Ross 1991). The decrease in acetylcholine in response to THC has also been related to an increase of slow-wave activity on EEG (Domino 1981). In vitro THC (1–100 nM) inhibited muscarinic receptor binding, which also ocurred with two nonpsychoactive cannabinoids (cannabidiol and cannabinol) (Ali et al. 1991). However, these effects were not observed in vivo.

Monoamines

Cannabinoid agonists produce dose-related activation of meso-prefrontal dopaminergic transmission, which depends upon the CB_1 receptor (Diana et al. 1998a). Conversely, withdrawal from chronic cannabinoid administration produces a reduction in mesolimbic dopaminergic transmission. Although THC stimulates the presynaptic activity of mesolimbic dopaminergic neurons, there is a decrease in postsynaptic sensitivity (Bonnin et al. 1993). Further, this effect is modulated by estrogen, but not estradiol. THC increases the firing rate and burst-pattern firing in the ventral tegmental area and substantia nigra, although the ventral tegmental area is more sensitive in this respect (French et al. 1997). In contrast, cannabidiol failed to have this effect. *In vivo* microdialysis, on the other hand, showed that THC has no effect on extracellular dopamine or 5-HT concentrations in the striatum or nucleus accumbens (Castaneda et al. 1991). However, this study also failed to show behavioral differences between drug and vehicle groups. Cannabinoids also induce increases in norepinephrine, but not 5-HT turnover in the prefrontal cortex (Jentsch et al. 1997).

Opioids

Cannabinoids are known to interact with opioid systems. This is particularly relevant to their analgesic effects and is discussed at length in chapter 8.

Neuroendocrine

Cannabis compounds interact with the endocrine system. THC reduces testicular production of testosterone, even though it enhances responsivity at neuroendocrine target sites to gonadotropins (Dalterio et al. 1985a, 1987) (table 10.5). The effects of THC on plasma gonadotropins may be mediated by effects on hypothalamic catecholamines and direct gonadal effects (Dalterio et al. 1985b; Murphy et al. 1994). THC also reduces male sexual behaviors in the presence of a receptive female, but the effects are reversible with time (Harclerode 1984).

Despite structrual similarity of cannabinoids to estrogens, they do not possess direct estrogenic activity (Abel 1981). Neither psychoactive nor nonpsychoactive cannabinoids acted as agonists in assays of the estrogen receptor (Ruh et al. 1997). THC does suppress secretion of luteinizing hormone and prolactin and is mediated through central and/or pituitary actions (Rettori et al. 1988; Murphy et al. 1991). The effects of cannabinoids on brain function may differ between the sexes (Rodriguez de Fonseca et al. 1994). For example, cannabinoid receptor affinity is higher in males than females in the limbic forebrain, although receptor density is the same. Sensitivity within females varies across the estrous cycle, where affinity is higher in diestrus and lower in estrus, but receptor density was unchanged. Direct effects occur on the ovulatory process and on steroid secretion from the corpus luteum and the preovulatory follicle (Tyrey 1984). Whether these effects have significant effects on physiological function remains to be seen. The CB_1 receptor is present in the uterus and chronic THC may act as a weak uterotrophic agent (Paria et al. 1994). In addition to sex effects, THC also had similar electrophysiological effects to 17-β-estradiol in the hippocampus, increasing field potentials at very low (picomolar) doses, but depressing function at higher (nanomolar) doses (Foy et al. 1982).

Cannabinoids interact with the adrenal axis also. Anandamide, similar to THC, activates the hypothalamic-pituitary-adrenal axis, increasing levels of adrenocorticotrophic hormone and corticosterone (Weidenfeld et al. 1994). THC interacts primarily with the type II class of glucocorticoid receptors (Eldridgde and Landfield 1990). Receptor down-regulation was noted after chronic (14 days) THC treatment, comparable to that seen in chronic stress or high corticosteroid administration. THC, but not cannabidiol, showed some noncompetitive agonist properties at glucocorticoid receptors (Eldridge et al. 1991). Withdrawal from chronic cannabis administration elevates corticotrophin-releasing factor (CRF) and gene transcription in the central nucleus amygdala with maximal increases corresponding to peak behavioral signs of withdrawal (Rodriguez de Fonseca et al. 1997).

Eicosanoids

THC has been shown to alter eicosanoid levels (Reichman et al. 1987). Psychoactive, but not nonpsychoactive constituents altered levels of prostaglandins (PGE and PGF). This effect was region-specific, altering levels in the striatum but not cerebellum.

Pharmacokinetics

Cannabis is most commonly consumed by smoking in a cigarette or pipe. Because the average cannabis cigarette contains 0.5 to 1 g of cannabis, and the usual THC content of cannabis is 4 to 5 percent, then the average cannabis cigarette would contain approximately 50 mg of THC (Julien 1998). Of this amount, 25–50% (12–25 mg) of the THC is available in the smoke. Accordingly, the amount of THC that is absorbed into the blood after smoking one cannabis cigarette is 0.4 to 10 mg. People appear to regulate their intake based on the potency of the cannabis being smoked by altering the length and depth of inhalation. Smoking topography measures revealed smaller puff and inhalation volumes and shorter puff duration for the high cannabis dose compared to the low dose (Heishman et al. 1989).

After smoking the first puff, the acute intoxication starts within 6 to 12 minutes, and maximum effects occur at 15 to 30 minutes. Effects typically last 2 to 4 hours. THC remains in fatty tissues and has a long half-life of 57 hours. The lungs and liver convert THC to the metabolite 11-OH-THC, which is also active. There is a recirculation of 10–15% of hepatic metabolites. 11-OH-THC is further converted by the liver to inactive metabolites, which are eliminated by the kidneys.

Although there is a high degree of binding to protein, both bound and unbound drug is metabolized. The estimated terminal half-life is relatively long at 1.24 days, and is apparently unaffected by enzyme induction. Tolerance may be due to a shift toward highly polar metabolites in the brain, rather than an increased elimination or decreased sensitivity of the brain tissue to THC (Magour et al. 1977).

Route of administration alters the effectiveness of cannabinoids. Orally administered THC has a slower and more erratic absorption. THC was found to be 45 times more effective for analgesia after intravenous than after subcutaneous administration (Martin 1985). The pharmacokinetics of different chemical constituents of cannabis vary (Consroe et al. 1991). The elimination half-life of cannabidiol is estimated to be about 2–5 days, with no differences between genders. Comparably, the elimination half-life of Δ^1-THC is approximately 4 days, and may be prolonged in chronic users (Johansson et al. 1988, 1989).

The central distribution of THC was studied in the primate brain using positron emission tomography (Charlambous et al. 1991). The THC analog, (–)-^{18}F-Δ^8-THC, was administered intravenously to baboons. Neuroanatomical distribution in the baboon brain was comparable to prior autoradiographic studies, with binding evident in the basal ganglia, thalamus, and cerebellum. Clearance was rapid from these areas.

General Effects

Subjective Effects

As with many other psychoactive drugs, the psychological effects of cannabis are variable, depending on the degree of prior use, as well as the expectations and personality of the user (Taylor 1998). The acute subjective effects of cannabis may include relaxation, mild euphoria, and giddiness (table 10.6). There is a heightening of sensory perceptions and time is perceived to pass more slowly. Adverse effects include a panic or anxiety reaction and are more common in novice users. Half of users report having experienced adverse effects at least once (O'Brien 1996). Other adverse effects may include dissociative symptoms such as derealization, the feeling that one's experiences are not real, or depersonalization, a feeling of detachment from oneself (Mathew et al. 1993). The best treatment for these experiences is supportive reassurance, or "talking down," although anxiolytic medication may be used in more extreme cases.

Table 10.6
Physiological effects of cannabis

Subjective Effects (vary with set and setting)
Relaxation
Mild euphoria
Giddiness
Heightened sensory perceptions
Stimulates appetite
Perceived slower passage of time
Panic or anxiety
Dissociative symptoms
Physiological Effects
Increases heart rate
Reduces body temperature
Slowed gastrointestinal function
Electrophysiology
Mixed excitation and inhibition, biphasic pattern
Increased theta activity (long-term use)
"Alpha hyperfrontality"
Increased slow-wave sleep, reduces REM sleep

See text for references.

Physiological Effects

THC produces dose-dependent increases in heart rate and reductions in body temperature after injection, maximizing after 2 to 3 hours (table 10.6) (Heishman et al. 1989). Similarly, anandamide creates hypothermia in mice after injection (Fride and Mechoulam 1993). The cognitive effects of THC are dissociable from the autonomic effects (Bachman et al. 1979).

Certain cannabinoids exert an inhibitory effect on gastrointestinal transit (Shook and Burks 1989). THC slows the rate of gastric emptying and small intestinal transit. Other cannabinoids ($\Delta^{9,11}$-THC, cannabinol, and nabilone) also inhibit transit through the small intestine in mice, but they have less effect on gastric emptying. In contrast, cannabidiol has no effect on gastric emptying or intestinal transit. Further, THC has a greater effect on transit in the small intestine than in the large intestine.

Cannabis use does not appear to induce a "hangover" syndrome like that produced with alcohol or sedative-hypnotics in terms of sleep effects, mood, psychomotor skills, or cognitive function (Chait 1990).

Hormonal and Reproductive Effects

The hormonal effects of smoking cannabis were examined in healthy male subjects (cigarettes with 2.8% THC) (Cone et al. 1986). Plasma luteinizing hormone levels were reduced and cortisol was significantly elevated. Nonsignificant depressions were seen in prolactin, FSH, and testosterone, as well as a nonsignificant elevation of GH. In female volunteers, smoking cannabis (1 g cigarette, 1.8% THC) caused a 30% suppression of plasma luteinizing hormone levels during the luteal phase of the menstrual cycle (Mendelson et al. 1986). The authors speculate that this could have adverse effects on reproductive function. Althogh cannabis usage does adversely affect sperm production, the physiological significance of these effects is unclear (Abel 1981). There is no evidence at this time that cannabis exposure reduces male fertility or increases risk for dominant lethal mutations in animals or humans.

Appetite and Ingestive Behavior

Animal studies support the reputation of cannabis for stimulating appetite, although this effect has not been universally reported (Graceffo and Robinson 1998). Sated rats showed substantial hyperphagia when administered THC at doses of 0.5, 1.0, and 2.0 mg/kg (Williams et al. 1998). This appetitive effect of THC was found in other species, such as dogs, whereas LSD, by contrast, produces anorexia (Vaupel and Morton 1982).

Conversely, food intake and body weight are reduced by the selective cannabinoid CB_1 antagonist SR 141716. Tolerance developed to the anorectic effect of SR 141716 within 5 days of chronic treatment, but body weight remained low throughout 14 days of treatment. In contrast, chronic THC treatment (15 days) suppresses intake of food and water (Drewnowski and Grinker 1978). This effect is of short duration, with no apparent rebound eating afterwards. However, this may be due to general low arousal rather than a specific appetite suppression.

Electrophysiology: Animal Studies

Electrophysiological responses to cannabinoids are complex. THC produces both CNS excitation and depression in several electrophysiological paradigms (Turkanis and Karler 1981). The effect produced depended on the cannabinoid dosage and paradigm used. In contrast to THC, cannabidiol generated no CNS excitation, and produced either depressant effects or no effects at all.

THC (0.75–4.0 mg/kg IP) produced a biphasic pattern on EEG in rhesus monkeys (Matsuzaki et al. 1987). The first phase consisted of high-voltage slow waves (HVSW) on the EEG, which appeared 20–30 minutes after drug administration and lasted for 3–4 hours. Spike-bursts occurred in frontal and temporal lobes and hypothalamus, theta waves ocurred in parietal and occipital lobes, and generalized HVSW ocurred in subcortical regions. Behavioral sedation, bradycardia, and hypothermia were also evident during this phase. Similarly, high-voltage EEG bursts were also seen in the rat after THC administration, which carried over into the initial subsequent REM sleep episodes (Buonamici et al. 1982). The second EEG/behavioral phase consisted of high-voltage fast waves on EEG, with decreased neocortical spike-bursts. These physiological, behavioral, and electroencephalographic changes correlated with THC levels and disposition in blood. EEG slowing has been related to the concomitant decrease in neocortical acetylcholine release (Domino 1981).

Electrophysiology: Human Studies

When long-term chronic cannabis users (i.e., daily use for 15–24 years) were compared to short-term users and nonusers, they were found to have elevated absolute power of theta activity over bilateral frontal-central cortex, as well as significantly increased interhemispheric coherence of theta activity across central and posterior regions (Struve et al. 1998). Concurrent reaction time studies also showed slowed cognitive processing in that group. Other work by this group has shown that in daily cannabis users, as contrasted with nonusers, there is an association between increased absolute and relative power and interhemispheric coherence of EEG alpha activity over the bilateral frontal-central cortex (termed "alpha hyperfrontality") (Struve et al. 1994).

These EEG changes have been related to effects of cannabis on motor functions and sleep. One study of occasional cannabis smokers had them report quantitative changes in their mood during EEG monitoring (Lukas et al. 1995). Mood elevations were reported during the first 15 minutes, which occurred while plasma THC levels were rising and EEG alpha power was significantly higher.

A few studies have been performed with event-related potentials (ERP) to examine the cognitive effects of THC. In subjects viewing emotionally valenced words (neutral, negative, or positive), THC produced a behavioral decrease in recognition rate (Leweke et al. 1998). The ERPs showed the typical difference between old and new words (enhanced positivity for old words beginning 250 milliseconds poststimulus), and THC enhanced the positivity in response to old words. This counterintuitive dissociation between ERPs and behavioral indices was interpreted as a reflection of implicit memory processes underlying the ERP effect.

Several studies of ERPs and brain function have produced mixed results due to methodological confounds. When subjects are screened for medical and psychiatric illness, and age effects were controlled, THC does not alter brain stem and auditory or visual P300 responses (Patrick et al. 1997). Despite daily cannabis use in subjects, the only finding consisted of an elevated auditory P50 amplitude.

Sleep

Anandamide increases slow-wave and REM sleep at the expense of wakefulness (Murillo-Rodriguez et al. 1998). In contrast, chronic THC treatment in nonhuman primates reduced the time spent in slow-wave sleep (Adams and Barratt 1975). The time spent in stage 1 increased with repeated treatment and remained elevated through recovery.

Cannabis has electrophysiological effects on human sleep as well. Daily doses (70 to 210 mg) of THC reduced REM sleep and increased stage 4 sleep (Feinberg et al. 1976, 1975). Abrupt withdrawal increased REM and reduced stage 4 to baseline levels.

Neuroimaging: Human Studies

A few studies have been done to determine the in vivo effects of cannabis on humans using functional neuroimaging. The effects of an acute dose of THC on cerebral blood flow (CBF) was examined in volunteers with prior histories of exposure to cannabis by using positron emission tomography (PET) (Mathew et al. 1997). THC increased CBF in the frontal regions bilaterally, insula and cingulate gyrus and subcortical regions with somewhat greater effects in the right hemisphere. The effects were significant at 60 minutes for the lower dose and at 30 minutes for the larger dose. There was also a highly significant change in the anterior/posterior ratio, reflecting minimal change in occipital regions but significant increases in frontal CBF. Ratings of subjective effects correlated most markedly with alterations in the right frontal region.

Another study examined the effects of THC on regional brain glucose metabolism (^{18}F-2-fluoro-2-deoxyglucose and PET) following an acute intravenous dose (Volkow et al. 1991). Changes in global glucose metabolism in response to THC were variable, and only the cerebellum consistently showed an increase in metabolic activity. Further, this cerebellar increase was correlated with subjective ratings of intoxication and plasma THC concentration. This finding is interesting in light of the high density of cannabinoid receptors in the cerebellum.

A third neuroimaging study using CBF (PET) and magnetic resonance imaging found a significant increase in cortical and cerebellar blood flow following THC administration, but again this effect was inconsistent across subjects (Mathew et al. 1998). The decrease in cerebellar CBF was related to alterations in time sense. This is interesting in light of the proposed role of the cerebellum as an internal timing system.

Motor Effects

The effects of THC on motor activity are dependent on dosage, species examined, and behavioral paradigm used. THC increases activity in mice but reduces social investigation and sexual behaviors (Evans et al. 1976; Cutler and Mackintosh 1984). Central administration of anandamide also increases locomotor activity in immobility and open-field tests (Murillo-Rodriguez et al. 1998). THC and other cannabinoids were shown to produce ataxia in dogs at doses as low as 2 μg/kg (Stark and Dews 1980).

The motor changes produced by THC may relate to altered nigrostriatal dopaminergic function (Navarro et al. 1993). An oral dose of THC reduced spontaneous motor activity and stereotypic behaviors (e.g., rearing and self-grooming) in the rat. These motor changes correlated with a low number of D_1 receptors in the striatum, but not other measures of dopamine or 5-HT activity. Anandamide motor inhibition also corresponded with reductions in nigrostriatal activity (Romero et al. 1995). High doses (10 mg/kg IP) produce catalepsy (Pertwee and Ross 1991).

Cognition: Animal Studies

Central administration (intracerebroventricular) of anandamide has been found to impair memory consolidation in animals (Murillo-Rodriguez et al. 1998). Both THC and anandamide impair recent memory in animals (Mallet and Beninger 1998). This effect was mediated by the CB_1 receptor in a working memory (delayed nonmatch to sample) paradigm. The impairment of working memory by cannabinoids may relate to the activation of mesoprefrontal dopaminergic transmission via CB_1 receptors, because overstimulation of dopamine receptors impairs working memory (Diana et al. 1998a; Jentsch et al. 1997). On the other hand, administration of dopamine (D_1 and D_2) agonists improved the memory impairment induced by anandamide on an inhibitory avoidance response (Castellano et al. 1997). Clearly, the experimental paradigm used, as well as endogenous versus exogenous ligands alters the results obtained. The effect of THC on a working memory measure (delayed-match-to-sample) was found to correspond to effects in the hippocampus (Heyser et al. 1993). However, these effects completely reversed within 24 hours of injection. Another possible mechanism for THC's effect on memory is inhibition of hippocampal long-term potentiation, although this has only been observed with synthetic cannabinoids (Collins et al. 1994).

Table 10.7
Sources of variability in cognitive studies of THC

Dosage/potency
Route of administration
Frequency of use
Acute vs. chronic effects
Subject population

See text for references.

Cognition: Human Studies

The effects of cannabis on cognition is a complicated issue. Numerous studies have been conducted to measure the mental effects of cannabis, but many of these are fraught with methodological problems. Several variables must be controlled in this type of research, including the dosage and potency of cannabis used, route of administration (e.g., smoking, oral, etc.), chronicity of dose, and the subject population (nonusers, occasional users, chronic users) employed (table 10.7). Population make-up has a large effect on outcome because there have been differences demonstrated between naive and experienced cannabis users (Murray 1986).

Impairment is observed in some studies on measures of concentration and attention (e.g., reaction time, digit span, and digit symbol tasks) (table 10.8). In some studies, the effect only occured at the higher (2.7%) but not lower (1.3%) dose of THC (Wilson et al. 1994). Some studies did not show an effect on divided-attention tasks, while other studies showed effects correlating with THC plasma levels for approximately 2 hours after smoking (Barnett et al. 1985; Heishman et al. 1989). The nature and complexity of the task may affect whether differences are found between cannabis and placebo groups. No effects are seen on simple measures of immediate or sustained attention (Rafaelsen et al. 1973; Waskow et al. 1970; Hooker and Jones 1987). Casual and heavy cannabis users did not differ on a simple vigilance task, but both were impaired on a goal directed serial alternation task, requiring mental calculations, working memory, and alternating attention (Casswell and Marks 1973a, 1973b). Cannabis (1.2% THC) increased the Stroop

Table 10.8
Cognitive effects of cannabis

Attention/concentration	Simple and sustained attention are unaffected Mild impairment of some forms of complex attention
Memory	Impairment of recent memory, consolidation Increased recognition false positive errors Remote memory unaffected
Perceptual and motor	Mild effects at low doses Hallucinations and catalepsy at high doses
Executive functions	Mild increase in perseverative responses with heavy use

Note: Effects of THC on cognition are likely to be dose and task dependent. See text for references.

effect, decreasing subjects' ability to inhibit automatic responses (Hooker and Jones 1987). Yet performance was not affected on the paced auditory serial attention test (PASAT), a demanding task requiring attention, working memory, and mental calculations.

The effects of cannabis on memory was examined in numerous studies, and again the results are variable. For example, fewer words are recalled from a list by subjects administered cannabis compared to placebo, but no effects were seen on a verbal paired-associate learning (Abel 1971; Hooker and Jones 1987).

Perhaps the most consistent effect of cannabis is consolidation of information from short-term memory (Dornbush et al 1971; Murray 1986). In contrast, cannabis does not appear to impair access to information already in long-term memory (Darley et al. 1977; Parker et al. 1980). While cannabis and placebo groups performed equally well on a word list recognition task, the cannabis group made more false positive errors (Abel 1970, 1971). Another effect on memory reported in severeal studies is increased intrusion of irrelevant material (Abel 1970, 1971; Clark et al. 1970; Tinklenberg et al. 1970; Pfefferbaum et al. 1977).

THC produced small but consistent detrimental effects and increased the variability of performance on a battery of sensory and perceptual-motor tests (Peters et al. 1976). This mild effect is in contrast to the profound subjective effects concurrently reported on subjective measures (the subjective drug effects questionnaire). Subjective changes reported in mood and perceptual experiences were more pronounced among occasional than frequent cannabis users. Although it has effects on motor performance, it appears that cannabis has little effect on eye movements (Stapleton et al. 1986; Baloh et al. 1979). No effects were observed on a controlled verbal fluency measure (controlled oral word associations) (Hooker and Jones 1987).

Chronic use has been associated with an "amotivational syndrome" characterized by loss of interest in social activities, school, work, or other goal-directed activities. Cannabis use is cited as the cause of this phenomenon, but there is no evidence to support any causal relationship. There is evidence, however, that the symptoms of the "amotivational syndrome" are secondary to depression (Musty and Kraback 1995). In contrast to ethanol, there is no evidence to support that cannabis causes an increase in violent behavior (Murray 1986). However, cannabis use may be contraindicated in those with preexisting psychiatric disturbances such as bipolar disorder or schizophrenia.

Cognitive Effects in Experienced Users

A study of experienced cannabis smokers tested them on cognitive measures using two doses (1.75% or 3.55%) and placebo (Wilson et al. 1994). The functions most sensitive to the effects of THC were mental processing speed (digit-symbol substitution) and reaction time. When compared with cannabis nonusers, chronic users of cannabis—with a mean duration of use of 6.76 years and an average daily intake of 150 mg of THC—were found to have slower reactions on perceptuo-motor tasks, but no differences on intelligence or memory tests (Varma et al. 1988).

Compared to infrequent (monthly) users of cannabis, regular (daily) users show decreases in attention and executive functions, such as greater perseverations on card sorting and reduced learning of word lists (Pope and Yurgelun-Todd 1996). However, studies comparing heavy users to occasional users or nonusers, although otherwise well-controlled, are plagued with the methodological problem of self-selecting groups. It may well be that people with executive and attentional dysfunctions are more prone to heavier cannabis use. Indeed, abstinent polysubstance users were found to have lesser grey matter in prefrontal cortex than nonusers (Liu et al. 1998).

In a study by Fletcher and colleagues (1996), long-term users tended to experience greater difficulty in complex tasks of memory and attention. However, it was concluded that these deficits are comparably subtle. The older long-term users were functional, employable, and did not show the degree of cognitive deficits that are associated with comparable use of alcohol. The physical health of the subjects was generally good.

THC and Ethanol

Comparisons have been made of the cognitive effects of THC and alcohol, alone and in combination. Separately, THC and alcohol were found to produce comparable impairments on the digit-symbol substitution test and word recall (Heishman et al. 1997). The interaction of THC and ethanol was studied in a signal detection paradigm (Marks and MacAvoy 1989). Cannabis users were less impaired in peripheral signal detection than nonusers while intoxicated by cannabis and/or alcohol. These findings suggest the development of tolerance and cross-tolerance in regular cannabis users and/or the ability to compensate for intoxication effects.

Both THC and ethanol increase reaction time, and produce decrements in standing steadiness and psychomotor coordination (Belgrave et al. 1979). Whereas the peak effects of ethanol appeared quickly and wore off quickly (after 280 minutes), THC's effects were slower in onset and longer in duration. The effects of combined THC and ethanol are additive and not synergistic, and THC did not alter blood-ethanol levels. Other studies have shown an interaction between ethanol and THC on psychomotor skills necessary for driving, although there were no interactions on the subjective "high," heart rate acceleration, or THC plasma concentration (Perez-Reyes et al. 1988).

Cognitive Effects of Cannabis: Conclusions

The cognitive effects of cannabis are mild, and have many variables (dosage, chronicity of use, cognitive task employed, etc.). Of prime importance in such studies is the usage (or misusage) of the term *impair-*

ment. Many studies label an *impairment* when they find statistically significant differences between users and nonusers, or various dosages of THC. While statistically significant, this does not address the size of the effect. Neuropsychologists use a cutoff of two standard deviations below the mean to signify impairment. While cannabis does create some subtle deficits, the test performances are often well within the normal range and would not be diagnosed as an impairment.

A comprehensive study by Wert and Raulin (1986) examined both American and cross-cultural studies, and pointed out methodological problems in the body of research on cannabis. It was concluded that cannabis use may produce subtle impairment, but there is no evidence that cannabis produces gross structural cerebral changes or functional impairment. Many cannabis users remain intelligent, functional, and productive members of society (Grinspoon 1999; Davidson 1999).

Tolerance, Dependence, and Addiction

A rapid tolerance to the acute effects of THC occurs in mice, which rapidly reverses as well (Hutcheson et al. 1998). Although chronic exposure to THC alters cannabinoid receptors, this effect is not irreversible (Westlake et al. 1991).

Pharmacokinetic tolerance to THC occurs, which parallels the development of psychological, cardiovascular, and hypothermic effects (Hunt and Jones 1980). These changes include altered metabolic clearance, distribution volume, urinary excretion, and slow elimination of metabolites. Low renal clearance indicated an accumulation of metabolites. Despite the pharmacokinetic tolerance evident here, it was concluded that this alone is not sufficient to account for tolerance to cardiovascular, psychological, and skin hypothermic effects, which are likely to involve central effects.

Cannabis has the potential to produce dependence (Taylor 1998). Like many drugs of abuse, cerebral dopamine is involved in the pleasurable effects of cannabis, and corticotrophin-releasing factor is involved in the unpleasant withdrawal phenomena. While central dopaminergic activity does not automatically make a drug addictive (e.g., neither the antidepressant bupropion nor the dopamine agonist bromocriptine appear to

Table 10.9
Cannabis withdrawal syndrome

Restlessness
Irritability
Insomnia
Nausea
Muscle cramping

See text for references.

be addictive), it does raise the potential. On the other hand, cannabis is less addictive and produces milder withdrawal symptoms compared to cocaine, alcohol, and heroin (Taylor 1998). Nonetheless, dependence to cannabis may develop after heavy chronic use, and the intensity of the withdrawal syndrome is related to the degree of use and tolerance.

Concurrent use with ethanol may alter the patterns of drug use. While low to moderate doses of ethanol do not influence the amount of cannabis self-administered by humans, there is evidence that chronic THC administration can increase ethanol intake (McMillan and Saodgrass 1991; Chait and Perry 1994).

Cannabis Withdrawal Syndrome

Cessation of chronic cannabis use is known to produce a withdrawal syndrome consisting of restlessness, irritability, insomnia, nausea, and muscle cramping (table 10.9) (O'Brien 1996). However, this syndrome is only seen in people who use high daily amounts and then suddenly stop (O'Brien 1996). These symptoms are not usually seen in clinical populations, and frequent users of cannabis are not driven by a fear to avoid a withdrawal syndrome as seen in opioid addiction.

In mice, somatic signs of withdrawal include wet dog shakes, front paw tremor, ataxia, hunched posture, tremor, ptosis, piloerection, mastication and decreased locomotor activity (Hutcheson et al. 1998). The CB_1 antagonist (SR141716A) has been used to precipitate a withdrawal state in THC-tolerant animals, and higher doses of THC produced a greater withdrawal syndrome (Aceto et al. 1995; Cook et al. 1998). Withdrawal from chronic cannabis use reduces mesolimbic dopaminergic transmission, which is also observed in other drugs of abuse (Diana et al. 1998b). Withdrawal from chronic cannabis administration elevates corticotrophin-releasing factor (CRF) and activity in the central nucleus amygdala (Rodriguez de Fonseca et al. 1997).

Abuse of Therapeutic Cannabinoids

Dronabinol (Marinol) is an oral form of THC indicated for treatment of AIDS and cancer chemotherapy (Calhoun et al. 1998). Because it is the active principle of cannabis, there has been some concern over its abuse potential. However, in a thorough study utilizing literature review, surveys, and interviews with medical and law enforcement personnel, it was concluded that dronabinol has very low abuse potential (Calhoun et al. 1998). There was no evidence of abuse or illegal diversion of dronabinol. Prescription data indicate usage within the therapeutic dosage range over time, and no instances of "script-chasing" or "doctor-shopping" were reported. As opposed to smoked cannabis, the onset of action in Dronabinol is slow and gradual. It seems at best weakly reinforcing, and many users report unappealing effects.

Therapeutic Uses of Cannabis and Cannabinoids

Cannabis shows promise for clinical treatment of many illnesses, including glaucoma, nausea and vomiting, analgesia, spasticity, multiple sclerosis, and AIDS wasting syndrome (table 10.10) (Taylor 1998). While the legality of treatment with cannabis varies from region to region, ballot initiatives in California and Arizona have recently made crude

Table 10.10
Potential therapeutic uses of cannabis and cannabinoids

Glaucoma
Nausea/emesis
Pain
Muscle spasticity
Multiple sclerosis
Appetite loss (e.g. AIDS wasting syndrome)

See text for references.

cannabis accessible to patients under certain circumstances (Voth and Schwartz 1997).

Antiemetic

THC was first used to control nausea and vomiting during chemotherapy in the 1970s (Vincent et al. 1983). Until the development of 5-HT_3 antagonists, dronabinol and cannabis were frequently used by cancer patients receiving chemotherapy (Taylor 1998). THC and synthetic cannabinoids have been effective in controlled clinical trials. THC is superior to placebo and as effective or superior to prochlorperazine. Although there are more drug-related effects associated with THC than prochlorperazine, they did not reduce the patients' preference for the drug (Ungerleider et al. 1982). The antiemetic effectiveness of THC correlates with the subjective high reported (Vincent et al. 1983). THC is effective in several chemotherapy regimens, including methotrexate and the doxorubicin/cyclophosphamide/fluorouracil combination. Cisplatin treatment, however, is more resistant. Side effects of THC are generally well tolerated, and use may be limited in the elderly or with higher doses. Nabilone is a synthetic cannabinoid that is more effective than prochlorperazine in chemotherapy-induced emesis, including cisplatin. Its side effects are similar to THC. Levonantradol is another synthetic cannabinoid with antiemetic effects, and may be administered orally or intramuscularly. The side effect of dysphoria may limit its use.

Appetite Stimulant

A review of evidence supported the use of pure THC preparations to treat nausea associated with cancer chemotherapy and to stimulate appetite (Voth and Schwartz 1997). In patients with anorexia due to advanced cancer, THC (2.5 mg PO tid) was effective in stimulating appetite and was well tolerated at low doses (Nelson et al. 1994).

Cannabinoids produced positive results for treatment of AIDS-related anorexia. Positive results of open trials were later confirmed with methodologically controlled studies. Dronabinol (2.5 mg PO twice daily) produced consistent and substantial improvement in appetite in patients with AIDS (Beal et al. 1995, 1997). Patients also reported improved mood and tended to maintain stable body weight for at least 7 months. Side effects reported were primarily psychoactive. Increases were seen in body fat (1%) and prealbumin (Struwe et al. 1993). There was also decreased symptom distress and improved appetite. There are reports that the psychotropic effects of dronabinol can be decreased by administration of prochlorperazine (Plasse et al. 1991).

Glaucoma

In the early 1970s, cannabis was noted to reduce intraocular pressure in people with glaucoma (Cooler and Gregg 1977). In a controlled study, THC decreased intraocular pressure an average of 37%, with maximum decreases at 51% of baseline. Concurrent increases in heart rate were also observed. The mechanism of this effect of THC is uncertain.

Spasticity

There are some antispasticity effects of THC (Petro and Ellenberger 1981). Animal studies have indicated that THC inhibits polysynaptic reflexes. In a controlled study, THC (10 mg) significantly reduced spasticity of various etiologies. However, no benefit was noted in patients with spasticity due to cerebellar disease. In a survey of multiple sclerosis patients, cannabis was reported to relieve spasticity, pain, and tremors (Consroe et al. 1997). A recent study in a mouse model of multiple sclerosis (chronic relapsing experimental encephalomyelitis) has provided more quantitative support along these lines (Baker et al. 2000). Cannabinoid receptor agonists improved tremor and spasticity in mice, which was dependent on the CB_2 and, to a greater degree, the CB_1 receptors.

Toxicity

Developmental Toxicity

Cannabinoids are teratogenic and should be avoided during pregnancy. Cannabis use during pregnancy is associated with lower gestational age at delivery, increased risk of prematurity, and reduction in birth weight (Abel et al. 1980; Walker, et al. 1999; Sherwood et al. 1999). There are also behavioral alterations in the development of spontaneous locomotion and exploration in rats (Navarro et al. 1995). Exposure to THC through gestational and lactational periods produces changes in response to novelty, social interactions, and sexual behavior. Primates exposed to THC in utero show an altered visual attention characterized by a reduced ability to disengage from novel stimuli (Golub et al. 1982).

Human newborns of mothers who smoke cannabis during pregnancy experience mild withdrawal symptoms and some autonomic disruption upon childbirth (Fried 1995a, 1995b). Although behavioral consequences are not apparent until 3 years of age, decrements in languange comprehension, sustained attention, memory, and behavior are related to in utero cannabis exposure.

Pulmonary Toxicity

One of the major toxicity issues in cannabis consumption relates to the fact that it is most often smoked. Cannabis and tobacco smoke, apart from having different psychoactive constituents, are actually very similar in their composition (Hoffman et al. 1975). Cannabis smoke is mutagenic, which gives it carcinogenic potential (Nahas and Latour 1992). Although no specific reports of lung cancer or emphysema from cannabis smoke exist, it is at least as harmful as tobacco smoke, containing three times as much tar and five times as much carbon monoxide (Wu et al. 1988). Cannabis smoke inflames the airways and reduces respiratory capacity. Airway obstruction and squamous metaplasias may also occur.

Cardiovascular

A common effect of THC is increased heart rate and blood pressure. Corneal blood vessels dilate, creating the red-eyed presentation that is commonly associated with cannabis. These effects are generally not dangerous because cannabis has a high therapeutic margin and no fatal dosages are known in humans. However, these effects may be a danger to those individuals with preexisting cardiovascular disease.

Immune System

The presence of cannabinoid receptors in the immune system has led to consideration of the effects of cannabis on its function. Cannabinoid receptors have been found in spleen cells (Kaminski et al. 1992). Activation of these receptors would inhibit their function in the immune response. Similar suppressant effects occur on lymphocytes (Diaz et al. 1993). THC and anandamide inhibit macrophage-mediated tumor necrosis (Cabral et al. 1995). Despite these effects, their functional significance remains to be determined. These effects are most likely subtle.

Neurotoxicity and Neuroprotection

Until recently, there was little clear evidence that cannabis use was toxic to neurons. Cannabinoids have been shown to have a mix of neurotoxic and neuroprotective effects and mixed results have been found in different studies. Scallet (1991) points out significant methodological differences in the existing studies that influence their outcomes. Critical determinants of neurotoxicity are both age during exposure and duration of exposure. For example, cannabinoid administration was required for at least three months (8–10% of a rat's lifespan) to produce neurotoxic effects in peripubertal rodents. This is comparable to about three years exposure in rhesus monkeys and seven to ten years in humans. Reports of neurotoxicity in primates were inconsistent, with up to 12 months of daily exposure. Longer exposures have not yet been studied (Scallet 1991).

A recent study showed THC to be toxic to hippocampal neurons, while sparing cortical neurons in concentrations likely to be reached in normal human doses (0.5 μM) (Chan et al. 1998). Apoptotic changes were noted in the hippocampus such as shrinkage of neuronal cell bodies and nuclei as well as DNA strand breaks. THC stimulates release of arachidonic acid, and it was hypothesized that this neurotoxic effect is mediated by cyclooxygenase pathways and free radical generation. In support of this, the toxicity is inhibited by nonsteroidal anti-inflammatory drugs, such as aspirin, and antioxidants such as vitamin E.

Cannabidiol and THC reduced neurotoxicty induced by glutamate in cortical neurons (Hampson et al. 1998). This result was effective for toxicity induced at both NMDA and AMPA/kainate receptors, and was independent of cannabinoid receptor activity. The mechanism of neuroprotection appears to be by their potent antioxidant activity. They were even more protective against glutamate neurotoxicity than either ascorbate or α-tocopherol.

Dexanabinol is a synthetic cannabinoid (devoid of psychoactive effects) that is being evaluated for neuroprotective effects (Brewster et al. 1997). It acts as a noncompetitive NMDA receptor antagonist and also as a D_1 agonist (Striem et al. 1997). Dexanabinol is also a potent scavenger of free radicals and protects cultured neurons from toxicity of radical generators (Biegon and Joseph 1995). Its neuroprotective effects are seen in models of ischemia and optic nerve crush. Dexanabinol inhibits production of brain tumor necrosis factor (TNFα) and nitric oxide after head injury and septic shock (Gallily et al. 1997).

Seizures and Epilepsy

Although cannabis does not induce seizures in normal doses, it may have negative effects on seizure disorders. The effects of cannabinoids on seizures are complex. Either inhibition or facilitation of seizures may occur depending on the cannabinoid used, dose, tolerance, and the experimental seizure paradigm used (Karler and Turkanis 1980). THC itself has mixed effects on seizures. Some researchers have reported antiseizure effects (Wada et al. 1975, 1976; Sofia et al. 1976). However, other studies have shown proseizure effects, such as increases in the frequency of focal potentials, generalized bursts of polyspikes, and frank convulsions in cobalt-induced seizures (Chiu et al. 1979). The major metabolite of THC, 11-OH-Δ^9-THC, also has excitatory effects. THC enhanced both electrical and chemical (pentylenetetrazol or picrotoxin) kindling in mice (Karler et al. 1984). In some cases, kindling was facilitated after withdrawal of the cannabinoid. The effect on kindling may be due to prolonged "rebound hyperexcitability," which occurs after THC administration (Karler and Turkanis 1981; Karler et al. 1986). The peak of this effect occurred at 24 hours after administration and lasted as long as 196 hours. This rebound hyperexcitability enhanced electrical seizure kindling and blocked the antiseizure effect of phenytoin. Thus, THC itself may inhibit seizure activity, but may leave in its wake a period of hyperexcitability that promotes seizures.

The chronicity of THC administration also influences its effects on seizures. Δ^8-THC and Δ^9-THC reduced cobalt-induced seizures, but tolerance to this effect developed after only two days (Colasanti et al. 1982). Additionally, even though seizures were suppressed, interictal spiking was enhanced. Studies that showed a preventive effect of cannabinoids on kindling also showed rapid development of tolerance to the effect (Corcoran et al. 1978). It was suggested that the initial anticonvulsant effect occurred by limiting the spread of epileptogenic activity originating from the focus (Colasanti et al. 1982).

Different cannabinoids have different effects on seizures. Cannabidiol may have the most therapeutic potential of the cannibinoids (Turkanis et al. 1979). Unlike THC, cannabidiol does not have excitatory effects and instead elevates the afterdischarge threshold. Similar to ethosuximide, it decreased the duration and amplitude of afterdischarges. Cannabidiol also lacks the CNS excitatory effects that THC produces. Lesser tolerance is observed with cannabidiol than other cannabinoids (Karler and Turkanis 1981).

The effects of cannabis on seizures is, at best, unpredictable. Although some cannabinoids have antiseizure effects, tolerance rapidly develops. Further, rebound hyperexcitability following THC administration may render these benefits impractical. Indeed, cannabinoids facilitate seizures and kindling in many studies. Certain isolated cannabinoids may eventually prove useful for treating seizures, but cannabis as a whole is not effective. In light of this, individuals with epilepsy are strongly recommended to avoid cannabis.

Behavioral Toxicity

There has been discussion in the clinical literature over whether chronic use of psychoactive substances can cause a lasting psychiatric disturbance, such as psychosis (Boutros and Bowers 1996). One review described 70 cases of cannabis-related psychoses, with only rare occasions where the effects persisted past the acute stage (Tunving 1985). Acute cannabis psychosis may have paranoid characteristics, but unlike paranoid schizophrenia, subjects respond quickly to antipsychotic medications and tend to recover completely. A distinction should be made between substance-induced and primary psychotic disorders. Cannabis may promote relapse into psychosis in individuals who have had prior psychotic episodes. There is little support to suggest that cannabis contributes to the development of schizophrenia, although controlled longitudinal studies are needed to state this with certainty (Grinspoon and Bakalar 1992; Boutros and Bowers 1996).

The amotivational syndrome discussed earlier has also been ascribed to chronic cannabis use, but there is no evidence for a causal relationship. Rather, it may be a manifestation of depression. College students who were occasional or heavy cannabis users were objectively compared in psychiatric functioning (DSM diagnoses). The two groups were found to be indistinguishable (Kouri et al. 1995). One aspect in which they did differ was use of other psychoactive drugs, in which the heavy users reported greater use. The correlational nature of this study does not permit one to conclude that heavier cannabis use causes polydrug use, because the directionality may be opposite, or underlying factors may govern both.

Conclusions

Cannabis has been used by humans for thousands of years for both psychoactive and nonpsychoactive purposes. It has long been known and remains in popular use for recreational purposes. Through the study of cannabis, we have discovered new chemical systems in the brain and body, and are just beginning to appreciate their functions. To be certain, cannabis is not an innocuous substance. Its chemical constituents potently act on the nervous system and other physiological systems. Several neurochemical systems in the brain are affected, with consequences in systems governing cognitive, motor, and emotional function.

Cannabis has definite effects on cognitive functioning, but these have been overstated in many cases. The acute, short-term effects on cognitive functioning are dose- and task-dependent, but they are relatively mild. Only with heavier chronic use do cognitive effects become more apparent. As with alcohol, cannabis should certainly not be used by adolescents or pregnant women due to potentially harmful effects on development. Also similar to alcohol, cannabis use is not appropriate when peak cognitive abilities are essential.

Cannabis carries some potential for dependence and addiction. Compared to cocaine, heroin, alcohol, and nicotine, cannabis has lesser addictive potential and withdrawal effects, but some users do develop compulsive and maladaptive use patterns that require treatment (Taylor 1998). Individuals with underlying psychopathology or tendencies for substance abuse should be particularly leery of using cannabis in the interests of avoiding compulsive use patterns.

Several potential therapeutic uses of cannabis have been discovered for such conditions as cancer, AIDS, multiple sclerosis, muscle spasticity, pain, and glaucoma. More controlled research is warranted in order for cannabis to become a legitimate treatment for these conditions. The Administrative Law Judge of the DEA, Francis J. Young, reviewed the evidence for medical use of cannabis in 1988 and stated that it met the standard for a schedule II drug, with acceptable safety under medical supervision. He also added that to conclude otherwise would be "unreasonable, arbitrary, and capricious" (Grinspoon 1999). However, political climate hampers the progress of research in the supervised medical use of cannabis through restricting the use of cannabinoids in research and the allocation of grant funding.

Ultimately, the cultivation, sale, and possession of cannabis is illegal at present in most places. Individuals who use it for whatever purpose in most areas carry the risk of arrest and prosecution. From the perspective of addictiveness, it seems inconsistent that cannabis use is prohibited, while the use of alcohol and nicotine are permitted. Apart from arguments about the recreational use of cannabis, resistance to its medical application is even more inconsistent. For example, the opioids carry some risk for dependence, but with medical supervision they are useful medications and their abuse is minimal (Joranson et al. 2000). Whether use of cannabis is to be permitted and for which purposes (medical or recreational) remains to be collectively decided by society and the legislators it appoints.

References

Chapter 1

American Botanical Council (English trans.). (1998). *The Complete German Commission E Monographs: Therapeutic Guide to Herbal Medicines.* Original source: German Commission E of the Federal Institute for Drugs and Medical Devices. Austin, TX: American Botanical Council.

Canadian Task Force on the Periodic Health Examination. (1979). The periodic health examination. *Can Med Assoc J.* 121: 1193–254.

Cupp MJ. (1999). Herbal remedies: adverse effects and drug interactions. *Am Fam Physician.* 59(5): 1239–45.

Darwin C. (1859). *On the Origin of Species.* Reprinted by Washington Square. New York: New York University Press, 1988.

Dietary Supplement Health and Education Act of 1994. (1994). Pub L No. 103–417.

Eisenberg DM. (1997). Advising patients who seek alternative medical therapies. *Ann Intern Med.* 127(1): 61–69.

Eisenberg DM, Davis RB, Ettner SL, Appel S, Wilkey S, Van Rompay M, Kessler RC. (1998). Trends in alternative medicine use in the United States, 1990–1997: results of a follow-up national survey. *JAMA.* 280(18): 1569–75.

Eisenberg DM, Kessler RC, Foster C, Norlock FE, Calkins DR, Delbanco TL. (1993). Unconventional medicine in the United States. Prevalence, costs, and patterns of use. *N Engl J Med.* 328(4): 246–52.

Hadley SK, Petry JJ. (1999). Medicinal herbs: a primer for primary care. *Hosp Pract (Off Ed).* 34(6): 105–6, 109–12, 115–16.

Hollister LE, Page IH, Pfeiffer CC, Visscher MB. (1968). The Kefauver-Harris amendments of 1962: a critical appraisal of the first five years. *J Clin Pharmacol J New Drugs.* 8(2): 69–73.

Heiligenstein E, Guenther G. (1998). Over-the-counter psychotropics: a review of melatonin, St John's wort, valerian, and kava-kava. *J Am Coll Health.* 46(6): 271–6.

Kaptchuk TJ, Eisenberg DM. (1998). The persuasive appeal of alternative medicine. *Ann Intern Med.* 129(12): 1061–65.

Lezak, MD. (1995). *Neuropsychological Assessment.* New York: Oxford University Press.

O'Hara M, Kiefer D, Farrell K, Kemper K. (1998). A review of 12 commonly used medicinal herbs. *Arch Fam Med.* 7(6): 523–36.

Onopa J. (1999). Complementary and alternative medicine (CAM): a review for the primary care physician. *Hawaii Med J.* 58(2): 9–19.

Page JE, Balza F, Nishida T, Towers GH. (1992). Biologically active diterpenes from Aspilia mossambicensis, a chimpanzee medicinal plant. *Phytochemistry.* 31(10): 3437–39.

Posner MI, Driver J. (1992). The neurobiology of selective attention. *Curr Opin Neurobiol.* 2(2): 165–69.

Ray OS, Ksir C. (1990). *Drugs, Society, and Human Behavior.* St. Louis: Times Mirror/Mosby.

Robbers JE, Speedie MK, Tyler VE. (1996). *Pharmacognosy and Pharmacobiotechnology.* Baltimore: Willams and Wilkins.

Rodriguez E, Aregullin M, Nishida T, Uehara S, Wrangham R, Abramowski Z, Finlayson A, Towers GH. (1985). Thiarubrine A, a bioactive constituent of Aspilia (Asteraceae) consumed by wild chimpanzees. *Experientia.* 41(3): 419–20.

Schacter DL. (1997). The cognitive neuroscience of memory: perspectives from neuroimaging research. *Philos Trans R Soc Lond B Biol Sci.* 352(1362): 1689–95.

Siahpush M. (1999). Why do people favour alternative medicine? *Aust N Z J Public Health.* 23(3): 266–71.

Sixma HJ, Spreeuwenberg PMM, van der Pasch MA. (1998). Patient satisfaction with the general practitioner: A two-level analysis. *Medical Care.* 36(2): 212–29.

Southwood TR. (1984). Insect-plant adaptations. *Ciba Found Symp.* 102: 138–51.

Spreen O, Strauss E. (1998). *A Compendium of Neuropsychological Tests: Administration, Norms, and Commentary.* New York: Oxford University Press.

Studdert DM, Eisenberg DM, Miller FH, Curto DA, Kaptchuk TJ, Brennan TA. (1998). Medical malpractice implications of alternative medicine. *JAMA.* 280(18): 1610–15.

Tyler V. (1994). *Herbs of Choice.* New York: Pharmaceutical Products Press.

Verfaellie M, Keane MM. (1997). The neural basis of aware and unaware forms of memory. *Semin Neurol.* 17(2): 153–61.

Wetzel MS, Eisenberg DM, Kaptchuk TJ. (1998). Courses involving complementary and alternative medicine at US medical schools. *JAMA.* 280(9): 784–87.

Wong AH, Smith M, Boon HS. (1998). Herbal remedies in psychiatric practice. *Arch Gen Psychiatry.* 55(11): 1033–44.

Woolf, SH. (1992). Practice guidelines, a new reality in medicine: II. Methods of developing guidelines. *Ann Intern Med.* 152: 946–52.

Chapter 2

Cooper JR, Bloom FE, Roth RH. (1996). *The Biochemical Basis of Neuropharmacology*, 7th ed. New York: Oxford University Press.

DeArmond SJ, Fusco MM, Dewey MM. (1989). *Structure of the Human Brain*, 3rd ed. New York: Oxford University Press.

Hall ZW. (1992). *Introduction to Molecular Neurobiology*. Sunderland, MA: Sinauer Associates.

Hardman JG, Gilman AG, Limbird LE, eds. (1996). *Goodman and Gilman's The Pharmacological Basis of Therapeutics*, 9th ed. New York: McGraw-Hill.

Hille B. (1992). *Ionic Channels of Excitable Membranes*, 2nd ed. Sunderland, MA: Sinauer Associates.

Kandel E, Schwartz JH, Jessel TM, eds. (1991). *Principles of Neural Science*, 3rd ed. Norwalk, CT: Appleton and Lange.

Kebabian JW, Neumeyer JL. (1994). *The RBI Handbook of Receptor Classification*. Natick, MA: Research Biochemicals International.

Parent A. (1996). *Carpenter's Human Neuroanatomy*, 9th ed. Baltimore: Williams and Wilkins.

Siegel GJ, Agranoff BW, Albers RW, Molinoff PB, eds. (1994). *Basic Neurochemistry: Molecular, Cellular, and Medical aspects*, 6th ed. New York: Lipincott-Raven.

Chapter 3

Clark WG, Brater DC, Johnson AR. (1992). *Goth's Medical Pharmacology*, 12th ed. St. Louis: Mosby, 1988.

Cooper JR, Bloom FE, Roth RH. (1996). *The Biochemical Basis of Neuropharmacology*, 7th ed. New York: Oxford University Press.

Hardman JG, Gilman AG, Limbird LE, eds. (1996). *Goodman and Gilman's The Pharmacological Basis of Therapeutics*, 9th ed. New York: McGraw-Hill.

Hille B. (1992). *Ionic Channels of Excitable Membranes*, 2nd ed. Sunderland, MA: Sinauer Associates.

Chapter 4

Abdulla FA, Bradbury E, Calaminici MR, Lippiello PM, Wonnacott S, Gray JA, Sinden JD. (1996). Relationship between up-regulation of nicotine binding sites in rat brain and delayed cognitive enhancement observed after chronic or acute nicotinic receptor stimulation. *Psychopharmacology (Berlin).* April 124(4): 323–31.

Albrecht AE, Marcus BH, Roberts M, Forman DE, Parisi AF. (1998). Effect of smoking cessation on exercise performance in female smokers participating in exercise training. *Am J Cardiol.* 82(8): 950–55.

Alm B, Milerad J, Wennergren G, Skjaerven R, Oyen N, Norvenius G, Daltveit AK, Helweg-Larsen K, Markestad T, Irgens LM. (1998). A case-control study of smoking and sudden infant death syndrome in the Scandinavian countries, 1992 to 1995. The Nordic Epidemiological SIDS Study. *Arch Dis Child.* 78(4): 329–34.

Arnold ME, Petros TV, Beckwith BE, Coons G, Gorman N. (1987). The effects of caffeine, impulsivity, and sex on memory for word lists. *Physiol Behav.* 41(1): 25–30.

Asthana S, Greig NH, Holloway HW, Raffaele KC, Berardi A, Schapiro MB, Rapoport SI, Soncrant TT. (1996). Clinical pharmacokinetics of arecoline in subjects with Alzheimer's disease. *Clin Pharmacol Ther.* 60(3): 276–82.

Asthana S, Raffaele KC, Greig NH, Berardi A, Morris PP, Schapiro MB, Rapoport SI, Blackman MR, Soncrant TT. (1995). Neuroendocrine responses to intravenous infusion of arecoline in patients with Alzheimer's disease. *Psychoneuroendocrinology.* 20(6): 623–36.

Avidor T, Clementi E, Schwartz L, Atlas D. (1994). Caffeine-induced transmitter release is mediated via ryanodine-sensitive channel. *Neurosci Lett.* 165(1–2): 133–36.

Baer RA. (1987). Effects of caffeine on classroom behavior, sustained attention, and a memory task in preschool children. *Appl Behav Analysis.* 20(3): 225–34.

Balfour DJ. (1994). Neural mechanisms underlying nicotine dependence. *Addiction.* 89(11): 1419–23.

Balfour DJ, Benwell ME, Birrell CE, Kelly RJ, Al-Aloul M. (1998). Sensitization of the mesoaccumbens dopamine response to nicotine. *Pharmacol Biochem Behav.* 59(4): 1021–30.

Barr HM, Streissguth A. (1991). Caffeine use during pregnancy and child outcome: a 7-year prospective study. *Neurotoxicol Teratol.* 13(4): 441–48.

Barry M. (1991). The influence of the U.S. tobacco industry on the health, economy, and environment of developing countries. *N Engl J Med.* 324(13): 917–20.

Baumann MH, Rothman RB. (1998). Alterations in serotonergic responsiveness during cocaine withdrawal in rats: similarities to major depression in humans. *Biol Psychiatry.* 44(7): 578–91.

Bek K, Tomac N, Delibas A, Tuna F, Tezic HT, Sungur M. (1999). The effect of passive smoking on pulmonary function during childhood. *Postgrad Med J.* 75(884): 339–41.

Belej T, Manji D, Sioutis S, Barros HM, Nobrega JN. (1996). Changes in serotonin and norepinephrine uptake sites after chronic cocaine: pre- vs. post-withdrawal effects. *Brain Res.* 736(1–2): 287–96.

Bennett TL. (1973). The effects of centrally blocking hippocampal theta activity on learning and retention. *Behav Biol.* 9(5): 541–52.

Benwell ME, Balfour DJ. (1998). The influence of lobeline on nucleus accumbens dopamine and locomotor responses to nicotine in nicotine-pretreated rats. *Br J Pharmacol.* 125(6): 1115–19.

Benwell ME, Balfour DJ, Birrell CE. (1995). Desensitization of the nicotine-induced mesolimbic dopamine responses during constant infusion with nicotine. *Br J Pharmacol.* 114(2): 454–60.

Berlin I, Said S, Spreux-Varoquaux O, Launay JM, Olivares R, Millet V, Lecrubier Y, Puech AJ. (1995). A reversible monoamine oxidase A inhibitor (moclobemide) facilitates smoking cessation and abstinence in heavy, dependent smokers. *Clin Pharmacol Ther.* 58(4): 444–52.

Bernstein GA, Carroll ME, Crosby RD, Perwien AR, Go FS, Benowitz NL. (1994). Caffeine effects on learning, performance, and anxiety in normal school-age children. *J Am Acad Child Adolesc Psychiatry.* 33(3): 407–15.

Bernstein GA, Carroll ME, Dean NW, Crosby RD, Perwien AR, Benowitz NL. (1998). Caffeine withdrawal in normal school-age children. *J Am Acad Child Adolesc Psychiatry.* 37(8): 858–65.

Berry J, van Gorp WG, Herzberg DS, Hinkin C, Boone K, Steinman L, Wilkins JN. (1993). Neuropsychological deficits in abstinent cocaine abusers: preliminary findings after two weeks of abstinence. *Drug Alcohol Depend.* 32(3): 231–37.

Berti C, Nistri A. (1983). Influence of caffeine and midazolam on gamma-aminobutyric acid-evoked responses in the frog spinal cord. *Neuropharmacology.* 22(12A): 1409–12.

Blumenthal M, King P. (1997). The Agony of the Ecstasy. *HerbalGram.* 37: 20–49.

Bolla KI, Cadet JL, London ED. (1998). The neuropsychiatry of chronic cocaine abuse. *J Neuropsychiatry Clin Neurosci.* 10(3): 280–89.

Boutros NN, Bowers MB. (1996). Chronic substance-induced psychotic disorders: state of the literature. *J Neuropsychiatry Clin Neurosci.* 8(3): 262–69.

Brenneisen R, Fisch HU, Koelbing U, Geisshüsler S, Kalix P. (1990). Amphetamine-like effects in humans of the khat alkaloid cathinone. *Br J Clin Pharmacol.* 30(6): 825–28.

Brenneisen R, Geisshüsler S, Schorno X. (1986). Metabolism of cathinone to (–)-norephedrine and (–)-norpseudoephedrine. *J Pharm Pharmacol.* 38(4): 298–300.

Briggs CA, McKenna DG. (1998). Activation and inhibition of the human alpha7 nicotinic acetylcholine receptor by agonists. *Neuropharmacology.* 37(9): 1095–102.

Brioni JD, Kim DJ, Brodie MS, Decker MW, Arneric SP. (1995). ABT-418: discriminative stimulus properties and effect on ventral tegmental cell activity. *Psychopharmacology (Berlin).* 119(4): 368–75.

Brioni JD, O'Neill AB, Kim DJ, Buckley MJ, Decker MW, Arneric SP. (1994). Anxiolytic-like effects of the novel cholinergic channel activator ABT-418. *J Pharmacol Exp Ther.* 271(1): 353–61.

Bryant CA, Farmer A, Tiplady B, Keating J, Sherwood R, Swift CG, Jackson SH. (1998). Psychomotor performance: investigating the dose-response relationship for caffeine and theophylline in elderly volunteers. *Eur J Clin Pharmacol.* 54(4): 309–13.

Buccafusco JJ, Jackson WJ, Gattu M, Terry AV Jr. (1995). Isoarecolone-induced enhancement of delayed matching to sample performance in monkeys: role of nicotinic receptors. *Neuroreport.* 6(8): 1223–27.

Bunker ML, McWilliams M. (1979). Caffeine content of common beverages. *J Am Diet Assoc.* 74(1): 28–32.

Cameron OG, Modell JG, Hariharan M. (1990). Caffeine and human cerebral blood flow: a positron emission tomography study. *Life Sci.* 47(13): 1141–46.

Carmody TP. (1989). Affect regulation, nicotine addiction, and smoking cessation. *J Psychoactive Drugs.* 21(3): 331–42.

Carter AJ, O'Connor WT, Carter MJ, Ungerstedt U. (1995). Caffeine enhances acetylcholine release in the hippocampus in vivo by a selective interaction with adenosine A1 receptors. *J Pharmacol Exp Ther.* 273(2): 637–42.

Cestari V, Castellano C. (1996). Caffeine and cocaine interaction on memory consolidation in mice. *Arch Int Pharmacodyn Ther.* 331(1): 94–104.

Chiang WT, Yang CC, Deng JF, Bullard M. (1998). Cardiac arrhythmia and betel nut chewing—is there a causal effect? *Vet Hum Toxicol.* 40(5): 287–89.

Chu NS. (1994a). Effect of betel chewing on performance reaction time. *J Formos Med Assoc.* 93(4): 343–45.

Chu NS. (1994b). Effects of betel chewing on electroencephalographic activity: spectral analysis and topographic mapping. *J Formos Med Assoc.* 93(2): 167–69.

Chu NS. (1995). Betel chewing increases the skin temperature: effects of atropine and propranolol. *Neurosci Lett.* 194(1–2): 130–32.

Clarke PB. (1990). Mesolimbic dopamine activation—the key to nicotine reinforcement? *Ciba Found Symp.* 152: 153–62; discussion 162–68.

Clarke PB, Reuben M. (1996). Release of [^{3}H]-noradrenaline from rat hippocampal synaptosomes by nicotine: mediation by different nicotinic receptor subtypes from striatal [^{3}H]-dopamine release. *Br J Pharmacol.* 117(4): 595–606.

Cohen C, Pickworth WB, Bunker EB, Henningfield JE. (1994). Caffeine antagonizes EEG effects of tobacco withdrawal. *Pharmacol Biochem Behav.* 47(4): 919–36.

Colom LV, Christie BR, Bland BH. (1988). Cingulate cell discharge patterns related to hippocampal EEG and their modulation by muscarinic and nicotinic agents. *Brain Res.* 460(2): 329–38.

Cone EJ. (1995). Pharmacokinetics and pharmacodynamics of cocaine. *J analytical Toxicol.* 19(6): 459–78.

Corrigall WA, Franklin KB, Coen KM, Clarke PB. (1992). The mesolimbic dopaminergic system is implicated in the reinforcing effects of nicotine. *Psychopharmacology (Berlin).* 107(2–3): 285–89.

Dackis C, Gold MS. (1985). Neurotransmitter and neuroendocrine abnormalities associated with cocaine use. *Psychiatr Med.* 3(4): 461–83.

Dager SR, Layton ME, Strauss W, Richards TL, Heide A, Friedman SD, Artru AA, Hayes CE, Posse S. (1999). Human brain metabolic response to caffeine and the effects of tolerance. *Am J Psychiatry.* 156(2): 229–37.

Dager SR, Rainey JM, Kenny MA, Artru AA, Metzger GD, Bowden DM. (1990). Central nervous system effects of lactate infusion in primates. *Biol Psychiatry.* 27(2): 193–204.

Damaj MI, Patrick GS, Creasy KR, Martin BR. (1997). Pharmacology of lobeline, a nicotinic receptor ligand. *J Pharmacol Exp Ther.* 282(1): 410–19.

D'Ambrosio SM. (1994). Evaluation of the genotoxicity data on caffeine. *Regul Toxicol Pharmacol.* 19(3): 243–81.

Davidson RA, Smith BD. (1991). Caffeine and novelty: effects on electrodermal activity and performance. *Physiol Behav.* 49(6): 1169–75.

Deahl M. (1989). Betel nut-induced extrapyramidal syndrome: an unusual drug interaction. *Mov Disord.* 4(4): 330–32.

Decker MW, Majchrzak MJ, Arneric SP. (1993). Effects of lobeline, a nicotinic receptor agonist, on learning and memory. *Pharmacol Biochem Behav.* 45(3): 571–76.

Decker MW, Brioni JD, Sullivan JP, Buckley MJ, Radek RJ, Raszkiewicz JL, Kang CH, Kim DJ, Giardina WJ, Wasicak JT, et al. (1994). (S)-3-methyl-5-(1-methyl-2-pyrrolidinyl)isoxazole (ABT 418): a novel cholinergic ligand with cognition-enhancing and anxiolytic activities: II. In vivo characterization. *J Pharmacol Exp Ther.* 270(1): 319–28.

Denissenko MF, Pao A, Tang M, Pfeifer GP. (1996). Preferential formation of benzo[a]pyrene adducts at lung cancer mutational hotspots in P53. *Science.* 274(5286): 430–32.

Di Benedetto G. (1995). Passive smoking in childhood. *J R Soc Health* 115(1): 13–6.

Dimpfel W, Schober F. (1993). The influence of caffeine on human EEG under resting conditions and during mental loads. *Clin Investig.* 71(3): 197–207.

Dodd SL, Herb RA, Powers SK. (1993). Caffeine and exercise performance. An update. *Sports Med.* 15(1): 14–23.

Domino EF, Matsuoka S. (1994). Effects of tobacco smoking on the topographic EEG-I. *Prog Neuropsychopharmacol Biol Psychiatry.* 18(5): 879–89.

Dougherty J, Miller D, Todd G, Kostenbauder HB. (1981). Reinforcing and other behavioral effects of nicotine. *Neurosci Biobehav Rev.* 5(4): 487–95.

Easton C, Bauer LO. (1997). Neuropsychological differences between alcohol-dependent and cocaine-dependent patients with or without problematic drinking. *Psychiatry Res.* 71(2): 97–103.

Edwards S, Brice C, Craig C, Penri-Jones R. (1996). Effects of caffeine, practice, and mode of presentation on Stroop task performance. *Pharmacol Biochem Behav.* 54(2): 309–15.

Ehlers CL, Somes C, Thomas J, Riley EP. (1997). Effects of neonatal exposure to nicotine on electrophysiological parameters in adult rats. *Pharmacol Biochem Behav.* 58(3): 713–20.

Elmi AS. (1983). The chewing of khat in Somalia. *J Ethnopharmacol.* 8(2): 163–76.

Epping-Jordan MP, Watkins SS, Koob GF, Markou A. (1998). Dramatic decreases in brain reward function during nicotine withdrawal. *Nature.* 393(6680): 76–79.

Farid P, Abate MA. (1998). Buspirone use for smoking cessation. *Ann Pharmacother.* 32(12): 1362–64.

Fedele E, Varnier G, Ansaldo MA, Raiteri M. (1998). Nicotine administration stimulates the in vivo N-methyl-D-aspartate receptor/nitric oxide/cyclic GMP pathway in rat hippocampus through glutamate release. *Br J Pharmacol.* 125(5): 1042–48.

Fisher JL, Pidoplichko VI, Dani JA. (1998). Nicotine modifies the activity of ventral tegmental area dopaminergic neurons and hippocampal GABAergic neurons. *J Physiol Paris.* 92(3–4): 209–13.

Foltin RW, Fischman MW, Levin FR. (1995). Cardiovascular effects of cocaine in humans: laboratory studies. *Drug Alcohol Depend.* 37(3): 193–210.

Ford RP, Schluter PJ, Mitchell EA, Taylor BJ, Scragg R, Stewart AW. (1998). Heavy caffeine intake in pregnancy and sudden infant death syndrome. New Zealand Cot Death Study Group. *Arch Dis Child.* 78(1): 9–13.

Foreman N, Barraclough S, Moore C, Mehta A, Madon M. (1989). High doses of caffeine impair performance of a numerical version of the Stroop task in men. *Pharmacol Biochem Behav.* 32(2): 399–403.

Forman HP, Levin S, Stewart B, Patel M, Feinstein S. (1989). Cerebral vasculitis and hemorrhage in an adolescent taking diet pills containing phenylpropanolamine: case report and review of literature. *Pediatrics.* 83(5): 737–41.

Foulds J, McSorley K, Sneddon J, Feyerabend C, Jarvis MJ, Russell MA. (1994). Effect of subcutaneous nicotine injections of EEG alpha frequency in non-smokers: a placebo-controlled pilot study. *Psychopharmacology (Berlin).* 115(1–2): 163–66.

Fowler JS, Volkow ND, Wang GJ, Pappas N, Logan J, MacGregor R, Alexoff D, Shea C, Schlyer D, Wolf AP, Warner D, Zezulkova I, Cilento R. (1996a). Inhibition of monoamine oxidase B in the brains of smokers. *Nature*. 379(6567): 733–6.

Fowler JS, Volkow ND, Wang GJ, Pappas N, Logan J, Shea C, Alexoff D, MacGregor RR, Schlyer DJ, Zezulkova I, Wolf AP. (1996b). Brain monoamine oxidase A inhibition in cigarette smokers. *Proc Natl Acad Sci USA*. 93(24): 14065–9.

Fowler JS, Volkow ND, Wang GJ, Pappas N, Logan J, MacGregor R, Alexoff D, Wolf AP, Warner D, Cilento R, Zezulkova I. (1998). Neuropharmacological actions of cigarette smoke: brain monoamine oxidase B (MAO B) inhibition. *J Addict Dis*. 17(1): 23–34.

Fox BS, Kantak KM, Edwards MA, Black KM, Bollinger BK, Botka AJ, French TL, Thompson TL, Schad VC, Greenstein JL, Gefter ML, Exley MA, Swain PA, Briner TJ. (1996). Efficacy of a therapeutic cocaine vaccine in rodent models. *Nat Med*. 2(10): 1129–32.

Franks HM, Hagedorn H, Hensley VR, Hensley WJ, Starmer GA. (1975). The effect of caffeine on human performance, alone and in combination with ethanol. *Psychopharmacologia*. 45(2): 177–81.

Franks P, Harp J, Bell B. (1989). Randomized, controlled trial of clonidine for smoking cessation in a primary care setting. *JAMA*. 262(21): 3011–13.

Frewer LJ. (1990). The effect of betel nut on human performance. *PNG Med J*. 33(2): 143–45.

Fryer JD, Lukas RJ. (1999). Noncompetitive functional inhibition at diverse, human nicotinic acetylcholine receptor subtypes by bupropion, phencyclidine, and ibogaine. *J Pharmacol Exp Ther*. 288(1): 88–92.

Fu Y, Matta SG, Sharp BM. (1999). Local alpha-bungarotoxin-sensitive nicotinic receptors modulate hippocampal norepinephrine release by systemic nicotine. *J Pharmacol Exp Ther*. 289(1): 133–39.

Fudala PJ, Iwamoto ET. (1986). Further studies on nicotine-induced conditioned place preference in the rat. *Pharmacol Biochem Behav*. 25(5): 1041–49.

Fukumoto M, Kubo H, Ogamo A. (1997). Determination of nicotine content of popular cigarettes. *Veterinary Hum Toxicol*. 39(4): 225–27.

Fung YK, Reed JA. (1988). Effect of nicotine on central GABAergic system. *Gen Pharmacol*. 19(4): 533–36.

Fuxe K, Everitt BJ, Hokfelt T. (1977). Enhancement of sexual behavior in the female rat by nicotine. *Pharmacol Biochem Behav*. 7(2): 147–51.

Gallardo KA, Leslie FM. (1998). Nicotine-stimulated release of [3H]norepinephrine from fetal rat locus coeruleus cells in culture. *J Neurochem*. 70(2): 663–70.

Garaschuk O, Yaari Y, Konnerth A. (1997). Release and sequestration of calcium by ryanodine-sensitive stores in rat hippocampal neurones. *J Physiol (London)*. 502(pt 1): 13–30.

Garfinkel BD, Webster CD, Sloman L. (1981). Responses to methylphenidate and varied doses of caffeine in children with attention deficit disorder. *Can J Psychiatry.* 26(6) 395–401.

Ghatan PH, Ingvar M, Eriksson L, Stone-Elander S, Serrander M, Ekberg K, Wahren J. (1998). Cerebral effects of nicotine during cognition in smokers and non-smokers. *Psychopharmacology (Berlin).* 136(2): 179–89.

Gilbert DG, Robinson JH, Chamberlin CL, Spielberger CD. (1989). Effects of smoking/nicotine on anxiety, heart rate, and lateralization of EEG during a stressful movie. *Psychophysiology.* 26(3): 311–20.

Gilbert RM, Marshman JA, Schwieder M, Berg R. (1976). Caffeine content of beverages as consumed. *Can Med Assoc J.* 114(3): 205–8.

Gioanni Y, Rougeot C, Clarke PB, Lepouse C, Thierry AM, Vidal C. (1999). Nicotinic receptors in the rat prefrontal cortex: increase in glutamate release and facilitation of mediodorsal thalamo-cortical transmission. *Eur J Neurosci.* 11(1): 18–30.

Glennon RA, Young R, Martin BR, Dal Cason TA. (1995). Methcathione ("cat"): an enantiomeric potency comparison. *Pharmacol Biochem Behav.* 50(4): 601–6.

Golding J. (1995). Reproduction and caffeine consumption—a literature review. *Early Hum Dev.* 43(1): 1–14.

Gori GB, Lynch CJ. (1985). Analytical cigarette yields as predictors of smoke bioavailability. *Regul Toxicol Pharmacol.* 5(3): 314–26.

Gourlay S, Forbes A, Marriner T, Kutin J, McNeil J. (1994). A placebo-controlled study of three clonidine doses for smoking cessation. *Clin Pharmacol Ther.* 55(1): 64–69.

Granek M, Shalev A, Weingarten AM. (1988). Khat-induced hypnagogic hallucinations. *Acta Psychiatr Scand.* 78(4): 458–61.

Grassi G, Seravalle G, Calhoun DA, Bolla GB, Giannattasio C, Marabini M, Del Bo A, Mancia G. (1994). Mechanisms responsible for sympathetic activation by cigarette smoking in humans. *Circulation.* 90(1): 248–53.

Gray R, Rajan AS, Radcliffe KA, Yakehiro M, Dani JA. (1996). Hippocampal synaptic transmission enhanced by low concentrations of nicotine. *Nature.* Oct. 24;383: 6602 713–16.

Grobbee DE, Rimm EB, Giovannucci E, Colditz G, Stampfer M, Willett W. (1990). Coffee, caffeine, and cardiovascular disease in men. *N Engl J Med.* 323(15): 1026–32.

Gruber AJ, Pope HG Jr. (1998). Ephedrine abuse among 36 female weightlifters. *Am J Addict.* 7(4): 256–61.

Gruenwald J, Brendler T, Jaenicke C. (1998). *PDR for Herbal Medicines*, 1st ed. Montvale, NJ: Medical Economics Company.

Grunberg NE, Bowen DJ, Winders SE. (1986). Effects of nicotine on body weight and food consumption in female rats. *Psychopharmacology (Berlin).* 90(1): 101–5.

Guantai AN, Maitai CK. (1983). Metabolism of cathinone to d-norpseudoephedrine in humans. *J Pharm Sci.* 72(10): 1217–18.

Guantai AN, Mwangi JW, Muriuki G, Kuria KA. (1987). Effects of the active constituents of Catha edulis on the neuromuscular junction. *Neuropharmacology.* 26(5): 401–5.

Haass M, Kubler W. (1997). Nicotine and sympathetic neurotransmission. *Cardiovasc Drugs Ther.* 10(6): 657–65.

Halket JM, Karasu Z, Murray-Lyon IM. (1995). Plasma cathinone levels following chewing khat leaves (Catha edulis Forsk.). *J Ethnopharmacol.* 49(2): 111–13.

Hall SM, Munoz RF, Reus VI, Sees KL. (1993). Nicotine, negative affect, and depression. *J Consult Clin Psychol.* 61(5): 761–67.

Hara T, Komiyama T, Yokoi F. (1993). Distribution of 11C-(R)nicotine in human brain measured by positron emission tomography: measurement of cerebral blood flow. *Yakubutsu Seishin Kodo.* 13(3): 175–81.

Hatsukami DK, Fischman MW. (1996). Crack cocaine and cocaine hydrochloride. Are the differences myth or reality? *JAMA.* 276(19): 1580–88.

Hilleman DE, Mohiuddin SM, Delcore MG, Lucas BD Jr. (1993). Randomized, controlled trial of transdermal clonidine for smoking cessation. *Ann Pharmacother.* 27(9): 1025–28.

Hindmarch I, Quinlan PT, Moore KL, Parkin C. (1998). The effects of black tea and other beverages on aspects of cognition and psychomotor performance. *Psychopharmacology (Berlin).* 139(3): 230–38.

Hoff AL, Riordan H, Morris L, Cestaro V, Wieneke M, Alpert R, Wang GJ, Volkow N. (1996). Effects of crack cocaine on neurocognitive function. *Psychiatry Res.* 60(2–3): 167–76.

Hoffmann D, Brunnemann KD, Prokopczyk B, Djordjevic MV. (1994). Tobacco-specific N-nitrosamines and Areca-derived N-nitrosamines: chemistry, biochemistry, carcinogenicity, and relevance to humans. *J Toxicol Environ Health.* 41(1): 1–52.

Homstedt B, Lindgren JE, Rivier L, Plowman T. (1979). Cocaine in blood of coca chewers. *J Ethnopharmacol.* 1(1): 69–78.

Houlihan ME, Pritchard WS, Robinson JH. (1996). Faster P300 latency after smoking in visual but not auditory oddball tasks. *Psychopharmacology (Berlin).* 123(3): 231–38.

Huang D, Wilson MC. (1986). Comparative discriminative stimulus properties of dl-cathinone, d-amphetamine, and cocaine in rats. *Pharmacol Biochem Behav.* 24(2): 205–10.

Hughes JR, Gust SW, Skoog K, Keenan RM, Fenwick JW. (1991). Symptoms of tobacco withdrawal. A replication and extension. *Arch Gen Psychiatry*. 48(1): 52–9.

Hung DZ, Deng JF. (1998). Acute myocardial infarction temporally related to betel nut chewing. *Veterinary Hum Toxicol*. 40(1): 25–28.

Hussain MA, Mollica JA. (1991). Intranasal absorption of physostigmine and arecoline. *J Pharm Sci*. 80(8): 750–51.

Islam MW, Tariq M, Ageel AM, el-Feraly FS, al-Meshal IA, Ashraf I. (1990). An evaluation of the male reproductive toxicity of cathinone. *Toxicology*. 60(3): 223–34.

James JE. (1998). Acute and chronic effects of caffeine on performance, mood, headache, and sleep. *Neuropsychobiology*. 38(1): 32–41.

Jarvis MJ. (1993). Does caffeine intake enhance absolute levels of cognitive performance? *Psychopharmacology (Berlin)*. 110(1–2): 45–52.

Jeng JH, Hahn LJ, Lin BR, Hsieh CC, Chan CP, Chang MC. (1999). Effects of areca nut, inflorescence piper betle extracts and arecoline on cytotoxicity, total and unscheduled DNA synthesis in cultured gingival keratinocytes. *J Oral Pathol Med*. 28(2): 64–71.

Johnston GA, Krogsgaard-Larsen P, Stephanson A. (1975). Betel nut constituents as inhibitors of gamma-aminobutyric acid uptake. *Nature*. 258(5536): 627–28.

Jorenby DE, Hatsukami DK, Smith SS, Fiore MC, Allen S, Jensen J, Baker TB. (1996). Characterization of tobacco withdrawal symptoms: transdermal nicotine reduces hunger and weight gain. *Psychopharmacology (Berlin)*. 128(2): 130–38.

Kalix P. (1980). A constituent of khat leaves with amphetamine-like releasing properties. *Eur J Pharmacol*. 68(2): 213–15.

Kalix P. (1981). Cathinone, an alkaloid from khat leaves with an amphetamine-like releasing effect. *Psychopharmacology (Berlin)*. 74(3): 269–70.

Kalix P. (1982). The amphetamine-like releasing effect of the alkaloid (–)cathinone on rat nucleus accumbens and rabbit caudate nucleus. *Prog Neuropsychopharmacol Biol Psychiatry*. 6(1): 43–49.

Kalix P. (1983). A comparison of the catecholamine releasing effect of the khat alkaloids (–)-cathinone and (+)-norpseudoephedrine. *Drug Alcohol Depend*. 11(3–4): 395–401.

Kalix P. (1984). Effect of the alkaloid (–)-cathinone on the release of radioactivity from rat striatal tissue prelabelled with 3H-serotonin. *Neuropsychobiology*. 12(2–3) 127–29.

Kalix P. (1988). Khat: a plant with amphetamine effects. *J Subst Abuse Treat*. 5(3): 163–69.

Kalix P. (1991). The pharmacology of psychoactive alkaloids from ephedra and catha. *J Ethnopharmacol*. 32(1–3): 201–8.

Kalix P. (1992). Cathinone, a natural amphetamine. *Pharmacol Toxicol.* 70(2): 77–86.

Kalix P. (1994). Khat, an amphetamine-like stimulant. *Psychoactive Drugs.* 26(1): 69–74.

Kalix P, Glennon RA. (1986). Further evidence for an amphetamine-like mechanism of action of the alkaloid cathinone. *Biochem Pharmacol.* 35(18): 3015–19.

Kaplan GB, Greenblatt DJ, Ehrenberg BL, Goddard JE, Cotreau MM, Harmatz JS, Shader RI. (1997). Dose-dependent pharmacokinetics and psychomotor effects of caffeine in humans. *J Clin Pharmacol.* 37(8): 693–703.

Karacan I, Thornby JI, Anch M, Booth GH, Williams RL, Salis PJ. (1976). Dose-related sleep disturbances induced by coffee and caffeine. *Clin Pharmacol Ther.* 20(6): 682–89.

Kardos J, Blandl T. (1994). Inhibition of a gamma aminobutyric acid A receptor by caffeine. *Neuroreport.* 5(10): 1249–52.

Kaye BR, Fainstat M. (1987). Cerebral vasculitis associated with cocaine abuse. *JAMA.* 258(15): 2104–6.

Kenemans JL, Verbaten MN. (1998). Caffeine and visuo-spatial attention. *Psychopharmacology (Berlin).* 135(4): 353–60.

Kennedy JG, Teague J, Rokaw W, Cooney E. (1983). A medical evaluation of the use of qat in North Yemen. *Soc Sci Med.* 17(12): 783–93.

Kiyatkin EA, Stein EA. (1995). Fluctuations in nucleus accumbens dopamine during cocaine self-administration behavior: an in vivo electrochemical study. *Neuroscience.* 64(3): 599–617.

Knott VJ, Harr A, Ilivitsky V, Mahoney C. (1998). The cholinergic basis of the smoking-induced EEG activation profile. *Neuropsychobiology.* 38(2): 97–107.

Kuitunen T, Karkkainen S, Ylitalo P. (1984). Comparison of the acute physical and mental effects of ephedrine, fenfluramine, phentermine and prolintane. *Methods Find Exp Clin Pharmacol.* 6(5): 265–70.

Kuo MY, Huang JS, Hsu HC, Chiang CP, Kok SH, Kuo YS, Hong CY. (1999). Infrequent p53 mutations in patients with areca quid chewing-associated oral squamous cell carcinomas in Taiwan. *J Oral Pathol Med.* 28(5): 221–25.

Lane JD, Phillips-Bute BG. (1998). Caffeine deprivation affects vigilance performance and mood. *Physiol Behav.* 65(1): 171–75.

Lane JD, Steege JF, Rupp SL, Kuhn CM. (1992). Menstrual cycle effects on caffeine elimination in the human female. *Eur J Clin Pharmacol.* 43(5): 543–46.

Langstrom B. (1997). Imaging of nicotinic and muscarinic receptors in Alzheimer's disease: effect of tacrine treatment. *Dement Geriatr Cogn Disord.* 8(2): 78–84.

Le Houezec J, Benowitz NL. (1991). Basic and clinical psychopharmacology of nicotine. *Clin Chest Med.* 12(4): 681–99.

LeBras M, Fretillere Y. (1965). Les aspects medicaux de la consommation habituelle du cath. *Méd Trop.* 25: 720–32.

Leech SL, Richardson GA, Goldschmidt L, Day NL. (1999). Prenatal substance exposure: effects on attention and impulsivity of 6-year-olds. *Neurotoxicol Teratol.* 21(2): 109–18.

Lelo A, Miners JO, Robson R, Birkett DJ. (1986). Assessment of caffeine exposure: caffeine content of beverages, caffeine intake, and plasma concentrations of methylxanthines. *Clin Pharmacol Ther.* 39(1): 54–59.

Léna C, Changeux JP. (1997). Role of Ca2+ ions in nicotinic facilitation of GABA release in mouse thalamus. *J Neurosci.* 17(2): 576–85.

Lendvai B, Sershen H, Lajtha A, Santha E, Baranyi M, Vizi ES. (1996). Differential mechanisms involved in the effect of nicotinic agonists DMPP and lobeline to release [^{3}H]5-HT from rat hippocampal slices. *Neuropharmacology.* 35(12): 1769–77.

Lerman C, Audrain J, Orleans CT, Boyd R, Gold K, Main D, Caporaso N. (1996). Investigation of mechanisms linking depressed mood to nicotine dependence. *Addict Behav.* 21(1): 9–19.

Leshner AI, Koob GF. (1999). Drugs of abuse and the brain. *Proc Assoc Am Physicians.* 111(2): 99–108.

Levin ED, Briggs SJ, Christopher NC, Rose JE. (1993). Prenatal nicotine exposure and cognitive performance in rats. *Neurotoxicol Teratol.* 15(4): 251–60.

Levine SR, Brust JC, Futrell N, Brass LM, Blake D, Fayad P, Schultz LR, Millikan CH, Ho KL, Welch KM. (1991). A comparative study of the cerebrovascular complications of cocaine: alkaloidal versus hydrochloride—a review. *Neurology.* 41(8): 1173–77.

Li X, Rainnie DG, McCarley RW, Greene RW. (1998). Presynaptic nicotinic receptors facilitate monoaminergic transmission. *J Neurosci.* 18(5): 1904–12.

Liachenko S, Tang P, Somogyi GT, Xu Y. (1999). Concentration-dependent isoflurane effects on depolarization-evoked glutamate and GABA outflows from mouse brain slices. *Br J Pharmacol.* 127(1): 131–38.

Lieberman HR, Wurtman RJ, Emde GG, Coviella IL. (1987). The effects of caffeine and aspirin on mood and performance. *J Clin Psychopharmacol.* 7(5): 315–20.

Lin Y, Phillis JW. (1990). Chronic caffeine exposure reduces the excitant action of acetylcholine on cerebral cortical neurons. *Brain Res.* 524(2): 316–18.

Linde L. (1995). Mental effects of caffeine in fatigued and non-fatigued female and male subjects. *Ergonomics.* 38(5): 864–85.

Linville DG, Williams S, Raszkiewicz JL, Arneric SP. (1993). Nicotinic agonists modulate basal forebrain control of cortical cerebral blood flow in anesthetized rats. *J Pharmacol Exp Ther.* 267(1): 440–48.

Lodge D, Johnston GA, Curtis DR, Brand SJ. (1977). Effects of the Areca nut constituents arecaidine and guvacine on the action of GABA in the cat central nervous system. *Brain Res.* 136(3): 513–22.

Loke WH. (1988). Effects of caffeine on mood and memory. *Physiol Behav.* 44(3): 367–72.

Loke WH, Meliska CJ. (1984). Effects of caffeine use and ingestion on a protracted visual vigilance task. *Psychopharmacology (Berlin).* 84(1): 54–57.

Lorist MM, Snel J, Kok A, Mulder G. (1994). Influence of caffeine on selective attention in well-rested and fatigued subjects. *Psychophysiology.* 31(6): 525–34.

Lorist MM, Snel J, Kok A, Mulder G. (1996). Acute effects of caffeine on selective attention and visual search processes. *Psychophysiology.* 33(4): 354–61.

Lorist MM, Snel J, Mulder G, Kok A. (1995). Aging, caffeine, and information processing: an event-related potential analysis. *Electroencephalogr Clin Neurophysiol.* 96(5): 453–67.

Maiese K, Holloway HH, Larson DM, Soncrant TT. (1994). Effect of acute and chronic arecoline treatment on cerebral metabolism and blood flow in the conscious rat. *Brain Res.* 641(1): 65–75.

Malloy MH, Kleinman JC, Land GH, Schramm WF. (1988). The association of maternal smoking with age and cause of infant death. *Am J Epidemiol.* 128(1): 46–55.

Mathew RJ, Barr DL, Weinman ML. (1983). Caffeine and cerebral blood flow. *Br J Psychiatry* 143: 604–8.

Mathew RJ, Wilson WH. (1985). Caffeine induced changes in cerebral circulation. *Stroke.* 16(5): 814–17.

McGehee DS, Heath MJ, Gelber S, Devay P, Role LW. (1995). Nicotine enhancement of fast excitatory synaptic transmission in CNS by presynaptic receptors. *Science.* 269(5231): 1692–96.

McNamara D, Larson DM, Rapoport SI, Soncrant TT. (1990). Preferential metabolic activation of subcortical brain areas by acute administration of nicotine to rats. *J Cereb Blood Flow Metab.* 10(1): 48–56.

Mereu GP, Pacitti C, Argiolas A. (1983). Effect of (–)-cathinone, a khat leaf constituent, on dopaminergic firing and dopamine metabolism in the rat brain. *Life Sci.* 32(12): 1383–89.

Meston CM, Heiman JR. (1998). Ephedrine-activated physiological sexual arousal in women. *Arch Gen Psychiatry.* 55(7): 652–56.

Mets B, Winger G, Cabrera C, Seo S, Jamdar S, Yang G, Zhao K, Briscoe RJ, Almonte R, Woods JH, Landry DW. (1998). A catalytic antibody against cocaine prevents cocaine's reinforcing and toxic effects in rats. *Proc Natl Acad Sci USA.* 95(17): 10176–81.

Metting TL, Burgio DE, Terry AV Jr, Beach JW, McCurdy CR, Allen DD. (1998). Inhibition of brain choline uptake by isoarecolone and lobeline derivatives: implications for potential vector-mediated brain drug delivery. *Neurosci Lett.* Dec. 11;258(1): 25–28.

Millar K, Wilkinson RT. (1981). The effects upon vigilance and reaction speed of the addition of ephedrine hydrochloride to chlorpheniramine maleate. *Eur J Clin Pharmacol.* 20(5): 351–57.

Mirza NR, Pei Q, Stolerman IP, Zetterstrom TS. (1996). The nicotinic receptor agonists (–)-nicotine and isoarecolone differ in their effects on dopamine release in the nucleus accumbens. *Eur J Pharmacol.* Jan. 11;295(2–3): 207–10.

Mitchell SN. (1993). Role of the locus coeruleus in the noradrenergic response to a systemic administration of nicotine. *Neuropharmacology.* Oct. 32(10): 937–49.

Molinengo L, Cassone MC, Orsetti M. (1986). Action of arecoline on the levels of acetylcholine, norepinephrine, and dopamine in the mouse central nervous system. *Pharmacol Biochem Behav.* 24(6): 1801–3.

Molinengo L, Orsetti M, Pastorello B, Scordo I, Ghi P. (1995). The action of arecoline on retrieval and memory storage evaluated in the staircase maze. *Neurobiol Learn Mem.* 63(2): 167–73.

Morgan ME, Vestal RE. (1989). Methylxanthine effects on caudate dopamine release as measured by in vivo electrochemistry. *Life Sci.* 45(21): 2025–39.

Morton JF. (1992). Widespread tannin intake via stimulants and masticatories, especially guarana, kola nut, betel vine, and accessories. *Basic Life Sci.* 59: 739–65.

Murdoch I, Perry EK, Court JA, Graham DI, Dewar D. (1998). Cortical cholinergic dysfunction after human head injury. *J Neurotrauma.* 15(5): 295–305.

Musto DF. (1991). Opium, cocaine and marijuana in American history. *Sci Am.* 265(1): 40–7.

Nanji AA, Filipenko JD. (1984). Asystole and ventricular fibrillation associated with cocaine intoxication. *Chest.* 85(1): 132–33.

Nanri M, Kasahara N, Yamamoto J, Miyake H, Watanabe H. (1998). A comparative study on the effects of nicotine and GTS-21, a new nicotinic agonist, on the locomotor activity and brain monoamine level. *Jpn J Pharmacol.* 78(3): 385–89.

Nehlig A, Lucignani G, Kadekaro M, Porrino LJ, Sokoloff L. (1984). Effects of acute administration of caffeine on local cerebral glucose utilization in the rat. *Eur J Pharmacol.* 101(1–2): 91–100.

Nehlig A, Pereira de Vasconcelos A, Dumont I, Boyet S. (1990). Effects of caffeine, L-phenylisopropyladenosine and their combination on local cerebral blood flow in the rat. *Eur J Pharmacol.* 179(3): 271–80.

Nelson CB, Wittchen HU. (1998). Smoking and nicotine dependence. Results from a sample of 14- to 24-year-olds in Germany. *Eur Addict Res.* 4(1–2): 42–49.

Nencini P, Amiconi G, Befani O, Abdullahi MA, Anania MC. (1984). Possible involvement of amine oxidase inhibition in the sympathetic activation induced by khat (Catha edulis) chewing in humans. *J Ethnopharmacol.* 11: 179–86.

Newton TF, Cook IA, Holschneider DP, Rosenblatt MR, Lindholm JE, Jarvik MM. (1983). Quantitative EEG effects of nicotine replacement by cigarette smoking. *Neuropsychobiology*. 37(2): 112–16.

Nil R. (1991). A psychopharmacological and psychophysiological evaluation of smoking motives. *Rev Environ Health*. 9(2): 85–115.

Nisell M, Nomikos GG, Svensson TH. (1995). Nicotine dependence, midbrain dopamine systems and psychiatric disorders. *Pharmacol Toxicol*. 76(3): 157–62.

Nordberg A, Lundqvist H, Hartvig P, Andersson J, Johansson M, Hellstrom-Lindahi E, Norton SA. (1998). Betel: consumption and consequences. *J Am Acad Dermatol*. 38(1): 81–88.

Nuotto E. (1983). Psychomotor, physiological, and cognitive effects of scopolamine and ephedrine in healthy man. *Eur J Clin Pharmacol*. 24(5): 603–9.

Nygård O, Refsum H, Ueland PM, Stensvold I, Nordrehaug JE, Kvåle G, Vollset SE. (1997). Coffee consumption and plasma total homocysteine: the Hordaland Homocysteine Study. *Am J Clin Nutr*. 65(1): 136–43.

O'Brien CP. (1996). Drug addiction and abuse. In: *Goodman and Gilman's The Pharmacological Basis of Therapeutics*, 9th ed. Hardman JG, Limbird LE, Molinoff PB, Ruddon RW, Goodman Gilman A, eds. New York: McGraw-Hill.

Okada M, Kawata Y, Murakami T, Wada K, Mizuno K, Kondo T, Kaneko S. (1999). Differential effects of adenosine receptor subtypes on release and reuptake of hippocampal serotonin. *Eur J Neurosci*. 11(1): 1–9.

O'Malley S, Adamse M, Heaton RK, Gawin FH. (1992). Neuropsychological impairment in chronic cocaine abusers. *Am J Drug Alcohol Abuse*. 18(2): 131–44.

Pantellis C, Hindler C, Taylor J. (1989). Use and abuse of khat: distribution, pharmacology, side effects, and description of psychosis attributed to khat chewing. *Psychological Med*. 19: 657–58.

Parker MJ, Beck A, Luetje CW. (1989). Neuronal nicotinic receptor beta2 and beta4 subunits confer large differences in agonist binding affinity. *Mol Pharmacol*. 54(6): 1132–39.

Pedata F, Pepeu G, Spignoli G. (1984). Biphasic effect of methylxanthines on acetylcholine release from electrically-stimulated brain slices. *Br J Pharmacol*. 83(1): 69–73.

Pehek EA, Schechter MD, Yamamoto BK. (1990). Effects of cathinone and amphetamine on the neurochemistry of dopamine in vivo. *Neuropharmacology*. 29(12): 1171–76.

Penetar D, McCann U, Thorne D, Kamimori G, Galinski C, Sing H, Thomas M, Belenky G. (1993). Caffeine reversal of sleep deprivation effects on alertness and mood. *Psychopharmacology (Berlin)*. 112(2–3): 359–65.

Perret G, Schluger JH, Unterwald EM, Kreuter J, Ho A, Kreek MJ. (1998). Downregulation of 5-HT1A receptors in rat hypothalamus and dentate gyrus after "binge" pattern cocaine administration. *Synapse*. 30(2): 166–71.

Pickworth WB, Fant RV, Butschky MF, Henningfield JE. (1996). Effects of transdermal nicotine delivery on measures of acute nicotine withdrawal. *J Pharmacol Exp Ther.* 279(2): 450–56.

Pickworth WB, Fant RV, Butschky MF, Henningfield JE. (1997). Effects of mecamylamine on spontaneous EEG and performance in smokers and non-smokers. *Pharmacol Biochem Behav.* 56(2): 181–87.

Pickworth WB, Herning RI, Henningfield JE. (1986). Electroencephalographic effects of nicotine chewing gum in humans. *Pharmacol Biochem Behav.* 25(4): 879–82.

Pickworth WB, Herning RI, Henningfield JE. (1989). Spontaneous EEG changes during tobacco abstinence and nicotine substitution in human volunteers. *J Pharmacol Exp Ther.* 251(3): 976–82.

Pidoplichko VI, DeBiasi M, Williams JT, Dani JA. (1997). Nicotine activates and desensitizes midbrain dopamine neurons. *Nature.* 390(6658): 401–4.

Piha T, Besselink E, Lopez AD. (1993). Tobacco or health. *World Health Stat Q.* 46(3): 188–94.

Pineda JA, Herrera C, Kang C, Sandler A. (1998). Effects of cigarette smoking and 12-h abstention on working memory during a serial-probe recognition task. *Psychopharmacology (Berlin).* 139(4): 311–21.

Pirich C, O'Grady J, Sinzinger H. (1993). Coffee, lipoproteins, and cardiovascular disease. *Wien Klin Wochenschr.* 105(1): 3–6.

Poli A, Lucchi R, Vibio M, Barnabei O. (1991). Adenosine and glutamate modulate each other's release from rat hippocampal synaptosomes. *J Neurochem.* 57(1): 298–306.

Pomerleau OF. (1992). Nicotine and the central nervous system: biobehavioral effects of cigarette smoking. *Am J Med.* 93(1A): 2S–7S.

Pomerleau OF, Fertig JB, Seyler LE, Jaffe J. (1983). Neuroendocrine reactivity to nicotine in smokers. *Psychopharmacology (Berlin).* 81(1): 61–67.

Pontieri FE, Passarelli F, Calo L, Caronti B. (1998). Functional correlates of nicotine administration: similarity with drugs of abuse. *J Mol Med.* 76(3–4): 193–201.

Porta M, Jick H, Habakangas JA. (1986). Follow-up study of pseudoephedrine users. *Ann Allergy.* 57(5): 340–42.

Pritchard WS, Houlihan ME, Guy TD, Robinson JH. (1999). Little evidence that "denicotinized" menthol cigarettes have pharmacological effects: an EEG/heart-rate/subjective-response study. *Psychopharmacology (Berlin).* 143(3): 273–79.

Radcliffe KA, Dani JA. (1998). Nicotinic stimulation produces multiple forms of increased glutamatergic synaptic transmission. *J Neurosci.* 18(18): 7075–83.

Raffaele KC, Asthana S, Berardi A, Haxby JV, Morris PP, Schapiro MB, Soncrant TT. (1996). Differential response to the cholinergic agonist arecoline among different cognitive modalities in Alzheimer's disease. *Neuropsychopharmacology.* 15(2): 163–70.

Raffaele KC, Berardi A, Asthana S, Morris P, Haxby JV, Soncrant TT. (1991). Effects of long-term continuous infusion of the muscarinic cholinergic agonist arecoline on verbal memory in dementia of the Alzheimer type. *Psychopharmacol Bull.* 27(3): 315–19.

Raj H, Singh VK, Anand A, Paintal AS. (1995). Sensory origin of lobeline-induced sensations: a correlative study in man and cat. *J Physiol (London).* 482(pt 1): 235–46.

Rao TS, Correa LD, Lloyd GK. (1997). Effects of lobeline and dimethylphenylpiperazinium iodide (DMPP) on N-methyl-D-aspartate (NMDA)-evoked acetylcholine release in vitro: evidence for a lack of involvement of classical neuronal nicotinic acetylcholine receptors. *Neuropharmacology.* 36(1): 39–50.

Rapoport JL, Berg CJ, Ismond DR, Zahn TP, Neims A. (1984). Behavioral effects of caffeine in children. Relationship between dietary choice and effects of caffeine challenge. *Arch Gen Psychiatry.* 41(11): 1073–79.

Rasmussen T, Swedberg MD. (1998). Reinforcing effects of nicotinic compounds: intravenous self-administration in drug-naive mice. *Pharmacol Biochem Behav.* 60(2): 567–73.

Reavill C, Walther B, Stolerman IP, Testa B. (1990). Behavioural and pharmacokinetic studies on nicotine, cytisine, and lobeline. *Neuropharmacology.* 29(7): 619–24.

Reeves RR, Struve FA, Patrick G. (1999). The effects of caffeine withdrawal on cognitive P300 auditory and visual evoked potentials. *Clin Electroencephalogr.* 30(1): 24–27.

Reichard CC, Elder ST. (1977). The effects of caffeine on reaction time in hyperkinetic and normal children. *Psychiatry.* 134(2): 144–48.

Reichart PA, Phillipsen HP. (1998). Betel chewer's mucosa—a review. *J Oral Pathol Med.* 27(6): 239–42.

Reith ME, Sershen H, Lajtha A. (1987). Effects of caffeine on monoaminergic systems in mouse brain. *Acta Biochim Biophys Hung.* 22(2–3): 149–63.

Reitstetter R, Lukas RJ, Gruener R. (1999). Dependence of nicotinic acetylcholine receptor recovery from desensitization on the duration of agonist exposure. *J Pharmacol Exp Ther.* 289(2): 656–60.

Ribeiro EB, Bettiker RL, Bogdanov M, Wurtman RJ. (1993). Effects of systemic nicotine on serotonin release in rat brain. *Brain Res.* 621(2): 311–18.

Richardson GA. (1998). Prenatal cocaine exposure. A longitudinal study of development. *Ann N Y Acad Sci.* 846: 144–52.

Richardson GA, Day NL, McGauhey PJ. (1993). The impact of prenatal marijuana and cocaine use on the infant and child. *Clin Obstet Gynecol.* 36(2): 302–18.

Richardson GA, Hamel SC, Goldschmidt L, Day NL. (1999). Growth of infants prenatally exposed to cocaine/crack: comparison of a prenatal care and a no prenatal care sample. *Pediatrics.* 104(2): e18.

Riedel W, Hogervorst E, Leboux R, Verhey F, van Praag H, Jolles J. (1995). Caffeine attenuates scopolamine-induced memory impairment in humans. *Psychopharmacology (Berlin)*. 122(2): 158–68.

Riekkinen M, Aroviita L, Kivipelto M, Taskila K, Riekkinen P Jr. (1996). Depletion of serotonin, dopamine, and noradrenaline in aged rats decreases the therapeutic effect of nicotine, but not of tetrahydroaminoacridine. *Eur J Pharmacol*. 308(3): 243–50.

Ritz MC, Lamb RJ, Goldberg SR, Kuhar MJ. (1987). Cocaine receptors on dopamine transporters are related to self-administration of cocaine. *Science*. 237(4819): 1219–23.

Robbers JE, Speedie MK, and Tyler VE. (1996). *Pharmacognosy and Pharmacobiotechnology*. Baltimore: Willams and Wilkins.

Rogers PJ, Dernoncourt C. (1998). Regular caffeine consumption: a balance of adverse and beneficial effects for mood and psychomotor performance. *Pharmacol Biochem Behav*. 59(4): 1039–45.

Rounsaville BJ, Anton SF, Carroll K, Budde D, Prusoff BA, Gawin F. (1991). Psychiatric diagnoses of treatment-seeking cocaine abusers. *Arch Gen Psychiatry*. 48(1): 43–51.

Roussinov KS, Yonkov DI. (1976). Cholinergic mechanisms in the learning and memory facilitating effect of caffeine. *Acta Physiol Pharmacol Bulg*. 2(3): 61–68.

Rudgley R. (1999). *The Encyclopaedia of Psychoactive Substances*. NY: St. Martin Press.

Rusted JM, Graupner L, Greenwood K. (1996). Methodological considerations in nicotine research: the use of "denicotinised" cigarettes as the control condition in smoking studies. *Psychopharmacology (Berlin)*. 125(2): 176–78.

Sachs DP, Leischow SJ. (1991). Pharmacologic approaches to smoking cessation. *Clin Chest Med*. 12(4): 769–91.

Sakurai Y, Takano Y, Kohjimoto Y, Honda K, Kamiya HO. (1982). Enhancement of [^{3}H]dopamine release and its [^{3}H]metabolites in rat striatum by nicotinic drugs. *Brain Res*. 242(1): 99–106.

Schechter MD. (1990). Rats become acutely tolerant to cathine after amphetamine or cathinone administration. *Psychopharmacology (Berlin)*. 101(1): 126–31.

Schechter MD. (1991). Effect of learned behavior upon conditioned place preference to cathinone. *Pharmacol Biochem Behav*. 38(1): 7–11.

Schechter MD. (1992). Effect of altering dopamine or serotonin neurotransmitters upon cathinone discrimination. *Pharmacol Biochem Behav*. 41(1): 37–41.

Schellscheidt J, Oyen N, Jorch G. (1997). Interactions between maternal smoking and other prenatal risk factors for sudden infant death syndrome (SIDS). *Acta Paediatr*. 86(8): 857–63.

Schilstrom B, Svensson HM, Svensson TH, Nomikos GG. (1998). Nicotine and food induced dopamine release in the nucleus accumbens of the rat: putative role of alpha7 nicotinic receptors in the ventral tegmental area. *Neuroscience*. 85(4): 1005–9.

Schlyer D, Wolf AP, Warner D, Zezulkova I, Cilento R. (1996). Inhibition of monoamine oxidase B in the brains of smokers. *Nature*. 379(6567): 733–36.

Schroeder H, Boyet S, Nehlig A. (1989). Effects of caffeine and doxapram perfusion on local cerebral glucose utilization in conscious rats. *Eur J Pharmacol*. 167(2): 245–54.

Sekkadde Kiyingi K, Saweri A. (1994). Betelnut chewing causes bronchoconstriction in some asthma patients. *PNG Med J*. 37(2): 90–99.

Selby MJ, Azrin RL. (1998). Neuropsychological functioning in drug abusers. *Drug Alcohol Depend*. 50(1): 39–45.

Serafin WE. (1996). Drugs used in the treatment of asthma. In: *Goodman and Gilman's The Pharmacological Basis of Therapeutics*, 9th ed. Hardman JG, Limbird LE, Molinoff PB, Ruddon RW, Goodman Gilman A, eds. New York: McGraw-Hill.

Sershen H, Balla A, Lajtha A, Vizi ES. (1997). Characterization of nicotinic receptors involved in the release of noradrenaline from the hippocampus. *Neuroscience*. 77(1): 121–30.

Shannon JR, Gottesdiener K, Jordan J, Chen K, Flattery S, Larson PJ, Candelore MR, Gertz B, Robertson D, Sun M. (1999). Acute effect of ephedrine on 24-h energy balance. *Clin Sci (Colch)*. 96(5): 483–91.

Shapira B, Lerer B, Gilboa D, Drexler H, Kugelmass S, Calev A. (1987). Facilitation of ECT by caffeine pretreatment. *Am J Psychiatry*. 144(9): 1199–202.

Shear MK. (1986). Pathophysiology of panic: a review of pharmacologic provocative tests and naturalistic monitoring data. *J Clin Psychiatry*. 47(suppl): 18–26.

Sherief HT, Carpentier RG. (1991). Electrophysiological mechanisms of cocaine-induced cardiac arrest. A possible cause of sudden cardiac death. *J Electrocardiol*. 24(3): 247–55.

Shiffman S, Paty JA, Gnys M, Kassel JD, Elash C. (1995). Nicotine withdrawal in chippers and regular smokers: subjective and cognitive effects. *Health Psychol*. 14(4): 301–9.

Shively CA, Tarka SM Jr. (1984). Methylxanthine composition and consumption patterns of cocoa and chocolate products. *Prog Clin Biol Res*. 158: 149–78.

Shoaib M. (1998). Is dopamine important in nicotine dependence? *J Physiol Paris*. 92(3–4): 229–33.

Sieb JP, Engel AG. (1993). Ephedrine: effects on neuromuscular transmission. *Brain Res*. 623(1): 167–71.

Sloan JW, Martin WR, Bostwick M, Hook R, Wala E. (1988). The comparative binding characteristics of nicotinic ligands and their pharmacology. *Pharmacol Biochem Behav*. 30(1): 255–67.

Smith A, Kendrick A, Maben A, Salmon J. (1994). Effects of breakfast and caffeine on cognitive performance, mood, and cardiovascular functioning. *Appetite.* 22(1): 39–55.

Smith BD, Davidson RA, Green RL. (1993). Effects of caffeine and gender on physiology and performance: further tests of a biobehavioral model. *Physiol Behav.* 54(3): 415–22.

Smith BD, Rafferty J, Lindgren K, Smith DA, Nespor A. (1992). Effects of habitual caffeine use and acute ingestion: testing a biobehavioral model. *Physiol Behav.* 51(1): 131–37.

Smith KM, Mitchell SN, Joseph MH. (1991). Effects of chronic and subchronic nicotine on tyrosine hydroxylase activity in noradrenergic and dopaminergic neurones in the rat brain. *J Neurochem.* 57(5): 1750–56.

Snyder SH, Sklar P. (1984). Behavioral and molecular actions of caffeine: focus on adenosine. *J Psychiatr Res.* 18(2): 91–106.

Sobrian SK, Burton LE, Robinson NL, Ashe WK, James H, Stokes DL, Turner LM. (1990). Neurobehavioral and immunological effects of prenatal cocaine exposure in rat. *Pharmacol Biochem Behav.* 35(3): 617–29.

Soncrant TT, Holloway HW, Rapoport SI. (1985). Arecoline-induced elevations of regional cerebral metabolism in the conscious rat. *Brain Res.* 347(2): 205–16.

Sopranzi N, De Feo G, Mazzanti G, Braghiroli L. (1991). [The biological and electrophysiological parameters in the rat chronically treated with Lobelia inflata L]. *Clin Ter.* 137(4): 265–68.

Spindel E. (1984). Action of the methylxanthines on the pituitary and pituitary-dependent hormones. *Prog Clin Biol Res.* 158: 355–63.

Spindel ER, Wurtman RJ, McCall A, Carr DB, Conlay L, Griffith L, Arnold MA. (1984). Neuroendocrine effects of caffeine in normal subjects. *Clin Pharmacol Ther.* 36(3): 402–7.

Spriet LL. (1995). Caffeine and performance. *Int J Sport Nutr.* 5(suppl): S84–99.

Stankov B, Cimino M, Marini P, Lucini V, Fraschini F, Clementi F. (1993). Identification and functional significance of nicotinic cholinergic receptors in the rat pineal gland. *Neurosci Lett.* 156(1–2): 131–34.

Stein MA, Krasowski M, Leventhal BL, Phillips W, Bender BG. (1996). Behavioral and cognitive effects of methylxanthines. A meta-analysis of theophylline and caffeine. *Arch Pediatr Adolesc Med.* 150(3): 284–8.

Stewart SH, Karp J, Pihl RO, Peterson RA. (1997). Anxiety sensitivity and self-reported reasons for drug use. *J Subst Abuse.* 9: 223–40.

Stoessl AJ, Young GB, Feasby TE. (1985). Intracerebral haemorrhage and angiographic beading following ingestion of catecholaminergics. *Stroke.* 16(4): 734–36.

Stolerman IP, Garcha HS, Mirza NR. (1995). Dissociations between the locomotor stimulant and depressant effects of nicotinic agonists in rats. *Psychopharmacology (Berlin).* 117(4): 430–37.

Stolerman IP, Shoaib M. (1991). The neurobiology of tobacco addiction. *Trends Pharmacol Sci.* 12(12): 467–73.

Stone WS, Croul CE, Gold PE. (1998). Attenuation of scopolamine-induced amnesia in mice. *Psychopharmacology (Berlin).* 96(3): 417–20.

Streufert S, Pogash R, Miller J, Gingrich D, Landis R, Lonardi L, Severs W, Roache JD. (1995). Effects of caffeine deprivation on complex human functioning. *Psychopharmacology (Berlin).* 118(4): 377–84.

Stricherz ME, Pratt P. (1976). Betel quid and reaction time. *Pharmacol Biochem Behav.* 4(5): 627–28.

Subarnas A, Oshima Y, Sidik, Ohizumi Y. (1992). An antidepressant principle of Lobelia inflata L. (Campanulaceae). *J Pharm Sci.* 81(7): 620–21.

Subarnas A, Tadano T, Kisara K, Ohizumi Y. (1993c). An alpha-adrenoceptor-mediated mechanism of hypoactivity induced by beta-amyrin palmitate. *J Pharm Pharmacol.* 45(11): 1006–8.

Subarnas A, Tadano T, Nakahata N, Arai Y, Kinemuchi H, Oshima Y, Kisara K, Ohizumi Y. (1993b). A possible mechanism of antidepressant activity of beta-amyrin palmitate isolated from Lobelia inflata leaves in the forced swimming test. *Life Sci.* 52(3): 289–96.

Subarnas A, Tadano T, Oshima Y, Kisara K, Ohizumi Y. (1993a). Pharmacological properties of beta-amyrin palmitate, a novel centrally acting compound, isolated from Lobelia inflata leaves. *J Pharm Pharmacol.* 45(6): 545–50.

Szendrei K. (1980). The chemistry of khat. *Bull Narc.* 32(3): 5–35.

Taha SA, Ageel AM, Islam MW, Ginawi OT. (1995). Effect of (–)-cathinone, a psychoactive alkaloid from khat (Catha edulis Forsk.) and caffeine on sexual behaviour in rats. *Pharmacol Res.* 31(5): 299–303.

Tani Y, Saito K, Imoto M, Ohno T. (1998). Pharmacological characterization of nicotinic receptor-mediated acetylcholine release in rat brain—an in vivo microdialysis study. *Eur J Pharmacol.* 351(2): 181–88.

Tani Y, Saito K, Tsuneyoshi A, Imoto M, Ohno T. (1997). Nicotinic acetylcholine receptor (nACh-R) agonist-induced changes in brain monoamine turnover in mice. *Psychopharmacology (Berlin).* 129(3): 225–32.

Targovnik JH. (1989). Nicotine, corticotropin, and smoking withdrawal symptoms: literature review and implications for successful control of nicotine addiction. *Clin Ther.* 11(6): 846–53.

Tariot PN, Cohen RM, Welkowitz JA, Sunderland T, Newhouse PA, Murphy DL, Tariq M, Islam MW, al-Meshal IA, el-Feraly FS, Ageel AM. (1989). Comparative study of cathinone and amphetamine on brown adipose thermogenesis. *Life Sci.* 44(14): 951–55.

Tariq M, Islam MW, al-Meshal IA, el-Feraly FS, Ageel AM. (1989). Comparative study of cathinone and amphetamine on brown adipose thermogenesis. *Life Sci.* 44(14): 951–5.

Taylor P. (1996) Agents acting at the neuromuscular junction and autonomic ganglia. In: *Goodman and Gilman's The Pharmacological Basis of Therapeutics*, 9th ed. Hardman JG, Limbird LE, Molinoff PB, Ruddon RW, Goodman Gilman A, eds. New York: McGraw-Hill.

Taylor RF, al-Jarad N, John LM, Conroy DM, Barnes NC. (1992). Betel-nut chewing and asthma. *Lancet.* 339(8802): 1134–36.

Teng L, Crooks PA, Dwoskin LP. (1998). Lobeline displaces [^{3}H]dihydrotetrabenazine binding and releases [^{3}H]dopamine from rat striatal synaptic vesicles: with d-amphetamine. *J Neurochem.* 71(1): 258–65.

Teng L, Crooks PA, Sonsalla PK, Dwoskin LP. (1997). Lobeline and nicotine evoke [^{3}H]overflow from rat striatal slices preloaded with [^{3}H]dopamine: differential inhibition of synaptosomal and vesicular [^{3}H]dopamine uptake. *J Pharmacol Exp Ther.* 280(3): 1432–44.

Terry AV Jr, Williamson R, Gattu M, Beach JW, McCurdy CR, Sparks JA, Pauly JR. (1998). Lobeline and structurally simplified analogs exhibit differential agonist activity and sensitivity to antagonist blockade when compared to nicotine. *Neuropharmacology.* 37(1): 93–102.

Terry WS, Phifer B. (1986). Caffeine and memory performance on the AVLT. *J Clin Psychol.* 42(6): 860–63.

Thurlbeck WM. (1984). The pathobiology and epidemiology of human emphysema. *J Toxicol Environ Health.* 13(2–3): 323–43.

Tongjaroenbuangam W, Meksuriyen D, Govitrapong P, Kotchabhakdi N, Baldwin BA. (1998). Drug discrimination analysis of pseudoephedrine in rats. *Pharmacol Biochem Behav.* 59(2): 505–10.

Toth PT, Vizi ES. (1998). Lobeline inhibits Ca2+ current in cultured neurones from rat sympathetic ganglia. *Eur J Pharmacol.* 363(1): 75–80.

Trivedy C, Warnakulasuriya S, Peters TJ. (1999). Areca nuts can have deleterious effects. *BMJ* 318: 1287.

Turchi J, Holley LA, Sarter M. (1995). Effects of nicotinic acetylcholine receptor ligands on behavioral vigilance in rats. *Psychopharmacology (Berlin).* 118(2): 195–205.

Tyler VE. (1994). *Herbs of Choice: The Theraputic Use of Phytomedicinals.* New York: Pharmaceutical Products Press.

U.S. Department of Health and Human Services. (1989). *Reducing the Health Consequences of Smoking: 25 Years of Progress. A Report of the Surgeon General.* Rockville, MD: U.S. Department of Health and Human Services.

Vidal C. (1996). Nicotinic receptors in the brain. Molecular biology, function, and therapeutics. *Mol Chem Neuropathol.* 28(1–3): 3–11.

Vidal C, Changeux JP. (1993). Nicotinic and muscarinic modulations of excitatory synaptic transmission in the rat prefrontal cortex in vitro. *Neuroscience.* 56(1): 23–32.

Vik T, Jacobsen G, Vatten L, Bakketeig LS. (1996). Pre- and post-natal growth in children of women who smoked in pregnancy. *Early Hum Dev.* 45(3): 245–55.

Volkow ND, Fowler JS, Wang GJ, Hitzemann R, Logan J, Schlyer DJ, Dewey SL, Wolf AP. (1993). Decreased dopamine D2 receptor availability is associated with reduced frontal metabolism in cocaine abusers. *Synapse.* 14(2): 169–77.

Volkow ND, Fowler JS, Wolf AP. (1991). Use of positron emission tomography to study cocaine in the human brain. *NIDA Res Monogr.* 112: 168–79.

Volkow ND, Mullani N, Gould KL, Adler S, Krajewski K. (1988). Cerebral blood flow in chronic cocaine users: a study with positron emission tomography. *Br J Psychiatry.* 152: 641–48.

Volkow ND, Wang GJ, Fowler JS, Hitzemann R, Angrist B, Gatley SJ, Logan J, Ding YS, Pappas N. (1999). Association of methylphenidate-induced craving with changes in right striato-orbitofrontal metabolism in cocaine abusers: implications in addiction. *Am J Psychiatry.* 156(1): 19–26.

Wagner GC, Preston K, Ricaurte GA, Schuster CR, Seiden LS. (1982). Neurochemical similarities between d,l-cathinone and d-amphetamine. *Drug Alcohol Depend.* 9(4): 279–84.

Wang H, Cui WY, Liu CG. (1996). Regulatory effects of acutely repeated nicotine treatment towards central muscarinic receptors. *Life Sci.* 59(17): 1415–21.

Warburton DM. (1995). Effects of caffeine on cognition and mood without caffeine abstinence. *Psychopharmacology (Berlin).* 119(1): 66–70.

Warnakulasuriya KAAS, Trivedy C, Maher R, Johnson NW. (1997). Aetiology of oral submucous fibrosis. *Oral Dis.* 3: 286–87.

Weil A, Rosen W. (1983) *Chocolate to Morphine.* Boston: Houghton Mifflin Company.

Weingartner H. (1988). Multiple-dose arecoline infusions in Alzheimer's disease. *Arch Gen Psychiatry.* 45(10): 901–5.

Wess J, Lambrecht G, Moser U, Mutschler E. (1987). Stimulation of ganglionic muscarinic M1 receptors by a series of tertiary arecaidine and isoarecaidine esters in the pithed rat. *Eur J Pharmacol.* 134(1): 61–67.

West R, Hajek P. (1997). What happens to anxiety levels on giving up smoking? *Am J Psychiatry.* 154(11): 1589–92.

White LM, Gardner SF, Gurley BJ, Marx MA, Wang PL, Estes M. (1997). Pharmacokinetics and cardiovascular effects of ma-huang (Ephedra sinica) in normotensive adults. *J Clin Pharmacol* 37(2): 116–22.

White SR, Obradovic T, Imel KM, Wheaton MJ. (1996). The effects of methylenedioxymethamphetamine (MDMA, "ecstasy") on monoaminergic neurotransmission in the central nervous system. *Prog Neurobiol.* 49(5): 455–79.

Wilder P, Mathys K, Brenneisen R, Kalix P, Fisch HU. (1994). Pharmacodynamics and pharmacokinetics of khat: a controlled study. *Clin Pharmacol Ther.* 55: 556–62.

Wilkinson JM, Pollard I. (1993). Accumulation of theophylline, theobromine, and paraxanthine in the fetal rat brain following a single oral dose of caffeine. *Brain Res Dev Brain Res.* 75(2): 193–99.

Winstock AR, Trivedy CR, Warnakulasuriya KAAS, Peters TJ. (In press). A dependency syndrome related to areca nut use: some medical and psychological aspects among areca nut users in the Gujarat community in the UK. *Addict Biol.*

Wolf-Pflugmann M, Lambrecht G, Wess J, Mutschler E. (1989). Synthesis and muscarinic activity of a series of tertiary and quaternary N-substituted guvacine esters structurally related to arecoline and arecaidine propargyl ester. *Arzneimittelforschung.* 39(5): 539–44.

Woolverton WL, Johanson CE. (1984). Preference in rhesus monkeys given a choice between cocaine and d,l-cathinone. *J Exp Analysis Behav.* 41(1): 35–43.

Woolverton WL, Johnson KM. (1992). Neurobiology of cocaine abuse. *Trends Pharmacol Sci.* 13(5): 193–200.

Wooten MR, Khangure MS, Murphy MJ. (1983). Intracerebral hemorrhage and vasculitis related to ephedrine abuse. *Ann Neurol.* 13(3): 337–40.

Wu JC, Bell K, Najafi A, Widmark C, Keator D, Tang C, Klein E, Bunney BG, Fallon J, Bunney WE. (1997). Decreasing striatal 6-FDOPA uptake with increasing duration of cocaine withdrawal. *Neuropsychopharmacology.* 17(6): 402–9.

Yamamoto J. (1998). Effects of nicotine, pilocarpine, and tetrahydroaminoacridine on hippocampal theta waves in freely moving rabbits. *Eur J Pharmacol.* 359(2–3): 133–37.

Yokoi F, Komiyama T, Ito T, Hayashi T, Lio M, Hara T. (1993). Application of carbon-11 labelled nicotine in the measurement of human cerebral blood flow and other physiological parameters. *Eur J Nucl Med.* 20(1): 46–52.

Young R, Glennon RA. (1998). Discriminative stimulus properties of (–)ephedrine. *Pharmacol Biochem Behav.* 60(3): 771–75.

Yu G, Maskray V, Jackson SH, Swift CG, Tiplady B. (1991). A comparison of the central nervous system effects of caffeine and theophylline in elderly subjects. *Br J Clin Pharmacol.* 32(3): 341–45.

Zelger JL, Carlini EA. (1980). Anorexigenic effects of two amines obtained from Catha edulis Forsk. (Khat) in rats. *Pharmacol Biochem Behav.* 12(5): 701–5.

Zuckerman M, Ball S, Black J. (1990). Influences of sensation seeking, gender, risk appraisal, and situational motivation on smoking. *Addict Behav.* 15(3): 209–20.

Zwyghuizen-Doorenbos A, Roehrs TA, Lipschutz L, Timms V, Roth T. (1990). Effects of caffeine on alertness. *Psychopharmacology (Berlin).* 100(1): 36–39.

Chapter 5

Abdulla FA, Bradbury E, Calaminici MR, Lippiello PM, Wonnacott S, Gray JA, Sinden JD. (1996). Relationship between up-regulation of nicotine binding sites in rat brain and delayed cognitive enhancement observed after chronic or acute nicotinic receptor stimulation. *Psychopharmacology (Berlin).* 124(4): 323–31.

Abe K, Cho SI, Nishiyama N, Saito H. (1994). Differential effects of ginsenoside Rb1 and malonylginsenoside Rb1 on long-term potentiation in the dentate gyrus. *Brain Res.* 649(1–2): 7–11.

Abe K, Fujimura H, Toyooka K, Sakoda S, Yorifuji S, Yanagihara T. (1997). Cognitive function in amyotrophic lateral sclerosis. *Neurol Sci.* 148(1): 95–100.

Acri JB, Morse DE, Popke EJ, Grunberg NE. (1994). Nicotine increases sensory gating measured as inhibition of the acoustic startle reflex in rats. *Psychopharmacology (Berlin).* 114(2): 369–74.

Adams RD, Victor M, Ropper AH. (1997). *Principles of Neurology.* New York: McGraw-Hill, Health Professions Division.

Aellig WH, Nuesch E. (1977). Comparative pharmacokinetic investigations with tritium-labeled ergot alkaloids after oral and intravenous administration in man. *Int J Clin Pharmacol Biopharmacy.* 15(3): 106–12.

Akisü M, Kültürsay N, Coker I, Hüseyinov A. (1998). Platelet-activating factor is an important mediator in hypoxic ischemic brain injury in the newborn rat. Flunarizine and Ginkgo biloba extract reduce PAF concentration in the brain. *Biol Neonate.* 74(6): 439–44.

Allain H, Raoul P, Lieury A, LeCoz F, Gandon JM, d'Arbigny P. (1993). Effect of two doses of ginkgo biloba extract (EGb 761) on the dual-coding test in elderly subjects. *Clin Ther.* 15(3): 549–58.

Amenta F, Cavallotti C, Franch F, Ricci A. (1989). Muscarinic cholinergic receptors in the hippocampus of the aged rat: effects of long-term Hydergine administration. *Arch Int Pharmacodyn Ther.* 297: 225–34.

American Psychiatric Association. (1994). *Diagnostic and Statistical Manual of Mental Disorders*, 4th ed. Washington DC: American Psychiatric Association.

Amri H, Drieu K, Papadopoulos V. (1997). Ex vivo regulation of adrenal cortical cell steroid and protein synthesis, in response to adrenocorticotropic hormone stimulation, by the Ginkgo biloba extract EGb 761 and isolated ginkgolide B. *Endocrinology.* 138(12): 5415–26.

Amri H, Ogwuegbu SO, Boujrad N, Drieu K, Papadopoulos V. (1996). In vivo regulation of peripheral-type benzodiazepine receptor and glucocorticoid synthesis by Ginkgo biloba extract EGb 761 and isolated ginkgolides. *Endocrinology.* 137(12): 5707–18.

Anderson DJ, Williams M, Pauly JR, Raszkiewicz JL, Campbell JE, Rotert G, Surber B, Thomas SB, Wasicak J, Arneric SP, et al. (1995). Characterization of [^{3}H]ABT-418: a novel cholinergic channel ligand. *J Pharmacol Exp Ther.* 273(3): 1434–41.

Arendash GW, Sanberg PR, Sengstock GJ. (1995a). Nicotine enhances the learning and memory of aged rats. *Pharmacol Biochem Behav.* 52(3): 517–23.

Arendash GW, Sengstock GJ, Sanberg PR, Kem WR. (1995b). Improved learning and memory in aged rats with chronic administration of the nicotinic receptor agonist GTS-21. *Brain Res.* 674(2): 252–9.

Arendt T. (1994). Impairment in memory function and neurodegenerative changes in the cholinergic basal forebrain system induced by chronic intake of ethanol. *J Neural Transm.* Supplement 44: 173–87.

Asthana S, Greig NH, Holloway HW, Raffaele KC, Berardi A, Schapiro MB, Rapoport SI, Soncrant TT. (1996). Clinical pharmacokinetics of arecoline in subjects with Alzheimer's disease. *Clin Pharmacol Ther.* 60(3): 276–82.

Aston-Jones G, Rajkowski J, Kubiak P, Alexinsky T. (1994). Locus coeruleus neurons in monkey are selectively activated by attended cues in a vigilance task. *J Neurosci.* 14(7): 4467–80.

Attele AS, Wu JA, Yuan CS. (1999). Ginseng pharmacology: multiple constituents and multiple actions. *Biochem Pharmacol.* 58(11): 1685–93.

Babikian VL, Wolfe N, Lin R, Knoefel JE, Albert ML. (1990). Cognitive changes in patients with multiple cerebral infarcts. *Stroke.* 21: 1013–18.

Barkats M, Venault P, Christen Y, Cohen-Salmon C. (1995). Effect of long-term treatment with EGb 761 on age-dependent structural changes in the hippocampi of three inbred mouse strains. *Life Sci.* 56(4): 213–22.

Baureithel KH, Buter KB, Engesser A, Burkard W, Schaffner W. (1997). Inhibition of benzodiazepine binding in vitro by amentoflavone, a constituent of various species of Hypericum. *Pharm Acta Helv.* 72(3): 153–7.

Bazan NG, Allan G. (1996). Platelet-activating factor in the modulation of excitatory amino acid neurotransmitter release and of gene expression. *J Lipid Mediators Cell Signalling.* 14(1–3): 321–30.

Becker K, Braquet P, Förster W. (1988). Influence of the specific antagonist of PAF-acether, BN 52021, and of Ginkgo extract on the rejection of murine tail skin allografts and the PAF-acether mortality in mice in particular consideration of the role of TXB2. *Biomedica Biochimica Acta.* 47: 10–11, S165–68.

Benishin CG. (1992). Actions of ginsenoside Rb1 on choline uptake in central cholinergic nerve endings. *Neurochem Int.* 21(1): 1–5.

Benishin CG, Lee R, Wang LC, Liu HJ. (1991). Effects of ginsenoside Rb1 on central cholinergic metabolism. *Pharmacology.* 42(4): 223–29.

Bhattacharya SK, Mitra SK. (1991). Anxiolytic activity of Panax ginseng roots: an experimental study. *J Ethnopharmacol.* 34(1): 87–92.

Biber A, Koch E. (1999). Bioavailability of ginkgolides and bilobalide from extracts of Ginkgo biloba using GC/MS. *Planta Med.* 65(2): 192–93.

Bolanos-Jimenez F, Manhaes de Castro R, Sarhan H, prudhomme N, Drieu K, Fillion G. (1995). Stress-induced 5-HT1A receptor desensitization: protective effects of Ginkgo biloba extract (EGb 761). *Fundam Clin Pharmacol.* 9(2): 169–74.

Boller F, Duyckaerts C. (1997). Alzheimer's disease: Clinical and anatomic aspects. In: *Behavioral Neurology and Neuropsychology*. Feinberg T, Farah MJ, eds. New York: McGraw-Hill.

Bourgain RH, Andries R, Braquet P. (1987). Effect of ginkgolide PAF-acether antagonists on arterial thrombosis. *Adv Prostaglandin, Thromboxane, Leukotriene Res.* 17B: 815–17.

Bourgain RH, Maes L, Andries R, Braquet P. (1986). Thrombus induction by endogenic PAF-acether and its inhibition by Ginkgo biloba extracts in the guinea pig. *Prostaglandins* 32(1): 142–44.

Bowler JV, Hachinski V. (1997). Vascular Dementia. In: *Behavioral Neurology and Neuropsychology*. Feinberg T, Farah MJ, eds. New York: McGraw-Hill.

Brailowsky S, Montiel T. (1997). Motor function in young and aged hemiplegic rats: effects of a Ginkgo biloba extract. *Neurobiol Aging*. 18(2): 219–27.

Braquet P, Hosford D. (1991). Ethnopharmacology and the development of natural PAF antagonists as therapeutic agents. *J Ethnopharmacol.* 32(1–3): 135–39.

Bratt AM, Kelly ME, Domeney AM, Naylor RJ, Costall B. (1996). Acute and chronic arecoline: effects on a scopolamine-induced deficit in complex maze learning. *Pharmacol Biochem Behav.* 53(3): 713–21.

Brown RG, Marsden CD. (1991). Dual task performance and processing resources in normal subjects and patients with Parkinson's disease. *Brain.* 114(pt 1A): 215–31.

Brunello N, Racagni G, Clostre F, Drieu K, Braquet P. (1985). Effects of an extract of Ginkgo biloba on noradrenergic systems of rat cerebral cortex. *Pharmacol Res Commun.* 17(11): 1063–72.

Bruno C, Cuppini R, Sartini S, Cecchini T, Ambrogini P, Bombardelli E. (1993). Regeneration of motor nerves in bilobalide-treated rats. *Planta Med.* 59(4): 302–7.

Buccafusco JJ, Jackson WJ, Terry AV Jr, Marsh KC, Decker MW, Arneric SP. (1995). Improvement in performance of a delayed matching-to-sample task by monkeys following ABT-418: a novel cholinergic channel activator for memory enhancement. *Psychopharmacology (Berlin).* 120(3): 256–66.

Burke DM, Mackay DG. (1997). Memory, language, and ageing. *Philos Trans R Soc Lond Br Biol Sci.* 352(1363): 1845–56.

Büyüköztürk A, Kanit L, Ersöz B, Mente G, Hariri NI. (1995). The effects of Hydergine on the MAO activity of the aged and adult rat brain. *Eur Neuropsychopharmacol.* 5(4): 527–29.

Cano-Cuenca B, Algarra JM, Perez Del Valle B, Pellicer P. (1995). [The effect of Gingko biloba on cochleovestibulary pathology of vascular origin]. *An Otorrinolaringol Ibero Am.* 22(6): 619–29.

Caso Marasco A, Vargas Ruiz R, Salas Villagomez A, Begoña Infante C. (1996). Double-blind study of a multivitamin complex supplemented with ginseng extract. *Drugs Exp Clin Res.* 22(6): 323–9.

Cesarani A, Meloni F, Alpini D, Barozzi S, Verderio L, Boscani PF. (1998). Ginkgo biloba (EGb 761) in the treatment of equilibrium disorders. *Adv Ther.* 15(5): 291–304.

Chen C, Wei T, Gao Z, Zhao B, Hou J, Xu H, Xin W, Packer L. (1999). Different effects of the constituents of EGb 761 on apoptosis in rat cerebellar granule cells induced by hydroxyl radicals. *Biochem Mol Biol Int.* 47(3): 397–405.

Chen SE, Sawchuk RJ, Staba EJ. (1980). American ginseng: III. Pharmacokinetics of ginsenosides in the rabbit. *Eur J Drug Metab Pharmacokinet.* 5(3): 161–68.

Chen X, Lee TJ. (1995). Ginsenosides-induced nitric oxide-mediated relaxation of the rabbit corpus cavernosum. *Br J Pharmacol.* 115(1): 15–18.

Chen X, Salwinski S, Lee TJ. (1997). Extracts of Ginkgo biloba and ginsenosides exert cerebral vasorelaxation via a nitric oxide pathway. *Clin Exp Pharmacol Physiol.* 24(12): 958–59.

Cheng D, Chen W, Yang X, Xiao X, Xu D. (1996). [Effects of ginkgo plus on hypoxic pulmonary hypertension in rats]. *Hua Hsi I Ko Ta Hsueh Hsueh Pao.* 27(4): 415–17.

Choi HK, and Seong DH. (1995). Effectiveness for erectile dysfunction after the administration of Korean red ginseng. *Korean J Ginseng Sci.* 19: 17–21.

Choi YD, Xin ZC, Choi HK. (1998). Effect of Korean red ginseng on the rabbit corpus cavernosal smooth muscle. *Int J Impot Res.* 10(1): 37–43.

Chopin P, Briley M. (1992). Effects of four non-cholinergic cognitive enhancers in comparison with tacrine and galanthamine on scopolamine-induced amnesia in rats. *Psychopharmacology (Berlin).* 106(1): 26–30.

Chu NS. (1994). Effect of betel chewing on performance reaction time. *J Formos Med Assoc.* 93(4): 343–5.

Cohen AJ, Bartlik B. (1998). Ginkgo biloba for antidepressant-induced sexual dysfunction. *J Sex Marital Ther.* 124(2): 139–43.

Cohen C, Pickworth WB, Bunker EB, Henningfield JE. (1994). Caffeine antagonizes EEG effects of tobacco withdrawal. *Pharmacol Biochem Behav.* 47(4): 919–36.

Cohen-Salmon C, Venault P, Martin B, Raffalli-Sebille MJ, Barkats M, Clostre F, Pardon MC, Christen Y, Chapouthier G. (1997). Effects of Ginkgo biloba extract (EGb 761) on learning and possible actions on aging. *J Physiol Paris.* Dec. 91(6): 291–300.

Cooper JR, Bloom FE, Roth RH. (1996). *The Biochemical Basis of Neuropharmacology*, 7th ed. New York: Oxford University Press.

Copeland RL Jr, Bhattacharyya AK, Aulakh CS, Pradhan SN. (1981). Behavioral and neurochemical effects of Hydergine in rats. *Arch Int Pharmacodyn Ther.* 252(1): 113–23.

Damaj MI, Creasy KR, Welch SP, Rosecrans JA, Aceto MD, Martin BR. (1995). Comparative pharmacology of nicotine and ABT-418, a new nicotinic agonist. *Psychopharmacology (Berlin).* 120(4): 483–90.

D'Angelo L, Grimaldi R, Caravaggi M, Marcoli M, Perucca E, Lecchini S, Frigo GM, Crema A. (1986). A double-blind, placebo-controlled clinical study on the effect of a standardized ginseng extract on psychomotor performance in healthy volunteers. *J Ethnopharmacol.* 16(1): 15–22.

de Kloet ER, Oitzl MS, Joels M. (1999). Stress and cognition: are corticosteroids good or bad guys? *Trends Neurosci.* 22(10): 422–26.

Decker MW, Pelleymounter MA, Gallagher M. (1988). Effects of training on a spatial memory task on high affinity choline uptake in hippocampus and cortex in young adult and aged rats. *J Neurosci.* 8(1): 90–9.

Delagarza VW. (1998). New drugs for Alzheimer's disease. *Am Fam Physician.* 58(5): 1175–82.

DeNoble VJ, Repetti SJ, Gelpke LW, Wood LM, Keim KL. (1986). Vinpocetine: nootropic effects on scopolamine-induced and hypoxia-induced retrieval deficits of a step-through passive avoidance response in rats. *Pharmacol Biochem Behav.* 24(4): 1123–28.

Didier A, Droy-Lefaix MT, Aurousseau C, Cazals Y. (1996). Effects of Ginkgo biloba extract (EGb 761) on cochlear vasculature in the guinea pig: morphometric measurements and laser Doppler flowmetry. *Eur Arch Otorhinolaryngol.* 253(1–2): 25–30.

Doly M, Braquet P, Bonhomme B, Meyniel G. (1987). Effects of PAF-acether on electrophysiological response of isolated retina. *Int J Tissue React.* 9(1): 33–37.

Dravid AR. (1983). Deficits in cholinergic enzymes and muscarinic receptors in the hippocampus and striatum of senescent rats: effect of chronic Hydergine treatment. *Arch Int Pharmacodyn Ther.* 264(2): 195–202.

Droy-Lefaix MT, Cluzel J, Menerath JM, Bonhomme B, Doly M. (1995). Antioxidant effect of a Ginkgo biloba extract (EGb 761) on the retina. *Int J Tissue React.* 17(3): 93–100.

Duche JC, Barre J, Guinot P, Duchier J, Cournot A, Tillement JP. (1989). Effect of Ginkgo biloba extract on microsomal enzyme induction. *Int J Clin Pharmacol Res.* 9(3): 165–68.

Duverger D, DeFeudis FV, Drieu K. (1995). Effects of repeated treatments with an extract of Ginkgo biloba (EGb 761) on cerebral glucose utilization in the rat: an autoradiographic study. *Gen Pharmacol.* 26(6): 1375–83.

Ernst E. (1996). [Ginkgo biloba in treatment of intermittent claudication. A systematic research based on controlled studies in the literature]. *Fortschr Med.* 114(8): 85–87.

Etou H, Sakata T, Fujimoto K, Terada K, Yoshimatsu H, Ookuma K, Hayashi T, Arichi S. (1988). [Ginsenoside-Rb1 as a suppressor in central modulation of feeding in the rat]. *Nippon Yakurigaku Zasshi.* 91(1): 9–15.

Fahim MS, Fahim Z, Harman JM, Clevenger TE, Mullins W, Hafez ES. (1982). Effect of Panax ginseng on testosterone level and prostate in male rats. *Arch Androl.* 8(4): 261–63.

Faraday MM, Rahman MA, Scheufele PM, Grunberg NE. (1998). Nicotine administration impairs sensory gating in Long-Evans rats. *Pharmacol Biochem Behav.* 61(3): 281–89.

Field B, Vadnal R. (1998). Ginkgo biloba and memory: an overview. *Nutr Neurosci.* 1: 2565–67.

Flood JF, Cherkin A. (1988). Effect of acute arecoline, tacrine, and arecoline + tacrine post-training administration on retention in old mice. *Neurobiol Aging.* 9(1): 5–8.

Flood JF, Smith GE, Cherkin A. (1985). Hydergine enhances memory in mice. *J Pharmacol.* 16(suppl 3): 39–49.

Flood JF, Smith GE, Cherkin A. (1988). Memory enhancement in mice: role of drug dose and training-testing interval. *Pharmacol Biochem Behav.* 29(3): 635–39.

Foulds J, Stapleton J, Swettenham J, Bell N, McSorley K, Russell MA. (1996). Cognitive performance effects of subcutaneous nicotine in smokers and never-smokers. *Psychopharmacology (Berlin).* 127(1): 31–38.

Fourtillan JB, Brisson AM, Girault J, Ingrand I, Decourt JP, Drieu K, Jouenne P, Biber A. (1995). [Pharmacokinetic properties of bilobalide and ginkgolides A and B in healthy subjects after intravenous and oral administration of Ginkgo biloba extract (EGb 761)]. *Therapie.* 50(2): 137–44.

Frewer LJ. (1990). The effect of betel nut on human performance. *PNG Med J.* 33(2): 143–5.

Gajewski A, Hensch SA. (1999). Ginkgo biloba and memory for a maze. *Psychol Rep.* 84(2): 481–84.

Garg RK, Nag D, Agrawal A. (1995). A double blind placebo controlled trial of Ginkgo biloba extract in acute cerebral ischaemia. *J Assoc Physicians India.* 43(11): 760–63.

Gessner B, Voelp A, Klasser M. (1985). Study of the long-term action of a Ginkgo biloba extract on vigilance and mental performance as determined by means of quantitative pharmaco-EEG and psychometric measurements. *Arzneimittelforschung.* 35(9): 1459–65.

Gibb WRG. (1998). The neuropathology of parkinsonian disorders. In: *Parkinson's Disease and Movement Disorders*, 3rd ed. Jankovic J, Tolosa E, ed. Baltimore: Williams and Wilkins.

Gillis CN. (1997). Panax ginseng pharmacology: a nitric oxide link? *Biochem Pharmacol.* 54(1): 1–8.

Gross TM, Jarvik ME, Rosenblatt MR. (1993). Nicotine abstinence produces content-specific Stroop interference. *Psychopharmacology (Berlin).* 110(3): 333–36.

Gruenwald J, Brendler T, Jaenicke C. (1998). *PDR for Herbal Medicines*, 1st ed. Montvale, NJ: Medical Economics.

Haase J, Halama P, Hörr R. (1996). [Effectiveness of brief infusions with Ginkgo biloba special extract EGb 761 in dementia of the vascular and Alzheimer type]. *Z Gerontol Geriatr.* 29(4): 302–9.

Haguenauer JP, Cantenot F, Koskas H, Pierart H. (1986). [Treatment of equilibrium disorders with Ginkgo biloba extract. A multicenter double-blind drug vs. placebo study]. *Presse Med* 15(31): 1569–72.

Han BH. (1986). Studies on the metabolic fates of ginsenosides. *Korean Biochem.* 19: 213–18.

Hara T, Komiyama T, Yokoi F. (1993). Distribution of 11C-(R)nicotine in human brain measured by positron emission tomography: measurement of cerebral blood flow. *Yakubutsu Seishin Kodo.* 13(3): 175–81.

Hatsukami D, Fletcher L, Morgan S, Keenan R, Amble P. (1989). The effects of varying cigarette deprivation duration on cognitive and performance tasks. *J Subst Abuse.* 1(4): 407–16.

Heishman SJ, Snyder FR, Henningfield JE. (1993). Performance, subjective, and physiological effects of nicotine in non-smokers. *Drug Alcohol Depend.* 34(1): 11–18.

Heiss WD, Podreka I. (1978). Assessment of pharmacological effects on cerebral blood flow. *Eur Neurol.* 17(suppl 1): 135–43.

Hiai S, Yokoyama H, Oura H, Yano S. (1979). Stimulation of pituitary-adrenocortical system by ginseng saponin. *Endocrinol Jpn.* 26(6): 661–65.

Himi T, Saito H, Nishiyama N. (1989). Effect of ginseng saponins on the survival of cerebral cortex neurons in cell cultures. *Chem Pharm Bull (Tokyo).* 37(2): 481–84.

Hindmarch I. (1986). [Activity of Ginkgo biloba extract on short-term memory]. *Presse Medicale.* 15(31): 1592–94.

Hindmarch I, Kerr JS, Sherwood N. (1990). Effects of nicotine gum on psychomotor performance in smokers and non-smokers. *Psychopharmacology (Berlin).* 100(4): 535–41.

Hironaka N, Ando K. (1996). Effects of cholinergic drugs on scopolamine-induced memory impairment in rhesus monkeys. *Nihon Shinkei Seishin Yakurigaku Zasshi.* 16(3): 103–8.

Hobbs, C. (1996). *Ginseng: The Energy Herb.* Loveland, CO: Botanica Press.

Holgers KM, Axelsson A, Pringle I. (1994). Ginkgo biloba extract for the treatment of tinnitus. *Audiology.* 33(2): 85–92.

Huang, KC. (1998). *The Pharmacology of Chinese Herbs.* Boca Raton, FL: CRC Press.

Huguet F, Drieu K, Piriou A. (1994). Decreased cerebral 5-HT1A receptors during ageing: reversal by Ginkgo biloba extract (EGb 761). *J Pharm Pharmacol.* 46(4): 316–18.

Huguet F, Tarrade T. (1992). Alpha 2-adrenoceptor changes during cerebral ageing. The effect of Ginkgo biloba extract. *J Pharm Pharmacol.* 44(1): 24–27.

Imperato A, Obinu MC, Dazzi L, Carta G, Mascia MS, Casu MA, Gessa GL. (1994). Co-dergocrine (Hydergine) regulates striatal and hippocampal acetylcholine release through D2 receptors. *Neuroreport.* 5(6): 674–76.

Inestrosa NC, Marzolo MP, Bonnefont AB. (1998). Cellular and molecular basis of estrogen's neuroprotection. Potential relevance for Alzheimer's disease. *Mol Neurobiol.* 17(1–3): 73–86.

Ishii K, Sakamoto S, Sasaki M, Kitagaki H, Yamaji S, Hashimoto M, Imamura T, Shimomura T, Hirono N, Mori E. (1998). Cerebral glucose metabolism in patients with frontotemporal dementia. *J Nucl Med.* 39(11): 1875–78.

Itil T, Martorano D. (1995). Natural substances in psychiatry (Ginkgo biloba in dementia). *Psychopharmacol Bull.* 31(1): 147–58.

Itil TM, Eralp E, Ahmed I, Kunitz A, Itil KZ. (1998). The pharmacological effects of ginkgo biloba, a plant extract, on the brain of dementia patients in comparison with tacrine. *Psychopharmacol Bull.* 34(3): 391–97.

Itoh T, Zang YF, Murai S, Saito H. (1989). Effects of Panax ginseng root on the vertical and horizontal motor activities and on brain monoamine-related substances in mice. *Planta Med.* 55(5): 429–33.

Iwangoff P, Enz A, Meier-Ruge W. (1978). Incorporation, after single and repeated application of radioactive labelled DH-ergot alkaloids in different organs of the cat, with special reference to the brain. *Gerontology.* 24(suppl 1): 126–38.

Izumiyama K, Kogure K. (1988). Effect of dihydroergotoxine mesylate (Hydergine) on delayed neuronal death in the gerbil hippocampus. *Acta Neurol Scand.* 78(3): 214–20.

Jacobs DM, Stern Y, Mayeux R. (1997). Dementia in Parkinson disease, Huntington disease, and other degenerative conditions. In: *Behavioral Neurology and Neuropsychology.* Feinberg T, Farah MJ, eds. New York: McGraw-Hill.

Jaggy H, Koch E. (1997). Chemistry and biology of alkylphenols from Ginkgo biloba L. *Pharmazie.* 52(10): 735–38.

Jagust WJ, Reed BR, Martin EM, Eberling JL, Nelson-Abbott RA. (1992). Cognitive function and regional cerebral blood flow in Parkinson's disease. *Brain.* 115(pt 2): 521–37.

Janssens D, Michiels C, Delaive E, Eliaers F, Drieu K, Remacle J. (1995). Protection of hypoxia-induced ATP decrease in endothelial cells by Ginkgo biloba extract and bilobalide. *Biochem Pharmacol.* 50(7): 991–99.

Jastreboff PJ, Zhou S, Jastreboff MM, Kwapisz U, Gryczynska U. (1997). Attenuation of salicylate-induced tinnitus by Ginkgo biloba extract in rats. *Audiol Neurootol.* 2(4): 197–212.

Jaton AL, Vigouret JM. (1985). Effects of Hydergine and its components on Lashley maze acquisition in rats. *J Pharmacol.* 16(suppl 3): 51–56.

Jimenez-Jimenez FJ, de Bustos F, Molina JA, Benito-Leon J, Tallon-Barranco A, Gasalla T, Orti-Pareja M, Guillamon F, Rubio JC, Arenas J, Enriquez-de-

Salamanca R. (1997). Cerebrospinal fluid levels of alpha-tocopherol (vitamin E) in Alzheimer's disease. *J Neural Transm.* 104(6–7): 703–10.

Joyce CA, Paller KA, McIsaac HK, Kutas M. (1998). Memory changes with normal aging: behavioral and electrophysiological measures. *Psychophysiology.* 35(6): 669–78.

Jung F, Mrowietz C, Kiesewetter H, Wenzel E. (1990). Effect of Ginkgo biloba on fluidity of blood and peripheral microcirculation in volunteers. *Arzneimittelforschung.* 40(5): 589–93.

Kaku T, Miyata T, Uruno T, Sako I, Kinoshita A. (1975). Chemico-pharmacological studies on saponins of Panax ginseng C. A. Meyer: II. Pharmacological part. *Arzneimittelforschung.* 25(4): 539–47.

Kang M, Yoshimatsu H, Oohara A, Kurokawa M, Ogawa R, Sakata T. (1995). Ginsenoside Rg1 modulates ingestive behavior and thermal response induced by interleukin-1 beta in rats. *Physiol Behav.* 57(2): 393–6.

Kanit L, Taskiran D, Furedy JJ, Kulali B, McDonald R, Pogun S. (1998). Nicotine interacts with sex in affecting rat choice between "look-out" and "navigational" cognitive styles in the Morris water maze place learning task. *Brain Res Bull.* 46(5): 441–45.

Kanowski S, Herrmann WM, Stephan K, Wierich W, Hörr R. (1996). Proof of efficacy of the Ginkgo biloba special extract EGb 761 in outpatients suffering from mild to moderate primary degenerative dementia of the Alzheimer type or multi-infarct dementia. *Pharmacopsychiatry.* 29(2): 47–56.

Karplus TM, Saag KG. (1998). Nonsteroidal anti-inflammatory drugs and cognitive function: do they have a beneficial or deleterious effect? *Drug Safety.* 19(6): 427–33.

Kassel JD. (1997). Smoking and attention: a review and reformulation of the stimulus-filter hypothesis. *Clin Psychol Rev.* 17(5): 451–78.

Kawas C, Resnick S, Morrison A, Brookmeyer R, Corrada M, Zonderman A, Bacal C, Lingle DD, Metter E. (1997). A prospective study of estrogen replacement therapy and the risk of developing Alzheimer's disease: the Baltimore longitudinal study of aging. *Neurology.* 48(6): 1517–21.

Keefover RW. (1998). Aging and cognition. *Neurol Clin.* 16(3): 635–48.

Kim C, Choi H, Kim CC, Kim JK, Kim MS. (1976). Influence of ginseng on mating behavior of male rats. *Am J Chin Med.* 4(2): 163–68.

Kim DH, Jung JS, Suh HW, Huh SO, Min SK, Son BK, Park JH, Kim ND, Kim YH, Song DK. (1998). Inhibition of stress-induced plasma corticosterone levels by ginsenosides in mice: involvement of nitric oxide. *Neuroreport.* 9(10): 2261–64.

Kim H, Chen X, Gillis N. (1992). Ginsenosides protect pulmonary vascular endothelium against free radical-induced injury. *Biochem Biophys Res Community.* 189: 670–72.

Kim HJ, Woo DS, Lee G, Kim JJ. (1998). The relaxation effects of ginseng saponin in rabbit corporal smooth muscle: is it a nitric oxide donor? *Br J Urology*. 82: 744–48.

Kim HS, Lee JH, Goo YS, Nah SY. (1998). Effects of ginsenosides on Ca2+ channels and membrane capacitance in rat adrenal chromaffin cells. *Brain Res Bull*. 46(3): 245–51.

Kim HS, Oh KW, Rheu HM, Kim SH. (1992). Antagonism of U-50,488H-induced antinociception by ginseng total saponins is dependent on serotonergic mechanisms. *Pharmacol Biochem Behav*. 42(4): 587–93.

Kim YS, Pyo MK, Park KM, Park PH, Hahn BS, Wu SJ, Yun-Choi HS. (1998). Antiplatelet and antithrombotic effects of a combination of ticlopidine and Ginkgo biloba ext (EGb 761). *Thromb Res*. 91(1): 33–38.

Kleijnen J, Knipschild P. (1992a). Ginkgo biloba. *Lancet*. 340(8828): 1136–39.

Kleijnen J, Knipschild P. (1992b). Ginkgo biloba for cerebral insufficiency. *Br J Clin Pharmacol*. 34(4): 352–58.

Klein J, Chatterjee SS, Loffelholz K. (1997). Phospholipid breakdown and choline release under hypoxic conditions: inhibition by bilobalide, a constituent of Ginkgo biloba. *Brain Res*. 755(2): 347–50.

Ko SR, Choi KJ, Kim YH. (1996). Comparative study on the essential oil componenets of the Panax species. *Korean J Ginseng Sci*. 20: 42–48.

Kobayashi K, Ishii S, Kume K, Takahashi T, Shimizu T, Manabe T. (1999). Platelet-activating factor receptor is not required for long-term potentiation in the hippocampal CA1 region. *Eur J Neurosci*. 11(4): 1313–16.

Kobuchi H, Droy-Lefaix MT, Christen Y, Packer L. (1997). Ginkgo biloba extract (EGb 761): inhibitory effect on nitric oxide production in the macrophage cell line RAW 264.7. *Biochem Pharmacol*. 53(6): 897–903.

Koc RK, Akdemir H, Kurtsoy A, Pasaoglu H, Kavuncu I, Pasaoglu A, Karakucuk I. (1995). Lipid peroxidation in experimental spinal cord injury. Comparison of treatment with Ginkgo biloba, TRH, and methylprednisolone. *Res Exp Med*. 195(2): 117–123.

Konno S, Meyer JS, Terayama Y, Margishvili GM, Mortel KF. (1997). Classification, diagnosis, and treatment of vascular dementia. *Drugs Aging*. 11(5): 361–73.

Kornhuber J, Quack G, Danysz W, Jellinger K, Danielczyk W, Gsell W, Riederer P. (1995). Therapeutic brain concentration of the NMDA receptor antagonist amantadine. *Neuropharmacology*. 34(7): 713–21.

Kowalchik C, Hylton WH, eds. (1987). *Rodale's Illustrated Encyclopedia of Herbs*. Emmaus, PA: Rodale Press.

Krall WJ, Sramek JJ, Cutler NR. (1999). Cholinesterase inhibitors: a therapeutic strategy for Alzheimer disease. *Ann Pharmacother*. 33(4): 441–50.

Krasowski MD, McGehee DS, Moss J. (1997). Natural inhibitors of cholinesterases: implications for adverse drug reactions. *Can J Anaesthesiol*. 44(5): 525–34.

Krieglstein J, Beck T, Seibert A. (1986). Influence of an extract of Ginkgo biloba on cerebral blood flow and metabolism. *Life Sci.* 39(24): 2327–34.

Kristofikova Z, Benesova O, Tejkalova H. (1992). Changes in high-affinity choline uptake in the hippocampus of old rats after long-term administration of two nootropic drugs (tacrine and Ginkgo biloba extract). *Dementia.* 3: 304–7.

Kristofikova Z, Klaschka J. (1997). In vitro effect of Ginkgo biloba extract (EGb 761) on the activity of presynaptic cholinergic nerve terminals in rat hippocampus. *Dementia Geriatr Cognitive Disord.* 8(1): 43–48.

Kunkel H. (1993). EEG profile of three different extractions of Ginkgo biloba. *Neuropsychobiology.* 27(1): 40–45.

Kurihara K, Wardlaw AJ, Moqbel R, Kay AB. (1989). Inhibition of platelet-activating factor (PAF)-induced chemotaxis and PAF binding to human eosinophils and neutrophils by the specific ginkgolide-derived PAF antagonist, BN 52021. *J Allergy Clin Immunol.* 83(1): 83–90.

Lacour M, Ez-Zaher L, Raymond J. (1991). Plasticity mechanisms in vestibular compensation in the cat are improved by an extract of Ginkgo biloba (EGb 761). *Pharmacol Biochem Behav.* 140(2): 367–79.

Lahiri DK, Farlow MR, Sambamurti K. (1998). The secretion of amyloid beta-peptides is inhibited in the tacrine-treated human neuroblastoma cells. *Brain Res Mol Brain Res.* 62(2): 131–40.

Lamant V, Mauco G, Braquet P, Chap H, Douste-Blazy L. (1987). Inhibition of the metabolism of platelet activating factor (PAF-acether) by three specific antagonists from Ginkgo biloba. *Biochem Pharmacol.* 36(17): 2749–52.

Lamour Y, Holloway HW, Rapoport SI, Soncrant TT. (1992). Ginkgo biloba extract decreases local glucose utilization in the adult rat brain. In *Effects of Ginkgo biloba extract (Egb 761) in the Central Nervous System.* Christen J, Costentin C, Lacour M, eds. Paris: Elsevier, pp 19–25.

Lasarova MB, Mosharrof AH, Petkov VD, Markovska VL, Petkov VV. (1987). Effect of piracetam and of standardized ginseng extract on the electroconvulsive shock-induced memory disturbances in "step-down" passive avoidance. *Acta Physiol Pharmacol Bulg.* 13(2): 11–17.

Lavoisier P, Aloui R, Schmidt MH, Watrelot A. (1995). Clitoral blood flow increases following vaginal pressure stimulation. *Arch Sex Behav.* 24(1): 37–45.

Lawrence AD, Sahakian BJ. (1995). Alzheimer disease, attention, and the cholinergic system. *Alzheimer Dis Assoc Disord.* 9(suppl 2): 43–49.

Lawrence AD, Sahakian BJ. (1998). The cognitive psychopharmacology of Alzheimer's disease: focus on cholinergic systems. *Neurochem Res.* 23(5): 787–94.

Le Bars PL, Katz MM, Berman N, Itil TM, Freedman AM, Schatzberg AF. (1997). A placebo-controlled, double-blind, randomized trial of an extract of Ginkgo biloba for dementia. North American EGb Study Group. *JAMA.* 278(16): 1327–32.

Lebert F, Pasquier F, Souliez L, Petit H. (1998). Tacrine efficacy in Lewy body dementia. *Int J Geriatr Psychiatry.* 13(8): 516–19.

Lee C, Frangou S, Russell MA, Gray JA. (1997). Effect of haloperidol on nicotine-induced enhancement of vigilance in human subjects. *J Psychopharmacol.* 11(3): 253–57.

Lee SP, Honda K, Rhee YH, Inoue S. (1990). Chronic intake of Panax ginseng extract stabilizes sleep and wakefulness in food-deprived rats. *Neurosci Lett.* 111(1–2): 217–21.

Lee YJ, Chung E, Lee KY, Lee YH, Huh B, Lee SK. (1997). Ginsenoside-Rg1, one of the major active molecules from Panax ginseng, is a functional ligand of glucocorticoid receptor. *Mol Cell Endocrinol.* 133(2): 135–40.

Le Houezec J. (1998). Nicotine: abused substance and therapeutic agent. *J Psychiatry Neurosci.* 23(2): 95–108.

Le Houezec J, Halliday R, Benowitz NL, Callaway E, Naylor H, Herzig K. (1994). A low dose of subcutaneous nicotine improves information processing in non-smokers. *Psychopharmacology (Berlin).* 114(4): 628–34.

Le Poncin-Lafitte M, Rapin JR, Duterte D, Galiez V, Lamproglou I. (1985). Learning and cholinergic neurotransmission in old animals: the effect of Hydergine. *J Pharmacol.* 16(suppl 3): 57–63.

Levin ED. (1992). Nicotinic systems and cognitive function. *Psychopharmacology (Berlin).* 108(4): 417–31.

Levin ED. (1997). Chronic haloperidol administration does not block acute nicotine-induced improvements in radial-arm maze performance in the rat. *Pharmacol Biochem Behav.* 58(4): 899–902.

Levin ED, Briggs SJ, Christopher NC, Rose JE. (1992). Persistence of chronic nicotine-induced cognitive facilitation. *Behav Neural Biol.* 58(2): 152–58.

Levin ED, Conners CK, Silva D, Hinton SC, Meck WH, March J, Rose JE. (1998). Transdermal nicotine effects on attention. *Psychopharmacology (Berlin).* 140(2): 135–41.

Levin ED, Rose JE. (1991). Nicotinic and muscarinic interactions and choice accuracy in the radial-arm maze. *Brain Res Bull.* 27(1): 125–28.

Levin ED, Simon BB. (1998). Nicotinic acetylcholine involvement in cognitive function in animals. *Psychopharmacology (Berlin).* 138(3–4): 217–30.

Lewis R, Wake G, Court G, Court JA, Pickering AT, Kim YC, Perry EK. (1994). Non-ginsenoside nicotinic activity in ginseng species. *Phytother Res.* 13(1): 59–64.

Li CL, Wong YY. (1997). The bioavailability of ginkgolides in Ginkgo biloba extracts. *Planta Med.* 63(6): 563–65.

Lim JH, Wen TC, Matsuda S, Tanaka J, Maeda N, Peng H, Aburaya J, Ishihara K, Sakanaka M. (1997). Protection of ischemic hippocampal neurons by ginsenoside Rb1, a main ingredient of ginseng root. *Neurosci Res.* 28(3): 191–200.

Liu M, Zhang JT. (1996). Effects of ginsenoside Rg1 on c-fos gene expression and cAMP levels in rat hippocampus. *Chung Kuo Yao Li Hsueh Pao*. 17(2): 171–74.

Lobstein-Guth A, Briancon-Scheid F, Victoire C, Haag-Berrurier M, Anton R. (1988). Isolation of amentoflavone from Ginkgo biloba. *Planta Med.* 54(6): 555–6.

Lugasi A, Horvahovich P, Dworschak E. (1999). Additional information to the in vitro antioxidant activity of Ginkgo biloba L. *Phytother Res.* 13(2): 160–62.

Lupien SJ, Nair NP, Briere S, Maheu F, Tu MT, Lemay M, McEwen BS, Meaney MJ. (1999). Increased cortisol levels and impaired cognition in human aging: implication for depression and dementia in later life. *Rev Neurosci.* 10(2): 117–39.

Ma TC, Yu QH. (1993). Effect of 20(S)-ginsenoside-Rg2 and cyproheptadine on two-way active avoidance learning and memory in rats. *Arzneimittelforschung*. 43(10): 1049–52.

Ma TC, Yu QH, Chen MH. (1991). Effects of ginseng stem-leaves saponins on one-way avoidance behavior in rats. *Chung Kuo Yao Li Hsueh Pao*. 12(5): 403–6.

Macovschi O, Prigent AF, Nemoz G, Pacheco H. (1987). Effects of an extract of Ginkgo biloba on the 3′,5′-cyclic AMP phosphodiesterase activity of the brain of normal and triethyltin-intoxicated rats. *J Neurochem.* 49(1): 107–14.

Maitra I, Marcocci L, Droy-Lefaix MT, Packer L. (1995). Peroxyl radical scavenging activity of Ginkgo biloba extract EGb 761. *Biochem Pharmacol.* 49(11): 1649–55.

Major RT. (1967). The ginkgo, the most ancient living tree. The resistance of Ginkgo biloba L. to pests accounts in part for the longevity of this species. *Science*. 157(794): 1270–3.

Manly JJ, Jacobs DM, Sano M, Bell K, Merchant CA, Small SA, Stern Y. (1999). Effect of literacy on neuropsychological test performance in nondemented, education-matched elders. *J Int Neuropsychol Soc.* 5(3): 191–202.

Marcilhac A, Dakine N, Bourhim N, Guillaume V, Grino M, Drieu K, Oliver C. (1998). Effect of chronic administration of Ginkgo biloba extract or ginkgolide on the hypothalamic-pituitary-adrenal axis in the rat. *Life Sci.* 62(25): 2329–40.

Marcocci L, Maguire JJ, Droy-Lefaix MT, Packer L. (1994). The nitric oxide-scavenging properties of Ginkgo biloba extract EGb 761. *Biochem Biophys Res Community*. 201(2): 748–55.

Markstein R. (1985). Hydergine: interaction with the neurotransmitter systems in the central nervous system. *J Pharmacol.* 16(suppl 3): 1–17.

Matsunaga H, Saita T, Nagumo F, Mori M, Katano M. (1995). A possible mechanism for the cytotoxicity of a polyacetylenic alcohol, panaxytriol: inhibition of mitochondrial respiration. *Cancer Chemother Pharmacol.* 35(4): 291–96.

Maurer K, Ihl R, Dierks T, Frolich L. (1997). Clinical efficacy of Ginkgo biloba special extract EGb 761 in dementia of the Alzheimer type. *J Psychiatr Res.* 31(6): 645–55.

McIntosh LJ, Trush MA, Troncoso JC. (1997). Increased susceptibility of Alzheimer's disease temporal cortex to oxygen free radical-mediated processes. *Free Radical Biol Med.* 23(2): 183–90.

Meguro K, Yamaguchi S, Arai H, Nakagawa T, Doi C, Yamada M, Ikarashi Y, Maruyama Y, Sasaki H. (1994). Nicotine improves cognitive disturbance in senescence-accelerated mice. *Pharmacol Biochem Behav.* 49(3): 769–72.

Mendis T, Suchowersky O, Lang A, Gauthier S. (1999). Management of Parkinson's disease: a review of current and new therapies. *Can J Neurol Sci.* 26(2): 89–103.

Meyer B. (1986a). [Multicenter randomized double-blind drug vs. placebo study of the treatment of tinnitus with Ginkgo biloba extract]. *Presse Med.* 15(31): 1562–64.

Meyer B. (1986b). [A multicenter study of tinnitus. Epidemiology and therapy]. *Ann Otolaryngol Chir Cervicofac.* 103(3): 185–88.

Mielke R, Kessler J, Szelies B, Herholz K, Wienhard K, Heiss WD. (1998). Normal and pathological aging—findings of positron-emission-tomography. *J Neural Transm.* 105(8–9): 821–37.

Mirza NR, Stolerman IP. (1998). Nicotine enhances sustained attention in the rat under specific task conditions. *Psychopharmacology (Berlin).* 138(3–4): 266–74.

Mitra SK, Chakraborti A, Bhattacharya SK. (1996). Neuropharmacological studies on Panax ginseng. *Indian J Exp Biol.* 34(1): 41–47.

Molinengo L, Orsetti M, Pastorello B, Scordo I, Ghi P. (1995). The action of arecoline on retrieval and memory storage evaluated in the staircase maze. *Neurobiol Learn Mem.* 63(2): 167–73.

Mondadori C, Hengerer B, Ducret T, Borkowski J. (1994). Delayed emergence of effects of memory-enhancing drugs: implications for the dynamics of long-term memory. *Proc Natl Acad Sci USA.* 91(6): 2041–45.

Murdoch I, Perry EK, Court JA, Graham DI, Dewar D. (1998). Cortical cholinergic dysfunction after human head injury. *J Neurotrauma.* 15(5): 295–305.

Murphy LL, Cadena RS, Chavez D, Ferraro JS. (1998). Effect of American ginseng (Panax quinquefolium) on male copulatory behavior in the rat. *Physiol Behav.* 64(4): 445–50.

Nah SY, McCleskey EW. (1994). Ginseng root extract inhibits calcium channels in rat sensory neurons through a similar path, but different receptor, as mu-type opioids. *J Ethnopharmacol.* 42(1): 45–51.

Nah SY, Park HJ, McCleskey EW. (1995). A trace component of ginseng that inhibits Ca2+ channels through a pertussis toxin-sensitive G protein. *Proc Natl Acad Sci USA.* 92(19): 8739–43.

Neary D, Snowden JS, Gustafson L, Passant U, Stuss D, Black S, Freedman M, Kertesz A, Robert PH, Albert M, et al. (1998). Frontotemporal lobar degeneration: a consensus on clinical diagnostic criteria. *Neurology.* 51(6): 1546–54.

Nebes RD. (1997). Alzheimer's disease: Cognitive neuropsychological aspects. In: *Behavioral Neurology and Neuropsychology.* Feinberg T, Farah MJ, eds. New York: McGraw-Hill.

Newhouse PA, Potter A, Levin ED. (1997). Nicotinic system involvement in Alzheimer's and Parkinson's diseases. Implications for therapeutics. *Drugs Aging.* 11(3): 206–28.

Nguyen TT, Matsumoto K, Yamasaki K, Watanabe H. (1997). Majonoside-R2 reverses social isolation stress-induced decrease in pentobarbital sleep in mice: possible involvement of neuroactive steroids. *Life Sciences.* 61(4): 395–402.

Ni Y, Zhao B, Hou J, Xin W. (1996). Preventive effect of Ginkgo biloba extract on apoptosis in rat cerebellar neuronal cells induced by hydroxyl radicals. *Neurosci Lett.* 214(2–3): 115–18.

Nil R. (1991). A psychopharmacological and psychophysiological evaluation of smoking motives. *Rev Environ Health.* 9(2): 85–115.

Nishiyama N, Cho SI, Kitagawa I, Saito H. (1994). Malonylginsenoside Rb1 potentiates nerve growth factor (NGF)-induced neurite outgrowth of cultured chick embryonic dorsal root ganglia. *Biol Pharm Bull.* 17(4): 509–13.

Nishiyama N, Chu PJ, Saito H. (1996). An herbal prescription, S-113m, consisting of biota, ginseng and schizandra, improves learning performance in senescence accelerated mouse. *Biol Pharm Bull.* 19(3): 388–93.

Nishiyama N, Wang YL, Saito H. (1995). Beneficial effects of S-113m, a novel herbal prescription, on learning impairment model in mice. *Biol Pharm Bull.* 18(11): 1498–503.

Nitta H, Matsumoto K, Shimizu M, Ni XH, Watanabe H. (1995). Panax ginseng extract improves the performance of aged Fischer 344 rats in radial maze task but not in operant brightness discrimination task. *Biol Pharm Bull.* 18(9): 1286–88.

Nordberg A. (1992). Neuroreceptor changes in Alzheimer disease. *Cerebrovasc Brain Metab Rev.* 4(4): 303–28.

Nordberg A. (1993). Clinical studies in Alzheimer patients with positron emission tomography. *Behav Brain Res.* 57(2): 215–24.

Nordberg A, Amberla K, Shigeta M, Lundqvist H, Viitanen M, Hellstrom-Lindahl E, Johansson M, Andersson J, Hartvig P, Lilja A, et al. (1998). Long-term tacrine treatment in three mild Alzheimer patients: effects on nicotinic receptors, cerebral blood flow, glucose metabolism, EEG, and cognitive abilities. *Alzheimer Dis Assoc Disord.* 12(3): 228–37.

Nordberg A, Lundqvist H, Hartvig P, Andersson J, Johansson M, Hellstrom-Lindahi E, Langstrom B. (1997). Imaging of nicotinic and muscarinic receptors in Alzheimer's disease: effect of tacrine treatment. *Dement Geriatr Cogn Disord.* 8(2): 78–84.

Nordberg A, Svensson AL. (1998). Cholinesterase inhibitors in the treatment of Alzheimer's disease: a comparison of tolerability and pharmacology. *Drug Safety*. 19(6): 465–80.

Nyenhuis DL, Gorelick PB. (1998). Vascular dementia: a contemporary review of epidemiology, diagnosis, prevention, and treatment. *J Am Geriatr Soc*. 46(11): 1437–48.

Odani T, Tanizawa H, Takino Y. (1983). Studies on the absorption, distribution, excretion, and metabolism of ginseng saponins: II. The absorption, distribution and excretion of ginsenoside Rg1 in the rat. *Chem Pharm Bull (Tokyo)*. 31(1): 292–98.

Odawara M, Tamaoka A, Yamashita K. (1997). Ginkgo biloba. *Neurology*. 48(3): 789–90.

Oken BS, Storzbach DM, Kaye JA. (1998). The efficacy of Ginkgo biloba on cognitive function in Alzheimer disease. *Arch Neurol*. 55(11): 1409–15.

Olanow CW. (1997). Attempts to obtain neuroprotection in Parkinson's disease. *Neurology*. 49(suppl 1): S26–33.

Olpe HR, Steinmann MW. (1982). The effect of vincamine, Hydergine, and piracetam on the firing rate of locus coeruleus neurons. *J Neural Transm*. 55(2): 101–9.

Olsen CG, Clasen ME. (1998). Senile dementia of the Binswanger's type. *Am Fam Physician* 58(9): 2068–74.

Owen AM, Doyon J, Dagher A, Sadikot A, Evans AC. (1998). Abnormal basal ganglia outflow in Parkinson's disease identified with PET. Implications for higher cortical functions. *Brain*. 121(pt 5): 949–65.

Oyama Y, Chikahisa L, Ueha T, Kanemaru K, Noda K. (1996). Ginkgo biloba extract protects brain neurons against oxidative stress induced by hydrogen peroxide. *Brain Res*. 712(2): 349–52.

Oyama Y, Fuchs PA, Katayama N, Noda K. (1994). Myricetin and quercetin, the flavonoid constituents of Ginkgo biloba extract, greatly reduce oxidative metabolism in both resting and Ca(2+)-loaded brain neurons. *Brain Res*. 635(1–2): 125–29.

Pachana NA, Boone KB, Miller BL, Cummings JL, Berman N. (1996). Comparison of neuropsychological functioning in Alzheimer's disease and frontotemporal dementia. *J Int Neuropsychol Soc*. 2(6): 505–10.

Paick JS, Lee JH. (1996). An experimental study of the effect of Ginkgo biloba extract on the human and rabbit corpus cavernosum tissue. *J Urology*. 156: 1876–80.

Papadopoulos V, Widmaier EP, Amri H, Zilz A, Li H, Culty M, Castello R, Philip GH, Sridaran R, Drieu K. (1998). In vivo studies on the role of the peripheral benzodiazepine receptor (PBR) in steroidogenesis. *Endocr Res*. 124(3–4): 479–87.

Peroutka, SJ. (1996). Drugs effective in the therapy of migraine. In: *Goodman and Gilman's The Pharmacological Basis of Therapeutics.* Hardman JG, Limbird LE, Molinoff PB, Ruddon RW, Goodman Gilman A, eds. New York: McGraw-Hill.

Perrig WJ, Perrig P, Stahelin HB. (1997). The relationship between antioxidants and memory performance in the old and very old. *J Am Geriatr Soc.* 45: 718–24.

Perry EK, Perry RH, Smith CJ, Purohit D, Bonham J, Dick DJ, Candy JM, Edwardson JA, Fairbairn A. (1986). Cholinergic receptors in cognitive disorders. *Can J Neurol Sci.* 13(4 suppl): 521–27.

Petkov VD, Cao Y, Todorov I, Lazarova M, Getova D, Stancheva S, Alova L. (1992). Behavioral effects of stem-leaves extract from Panax ginseng C.A. Meyer. *Acta Physiol Pharmacol Bulg.* 18(2): 41–48.

Petkov VD, Getova D, Mosharrof AH. (1987). A study of nootropic drugs for anti-anxiety action. *Acta Physiol Pharmacol Bulg.* 13(4): 25–30.

Petkov VD, Kehayov R, Belcheva S, Konstantinova E, Petkov VV, Getova D, Markovska V. (1993b). Memory effects of standardized extracts of Panax ginseng (G115), Ginkgo biloba (GK 501) and their combination Gincosan (PHL-00701). *Planta Med.* 59(2): 106–14.

Petkov VD, Mosharrof AH. (1987). Effects of standardized ginseng extract on learning, memory, and physical capabilities. *Am J Chin Med.* 15(1–2): 19–29.

Petkov VD, Mosharrof AH, Petkov VV, Kehayov RA. (1990). Age-related differences in memory and in the memory effects of nootropic drugs. *Acta Physiol Pharmacol Bulg.* 16(2): 28–36.

Petrie RX, Deary IJ. (1989). Smoking and human information processing. *Psychopharmacology (Berlin).* 99(3): 393–96.

Pfeffer A, Luczywek E, Golebiowski M, Czyzewski K, Barcikowska M. (1999). Frontotemporal Dementia: An Attempt at Clinical Characteristics. *Dement Geriatr Cogn Disord.* 10(3): 217–20.

Pickworth WB, Fant RV, Butschky MF, Henningfield JE. (1997). Effects of mecamylamine on spontaneous EEG and performance in smokers and non-smokers. *Pharmacol Biochem Behav.* 56(2): 181–87.

Pidoux B. (1986). [Effects of Ginkgo biloba extract on functional brain activity. An assessment of clinical and experimental studies]. *Presse Med.* 15(31): 1588–91.

Pierre S, Jamme I, Droy-Lefaix MT, Nouvelot A, Maixent JM. (1999). Ginkgo biloba extract (EGb 761) protects Na,K-ATPase activity during cerebral ischemia in mice. *Neuroreport.* 10(1): 47–51.

Pietri S, Maurelli E, Drieu K, Culcasi M. (1997). Cardioprotective and antioxidant effects of the terpenoid constituents of Ginkgo biloba extract (EGb 761). *J Mol Cell Cardiol.* 29(2): 733–42.

Pietta PG, Gardana C, Mauri PL. (1997). Identification of Gingko biloba flavonol metabolites after oral administration to humans. *J Chromatogr B Biomed Sci Appl.* 693(1): 249–55.

Pomerleau CS, Teuscher F, Goeters S, Pomerleau OF. (1994). Effects of nicotine abstinence and menstrual phase on task performance. *Addict Behav.* 19(4): 357–62.

Price DL, Wong PC, Borchelt DR, Pardo CA, Thinakaran G, Doan AP, Lee MK, Martin LJ, Sisodia SS. (1997). Amyotrophic lateral sclerosis and Alzheimer disease. Lessons from model systems. *Rev Neurol (Paris).* 153(8–9): 484–95.

Pritchard WS, Robinson JH, deBethizy JD, Davis RA, Stiles MF. (1995). Caffeine and smoking: subjective, performance, and psychophysiological effects. *Psychophysiology.* 32(1): 19–27.

Qizilbash N, Whitehead A, Higgins J, Wilcock G, Schneider L, Farlow M. (1998). Cholinesterase inhibition for Alzheimer disease: a meta-analysis of the tacrine trials. Dementia Trialists' Collaboration. *JAMA.* 280(20): 1777–82.

Quartermain D, Leo P. (1988). Alleviation of scopolamine amnesia by different retrieval enhancing treatments. *Pharmacol Biochem Behav.* 30(4): 1093–96.

Rabey JM, Vered Y, Shabtai H, Graff F, Harsat A, Korczyn AD. (1993). Broad bean (Vicia faba) consumption and Parkinson's disease. *Adv Neurol.* 60: 681–84.

Rabey JM, Vered Y. Shabtai H, Graff F, Korczyn AD. (1992). Improvement of parkinsonian features correlate with high plasma levodopa values after broad bean (Vicia faba) consumption. *J Neurol Neurosurg Psychiatry.* 55(8): 725–27.

Raffaele KC, Asthana S, Berardi A, Haxby JV, Morris PP, Schapiro MB, Soncrant TT. (1996). Differential response to the cholinergic agonist arecoline among different cognitive modalities in Alzheimer's disease. *Neuropsychopharmacology.* 15(2): 163–70.

Rajfer J, Aronson WJ, Bush PA, Dorey FJ, Ignarro LJ. (1992). Nitric oxide as a mediator of relaxation of the corpus cavernosum in response to noradrenergic, noncholinergic neurotransmission. *New Engl J Med.* 326: 90–94.

Ramassamy C, Christen Y, Clostre F, Costentin J. (1992). The Ginkgo biloba extract, EGb 761, increases synaptosomal uptake of 5-hydroxytryptamine: in-vitro and ex-vivo studies. *J Pharm Pharmacol.* 44(11): 943–45.

Ramassamy C, Clostre F, Christen Y, Costentin J. (1990). Prevention by a Ginkgo biloba extract (GBE 761) of the dopaminergic neurotoxicity of MPTP. *J Pharm Pharmacol.* 42(11): 785–89.

Rapin JR, Lamproglou I, Drieu K, DeFeudis FV. (1994). Demonstration of the "anti-stress" activity of an extract of Ginkgo biloba (EGb 761) using a discrimination learning task. *Gen Pharmacol.* 25(5): 1009–16.

Raskin SA, Borod JC, Tweedy JR. (1992). Set-shifting and spatial orientation in patients with Parkinson's disease. *J Clin Exp Neuropsychol.* 14(5): 801–21.

Raymond J. (1986). [Effects of Ginkgo biloba extract on the morphological preservation of vestibular sensory epithelia in mice]. *Presse Med.* 15(31): 1484–87.

Rich JB, Rasmusson DX, Folstein MF, Carson KA, Kawas C, Brandt J. (1995). Nonsteroidal anti-inflammatory drugs in Alzheimer's disease. *Neurology.* 45(1): 51–55.

Robbins TW, McAlonan G, Muir JL, Everitt BJ. (1997). Cognitive enhancers in theory and practice: studies of the cholinergic hypothesis of cognitive deficits in Alzheimer's disease. *Behav Brain Res.* 83(1–2): 15–23.

Robbers JE, Speedie MK, Tyler VE. (1996). *Pharmacognosy and Pharmacobiotechnology.* Baltimore: Willams and Wilkins.

Rodriguez de Turco EB, Droy-Lefaix MT, Bazan NG. (1993). Decreased electroconvulsive shock-induced diacylglycerols and free fatty acid accumulation in the rat brain by Ginkgo biloba extract (EGb 761): selective effect in hippocampus as compared with cerebral cortex. *J Neurochem.* 61(4): 1438–44.

Rogers SL, Farlow MR, Doody RS, Mohs R, Friedhoff LT. (1998). A 24-week, double-blind, placebo-controlled trial of donepezil in patients with Alzheimer's disease. Donepezil Study Group. *Neurology.* 50(1): 136–45.

Rosenblatt M, Mindel J. (1997). Spontaneous hyphema associated with ingestion of Ginkgo biloba extract. *N Engl J Med.* 336(15): 1108.

Rowland LP. (1998). Diagnosis of amyotrophic lateral sclerosis. *J Neurol Sci.* 160(suppl 1): S6–24.

Rowin J, Lewis SL. (1996). Spontaneous bilateral subdural hematomas associated with chronic Ginkgo biloba ingestion. *Neurology.* 46(6): 1775–6.

Salim KN, McEwen BS, Chao HM. (1997). Ginsenoside Rb1 regulates ChAT, NGF, and trkA mRNA expression in the rat brain. *Brain Res Mol Brain Res.* 47(1–2): 177–82.

Salvati G, Genovesi G, Marcellini L, Paolini P, De Nuccio I, Pepe M, Re M. (1996). Effects of Panax ginseng C.A. Meyer saponins on male fertility. *Panminerva Med.* 38(4): 249–54.

Samuel W, Galasko D, Thal LJ. (1997). Alzheimer disease: biochemical and pharmacologic aspects. In: *Behavioral Neurology and Neuropsychology.* Feinberg T, Farah MJ, eds. New York: McGraw-Hill.

Sano M, Ernesto C, Thomas RG, Klauber MR, Schafer K, Grundman M, Woodbury P, Growdon J, Cotman CW, Pfeiffer E, et al. (1997). A controlled trial of selegiline, alpha-tocopherol, or both as treatment for Alzheimer's disease. The Alzheimer's Disease Cooperative Study. *N Engl J Med.* 336(17): 1216–22.

Saponara R, Bosisio E. (1998). Inhibition of cAMP-phosphodiesterase by biflavones of Ginkgo biloba in rat adipose tissue. *J Nat Prod.* 61(11): 1386–87.

Sasaki H, Yanai M, Meguro K, Sekizawa K, Ikarashi Y, Maruyama Y, Yamamoto M, Matsuzaki Y, Takishima T. (1991). Nicotine improves cognitive disturbance in rodents fed with a choline-deficient diet. *Pharmacol Biochem Behav.* 138(4): 921–25.

Sasaki K, Hatta S, Haga M, Ohshika H. (1999). Effects of bilobalide on gamma-aminobutyric acid levels and glutamic acid decarboxylase in mouse brain. *Eur J Pharmacol.* 367(2–3): 165–73.

Sastre J, Millan A, Garcia de la Asuncion J, Pla R, Juan G, Pallardo FV, O'Connor E, Martin JA, Droy-Lefaix MT, Vina J. (1998). A Ginkgo biloba extract (EGb 761) prevents mitochondrial aging by protecting against oxidative stress. *Free Radic Biol Med.* 24(2): 298–304.

Satyan KS, Jaiswal AK, Ghosal S, Bhattacharya SK. (1998). Anxiolytic activity of ginkgolic acid conjugates from Indian Ginkgo biloba. *Psychopharmacology (Berlin).* 136(2): 148–52.

Schneider B. (1992). [Ginkgo biloba extract in peripheral arterial diseases. Meta-analysis of controlled clinical studies]. *Arzneimittelforschung.* 42(4): 428–36.

Schneider LS, Olin JT. (1994). Overview of clinical trials of Hydergine in dementia. *Arch Neurol.* 51: 787–97.

Schroder J, Kratz B, Pantel J, Minnemann E, Lehr U, Sauer H. (1998). Prevalence of mild cognitive impairment in an elderly community sample. *J Neural Transm.* (Suppl) 54: 51–59.

Seif-El-Nasr M, El-Fattah AA. (1995). Lipid peroxide, phospholipids, glutathione levels and superoxide dismutase activity in rat brain after ischaemia: effect of Ginkgo biloba extract. *Pharmacol Res.* 32(5): 273–78.

Semlitsch HV, Anderer P, Saletu B, Binder GA, Decker KA. (1995). Cognitive psychophysiology in nootropic drug research: effects of Ginkgo biloba on event-related potentials (P300) in age-associated memory impairment. *Pharmacopsychiatry.* 28(4): 134–42.

Sheline YI, Wang PW, Gado MH, Csernansky JG, Vannier MW. (1996). Hippocampal atrophy in recurrent major depression. *Proc Natl Acad Sci USA.* 93(9): 3908–13.

Sherwood N. (1995). Effects of cigarette smoking on performance in a simulated driving task. *Neuropsychobiology.* 32(3): 161–65.

Shiffman S, Paty JA, Gnys M, Kassel JD, Elash C. (1995). Nicotine withdrawal in chippers and regular smokers: subjective and cognitive effects. *Health Psychol.* 14(4): 301–9.

Shigeta M, Persson A, Viitanen M, Winblad B, Nordberg A. (1993). EEG regional changes during long-term treatment with tetrahydroaminoacridine (THA) in Alzheimer's disease. *Acta Neurol Scand Suppl.* 149: 58–61.

Shintani EY, Uchida KM. (1997). Donepezil: an anticholinesterase inhibitor for Alzheimer's disease. *Am J Health Syst Pharm.* 54(24): 2805–10.

Siegel RK. (1979). Ginseng abuse syndrome. Problems with the panacea. *JAMA.* 241(15): 1614–15.

Simon MF, Chap H, Braquet P, Douste-Blazy L. (1987). Effect of BN 52021, a specific antagonist of platelet activating factor (PAF-acether), on calcium movements and phosphatidic acid production induced by PAF-acether in human platelets. *Thromb Res.* 45(4): 299–309.

Sitaram N, Weingartner H, Gillin JC. (1978). Human serial learning: enhancement with arecholine and choline impairment with scopolamine. *Science.* 201(4352): 274–6.

Skoog I. (1979). Status of risk factors for vascular dementia. *Neuroepidemiology.* 17(1): 2–9.

Sliwinski M, Buschke H. (1999). Cross-sectional and longitudinal relationships among age, cognition, and processing speed. *Psychol Aging.* 14(1): 18–33.

Smith PF, Darlington CL. (1994). Can vestibular compensation be enhanced by drug treatment? A review of recent evidence. *J Vestib Res.* 4(3): 169–79.

Snaedal J, Johannesson T, Jonsson JE, Gylfadottir G. (1996). The effects of nicotine in dermal plaster on cognitive functions in patients with Alzheimer's disease. *Dementia.* 7(1): 47–52.

Snyder FR, Davis FC, Henningfield JE. (1989). The tobacco withdrawal syndrome: performance decrements assessed on a computerized test battery. *Drug Alcohol Depend.* 23(3): 259–66.

Snyder FR, Henningfield JE. (1989). Effects of nicotine administration following 12 h of tobacco deprivation: assessment on computerized performance tasks. *Psychopharmacology (Berlin).* 97(1): 17–22.

Socci DJ, Sanberg PR, Arendash GW. (1995). Nicotine enhances Morris water maze performance of young and aged rats. *Neurobiol Aging.* 16(5): 857–60.

Soholm B. (1998). Clinical improvement of memory and other cognitive functions by Ginkgo biloba: review of relevant literature. *Adv Ther.* 15(1): 54–65.

Sommese T, Patterson JC. (1995). Acute effects of cigarette smoking withdrawal: a review of the literature. *Aviat Space Environ Med.* 66(2): 164–67.

Sözmen EY, Kanit L, Kutay FZ, Hariri NI. (1998). Possible supportive effects of co-dergocrine mesylate on antioxidant enzyme systems in aged rat brain. *Eur Neuropsychopharmacol.* 8(1): 13–16.

Spengos M, Vassilopoulos D. (1988). Improvement of Parkinson's disease after Vicia faba consumption. Ninth International Symposium on Parkinson's disease. Jerusalem, Isreal. Abs. 46.

Spinnewyn B, Blavet N, Clostre F, Bazan N, Braquet P. (1987). Involvement of platelet-activating factor (PAF) in cerebral post-ischemic phase in Mongolian gerbils. *Prostaglandins.* 34(3): 337–49.

Standaert DG, Young AB. (1996). Treatment of central nervous system degenerative disorders. In: *Goodman and Gilman's The Pharmacological Basis of Therapeutics.* Hardman JG, Limbird LE, Molinoff PB, Ruddon RW, Goodman Gilman A, eds. New York: McGraw-Hill.

Stein EA, Pankiewicz J, Harsch HH, Cho JK, Fuller SA, Hoffmann RG, Hawkins M, Rao SM, Bandettini PA, Bloom AS. (1998). Nicotine-induced limbic cortical activation in the human brain: a functional MRI study. *Am J Psychiatry.* 155(8): 1009–15.

Stevens A, Kircher T. (1998). Cognitive decline unlike normal aging is associated with alterations of EEG temporo-spatial characteristics. *Eur Arch Psychiatry Clin Neurosci.* 248(5): 259–66.

Stewart WF, Kawas C, Corrada M, Metter EJ. (1997). Risk of Alzheimer's disease and duration of NSAID use. *Neurology*. 48(3): 626–32.

Stoll S, Scheuer K, Pohl O, Muller WE. (1996). Ginkgo biloba extract (EGb 761) independently improves changes in passive avoidance learning and brain membrane fluidity in the aging mouse. *Pharmacopsychiatry*. 29(4): 144–49.

Stoof JC, Booji J, Drukarch B. (1992). Amantadine as *N*-methyl-D-aspartic acid receptor antagonist: new possibilities for therapeutic applications? *Clin Neurol Neurosurg*. 94(suppl): S4–6.

Stough C, Mangan G, Bates T, Frank N, Kerkin B, Pellett O. (1995). Effects of nicotine on perceptual speed. *Psychopharmacology (Berlin)*. 119(3): 305–10.

Stough C, Mangan G, Bates T, Pellett O. (1994). Smoking and Raven IQ. *Psychopharmacology (Berlin)*. 116(3): 382–84.

Stücker O, Pons C, Duverger JP, Drieu K. (1996). Effects of Ginkgo biloba extract (EGb 761) on arteriolar spasm in a rat cremaster muscle preparation. *Int J Microcirc Clin Exp*. 16(2): 98–104.

Subhan Z, Hindmarch I. (1984). The psychopharmacological effects of Ginkgo biloba extract in normal healthy volunteers. *Int J Clin Pharmacol Res*. 4(2): 89–93.

Sunderland T, Tariot PN, Newhouse PA. (1988). Differential responsivity of mood, behavior, and cognition to cholinergic agents in elderly neuropsychiatric populations. *Brain Res*. 472(4): 371–89.

Tachikawa E, Kudo K, Harada K, Kashimoto T, Miyate Y, Kakizaki A, Takahashi E. (1999). Effects of ginseng saponins on responses induced by various receptor stimuli. *Eur J Pharmacol* 369(1): 23–32.

Tagami M, Ikeda K, Yamagata K, Nara Y, Fujino H, Kubota A, Numano F, Yamori Y. (1999). Vitamin E prevents apoptosis in hippocampal neurons caused by cerebral ischemia and reperfusion in stroke-prone spontaneously hypertensive rats. *Lab Invest*. 79(5): 609–15.

Taillandier J, Ammar A, Rabourdin JP, Ribeyre JP, Pichon J, Niddam S, Pierart H. (1986). [Treatment of cerebral aging disorders with Ginkgo biloba extract. A longitudinal multicenter double-blind drug vs. placebo study]. *Presse Med*. 15(31): 1583–87.

Takino Y, Odani T, Tanizawa H, Hayashi T. (1982). Studies on the absorption, distribution, excretion, and metabolism of ginseng saponins: I. Quantitative analysis of ginsenoside Rg1 in rats. *Chem Pharm Bull (Tokyo)*. 30(6): 2196–201.

Tariot PN, Cohen RM, Welkowitz JA, Sunderland T, Newhouse PA, Murphy DL, Weingartner H. (1988). Multiple-dose arecoline infusions in Alzheimer's disease. *Arch Gen Psychiatry*. 45(10): 901–5.

Taylor AE, Saint-Cyr JA, Lang AE. (1986). Frontal lobe dysfunction in Parkinson's disease. The cortical focus of neostriatal outflow. *Brain*. Oct. 109(pt 5): 845–83.

Taylor JE. (1986). [Neuromediator binding to receptors in the rat brain. The effect of chronic administration of Ginkgo biloba extract]. *Presse Med.* 15: 1491–93.

Terry AV Jr, Buccafusco JJ, Jackson WJ. (1993). Scopolamine reversal of nicotine enhanced delayed matching-to-sample performance in monkeys. *Pharmacol Biochem Behav.* 45(4): 925–29.

Tighilet B, Lacour M. (1995). Pharmacological activity of the Ginkgo biloba extract (EGb 761) on equilibrium function recovery in the unilateral vestibular neurectomized cat. *J Vestib Res.* 5(3): 187–200.

Turchi J, Holley LA, Sarter M. (1995). Effects of nicotinic acetylcholine receptor ligands on behavioral vigilance in rats. *Psychopharmacology (Berlin).* 118(2): 195–205.

Tyler, VE. (1994) *Herbs of Choice.* New York: Pharmaceutical Products Press.

Unger JM, van Belle G, Heyman A. (1999). Cross-sectional versus longitudinal estimates of cognitive change in nondemented older people: a CERAD study. Consortium to Establish a Registry for Alzheimer's Disease. *J Am Geriatr Soc.* 47(5): 559–63.

van Dongen PWJ, de Groot ANJA. (1995). History of ergot alkaloids frmo ergotism to ergometrine. *Eur J Obstet Gynecol Reprod Biol.* 60: 109–116.

Varma AR, Snowden JS, Lloyd JJ, Talbot PR, Mann DM, Neary D. (1999). Evaluation of the NINCDS-ADRDA criteria in the differentiation of Alzheimer's disease and frontotemporal dementia. *J Neurol Neurosurg Psychiatry.* 66(2): 184–88.

Vercelletto M, Ronin M, Huvet M, Magne C, Feve JR. (1999). Frontal type dementia preceding amyotrophic lateral sclerosis: a neuropsychological and SPECT study of five clinical cases. *Eur J Neurol.* 6(3): 295–99.

Vered Y, Grosskopf I, Palevitch D, Harsat A, Charach G, Weintraub MS, Graff F. (1997). The influence of Vicia faba (broad bean) seedlings on urinary sodium excretion. *Planta Med.* 63(3): 237–40.

Vidal C. (1996). Nicotinic receptors in the brain. Molecular biology, function, and therapeutics. *Mol Chem Neuropathol.* 28(1–3): 3–11.

Wada K, Sasaki K, Miura K, Yagi M, Kubota Y, Matsumoto T, Haga M. (1993). Isolation of bilobalide and ginkgolide A from Ginkgo biloba L. shorten the sleeping time induced in mice by anesthetics. *Biol Pharm Bull.* 16(2): 210–12.

Wang A, Cao Y, Wang Y, Zhao R, Liu C. (1995). [Effects of Chinese ginseng root and stem-leaf saponins on learning, memory, and biogenic monoamines of brain in rats]. *Chung Kuo Chung Yao Tsa Chih.* 20(8): 493–95.

Wang H, Cui WY, Liu CH. (1996). Modulation by nicotine on binding of cerebral muscarinic receptors with muscarinic agonist and antagonist. *Chung Kuo Yao Li Hsueh Pao.* 17(6): 497–9.

Wang J. (1982). [Quantitative determination of saponins in the roots of Panax notoginseng, P. ginseng, and P. quinquefolius.] *Yaozue Tongbao.* 17: 244–45.

Warburton DM. (1986). [Clinical psychopharmacology of Ginkgo biloba extract]. *Presse Med.* 15(31): 1595–604.

Warburton DM. (1992). Nicotine as a cognitive enhancer. *Prog Neuropsychopharmacol Biol Psychiatry.* 16(2): 181–91.

Warot D, Lacomblez L, Danjou P, Weiller E, Payan C, Puech AJ. (1991). [Comparative effects of Ginkgo biloba extracts on psychomotor performances and memory in healthy subjects]. *Therapie.* 46(1): 33–36.

Watanabe H, Ohta H, Imamura L, Asakura W, Matoba Y, Matsumoto K. (1991). Effect of Panax ginseng on age-related changes in the spontaneous motor activity and dopaminergic nervous system in the rat. *Jpn J Pharmacol.* 55(1): 51–56.

Wen TC, Yoshimura H, Matsuda S, Lim JH, Sakanaka M. (1996). Ginseng root prevents learning disability and neuronal loss in gerbils with 5-minute forebrain ischemia. *Acta Neuropathol (Berlin).* 91(1): 15–22.

White HK, Levin ED. (1999). Four-week nicotine skin patch treatment effects on cognitive performance in Alzheimer's disease. *Psychopharmacology (Berlin).* 143(2): 158–65.

White HL, Scates PW, Cooper BR. (1996). Extracts of Ginkgo biloba leaves inhibit monoamine oxidase. *Life Sci.* 58(16): 1315–21.

Wieraszko A, Li G, Kornecki E, Hogan MV, Ehrlich YH. (1993). Long-term potentiation in the hippocampus induced by platelet-activating factor. *Neuron.* 10(3): 553–57.

Wilson AL, Langley LK, Monley J, Bauer T, Rottunda S, McFalls E, Kovera C, McCarten JR. (1995). Nicotine patches in Alzheimer's disease: pilot study on learning, memory, and safety. *Pharmacol Biochem Behav.* 51(2–3): 509–14.

Winter JC. (1998). The effects of an extract of Ginkgo biloba, EGb 761, on cognitive behavior and longevity in the rat. *Physiol Behav.* 63(3): 425–33.

Winter JC, Timineri D. (1999). The discriminative stimulus properties of EGb 761, an extract of Ginkgo biloba. *Pharmacol Biochem Behav.* 62(3): 543–47.

Winther K, Randlov C, Rein E, Mehlsen J. (1998). Effects of Ginkgo biloba extract on cognitive function and blood pressure in elderly subjects. *Curr Therapeutic Res.* 59(12): 881–88.

Wójcicki J, Gawroska-Szklarz B, Bieganowski W, Patalan M, Smulski HK, Samochowiec L, Zakrzewski J. (1995). Comparative pharmacokinetics and bioavailability of flavonoid glycosides of Ginkgo biloba after a single oral administration of three formulations to healthy volunteers. *Materia Med Polona.* 27(4): 141–46.

Yabe T, Chat M, Malherbe E, Vidal PP. (1995). Effects of Ginkgo biloba extract (EGb 761) on the guinea pig vestibular system. *Pharmacol Biochem Behav.* 42(4): 595–604.

Yamada K, Tanaka T, Han D, Senzaki K, Kameyama T, Nabeshima T. (1999). Protective effects of idebenone and alpha-tocopherol on beta-amyloid-(1-42)-

induced learning and memory deficits in rats: implication of oxidative stress in beta-amyloid-induced neurotoxicity in vivo. *Eur J Neurosci.* 11(1): 83–90.

Yamamoto J. (1998). Effects of nicotine, pilocarpine, and tetrahydroaminoacridine on hippocampal theta waves in freely moving rabbits. *Eur J Pharmacol.* 359(2–3): 133–37.

Yatin SM, Yatin M, Aulick T, Ain KB, Butterfield DA. (1999). Alzheimer's amyloid beta-peptide associated free radicals increase rat embryonic neuronal polyamine uptake and ornithine decarboxylase activity: protective effect of vitamin E. *Neurosci Lett.* 263(1): 17–20.

Yokoi F, Komiyama T, Ito T, Hayashi T, Lio M, Hara T. (1993). Application of carbon-11 labelled nicotine in the measurement of human cerebral blood flow and other physiological parameters. *Eur J Nuc Med.* 20(1): 46–52.

Yoshimura H, Watanabe K, Ogawa N. (1988a). Psychotropic effects of ginseng saponins on agonistic behavior between resident and intruder mice. *Eur J Pharmacol.* 146(2–3): 291–97.

Yoshimura H, Watanabe K, Ogawa N. (1988b). Acute and chronic effects of ginseng saponins on maternal aggression in mice. *Eur J Pharmacol.* 150(3): 319–24.

Yuan CS, Attele AS, Wu JA, Liu D. (1998). Modulation of American ginseng on brainstem GABAergic effects in rats. *J Ethnopharmacol.* 62(3): 215–22.

Zhang JT, Qu ZW, Liu Y, Deng HL. (1990). Preliminary study on antiamnestic mechanism of ginsenoside Rg1 and Rb1. *Chin Med J (Engl).* 103(11): 932–38.

Zhang Y, Saito H, Nishiyama N, Abe K. (1994). Effects of DX-9386, a traditional Chinese medicinal prescription, on long-term potentiation in the dentate gyrus in rats. *Biol Pharm Bull* 17(10): 1337–40.

Zhao R, McDaniel WF. (1998). Ginseng improves strategic learning by normal and brain-damaged rats. *Neuroreport.* 9(7): 1619–24.

Zhu L, Wu J, Liao H, Gao J, Zhao XN, Zhang ZX. (1997). Antagonistic effects of extract from leaves of Ginkgo biloba on glutamate neurotoxicity. *Chung Kuo Yao Li Hsueh Pao.* 18(4): 344–47.

Zierer R. (1991). Prolonged infusion of Panax ginseng saponins into the rat does not alter the chemical and kinetic profile of hormones from the posterior pituitary. *J Ethnopharmacol.* 34(2–3): 269–74.

Chapter 6

Adam K, Tomeny M, Oswald I. (1986). Physiological and psychological differences between good and poor sleepers. *J Psychiatr Res.* 20(4): 301–16.

Almeida JC, Grimsley EW. (1996). Coma from the health food store: interaction between kava and alprazolam. *Ann Intern Med.* 125(11): 940–1.

American Psychiatric Association. (1994). *Diagnostic and Statistical Manual of Mental Disorders*, 4th ed. Washington, DC: American Psychiatric Association.

Aston-Jones G, Rajkowski J, Kubiak P, Alexinsky T. (1994). Locus coeruleus neurons in monkey are selectively activated by attended cues in a vigilance task. *J Neurosci.* 14(7): 4467–80.

Backhauss C, Krieglstein J. (1992). Extract of kava (Piper methysticum) and its methysticin constituents protect brain tissue against ischemic damage in rodents. *Eur J Pharmacol.* 215(2–3): 265–69.

Balderer G, Borbely AA. (1985). Effect of valerian on human sleep. *Psychopharmacology (Berlin).* 87(4): 406–9.

Basbaum AI, Fields HL. (1984). Endogenous pain control systems: brainstem spinal pathways and endorphin circuitry. *Annu Rev Neurosci.* 7: 309–38.

Baum SS, Hill R, Rommelspacher H. (1998). Effect of kava extract and individual kavalactones on neurotransmitter levels in the nucleus accumbens of rats. *Prog Neuropsychopharmacol Biol Psychiatry.* 22(7): 1105–20.

Bhate H, Gerster G, Gracza E. (1989). Orale pramedikation mit Zubereitungen aus Piper methysticum bei operativen Eingriffen in Epiduralanasthesie. *Erfahrungsheilkunde.* 6: 339–45.

Boonen G, Beck MA, Häberlein H. (1997). Contribution to the quantitative and enantioselective determination of kavalactones by high-performance liquid chromatography on ChiraSpher NT material. *J Chromatogr B Biomed Sci Appl.* 702(1–2): 240–44.

Boonen G, Ferger B, Kuschinsky K, Haberlein H. (1998). In vivo effects of the kavalactones (+)-dihydromethysticin and (+/−)-kavain on dopamine, 3,4-dihydroxyphenylacetic acid, serotonin and 5-hydroxyindoleacetic acid levels in striatal and cortical brain regions. *Planta Med.* 64(6): 507–10.

Boonen G, Haberlein H. (1998). Influence of genuine kavalactone enantiomers on the GABA-A binding site. *Planta Med.* 64(6): 504–6.

Bourdet C, Goldenberg F. (1994). Insomnia in anxiety: sleep EEG changes. *J Psychosom Res.* 38(suppl 1): 93–104.

Bourin M, Bougerol T, Guitton B, Broutin E. (1997). A combination of plant extracts in the treatment of outpatients with adjustment disorder with anxious mood: controlled study versus placebo. *Fundam Clin Pharmacol.* 11(2): 127–32.

Buchbauer G, Jager W, Jirovetz L, Meyer F, Dietrich H. (1992). [Effects of valerian root oil, borneol, isoborneol, bornyl acetate and isobornyl acetate on the motility of laboratory animals (mice) after inhalation]. *Pharmazie.* 1992 Aug. 47(8): 620–2.

Capasso A, Piacente S, Pizza C, Sorrentino L. (1998). Flavonoids reduce morphine withdrawal in-vitro. *J Pharm Pharmacol.* May 50: 5 561–64.

Cavadas C, Araujo I, Cotrim MD, Amaral T, Cunha AP, Macedo T, Ribeiro CF. (1995). In vitro study on the interaction of Valeriana officinalis L. extracts and their amino acids on GABAA receptor in rat brain. *Arzneimittelforschung.* 45(7): 753–5.

Chan TY, Tang CH, Critchley JA. (1995). Poisoning due to an over-the-counter hypnotic, Sleep-Qik (hyoscine, cyproheptadine, valerian). *Postgrad Med J.* 71(834): 227–8.

Chavadej S, Becker H, Weberling F. (1985). Further investigations of valepotriates in the Valerianaceae. *Pharm Weekbl Sci.* 7(4): 167–8.

Cooper JR, Bloom FE, Roth RH. (1996). *The Biochemical Basis of Neuropharmacology*, 7th ed. New York: Oxford University Press.

Cott J. (1995). NCDEU update. Natural product formulations available in europe for psychotropic indications. *Psychopharmacol Bull.* 31(4): 745–51.

Davidson RJ, Abercrombie H, Nitschke JB, Putnam K. (1999). Regional brain function, emotion, and disorders of emotion. *Curr Opin Neurobiol.* 9(2): 228–34.

Davies LP, Drew CA, Duffield P, Johnston GA, Jamieson DD. (1992). Kava pyrones and resin: studies on GABAA, GABAB and benzodiazepine binding sites in rodent brain. *Pharmacol Toxicol.* 71(2): 120–26.

Davis M, Rainnie D, Cassell M. (1994). Neurotransmission in the rat amygdala related to fear and anxiety. *Trends Neurosci.* 17(5): 208–14.

Della Logia R, Tubaro A, Redaelli C. (1981). [Evaluation of the activity on the mouse CNS of several plant extracts and a combination of them]. *Riv Neurol.* 51(5): 297–310.

Duffield AM, Jamieson DD, Lidgard RO, Duffield PH, Bourne DJ. (1989). Identification of some human urinary metabolites of the intoxicating beverage kava. *J Chromatogr.* 475: 273–81.

Duffield PH, Jamieson D. (1991). Development of tolerance to kava in mice. *Clin Exp Pharmacol Physiol.* 18(8): 571–8.

Dunaev VV, Trzhetsinskii SD, Tishkin VS, Fursa NS, Linenko VI. (1987). [Biological activity of the sum of the valepotriates isolated from Valeriana alliariifolia]. *Farmakol Toksikol.* 50(6): 33–37.

Eddy M, Walbroehl GS. (1999). Insomnia. *Am Fam Physician.* 59(7): 1911–16, 1918.

Faulhaber J, Steiger A, Lancel M. (1997). The $GABA_A$ agonist THIP produces slow wave sleep and reduces spindling activity in NREM sleep in humans. *Psychopharmacology (Berlin).* 130(3): 285–91.

Ferger B, Boonen G, Häberlein H, Kuschinsky K. (1998). In vivo microdialysis study of (+/–)-kavain on veratridine-induced glutamate release. *Eur J Pharmacol.* 347(2–3): 211–14.

Foo H, Lemon J. (1997). Acute effects of kava, alone or in combination with alcohol, on subjective measures of impairment and intoxication and on cognitive performance. *Drug Alcohol Rev.* 16(2): 147–55.

Frey R. (1991). [Demonstration of the central effects of D,L-kawain with EEG brain mapping]. *Fortschr Med.* 109(25): 505–58.

Friese J, Gleitz J. (1998). Kavain, dihydrokavain, and dihydromethysticin noncompetitively inhibit the specific binding of [^{3}H]-batrachotoxinin-A 20-alpha-benzoate to receptor site 2 of voltage-gated Na+ channels. *Planta Med.* 64(5): 458–59.

Geahlen RL, Koonchanok NM, McLaughlin JL, Pratt DE. (1989). Inhibition of protein-tyrosine kinase activity by flavonoids and related compounds. *J Nat Prod.* 52(5): 982–86.

Gerhard U, Hobi V, Kocher R, König C. (1991). [Acute sedative effect of an herbal relaxation tablet as compared to that of bromazepam]. *Schweiz Rundsch Med Prax.* 80(52): 1481–86.

Gerhard U, Linnenbrink N, Georghiadou C, Hobi V. (1996). [Vigilance-decreasing effects of 2 plant-derived sedatives]. *Schweiz Rundsch Med Prax.* 85(15): 473–81.

Gessner B, Klasser M. (1984). [Studies on the effect of Harmonicum Much on sleep using polygraphic EEG recordings]. *EEG EMG Z Elektroenzephalogr Verwandte Geb.* 15(1): 45–51.

Gleitz J, Beile A, Peters T. (1995). (+/–)-Kavain inhibits veratridine-activated voltage-dependent Na(+)-channels in synaptosomes prepared from rat cerebral cortex. *Neuropharmacology.* 34(9): 1133–38.

Gleitz J, Friese J, Beile A, Ameri A, Peters T. (1996a). Anticonvulsive action of (+/–)-kavain estimated from its properties on stimulated synaptosomes and Na+ channel receptor sites. *Eur J Pharmacol.* Nov. 7. 315(1): 89–97.

Gleitz J, Tosch C, Beile A, Peters T (1996b). The protective action of tetrodotoxin and (+/–)-kavain on anaerobic glycolysis, ATP content, and intracellular Na+ and Ca2+ of anoxic brain vesicles. *Neuropharmacology.* 35(12): 1743–52.

Gleitz J, Beile A, Wilkens P, Ameri A, Peters T. (1997). Antithrombotic action of the kava pyrone (+)-kavain prepared from Piper methysticum on human platelets. *Planta Med.* 63(1): 27–30.

Grella B, Dukat M, Young R, Teitler M, Herrick-Davis K, Gauthier CB, Glennon RA. (1998). Investigation of hallucinogenic and related beta-carbolines. *Drug Alcohol Depend.* 50(2): 99–107.

Gruenwald J, Brendler T, Jaenicke C. (1998). *PDR for Herbal Medicines*, 1st ed. Montvale, NJ: Medical Economics.

Halpern M. (1987). The organization and function of the vomeronasal system. *Annu Rev Neurosci.* 10: 325–62.

Hänsel R, Wagener HH. (1967). [Attempts to identify sedative-hypnotic active substances in hops]. *Arzneimittelforschung.* 17(1): 79–81.

Hänsel R, Wohlfart R, Coper H. (1980). [Sedative-hypnotic compounds in the exhalation of hops, II]. *Z Naturforsch.* 35(11–12): 1096–7.

Harney JW, Barofsky IM, Leary JD. (1978). Behavioral and toxicological studies of cyclopentanoid monoterpenes from Nepeta cataria. *Lloydia.* 41(4): 367–74.

Hart BL, Leedy MG. (1985). Analysis of the catnip reaction: mediation by olfactory system, not vomeronasal organ. *Behav Neural Biol.* 44(1): 38–46.

Hazelhoff B, Malingre TM, Meijer DK. (1982). Antispasmodic effects of valeriana compounds: an in-vivo and in-vitro study on the guinea-pig ileum. *Arch Int Pharmacodyn Ther.* 257(2): 274–87.

Heinze HJ, Münthe TF, Steitz J, Matzke M. (1994). Pharmacopsychological effects of oxazepam and kava-extract in a visual search paradigm assessed with event-related potentials. *Pharmacopsychiatry.* Nov. 27(6): 224–30.

Hille B. (1992). *Ionic Channels of Excitable membranes*, 2nd ed. Sunderland, MA: Sinauer.

Hiller KO, Zetler G. (1996). Neuropharmacological studies on ethanol extracts of Valeriana officinalis L.: behavioural and anticonvulsant properties. *Phytother Res.* 10(2): 145–151.

Hobbs WR, Rall TW, Verdoon TA. (1996). Hypnotics and Sedatives: Ethanol. In: *Goodman and Gilman's The Pharmacological Basis of Therapeutics.* Hardman JG, Limbird LE, Molinoff PB, Ruddon RW, Goodman Gilman A, eds. New York: McGraw-Hill.

Holm E, Staedt U, Heep J, Kortsik C, Behne F, Kaske A, Mennicke I. (1991). [The action profile of D,L-kavain. Cerebral sites and sleep-wakefulness-rhythm in animals]. *Arzneimittelforschung.* July 41(7): 673–83.

Hölzl J, Fink C. (1984). [Effect of valeprotriate on spontaneous motor activity in mice]. *Arzneimittelforschung.* 34(1): 44–47.

Houghton PJ. (1988). The biological activity of Valerian and related plants. *J Ethnopharmacol.* 22(2): 121–42.

Houghton PJ. (1999). The scientific basis for the reputed activity of valerian. *J Pharm Pharmacol.* 51(5): 505–12.

Jamieson DD, Duffield PH. (1990). Positive interaction of ethanol and kava resin in mice. *Clin Exp Pharmacol Physiol.* 17(7): 509–14.

Jamieson DD, Duffield PH, Cheng D, Duffield AM. (1989). Comparison of the central nervous system activity of the aqueous and lipid extract of kava (Piper methysticum). *Arch Int Pharmacodyn Ther.* Sept.–Oct. 301: 66–80.

Juhász G, Emri Z, Kékesi KA, Salfay O, Crunelli V. (1994). Blockade of thalamic GABAB receptors decreases EEG synchronization. *Neurosci Lett.* 172(1–2): 155–58.

Julien, RM. (1997). *A Primer of Drug Action: A Concise, Nontechnical Guide to the Actions, Uses, and Side Effects of Psychoactive Drugs.* New York: W. H. Freeman.

Jussofie A, Schmiz A, Hiemke C. (1994). Kavapyrone enriched extract from Piper methysticum as modulator of the GABA binding site in different regions of rat brain. *Psychopharmacology (Berlin).* 116(4): 469–74.

Kandel E, Schwartz JH, Jessel TM, eds. (1991). *Principles of Neural Science*, 3rd ed. Norwalk, CT: Appleton and Lange.

Keledjian J, Duffield PH, Jamieson DD, Lidgard RO, Duffield AM. (1988). Uptake into mouse brain of four compounds present in the psychoactive beverage kava. *J Pharm Sci.* 77(12): 1003–6.

Kellis JT Jr, Vickery LE. (1984). Inhibition of human estrogen synthetase (aromatase) by flavones. *Science.* 225(4666): 1032–34.

Kim KY, McCartney JR, Kaye W, Boland RJ, Niaura R. (1996). The effect of cimetidine and ranitidine on cognitive function in postoperative cardiac surgical patients. *Int J Psychiatry Med.* 26(3): 295–307.

Ko FN, Huang TF, Teng CM. (1991). Vasodilatory action mechanisms of apigenin isolated from Apium graveolens in rat thoracic aorta. *Biochim Biophys Acta.* 1115(1): 69–74.

Kowalchik C, Hylton WH, eds. (1987). *Rodale's Illustrated Encyclopedia of Herbs.* Emmaus, PA: Rodale Press.

Kretzschmar R, Meyer HJ. (1968). Der Einfluß naturlicher 5,6-hydrierter Kava-Pyrone auf isolierte Herzpraparate und irhe antifibrallatorische Wirkung am Ganztier. *Arch Int Pharmacodyn Ther.* 177: 261–77.

Kretzschmar R, Meyer HJ, Teschendorf HJ, Zöllner B (1969). [Antagonistic action of natural 5,6-hydrogenated kava pyrones against strychnine poisoning and experimental local tetanus]. *Arch Int Pharmacodyn Ther.* Dec. 182(2): 251–68.

Kuiper GG, Lemmen JG, Carlsson B, Corton JC, Safe SH, van der Saag PT, van der Burg B, Gustafsson JA. (1998). Interaction of estrogenic chemicals and phytoestrogens with estrogen receptor beta. *Endocrinology.* 139(10): 4252–63.

Kupfer DJ, Foster FG, Reich L, Thompson SK, Weiss B. (1976). EEG sleep changes as predictors in depression. *Am J Psychiatry.* 133(6): 622–26.

Lancel M, Crönlein TA, Faulhaber J. (1996). Role of $GABA_A$ receptors in sleep regulation. Differential effects of muscimol and midazolam on sleep in rats. *Neuropsychopharmacology.* 15(1): 63–74.

Lancel M, Faulhaber J. (1996). The $GABA_A$ agonist THIP (gaboxadol) increases non-REM sleep and enhances delta activity in the rat. *Neuroreport.* 7(13): 2241–45.

Lancel M, Faulhaber J, Deisz RA. (1998). Effect of the GABA uptake inhibitor tiagabine on sleep and EEG power spectra in the rat. *Br J Pharmacol.* 123(7): 1471–77.

Langosch JM, Normann C, Schirrmacher K, Berger M, Walden J. (1998). The influence of (+/–)-kavain on population spikes and long-term potentiation in guinea pig hippocampal slices. *Comp Biochem Physiol A Mol Integr Physiol.* July 120(3): 545–49.

Leathwood PD, Chauffard F. (1982–3). Quantifying the effects of mild sedatives. *J Psychiatr Res.* 17(2): 115–22.

Leathwood PD, Chauffard F. (1985). Aqueous extract of valerian reduces latency to fall asleep in man. *Planta Med.* 2: 144–48.

Leathwood PD, Chauffard F, Heck E, Munoz-Box R. (1982). Aqueous extract of valerian root (Valeriana officinalis L.) improves sleep quality in man. *Pharmacol Biochem Behav.* 17(1): 65–71.

Lebot V, Merlin M, Lindstrom L. (1997). *Kava—the Pacific Elixir: The Definitive Guide to Its Ethnobotany, History, and Chemistry.* Rochester, VT: Healing Arts Press. [Originally published: New Haven: Yale University Press, 1992.]

Lehmann E, Klieser E, Klimke A, Krach H, Spatz R. (1989). The efficacy of Cavain in patients suffering from anxiety. *Pharmacopsychiatry.* 22(6): 258–62.

Leuschner J, Müller J, Rudmann M. (1993). Characterisation of the central nervous depressant activity of a commercially available valerian root extract. *Arzneimittelforschung.* 43(6): 638–41.

Leyel CF, ed. (1994). *A Modern Herbal.* NY: Dorset Press.

Li B, Robinson DH, Birt DF. (1997). Evaluation of properties of apigenin and [G-^{3}H]apigenin and analytic method development. *J Pharm Sci.* 86(6): 721–5.

Lindahl O, Lindwall L. (1989). Double blind study of a valerian preparation. *Pharmacol Biochem Behav.* 32(4): 1065–66.

Lindenberg D, Pitule-Schodel H. (1990). [D,L-kavain in comparison with oxazepam in anxiety disorders. A double-blind study of clinical effectiveness]. *Fortschr Med.* 108(2): 49–50, 53–54.

Lorenzo PS, Rubio MC, Medina JH, Adler-Graschinsky E. (1996). Involvement of monoamine oxidase and noradrenaline uptake in the positive chronotropic effects of apigenin in rat atria. *Eur J Pharmacol.* 312(2): 203–7.

Loring DW, Meador KJ. (1989). Central nervous system effects of antihistamines on evoked potentials. *Ann Allergy.* 63(6): Pt 2 604–8.

Magura EI, Kopanitsa MV, Gleitz J, Peters T, Krishtal OA. (1997). Kava extract ingredients, (+)-methysticin and (+/–)-kavain inhibit voltage-operated Na(+)-channels in rat CA1 hippocampal neurons. *Neuroscience.* 81(2): 345–51.

Maluf E, Baros HMT, Frochtengarten ML, Benti R, Leite JR. (1991). Assessment of the hypnotic/sedative effects and toxicity of Passiflora edulis aqueous extract in rodents and humans. *Phytother Res.* 5(6): 262–66.

Manolov P, Petkov VD, Ivancheva S. (1977). Studies on the central depressive action of methanol extract from Geranium macrorrhizum L. *Dokl Bolg Akad Nauk.* 30(11): 1657–59.

Massoco CO, Silva MR, Gorniak SL, Spinosa MS, Bernardi MM. (1995). Behavioral effects of acute and long-term administration of catnip (Nepeta cataria) in mice. *Vet Hum Toxicol.* 37(6): 530–33.

Meier B. (1995). Passiflora incarnata L.—Passion flower. *Zeitschrift fur Phytotherapie.* 16(2): 115–26.

Medina JH, Paladini AC, Wolfman C, Levi de Stein M, Calvo D, Diaz LE, Pena C. (1990). Chrysin (5,7-di-OH-flavone), a naturally-occurring ligand for benzodiazepine receptors, with anticonvulsant properties. *Biochem Pharmacol.* 40(10): 2227–31.

Medina JH, Viola H, Wolfman C, Marder M, Wasowski C, Calvo D, Paladini AC. (1997). Overview—flavonoids: a new family of benzodiazepine receptor ligands. *Neurochem Res.* 22(4): 419–25.

Menghini A, Mancini LA. (1988). TLC determination of flavonoid accumulation in clonal populations of Passiflora incarnata L. *Pharmacol Res Commun.* 20(suppl 5): 113–16.

Middleton E Jr, Drzewiecki G. (1984). Flavonoid inhibition of human basophil histamine release stimulated by various agents. *Biochem Pharmacol.* 33(21): 3333–38.

Morisson F, Lavigne G, Petit D, Nielsen T, Malo J, Montplaisir J. (1998). Spectral analysis of wakefulness and REM sleep EEG in patients with sleep apnoea syndrome. *Eur Respir J.* 11(5): 1135–40.

Morita K, Hamano S, Oka M, Teraoka K. (1990). Stimulatory actions of bioflavonoids on tyrosine uptake into cultured bovine adrenal chromaffin cells. *Biochem Biophys Res Commun.* 171(3): 1199–204.

Muller-Limmroth W, Ehrenstein W. (1977). [Experimental studies of the effects of Seda-Kneipp on the sleep of sleep disturbed subjects; implications for the treatment of different sleep disturbances]. *Med Klin.* 72(25): 1119–25.

Münte TF, Heinze HJ, Matzke M, Steitz J. (1993). Effects of oxazepam and an extract of kava roots (Piper methysticum) on event-related potentials in a word recognition task. *Neuropsychobiology.* 27(1): 46–53.

Norton SA, Ruze P. (1994). Kava dermopathy. *J Am Acad Dermatol.* 31(1): 89–97.

Ortiz JG, Nieves-Natal J, Chavez P. (1999). Effects of Valeriana officinalis extracts on [^{3}H]flunitrazepam binding, synaptosomal [^{3}H]GABA uptake, and hippocampal [^{3}H]GABA release. *Neurochem Res.* 24(11): 1373–78.

Osterhoudt KC, Lee SK, Callahan JM, Henretig FM. (1997). Catnip and the alteration of human consciousness. *Vet Hum Toxicol.* 39(6): 373–75.

Pittler MH, Ernst E. (2000). Efficacy of kava extract for treating anxiety: systematic review and meta-analysis. *J Clin Psychopharmacol.* (1): 84–89.

Rajkowski J, Kubiak P, Aston-Jones G. (1994). Locus coeruleus activity in monkey: phasic and tonic changes are associated with altered vigilance. *Brain Res Bull.* 35(5–6): 607–16.

Riedel E, Hansel R, Ehrke G. (1982). [Inhibition of gamma-aminobutyric acid catabolism by valerenic acid derivatives]. *Planta Med.* 46(4): 219–20.

Robbers JE, Speedie MK, Tyler VE. (1996). *Pharmacognosy and Pharmacobiotechnology.* Baltimore: Williams & Wilkins.

Ruze P. (1990). Kava-induced dermopathy: a niacin deficiency? *Lancet.* 335(8703): 1442–5.

Rylski M, Duriasz-Rowinska H, Rewerski W. (1979). The analgesic action of some flavonoids in the hot plate test. *Acta Physiol Pol.* 30(3): 385–8.

Sakamoto T, Mitani Y, Nakajima K. (1992). Psychotropic effects of Japanese valerian root extract. *Chem Pharm Bull (Tokyo)*. 40(3): 758–61.

Salgueiro JB, Ardenghi P, Dias M, Ferreira MB, Izquierdo I, Medina JH. (1997). Anxiolytic natural and synthetic flavonoid ligands of the central benzodiazepine receptor have no effect on memory tasks in rats. *Pharmacol Biochem Behav*. 58(4): 887–91.

Sanders SK, Shekhar A. (1995). Regulation of anxiety by $GABA_A$ receptors in the rat amygdala. *Pharmacol Biochem Behav*. Dec 52(4): 701–6.

Santos MS, Ferreira F, Cunha AP, Carvalho AP, Ribeiro CF, Macedo T. (1994a). Synaptosomal GABA release as influenced by valerian root extract—involvement of the GABA carrier. *Arch Int Pharmacodyn Ther*. 327(2): 220–31.

Santos MS, Ferreira F, Cunha AP, Carvalho AP, Macedo T. (1994b). An aqueous extract of valerian influences the transport of GABA in synaptosomes. *Planta Med*. 60(3): 278–79.

Santos MS, Ferreira F, Faro C, Pires E, Carvalho AP, Cunha AP, Macedo T. (1994c). The amount of GABA present in aqueous extracts of valerian is sufficient to account for [^{3}H]GABA release in synaptosomes. *Planta Med*. 60(5): 475–76.

Schelosky L, Raffauf C, Jendroska K, Poewe W. (1995). Kava and dopamine antagonism [letter]. *J Neurol Neurosurg Psychiatry*. 58(5): 639–40.

Schirrmacher K, Busselberg D, Langosch JM, Walden J, Winter U, Bingmann D. (1999). Effects of (+/–)-kavain on voltage-activated inward currents of dorsal root ganglion cells from neonatal rats. *Eur Neuropsychopharmacol*. 9(1–2): 171–6.

Schulz H, Stolz C, Müller J. (1994). The effect of valerian extract on sleep polygraphy in poor sleepers: a pilot study. *Pharmacopsychiatry*. 27(4): 147–51.

Schwartz-Bloom RD, Cook TA, Yu X. (1996). Inhibition of GABA-gated chloride channels in brain by the arachidonic acid metabolite, thromboxane A2. *Neuropharmacology*. 35(9–10): 1347–53.

Seitz U, Schule A, Gleitz J. (1997). [^{3}H]-monoamine uptake inhibition properties of kava pyrones. *Planta Med*. 63(6): 548–49.

Sherry CJ, Hunter PS. (1979). The effect of an ethanol extract of catnip (Nepeta cataria) on the behavior of the young chick. *Experientia*. 35(2): 237–38.

Siegel RK. (1989). *Intoxication: Life in Pursuit of Artificial Paradise*. New York: Pocket Books.

Smith GW, Chalmers TM, Nuki G. (1993). Vasculitis associated with herbal preparation containing Passiflora extract [letter]. *Br J Rheumatol*. 32(1): 87–88.

Sopranzi N, De Feo G, Mazzanti G, Tolu L. (1990). [Biological and electroencephalographic parameters in rats in relation to Passiflora incarnata L.] *Clin Ter*. 132(5): 329–33.

Soulimani R, Fleurentin J, Mortier F, Misslin R, Derrieu G, Pelt JM. (1991). Neurotropic action of the hydroalcoholic extract of Melissa officinalis in the mouse. *Planta Med.* 57(2): 105–9.

Soulimani R, Younos C, Jarmouni S, Bousta D, Misslin R, Mortier F. (1997). Behavioural effects of Passiflora incarnata L. and its indole alkaloid and flavonoid derivatives and maltol in the mouse. *J Ethnopharmacol.* 57(1): 11–20.

Speroni E, Minghetti A. (1988). Neuropharmacological activity of extracts from Passiflora incarnata. *Planta Med.* 54(6): 488–91.

Subiza J, Subiza JL, Alonso M, Hinojosa M, Garcia R, Jerez M, Subiza E. (1990). Allergic conjunctivitis to chamomile tea. *Ann Allergy.* 65(2): 127–32.

Tasev T, Toléva P, Balabanova V. (1969). [Neurophysical effect of Bulgarian essential oils from rose, lavender, and geranium]. *Folia Med (Plovdiv).* 11(5): 307–17.

Temkin O. (1971). *The Falling Sickness: A History of Epilepsy from the Greeks to the Beginnings of Modern Neurology.* Baltimore: Johns Hopkins University Press.

Tyler VE. (1994). *Herbs of Choice.* New York: Pharmaceutical Products Press.

Uebelhack R, Franke L, Schewe HJ. (1998). Inhibition of platelet MAO-B by kava pyrone-enriched extract from Piper methysticum Forster (kava-kava). *Pharmacopsychiatry.* 31(5): 187–92.

Viola H, Wasowski C, Levi de Stein M, Wolfman C, Silveira R, Dajas F, Medina JH, Paladini AC. (1995). Apigenin, a component of Matricaria recutita flowers, is a central benzodiazepine receptors-ligand with anxiolytic effects. *Planta Med.* 61(3): 213–16.

Volz HP, Kieser M. (1997). Kava-kava extract WS 1490 versus placebo in anxiety disorders—a randomized placebo-controlled 25-week outpatient trial. *Pharmacopsychiatry.* 30(1): 1–5.

von der Hude W, Scheutwinkel-Reich M, Braun R. (1986). Bacterial mutagenicity of the tranquilizing constituents of Valerianaceae roots. *Mutat Res.* 169(1–2): 23–7.

Walden J, von Wegerer J, Winter U, Berger M, Grunze H. (1997). Effects of kawain and dihydromethysticin on field potential changes in the hippocampus. *Prog Neuropsychopharmacol Biol Psychiatry.* 21(4): 697–706.

Wolfman C, Viola H, Paladini A, Dajas F, Medina JH. (1994). Possible anxiolytic effects of chrysin, a central benzodiazepine receptor ligand isolated from Passiflora coerulea. *Pharmacol Biochem Behav.* 47(1): 1–4.

Wong AHC, Smith M, Boon H. (1998). Herbal remedies in psychiatric practice. *Arch Gen Psychiatry.* Nov. 55: 1033–44.

Woolf, SH. (1992). Practice guidelines, a new reality in medicine: II. Methods of developing guidelines. *Ann Intern Med.* 152: 946–52.

Chapter 7

Abi-Dargham A, Laruelle M, Wong DT, Robertson DW, Weinberger DR, Kleinman JE. (1993). Pharmacological and regional characterization of [^{3}H]LY278584 binding sites in human brain. *J Neurochem*. 60(2): 730–37.

Agostinis P, Vandenbogaerde A, Donella-Deana A, Pinna LA, Lee KT, Goris J, Merlevede W, Vandenheede JR, De Witte P. (1995). Photosensitized inhibition of growth factor-regulated protein kinases by hypericin. *Biochem Pharmacol*. 49(11): 1615–22.

Akbarian S, Sucher NJ, Bradley D, Tafazzoli A, Trinh D, Hetrick WP, Potkin SG, Sandman CA, Bunney WE Jr, Jones EG. (1996). Selective alterations in gene expression for NMDA receptor subunits in prefrontal cortex of schizophrenics. *J Neurosci*. 16(1): 19–30.

Alvarez-Guerra M, d'Alche-Biree F, Wolf WA, Vargas F, Dib M, Garay RP. (2000). 5-HT3- and 5-HT2C-antagonist properties of cyamemazine: significance for its clinical anxiolytic activity. *Psychopharmacology (Berlin)*. 147(4): 412–17.

American Psychiatric Association. (1994). *Diagnostic and Statistical Manual of Mental Disorders*, 4th ed. Washington, DC: American Psychiatric Association.

Amri H, Drieu K, Papadopoulos V. (1997). Ex vivo regulation of adrenal cortical cell steroid and protein synthesis, in response to adrenocorticotropic hormone stimulation, by the Ginkgo biloba extract EGb 761 and isolated ginkgolide B. *Endocrinology*. 138(12): 5415–26.

Amri H, Ogwuegbu SO, Boujrad N, Drieu K, Papadopoulos V. (1996). In vivo regulation of peripheral-type benzodiazepine receptor and glucocorticoid synthesis by Ginkgo biloba extract EGb 761 and isolated ginkgolides. *Endocrinology*. 137(12): 5707–18.

Apparsundaram S, Schroeter S, Giovanetti E, Blakely RD. (1998). Acute regulation of norepinephrine transport: II. PKC-modulated surface expression of human norepinephrine transporter proteins. *J Pharmacol Exp Ther*. 287(2): 744–51.

Arborelius L, Owens MJ, Plotsky PM, Nemeroff CB. (1999). The role of corticotropin-releasing factor in depression and anxiety disorders. *J Endocrinol*. 160(1): 1–12.

Arfeen Z, Owen H, Plummer JL, Ilsley AH, Sorby-Adams RA, Doecke CJ. (1995). A double-blind randomized controlled trial of ginger for the prevention of postoperative nausea and vomiting. *Anaesth Intensive Care*. 23(4): 449–52.

Armario A, Marti O, Molina T, de Pablo J, Valdes M. (1996). Acute stress markers in humans: response of plasma glucose, cortisol, and prolactin to two examinations differing in the anxiety they provoke. *Psychoneuroendocrinology*. 21(1): 17–24.

Artigas F, Romero L, de Montigny C, Blier P. (1996). Acceleration of the effect of selected antidepressant drugs in major depression by 5-HT_{1A} antagonists. *Trends Neurosci.* 19(9): 378–83.

Asakura T, Matsuda M. (1984). Efflux of gamma-aminobutyric acid from and appearance of free arachidonic acid inside synaptosomes. *Biochim Biophys Acta.* 773(2): 301–7.

Avery DH, Osgood TB, Ishiki DM, Wilson LG, Kenny M, Dunner DL. (1985). The DST in psychiatric outpatients with generalized anxiety disorder, panic disorder, or primary affective disorder. *Am J Psychiatry.* 142(7): 844–48.

Baba-Aïssa F, Raeymaekers L, Wuytack F, Dode L, Casteels R. (1998). Distribution and isoform diversity of the organellar Ca^{2+} pumps in the brain. *Mol Chem Neuropathol.* 33(3): 199–208.

Bagdy G, Perenyi A, Frecska E, Seregi A, Fekete MI, Tothfalusi L, Magyar K, Bela A, Arato M. (1988). Effect of adjuvant reserpine treatment on catecholamine metabolism in schizophrenic patients under long-term neuroleptic treatment. *J Neural Transm.* 71(1): 73–78.

Baldessarini, R. (1996). Drugs and the Treatment of Psychiatric Disorders. In: *Goodman and Gilman's The Pharmacological Basis of Therapeutics.* Hardman JG, Limbird LE, Molinoff PB, Ruddon RW, Goodman Gilman A, eds. New York: McGraw-Hill.

Baureithel KH, Buter KB, Engesser A, Burkard W, Schaffner W. (1997). Inhibition of benzodiazepine binding in vitro by amentoflavone, a constituent of various species of hypericum. *Pharm Acta Helv.* 72(3): 153–57.

Bennett DA Jr, Phun L, Polk JF, Voglino SA, Zlotnik V, Raffa RB. (1998). Neuropharmacology of St. John's Wort (Hypericum). *Ann Pharmacother.* 32(11): 1201–8.

Berendsen HH, Broekkamp CL. (1997). Indirect in vivo 5-HT1A-agonistic effects of the new antidepressant mirtazapine. *Psychopharmacology (Berlin).* 133(3): 275–82.

Bhattacharya SK, Chakrabarti A, Chatterjee SS. (1998). Activity profiles of two hyperforin-containing hypericum extracts in behavioral models. *Pharmacopsychiatry.* 31(suppl 1): 22–29.

Biber A, Fischer H, Romer A, Chatterjee SS. (1998). Oral bioavailability of hyperforin from hypericum extracts in rats and human volunteers. *Pharmacopsychiatry.* 31(suppl 1): 36–43.

Bladt S, Wagner H. (1994). Inhibition of MAO by fractions and constituents of hypericum extract. *J Geriatr Psychiatry Neurol.* 7(suppl 1): S57–59.

Blakely RD, Ramamoorthy S, Schroeter S, Qian Y, Apparsundaram S, Galli A, DeFelice LJ. (1998). Regulated phosphorylation and trafficking of antidepressant-sensitive serotonin transporter proteins. *Biol Psychiatry.* 44(3): 169–78.

Blazer DG, Kessler RC, McGonagle KA, Swartz MS. (1994). The prevalence and distribution of major depression in a national community sample: the National Comorbidity Survey. *Am J Psychiatry.* July 151: 7979–86.

Bloom FE, Morales M. (1998). The central 5-HT3 receptor in CNS disorders. *Neurochem Res.* 23(5): 653–59.

Bodkin JA, Zornberg GL, Lukas SE, Cole JO. (1995). Buprenorphine treatment of refractory depression. *J Clin Psychopharmacol.* 15(1): 49–57.

Bogerts B. (1997). The temporolimbic system theory of positive schizophrenic symptoms. *Schizophr Bull.* 23(3): 423–35.

Bolanos-Jimenez F, Manhaes de Castro R, Sarhan H, Prudhomme N, Drieu K, Fillion G. (1995). Stress-induced 5-HT1A receptor desensitization: protective effects of Ginkgo biloba extract (EGb 761). *Fundam Clin Pharmacol.* 9(2): 169–74.

Bolden-Watson C, Richelson E. (1993). Blockade by newly-developed antidepressants of biogenic amine uptake into rat brain synaptosomes. *Life Sci.* 52(12): 1023–29.

Bone ME, Wilkinson DJ, Young JR, McNeil J, Charlton S. (1990). Ginger root—a new antiemetic. The effect of ginger root on postoperative nausea and vomiting after major gynaecological surgery. *Anaesthesia.* 45(8): 669–71.

Bonhomme N, Esposito E. (1998). Involvement of serotonin and dopamine in the mechanism of action of novel antidepressant drugs: a review. *J Clin Psychopharmacol.* 18(6): 447–54.

Bouwer C, Stein DJ. (1997). Buspirone is an effective augmenting agent of serotonin selective re-uptake inhibitors in severe treatment-refractory depression. *South Afr Med J.* 87(4 suppl): 534–37, 540.

Brockmöller J, Reum T, Bauer S, Kerb R, Hübner WD, Roots I. (1997). Hypericin and pseudohypericin: pharmacokinetics and effects on photosensitivity in humans. *Pharmacopsychiatry.* 30(suppl 2): 94–101.

Brogden RN, Heel RC, Speight TM, Avery GS. (1978). Mianserin: a review of its pharmacological properties and therapeutic efficacy in depressive illness. *Drugs.* 16(4): 273–301.

Butterweck V, Wall A, Lieflander-Wulf U, Winterhoff H, Nahrstedt A. (1997). Effects of the total extract and fractions of Hypericum perforatum in animal assays for antidepressant activity. *Pharmacopsychiatry.* 30(suppl. 2): 117–24.

Carlsson A. (1978). Antipsychotic drugs, neurotransmitters, and schizophrenia. *Am J Psychiatry* 135(2): 165–73.

Carroll BJ, Feinberg M, Greden JF, Tarika J, Albala AA, Haskett RF, James NM, Kronfol Z, Lohr N, Steiner M, et al. (1981). A specific laboratory test for the diagnosis of melancholia. Standardization, validation, and clinical utility. *Arch Gen Psychiatry.* 38(1): 15–22.

Casanova MF. (1997). The temporolimbic system theory of paranoid schizophrenia. *Schizophr Bull.* 23(3): 513–15.

Charney DS. (1998). Monoamine dysfunction and the pathophysiology and treatment of depression. *J Clin Psychiatry.* 59(suppl 14): 11–14.

Chatterjee SS, Bhattacharya SK, Wonnemann M, Singer A, Muller WE. (1998a). Hyperforin as a possible antidepressant component of hypericum extracts. *Life Sci.* 63(6): 499–510.

Chatterjee SS, Noldner M, Koch E, Erdelmeier C. (1998b). Antidepressant activity of hypericum perforatum and hyperforin: the neglected possibility. *Pharmacopsychiatry.* 31(suppl 1): 7–15.

Chermat R, Brochet D, DeFeudis FV, Drieu K. (1997). Interactions of Ginkgo biloba extract (EGb 761), diazepam and ethyl beta-carboline-3-carboxylate on social behavior of the rat. *Pharmacol Biochem Behav.* 56(2): 333–9.

Clifford DB. (1985). Treatment of pain with antidepressants. *Am Fam Physician.* 31(2): 181–5.

Cooper JR, Bloom FE, Roth RH. (1996). *The Biochemical Basis of Neuropharmacology*, 7th ed. New York: Oxford.

Costall B, Naylor RJ. (1992). Neuropharmacology of emesis in relation to clinical response. *Br J Cancer.* 19: S2–7, discussion S7–8.

Costall B, Naylor RJ, Tyers MB. (1990). The psychopharmacology of 5-HT3 receptors. *Pharmacol Ther.* 47(2): 181–202.

Cott JM. (1997). In vitro receptor binding and enzyme inhibition by Hypericum perforatum extract. *Pharmacopsychiatry.* 30(suppl 2): 108–12.

Couldwell WT, Gopalakrishna R, Hinton DR, He S, Weiss MH, Law RE, Apuzzo ML, Law RE. (1994). Hypericin: a potential antiglioma therapy. *Neurosurgery.* 35(4): 705–9.

Cudd TA. (1998). Thromboxane A2 acts on the brain to mediate hemodynamic, adrenocorticotropin, and cortisol responses. *Am J Physiol.* 274(5 Pt 2): R1353–60.

Deakin JF. (1988). 5HT2 receptors, depression and anxiety. *Pharmacol Biochem Behav.* 29(4): 819–20.

Dimpfel W, Hofmann R. (1995). Pharmacodynamic effects of St. John's Wort on rat intracerebral field potentials. *Eur J Med Res.* 1(3): 157–67.

Dimpfel W, Schober F, Mannel M. (1998). Effects of a methanolic extract and a hyperforin-enriched CO2 extract of St. John's Wort (Hypericum perforatum) on intracerebral field potentials in the freely moving rat (Tele-Stereo-EEG). *Pharmacopsychiatry.* 31(suppl 1): 30–5.

Ding GH, Naora K, Hayashibara M, Katagiri Y, Kano Y, Iwamoto K. (1991). Pharmacokinetics of [6]-gingerol after intravenous administration in rats. *Chem Pharm Bull (Tokyo).* 39(6): 1612–14.

Dziedzicka-Wasylewska M, Willner P, Papp M. (1997). Changes in dopamine receptor mRNA expression following chronic mild stress and chronic antidepressant treatment. *Behav Pharmacol.* 8(6–7): 607–18.

Eison AS. (1990). Azapirones: history of development. *J Clin Psychopharmacol.* 10(3): Suppl 2S–5S.

Eison MS. (1990). Serotonin: a common neurobiologic substrate in anxiety and depression. *J Clin Psychopharmacol.* 10(3): Suppl 26S–30S.

Enns MW, Cox BJ, Parker JD, Guertin JE. (1998). Confirmatory factor analysis of the Beck anxiety and depression inventories in patients with major depression. *J Affective Disord.* 47(1–3): 195–200.

Erdelmeier CA. (1998). Hyperforin, possibly the major non-nitrogenous secondary metabolite of Hypericum perforatum L. *Pharmacopsychiatry.* 31(suppl 1): 2–6.

Ernst E. (1999). Second thoughts about safety of St. John's wort. *Lancet.* 354(9195): 2014–16.

Ernst E, Rand JI, Barnes J, Stevinson C. (1998). Adverse effects profile of the herbal antidepressant St. John's wort (Hypericum perforatum L.). *Eur J Clin Pharmacol.* 54(8): 589–94.

Fabre LF. (1990). Buspirone in the management of major depression: a placebo-controlled comparison. *J Clin Psychiatry.* 51(suppl): 55–61.

File SE, Gonzalez LE, Andrews N. (1996). Comparative study of pre- and post-synaptic 5-HT1A receptor modulation of anxiety in two ethological animal tests. *J Neurosci.* 16(15): 4810–15.

Fischer P, Tauscher J, Kufferle B, Kasper S. (1998). Weak antidepressant response after buspirone augmentation of serotonin reuptake inhibitors in refractory severe depression. *Int Clin Psychopharmacol.* 13(2): 83–86.

Fischer-Rasmussen W, Kjaer SK, Dahl C, Asping U. (1991). Ginger treatment of hyperemesis gravidarum. *Eur J Obstet Gynecol Reprod Biol.* 38(1): 19–24.

Flint AJ. (1994). Epidemiology and comorbidity of anxiety disorders in the elderly. *Am J Psychiatry.* 151(5): 640–49.

Flynn DL, Rafferty MF, Boctor AM. (1986). Inhibition of human neutrophil 5-lipoxygenase activity by gingerdione, shogaol, capsaicin and related pungent compounds. *Prostaglandins Leukot Med.* 24(2–3): 195–98.

Fortney JT, Gan TJ, Graczyk S, Wetchler B, Melson T, Khalil S, McKenzie R, Parrillo S, Glass PS, Moote C, Wermeling D, Parasuraman TV, Duncan B, Creed MR. (1998). A comparison of the efficacy, safety, and patient satisfaction of ondansetron versus droperidol as antiemetics for elective outpatient surgical procedures. S3A-409 and S3A-410 Study Groups. *Anesth Analg.* 86(4): 731–8.

Fossier P, Baux G, Tauc L. (1998). Role of different types of Ca^{2+} channels and a reticulum-like Ca^{2+} pump in neurotransmitter release. *J Physiol Paris.* 87(1): 3–14.

Fowler JS, Wang GJ, Volkow ND, Logan J, Franceschi D, Franceschi M, MacGregor R, Shea C, Garza V, Liu N, Ding YS. (2000). Evidence that Gingko biloba extract does not inhibit MAO A and B in living human brain. *Life Sci.* 66(9): PL141–46.

Gerlach J. (1991). New antipsychotics: classification, efficacy, and adverse effects. *Schizophr Bull.* 17(2): 289–309.

Gerra G, Calbiani B, Zaimovic A, Sartori R, Ugolotti G, Ippolito L, Delsignore R, Rustichelli P, Fontanesi B. (1998). Regional cerebral blood flow and comorbid diagnosis in abstinent opioid addicts. *Psychiatry Res.* 83(2): 117–26.

Goldberg HL, Finnerty RJ. (1979). The comparative efficacy of buspirone and diazepam in the treatment of anxiety. *Am J Psychiatry.* 136(9): 1184–87.

Goodwin DW, Guze SB. (1996). *Psychiatric Diagnosis.* New York: Oxford University Press.

Gordon JB. (1998). SSRIs and St. John's Wort: possible toxicity? *Am Fam Physician.* 57(5): 950–51.

Gorman JM. (1996–97). Comorbid depression and anxiety spectrum disorders. *Depression Anxiety.* 4(4): 160–68.

Govindarajan VS. (1982a). Ginger—chemistry, technology, and quality evaluation: part 1. *Crit Rev Food Sci Nutr.* 17(1): 1–96.

Govindarajan VS. (1982b). Ginger—chemistry, technology, and quality evaluation: part 2. *Crit Rev Food Sci Nutr.* 17(3): 189–258.

Graeff FG, Guimaraes FS, De Andrade TG, Deakin JF. (1996). Role of 5-HT in stress, anxiety, and depression. *Pharmacol Biochem Behav.* 54(1): 129–41.

Granier F, Girard M, Schmitt L, Boscredon J, Oules J, Escande M. (1985). Depression and anxiety: mianserin and nomifensine compared in a double-blind multicentre trial. *Acta Psychiatr Scand,* 320(suppl): 67–74.

Greenshaw AJ. (1993). Behavioural pharmacology of 5-HT3 receptor antagonists: a critical update on therapeutic potential. *Trends Pharmacol Sci.* 14(7): 265–70.

Greenshaw AJ, Silverstone PH. (1997). The non-antiemetic uses of serotonin 5-HT_3 receptor antagonists. Clinical pharmacology and therapeutic applications. *Drugs.* 53(1): 20–39.

Grontved A, Hentzer E. (1986). Vertigo-reducing effect of ginger root. A controlled clinical study. *ORL J Otorhinolaryngol Relat Spec.* 48(5): 282–6.

Grontved A, Brask T, Kambskard J, Hentzer E. (1988). Ginger root against seasickness. A controlled trial on the open sea. *Acta Otolaryngol.* 105(1–2): 45–9.

Gruenwald J, Brendler T, Jaenicke C. (1998). *PDR for Herbal Medicines,* 1st ed. Montvale, NJ: Medical Economics.

Haddjeri N, Blier P, de Montigny C. (1998). Long-term antidepressant treatments result in a tonic activation of forebrain 5-HT1A receptors. *J Neurosci.* 18(23): 10150–56.

Hansgen KD, Vesper J, Ploch M. (1994). Multicenter double-blind study examining the antidepressant effectiveness of the hypericum extract LI 160. *J Geriatr Psychiatry Neurol.* 7(suppl 1): S15–8.

Harrer G, Hubner WD, Podzuweit H. (1994). Effectiveness and tolerance of the hypericum extract LI 160 compared to maprotiline: a multicenter double-blind study. *J Geriatr Psychiatry Neurol.* 7(suppl 1): S24–28.

Harris MS, Sakamoto T, Kimura H, He S, Spee C, Gopalakrishna R, Gundimeda U, Yoo JS, Hinton DR, Ryan SJ. (1996). Hypericin inhibits cell growth and induces apoptosis in retinal pigment epithelial cells: possible involvement of protein kinase C. *Curr Eye Res.* 15(3): 255–62.

Hasenohrl RU, Nichau CH, Frisch CH, De Souza Silva MA, Huston JP, Mattern CM, Hacker R. (1996). Anxiolytic-like effect of combined extracts of Zingiber officinale and Ginkgo biloba in the elevated plus-maze. *Pharmacol Biochem Behav.* 53(2): 271–5.

Hasenohrl RU, Topic B, Frisch C, Hacker R, Mattern CM, Huston JP. (1998). Dissociation between anxiolytic and hypomnestic effects for combined extracts of zingiber officinale and ginkgo biloba, as opposed to diazepam. *Pharmacol Biochem Behav.* 59(2): 527–35.

Heiligenstein E, Guenther G. (1998). Over-the-counter psychotropics: a review of melatonin, St. John's wort, valerian, and kava-kava. *J Am Coll Health.* 46(6): 271–76.

Heninger GR, Delgado PL, Charney DS. (1996). The revised monoamine theory of depression: a modulatory role for monoamines, based on new findings from monoamine depletion experiments in humans. *Pharmacopsychiatry.* 29(1): 2–11.

Huang QR, Iwamoto M, Aoki S, Tanaka N, Tajima K, Yamahara J, Takaishi Y, Yoshida M, Tomimatsu T, Tamai Y. (1991). Anti-5-hydroxytryptamine3 effect of galanolactone, diterpenoid isolated from ginger. *Chem Pharm Bull (Tokyo).* 39(2): 397–9.

Huang Q, Matsuda H, Sakai K, Yamahara J, Tamai Y. (1990). [The effect of ginger on serotonin induced hypothermia and diarrhea]. *Yakugaku Zasshi.* 110(12): 936–42.

Hubner WD, Lande S, Podzuweit H. (1994). Hypericum treatment of mild depressions with somatic symptoms. *J Geriatr Psychiatry Neurol.* 7(suppl 1): S12–4.

Huguet F, Drieu K, Piriou A. (1994). Decreased cerebral 5-HT1A receptors during ageing: reversal by Ginkgo biloba extract (EGb 761). *J Pharm Pharmacol.* 46(4): 316–18.

Huguet F, Tarrade T. (1992). Alpha 2-adrenoceptor changes during cerebral ageing. The effect of Ginkgo biloba extract. *J Pharm Pharmacol.* 44(1): 24–27.

Hrdina P, Faludi G, Li Q, Bendotti C, Tekes K, Sotonyi P, Palkovits M. (1998). Growth-associated protein (GAP-43), its mRNA, and protein kinase C (PKC) isoenzymes in brain regions of depressed suicides. *Mol Psychiatry.* 3(5): 411–8.

Jahan MS, Farooque AI, Wahid Z. (1992). Neuroleptic malignant syndrome. *J Natl Med Assoc.* 84(11): 966–70.

Janssen PL, Meyboom S, van Staveren WA, de Vegt F, Katan MB. (1996). Consumption of ginger (Zingiber officinale roscoe) does not affect ex vivo platelet thromboxane production in humans. *Eur J Clin Nutr.* 50(11): 772–4.

Jenck F, Moreau JL, Berendsen HH, Boes M, Broekkamp CL, Martin JR, Wichmann J, Van Delft AM. (1998). Antiaversive effects of 5HT2C receptor agonists and fluoxetine in a model of panic-like anxiety in rats. *Eur Neuropsychopharmacol.* 8(3): 161–68.

Jenkins SW, Robinson DS, Fabre LF Jr, Andary JJ, Messina ME, Reich LA. (1990). Gepirone in the treatment of major depression. *J Clin Psychopharmacol.* Suppl 10(3): 77S–85S.

Johne A, Brockmoller J, Bauer S, Maurer A, Langheinrich M, Roots I. (1999). Pharmacokinetic interaction of digoxin with an herbal extract from St. John's wort (Hypericum perforatum). *Clin Pharmacol Ther.* 66(4): 338–45.

Johnson D, Ksciuk H, Woelk H, Sauerwein-Giese E, Frauendorf A. (1994). Effects of hypericum extract LI 160 compared with maprotiline on resting EEG and evoked potentials in 24 volunteers. *J Geriatr Psychiatry Neurol.* 7(suppl 1): S44–6.

Johnson KM, Jones SM. (1990). Neuropharmacology of phencyclidine: basic mechanisms and therapeutic potential. *Ann Rev Pharmacol Toxicol.* 30: 707–50.

Johnson RJ, Pyun HY, Lytton J, Fine RE. (1993). Differences in the subcellular localization of calreticulin and organellar $Ca(^{2+})$-ATPase in neurons. *Brain Res Mol Brain Res.* 17(1–2): 9–16.

Jones RS, Olpe HR. (1984). An increase in sensitivity of rat cingulate cortical neurones to substance P occurs following withdrawal of chronic administration of antidepressant drugs. *Br J Pharmacol.* 81(4): 659–64.

Kasper S. (1997). Treatment of seasonal affective disorder (SAD) with hypericum extract. *Pharmacopsychiatry.* 30(suppl 2): 89–93.

Kerb R, Brockmoller J, Staffeldt B, Ploch M, Roots I. (1996). Single-dose and steady-state pharmacokinetics of hypericin and pseudohypericin. *Antimicrob Agents Chemother.* 40(9): 2087–93.

Kim HL, Streltzer J, Goebert D. (1999). St. John's wort for depression: a meta-analysis of well-defined clinical trials. *J Nerv Ment Dis.* 187(9): 532–38.

Kiuchi F, Iwakami S, Shibuya M, Hanaoka F, Sankawa U. (1992). Inhibition of prostaglandin and leukotriene biosynthesis by gingerols and diarylheptanoids. *Chem Pharm Bull (Tokyo).* 40(2): 387–91.

Kobayashi M, Shoji N, Ohizumi Y. (1987). Gingerol, a novel cardiotonic agent, activates the Ca^{2+}-pumping ATPase in skeletal and cardiac sarcoplasmic reticulum. *Biochim Biophys Acta.* 903(1): 96–102.

Koivuranta M, Laara E, Ranta P, Ravaska P, Alahuhta S. (1997). Comparison of ondansetron and droperidol in the prevention of postoperative nausea and vomiting after laparoscopic surgery in women. A randomised, double-blind, placebo-controlled trial. *Acta Anaesthesiol Scand.* 41(10): 1273–9.

Kowalchik C, Hylton WH, eds. (1987). *Rodale's Illustrated Encyclopedia of Herbs*. Emmaus, PA: Rodale Press.

Kramer MS, Cutler N, Feighner J, Shrivastava R, Carman J, Sramek JJ, Reines SA, Liu G, Snavely D, Wyatt-Knowles E, et al. (1998). Distinct mechanism for antidepressant activity by blockade of central substance P receptors. *Science*. 281(5383): 1640–45.

Krummel S, Kathol RG. (1987). Buspirone: a new treatment for anxiety. *Iowa Med*. 77(6): 292–93, 295.

Laakmann G, Schule C, Baghai T, Kieser M. (1998). St. John's wort in mild to moderate depression: the relevance of hyperforin for the clinical efficacy. *Pharmacopsychiatry*. 31(suppl 1): 54–59.

Le Poul E, Laaris N, Hamon M, Lanfumey L. (1997). Fluoxetine-induced desensitization of somatodendritic 5-HT1A autoreceptors is independent of glucocorticoid(s). *Synapse*. 27(4): 303–12.

Leyel CF, ed. (1994). *A Modern Herbal*. NY: Dorset Press.

Lickey ME, Gordon B. (1991). *Medicine and Mental Illness*. New York: W. H. Freeman and Company.

Linde K, Ramirez G, Mulrow CD, Pauls A, Weidenhammer W, Melchart D. (1996). St. John's wort for depression—an overview and meta-analysis of randomised clinical trials. *BMJ*. 313(7052): 253–58.

Lingjaerde O, Foreland AR, Magnusson A. (1999). Can winter depression be prevented by Ginkgo biloba extract? A placebo-controlled trial. *Acta Psychiatr Scand*. 100(1): 62–66.

Lobstein-Guth A, Briancon-Scheid F, Victoire C, Haag-Berrurier M, Anton R. (1988). Isolation of amentoflavone from Ginkgo biloba. *Planta Med*. 54(6): 555–56.

Lumb AB. (1994). Effect of dried ginger on human platelet function. *Thromb Haemost*. 71(1): 110–1.

Maione S, Palazzo E, Pallotta M, Leyva J, Berrino L, Rossi F. (1997). Effects of imipramine on raphe nuclei and prefrontal cortex extracellular serotonin levels in the rat. *Psychopharmacology (Berlin)*. 134(4): 401–5.

Maisenbacher P, Kovar KA. (1992). Analysis and stability of Hyperici oleum. *Planta Med*. 58(4): 351–54.

Marcilhac A, Dakine N, Bourhim N, Guillaume V, Grino M, Drieu K, Oliver C. (1998). Effect of chronic administration of Ginkgo biloba extract or Ginkgolide on the hypothalamic-pituitary-adrenal axis in the rat. *Life Sci*. 62(25): 2329–40.

Martin P, Gozlan H, Puech AJ. (1992). 5-HT3 receptor antagonists reverse helpless behaviour in rats. *Eur J Pharmacol*. 212(1): 73–78.

Martin P, Lemonnier F. (1994). [The role of type 2 serotonin receptors, 5-HT2A and 5-HT2C, in depressive disorders: effect of medifoxamine]. *Encephale*. 20(4): 427–35.

Martin WR, Eades CG, Thompson JA, Huppler RE, Gilber PE. (1976). The effects of morphine-like drugs in the morphine-dependent chronic spinal dog. *J Pharmacol Exp Ther.* 197(3): 517–32.

Mascolo N, Jain R, Jain SC, Capasso F. (1989). Ethnopharmacologic investigation of ginger (Zingiber officinale). *J Ethnopharmacol.* 27(1–2): 129–40.

Mattson DT, Berk M, Lucas MD. (1997). A neuropsychological study of prefrontal lobe function in the positive and negative subtypes of schizophrenia. *J Genet Psychol.* 158(4): 487–94.

McGrath C, Norman TR. (1998). The effect of venlafaxine treatment on the behavioural and neurochemical changes in the olfactory bulbectomised rat. *Psychopharmacology (Berlin).* 136(4): 394–401.

Melzer R, Fricke U, Hölzl J. (1991). Vasoactive properties of procyanidins from Hypericum perforatum L. in isolated porcine coronary arteries. *Arzneimittelforschung.* 41(5): 481–3.

Menard J, Treit D. (1999). Effects of centrally administered anxiolytic compounds in animal models of anxiety. *Neurosci Biobehav Rev.* 23(4): 591–613.

Montgomery SA. (1983). Anxiety as part of depression. *Acta Psychiatr Scand.* Suppl 308: 171–74.

Morgan JP, Tulloss TC. (1976). The Jake Walk Blues. A toxicologic tragedy mirrored in American popular music. *Ann Intern Med.* 85(6): 804–8.

Morgan JP, Penovich P. (1978). Jamaica ginger paralysis. Forty-seven-year follow-up. *Arch Neurol.* 35(8): 530–2.

Muldner H, Zollner M. (1984). Antidepressive wirkung eines auf dem Wirkstoffkomplex Hypericin starndardisierten Hypericum-Extraktes. *Arneimittelforschung.* 34: 918–20.

Muller WE, Rossol R. (1994). Effects of hypericum extract on the expression of serotonin receptors. *J Geriatr Psychiatry Neurol.* 7(suppl 1): S63–64.

Muller WE, Rolli M, Schafer C, Hafner U. (1997). Effects of hypericum extract (LI 160) in biochemical models of antidepressant activity. *Pharmacopsychiatry.* 30(suppl 2): 102–7.

Muller WE, Singer A, Wonnemann M, Hafner U, Rolli M, Schafer C. (1998). Hyperforin represents the neurotransmitter reuptake inhibiting constituent of hypericum extract. *Pharmacopsychiatry.* 31(suppl 1): 16–21.

Murphy JE. (1978). Mianserin in the treatment of depressive illness and anxiety states in general practice. *Br J Clin Pharmacol.* 5(suppl 1): 81S–85S.

Mustafa T, Srivastava KC, Jensen KB. (1993). Pharmacology of ginger, Zingiber officinale. *J Drug Dev.* 6(1): 25–39.

Nagano T, Oyama Y, Kajita N, Chikahisa L, Nakata M, Okazaki E, Masuda T. (1997). New curcuminoids isolated from Zingiber cassumunar protect cells suffering from oxidative stress: a flow-cytometric study using rat thymocytes and H_2O_2. *Jpn J Pharmacol.* 75(4): 363–70.

Nahrstedt A, Butterweck V. (1997). Biologically active and other chemical constituents of the herb of Hypericum perforatum L. *Pharmacopsychiatry.* 30(suppl 2): 129–34.

Naora K, Ding G, Hayashibara M, Katagiri Y, Kano Y, Iwamoto K. (1992). Pharmacokinetics of [6]-gingerol after intravenous administration in rats with acute renal or hepatic failure. *Chem Pharm Bull (Tokyo).* 40(5): 1295–98.

Nebel A, Schneider BJ, Baker RK, Kroll DJ. (1999). Potential metabolic interaction between St. John's wort and theophylline. *Ann Pharmacother.* 33(4): 502.

Nielsen M, Frokjaer S, Braestrup C. (1988). High affinity of the naturally-occurring biflavonoid, amentoflavon, to brain benzodiazepine receptors in vitro. *Biochem Pharmacol.* 37(17): 3285–87.

Nutt D. (1997). Mirtazapine: pharmacology in relation to adverse effects. *Acta Psychiatr Scand.* Suppl 391: 31–37.

Oates J. (1996) Antihypertensive agents and the drug therapy of hypertension. In: *Goodman and Gilman's The Pharmacological Basis of Therapeutics.* Hardman JG, Limbird LE, Molinoff PB, Ruddon RW, Goodman Gilman A, eds. New York: McGraw-Hill.

O'Breasail AM, Argouarch S. (1998). Hypomania and St. John's Wort. *Can J Psychiatry.* 43(7): 746–47.

Okpanyi SN, Weischer ML. (1987). [Animal experiments on the psychotropic action of a Hypericum extract]. *Arzneimittelforschung.* 37(1): 10–13.

Onogi T, Minami M, Kuraishi Y, Satoh M. (1992). Capsaicin-like effect of (6)-shogaol on substance P-containing primary afferents of rats: a possible mechanism of its analgesic action. *Neuropharmacology.* 31(11): 1165–9.

Ostrowski E. (1988). *Untersuchung zur analytik, 14-Cmarkierung and pharmakokinetic phenolischer inhaltssoffe von Hypericum perforatum L.* Dissertation. Marburg, FRG. P. 18 ff.

Ozturk Y. (1997). Testing the antidepressant effects of Hypericum species on animal models. *Pharmacopsychiatry.* 30(suppl 2): 125–28.

Papadopoulos V, Widmaier EP, Amri H, Zilz A, Li H, Culty M, Castello R, Philip GH, Sridaran R, Drieu K. (1998). In vivo studies on the role of the peripheral benzodiazepine receptor (PBR) in steroidogenesis. *Endocr Res.* 24(3–4): 479–87.

Panfoli I, Musante L, Morelli A, Thellung S, Cupello A. (1997). $Ca(^{2+})$-ATPase pump forms and an endogenous inhibitor in bovine brain synaptosomes. *Neurochem Res.* 22(3): 297–304.

Parker RM, Barnes JM, Ge J, Barber PC, Barnes NM. (1996). Autoradiographic distribution of $[^3H]$-(S)-zacopride-labelled 5-HT3 receptors in human brain. *J Neurol Sci.* 144(1–2): 119–27.

Paul SM. (1988). Anxiety and depression: a common neurobiological substrate? *J Clin Psychiatry.* 49(suppl): 13–16.

Phillips S, Hutchinson S, Ruggier R. (1993). Zingiber officinale does not affect gastric emptying rate. A randomised, placebo-controlled, crossover trial. *Anaesthesia.* 48(5): 393–5.

Piazza LA, Markowitz JC, Kocsis JH, Leon AC, Portera L, Miller NL, Adler D. (1997). Sexual functioning in chronically depressed patients treated with SSRI antidepressants: a pilot study. *Am J Psychiatry.* 154(12): 1757–59.

Piccirillo G, Fimognari FL, Infantino V, Monteleone G, Fimognari GB, Falletti D, Marigliano V. (1994). High plasma concentrations of cortisol and thromboxane B2 in patients with depression. *Am J Med Sci.* 307(3): 228–32.

Pigott TA, Seay SM. (1999). A review of the efficacy of selective serotonin reuptake inhibitors in obsessive-compulsive disorder. *J Clin Psychiatry.* 60(2): 101–6.

Porsolt RD, Martin P, Lenegre A, Fromage S, Drieu K. (1990). Effects of an extract of Ginkgo biloba (EGB 761) on "learned helplessness" and other models of stress in rodents. *Pharmacol Biochem Behav.* 36(4): 963–71.

Preskorn S. (1997). Clinically relevant pharmacology of selective serotonin reuptake inhibitors. *Clinical Pharmacokinetics.* 32: 1–21.

Qian DS, Liu ZS. (1992). [Pharmacologic studies of antimotion sickness actions of ginger]. *Chung Kuo Chung Hsi I Chieh Ho Tsa Chih.* 12(2): 95–8, 70.

Quirion R, Shults CW, Moody TW, Pert CB, Chase TN, O'Donohue TL. (1983). Autoradiographic distribution of substance P receptors in rat central nervous system. *Nature.* 303(5919): 714–16.

Raffa RB. (1998). Screen of receptor and uptake-site activity of hypericin component of St. John's wort reveals sigma receptor binding. *Life Sci.* 62(16): PL265–70.

Ramassamy C, Christen Y, Clostre F, Costentin J. (1992). The Ginkgo biloba extract, EGb 761, increases synaptosomal uptake of 5-hydroxytryptamine: in-vitro and ex-vivo studies. *J Pharm Pharmacol.* 44(11): 943–45.

Rapin JR, Lamproglou I, Drieu K, DeFeudis FV. (1994). Demonstration of the "anti-stress" activity of an extract of Ginkgo biloba (EGb 761) using a discrimination learning task. *Gen Pharmacol.* 25(5): 1009–16.

Reddy DS, Kaur G, Kulkarni SK. (1998). Sigma (sigmal) receptor mediated anti-depressant-like effects of neurosteroids in the Porsolt forced swim test. *Neuroreport.* 9(13): 3069–73.

Rickels K, Amsterdam JD, Clary C, Puzzuoli G, Schweizer E. (1991). Buspirone in major depression: a controlled study. *J Clin Psychiatry.* 52(1): 34–38.

Rickels K, Downing R, Schweizer E, Hassman H. (1993). Antidepressants for the treatment of generalized anxiety disorder. A placebo-controlled comparison of imipramine, trazodone, and diazepam. *Arch Gen Psychiatry.* 50(11): 884–95.

Robbers JE, Speedie MK, Tyler VE. (1996). *Pharmacognosy and Pharmacobiotechnology.* Baltimore: Willams and Wilkins.

Rocha L, Marston A, Kaplan MA, Stoeckli-Evans H, Thull U, Testa B, Hostettmann K. (1994). An antifungal gamma-pyrone and xanthones with monoamine oxidase inhibitory activity from Hypericum brasiliense. *Phytochemistry.* 36(6): 1381–85.

Rodney J, Prior N, Cooper B, Theodoros M, Browning J, Steinberg B, Evans L. (1997). The comorbidity of anxiety and depression. *Aust N Z J Psychiatry.* 31(5): 700–3.

Rosen RC, Lane RM, Menza M. (1999). Effects of SSRIs on sexual function: a critical review. *J Clin Psychopharmacol.* 19(1): 67–85.

Ruschitzka F, Meier PJ, Turina M, Luscher TF, Noll G. (2000). Acute heart transplant rejection due to Saint John's wort. *Lancet.* 355(9203): 548–49.

Salmon P, Evans R, Humphrey DE. (1986). Anxiety and endocrine changes in surgical patients. *Br J Clin Psychol.* 25(pt 2): 135–41.

Satyan KS, Jaiswal AK, Ghosal S, Bhattacharya SK. (1998). Anxiolytic activity of ginkgolic acid conjugates from Indian Ginkgo biloba. *Psychopharmacology (Berlin).* 136(2): 148–52.

Schellenberg R, Sauer S, Dimpfel W. (1998). Pharmacodynamic effects of two different hypericum extracts in healthy volunteers measured by quantitative EEG. *Pharmacopsychiatry.* 31(suppl 1): 44–53.

Schmidt U, Sommer H. (1993). [St. John's wort extract in the ambulatory therapy of depression. Attention and reaction ability are preserved]. *Fortschr Med.* 111(19): 339–42.

Schulz H, Jobert M. (1994). Effects of hypericum extract on the sleep EEG in older volunteers. *J Geriatr Psychiatry Neurol.* 7(suppl 1): S39–43.

Schwartz RD, Yu X. (1992). Inhibition of GABA-gated chloride channel function by arachidonic acid. *Brain Res.* 585(1–2): 405–10.

Schwartz-Bloom RD, Cook TA, Yu X. (1996). Inhibition of GABA-gated chloride channels in brain by the arachidonic acid metabolite, thromboxane A2. *Neuropharmacology.* 35(9–10): 1347–53.

Schweizer E, Rickels K, Hassman H, Garcia-Espana F. (1998). Buspirone and imipramine for the treatment of major depression in the elderly. *J Clin Psychiatry.* 59(4): 175–83.

Seeman P. (1987). Dopamine receptors and the dopamine hypothesis of schizophrenia. *Synapse.* 1(2): 133–52.

Sharma SS, Gupta YK. (1998). Reversal of cisplatin-induced delay in gastric emptying in rats by ginger (Zingiber officinale). *J Ethnopharmacol.* 62(1): 49–55.

Sharma SS, Kochupillai V, Gupta SK, Seth SD, Gupta YK. (1997). Antiemetic efficacy of ginger (Zingiber officinale) against cisplatin-induced emesis in dogs. *J Ethnopharmacol.* 57(2): 93–6.

Sharpley AL, McGavin CL, Whale R, Cowen PJ. (1998). Antidepressant-like effect of Hypericum perforatum (St. John's wort) on the sleep polysomnogram. *Psychopharmacology (Berlin).* Oct. 139(3): 286–87.

Sheline YI, Wang PW, Gado MH, Csernansky JG, Vannier MW. (1996). Hippocampal atrophy in recurrent major depression. *Proc Natl Acad Sci USA*. 93(9): 3908–13.

Shirayama Y, Mitsushio H, Takashima M, Ichikawa H, Takahashi K. (1996). Reduction of substance P after chronic antidepressants treatment in the striatum, substantia nigra, and amygdala of the rat. *Brain Res*. 739(1–2): 70–78.

Simmen U, Schweitzer C, Burkard W, Schaffner W, Lundstrom K. (1998). Hypericum perforatum inhibited the binding of mu- and kappa-opioid receptor expressed with the Semliki Forest virus system. *Pharm Acta Helv*. 73: 53–56.

Solon EN. (1996). Risperidone-reserpine combination in refractory psychosis. *Schizophr Res*. 22(3): 265–66.

Sommer H, Harrer G. (1994). Placebo-controlled double-blind study examining the effectiveness of an hypericum preparation in 105 mildly depressed patients. *J Geriatr Psychiatry Neurol*. 7(suppl 1): S9–11.

Srivastava KC. (1984). Aqueous extracts of onion, garlic and ginger inhibit platelet aggregation and alter arachidonic acid metabolism. *Biomed Biochim Acta*. 43(8–9): S335–46.

Srivastava KC. (1989). Effect of onion and ginger consumption on platelet thromboxane production in humans. *Prostaglandins Leukot Essent Fatty Acids*. 35(3): 183–5.

Srivastava KC. (1986). Isolation and effects of some ginger components of platelet aggregation and eicosanoid biosynthesis. *Prostaglandins Leukot Med*. 25(2–3): 187–98.

Staffeldt B, Kerb R, Brockmoller J, Ploch M, Roots I. (1994). Pharmacokinetics of hypericin and pseudohypericin after oral intake of the hypericum perforatum extract LI 160 in healthy volunteers. *J Geriatr Psychiatry Neurol*. 7(suppl 1): S47–53.

Stahl SM. (1998). Basic psychopharmacology of antidepressants, part 1: antidepressants have seven distinct mechanisms of action. *J Clin Psychiatry*. 59(suppl 4): 5–14.

Stahl SM, Davis KL, Berger PA. (1982). The neuropharmacology of tardive dyskinesia, spontaneous dyskinesia, and other dystonias. *J Clin Psychopharmacol*. 2(5): 321–28.

Steiger A, von Bardeleben U, Herth T, Holsboer F. (1989). Sleep EEG and nocturnal secretion of cortisol and growth hormone in male patients with endogenous depression before treatment and after recovery. *J Affect Disord*. 16(2–3): 189–95.

Suekawa M, Ishige A, Yuasa K, Sudo K, Aburada M, Hosoya E. (1984). Pharmacological studies on ginger. I. Pharmacological actions of pungent constitutents, (6)-gingerol and (6)-shogaol. *J Pharmacobiodyn*. 7(11): 836–48.

Suekawa M, Aburada M, Hosoya E. (1986). Pharmacological studies on ginger. II. Pressor action of (6)-shogaol in anesthetized rats, or hindquarters, tail and mesenteric vascular beds of rats. *J Pharmacobiodyn*. 9(10): 842–52.

Surh YJ, Lee SS. (1992). Enzymatic reduction of shogaol: a novel biotransformation pathway for the alpha, beta-unsaturated ketone system. *Biochem Int.* 27(1): 179–87.

Sussman N. (1998). Anxiolytic antidepressant augmentation. *J Clin Psychiatry.* 59(suppl 5): 42–48.

Tadokoro C, Kiuchi Y, Yamazaki Y, Oguchi K, Kamijima K. (1998). Effects of imipramine and sertraline on protein kinase activity in rat frontal cortex. *Eur J Pharmacol.* 342(1): 51–4.

Takahashi I, Nakanishi S, Kobayashi E, Nakano H, Suzuki K, Tamaoki T. (1989). Hypericin and pseudohypericin specifically inhibit protein kinase C: possible relation to their antiretroviral activity. *Biochem Biophys Res Commun.* 165(3): 1207–12.

Tejedor-Real P, Mico JA, Maldonado R, Roques BP, Gibert-Rahola J. (1995). Implication of endogenous opioid system in the learned helplessness model of depression. *Pharmacol Biochem Behav.* 52(1): 145–52.

Thiede HM, Walper A. (1994). Inhibition of MAO and COMT by hypericum extracts and hypericin. *J Geriatr Psychiatry Neurol.* 7(suppl 1): S54–56.

Thiele B, Brink I, Ploch M. (1994). Modulation of cytokine expression by hypericum extract. *J Geriatr Psychiatry Neurol.* 7(suppl 1): S60–62.

Tronche F, Kellendonk C, Kretz O, Gass P, Anlag K, Orban PC, Bock R, Klein R, Schutz G. (1999). Disruption of the glucocorticoid receptor gene in the nervous system results in reduced anxiety. *Nat Genet.* 23(1): 99–103.

Tyler V. (1994). *Herbs of Choice.* New York: Pharmaceutical Products Press.

Visalyaputra S, Petchpaisit N, Somcharoen K, Choavaratana R. (1998). The efficacy of ginger root in the prevention of postoperative nausea and vomiting after outpatient gynaecological laparoscopy. *Anaesthesia.* 53(5): 506–10.

Volz HP. (1997). Controlled clinical trials of hypericum extracts in depressed patients—an overview. *Pharmacopsychiatry.* 30(suppl 2): 72–6.

Vorbach EU, Arnoldt KH, Hubner WD. (1997). Efficacy and tolerability of St. John's wort extract LI 160 versus imipramine in patients with severe depressive episodes according to ICD-10. *Pharmacopsychiatry.* 30(suppl 2): 81–85.

Vorbach EU, Hubner WD, Arnoldt KH. (1994). Effectiveness and tolerance of the hypericum extract LI 160 in comparison with imipramine: randomized double-blind study with 135 outpatients. *J Geriatr Psychiatry Neurol.* 7(suppl 1): S19–23.

Wagner H, Bladt S. (1994). Pharmaceutical quality of hypericum extracts. *J Geriatr Psychiatry Neurol.* 7(suppl 1): S65–68.

Walker DJ, Zacny JP. (1998). Subjective, psychomotor, and analgesic effects of oral codeine and morphine in healthy volunteers. *Psychopharmacology (Berlin).* 140(2): 191–201.

Weinberger DR. (1996). On the plausibility of "the neurodevelopmental hypothesis" of schizophrenia. *Neuropsychopharmacology.* 14(3 suppl): 1S–11S.

White HL, Scates PW, Cooper BR. (1996). Extracts of Ginkgo biloba leaves inhibit monoamine oxidase. *Life Sci.* 58(16): 1315–21.

Wieland S, Lucki I. (1990). Antidepressant-like activity of 5-HT1A agonists measured with the forced swim test. *Psychopharmacology (Berlin).* 101: 4497–504.

Winter JC, Timineri D. (1996). The discriminative stimulus properties of EGb 761, an extract of Ginkgo biloba. *Pharmacol Biochem Behav.* 62(3): 543–47.

Wolkowitz OM. (1993). Rational polypharmacy in schizophrenia. *Ann Clin Psychiatry.* 5(2): 79–90.

Woolf AD. (1995). Ginger Jake and the blues: a tragic song of poisoning. *Vet Hum Toxicol.* 37(3): 252–4.

Wu H, Ye D, Bai Y, Zhao Y. (1990). [Effect of dry ginger and roasted ginger on experimental gastric ulcers in rats]. *Chung Kuo Chung Yao Tsa Chih.* 15(5): 278–80, 317–8.

Wu H, Ye DJ, Zhao YZ, Wang SL. (1993). [Effect of different preparations of ginger on blood coagulation time in mice]. *Chung Kuo Chung Yao Tsa Chih.* 18(3): 147–9, 190.

Ye DJ, Ding AW, Guo R. (1989). [A research on the constituents of ginger in various preparations]. *Chung Kuo Chung Yao Tsa Chih.* 14(5): 278–80.

Yocca FD. (1990). Neurochemistry and neurophysiology of buspirone and gepirone: interactions at presynaptic and postsynaptic 5-HT1A receptors. *J Clin Psychopharmacol.* Suppl 10(3): 6S–12S.

Young EA, Haskett RF, Murphy-Weinberg V, Watson SJ, Akil H. (1991). Loss of glucocorticoid fast feedback in depression. *Arch Gen Psychiatry.* 48(8): 693–99.

Yue QY, Bergquist C, Gerden B. (2000). Safety of St. John's wort. *Lancet.* 355(9203): 576–77.

Zhang W, Law RE, Hinton DR, Couldwell WT. (1997). Inhibition of human malignant glioma cell motility and invasion in vitro by hypericin, a potent protein kinase C inhibitor. *Cancer Lett.* 120(1): 31–8.

Chapter 8

Adams IB, Compton DR, Martin BR. (1998). Assessment of anandamide interaction with the cannabinoid brain receptor: SR 141716A antagonism studies in mice and autoradiographic analysis of receptor binding in rat brain. *J Pharmacol Exp Ther.* 284(3): 1209–17.

Ahlijanian MK, Takemori AE. (1986). The effect of chronic administration of caffeine on morphine-induced analgesia, tolerance and dependence in mice. *Eur J Pharmacol.* 120(1): 25–32.

Albuquerque ML, Kurth CD. (1993). Cocaine constricts immature cerebral arterioles by a local anesthetic mechanism. *Eur J Pharmacol.* 249(2): 215–20.

Alhaider AA. (1991). Antinociceptive effect of ketanserin in mice: involvement of supraspinal 5-HT2 receptors in nociceptive transmission. *Brain Res.* 543(2): 335–40.

Bandler R, Shipley MT. (1994). Columnar organization in the midbrain periaqueductal gray: modules for emotional expression? *Trends Neurosci.* 17: 379–89.

Bannon AW, Decker MW, Holladay MW, Curzon P, Donnelly-Roberts D, Puttfarcken PS, Bitner RS, Diaz A, Dickenson AH, Porsolt RD, Williams M, Arneric SP. (1998). Broad-spectrum, non-opioid analgesic activity by selective modulation of neuronal nicotinic acetylcholine receptors. *Science.* 279: 77–81.

Barsby RW, Salan U, Knight DW, Hoult JR. (1993). Feverfew and vascular smooth muscle: extracts from fresh and dried plants show opposing pharmacological profiles, dependent upon sesquiterpene lactone content. *Planta Med.* 59(1): 20–25.

Basbaum AI, Fields HL. (1978). Endogenous pain control mechanisms: review and hypothesis. *Ann Neurol.* 4: 451–62.

Basbaum AI, Fields HL. (1984). Endogenous pain control systems: brainstem spinal pathways and endorphin circuitry. *Ann Rev Neurosci.* 7: 309–38.

Beitz AJ. (1982). The sites of origin of brainstem neurotensin and serotonin projections to the rodent nucleus raphe magnus. *J Neurosci.* 2: 829–42.

Belay ED, Bresee JS, Holman RC, Khan AS, Shahriari A, Schonberger LB. (1999). Reye's syndrome in the United States from 1981 through 1997. *N Engl J Med.* 340(18): 1377–82.

Bilsky EJ, Inturrisi CE, Sad e W, Hruby VJ, Porreca F. (1996). Competitive and non-competitive NMDA antagonists block the development of antinociceptive tolerance to morphine, but not to selective mu or delta opioid agonists in mice. *Pain.* 68(2–3): 229–37.

Bloom AS, Dewey WL. (1978). A comparison of some pharmacological actions of morphine and delta9-tetrahydrocannabinol in the mouse. *Psychopharmacology (Berlin).* 57(3): 243–48.

Bloom FE, Rossier J, Battenberg EL, Bayon A, French E, Henriksen SJ, Siggins GR, Segal D, Browne R, Ling N, Guillemin R. (1978). Beta-endorphin: cellular localization, electrophysiological and behavioral effects. *Adv Biochem Psychopharmacol.* 18: 89–109.

Bodnar RJ. (1996). Opioid receptor subtype antagonists and ingestion. In *Drug Receptor Subtypes and Ingestive Behavior*, Cooper SG, Clifton PG, eds. London: Academic Press, pp. 127–46.

Bodnar RJ, Paul D, Pasternak GW. (1991). Synergistic analgesic interactions between the periaqueductal gray and the locus coeruleus: studies with the partial mu-1 agonist ethylketocyclazocine. *Brain Res.* 558: 224–30.

Bodnar RJ, Williams CL, Lee SJ, Pasternak GW. (1988). Role of mu1 opiate receptors in supraspinal opiate analgesia: a microinjection study. *Brain Res.* 447: 25–34.

Braida D, Gori E, Sala M. (1994). Relationship between morphine and etonitazene-induced working memory impairment and analgesia. *Eur J Pharmacol.* 271(2–3): 497–504.

Brodin P, Røed A. (1984). Effects of eugenol on rat phrenic nerve and phrenic nerve-diaphragm preparations. *Arch Oral Biol.* 29(8): 611–15.

Burstein SH, Hull K, Hunter SA, Latham V. (1988). Cannabinoids and pain responses: a possible role for prostaglandins. *FASEB J.* 2(14): 3022–26.

Butterworth JF 4th, Moran JR, Whitesides GM, Strichartz GR. (1987). Limited nerve impulse blockade by "leashed" local anesthetics. *J Med Chem.* 30(8): 1295–302.

Calignano A, La Rana G, Giuffrida A, Piomelli D. (1998). Control of pain initiation by endogenous cannabinoids. *Nature.* 394(6690): 277–81.

Capasso F. (1986). The effect of an aqueous extract of Tanacetum parthenium L. on arachidonic acid metabolism by rat peritoneal leucocytes. *J Pharm Pharmacol.* 38(1): 71–72.

Cassella G, Wu AH, Shaw BR, Hill DW. (1997). The analysis of thebaine in urine for the detection of poppy seed consumption. *J Analytical Toxicol.* 21(5): 376–83.

Castellano C, Cestari V, Cabib S, Puglisi-Allegra S. (1994). The effects of morphine on memory consolidation in mice involve both D1 and D2 dopamine receptors. *Behav Neural Biol.* 61(2): 156–61.

Catterall WA, Mackie K. (1996). Local Anesthetics. In: *Goodman and Gilman's The Pharmacological Basis of Therapeutics.* Hardman JG, Limbird LE, Molinoff PB, Ruddon RW, Goodman Gilman A, eds. New York: McGraw-Hill.

Clark FM, Proudfit HK. (1991). Projections of neurons in the ventromedial medulla to pontine catecholamine cell groups involved in the modulation of nociception. *Brain Res.* 540: 105–115.

Clark GC. (1989). Comparison of the inhalation toxicity of kretek (clove cigarette) smoke with that of American cigarette smoke: I. One day exposure. *Arch Toxicol.* 63(1): 1–6.

Clements JR, Beitz AJ, Fletcher TF, Mullett MA. (1985). Immunocytochemical localization of serotonin in the rat periaqueductal gray: a quantitative light and electron microscopic study. *J Comp Neurol.* 236: 60–70.

Clements JR, Madl JE, Johnson RL, Larson AA, Beitz AJ. (1987). Localization of glutamate, glutaminase, aspartate, and aspartate aminotransferase in the rat midbrain periaqueductal gray. *Exp Brain Res.* 67: 594–602.

Cook SA, Welch SP, Lichtman AH, Martin BR. (1995). Evaluation of cAMP involvement in cannabinoid-induced antinociception. *Life Sci.* 56(23–24): 2049–56.

Cortés R, Palacios JM. (1986). Muscarinic cholinergic receptor subtypes in the rat brain. I. Quantitative autoradiographic studies. *Brain Res.* 362: 227–38.

Council on Scientific Affairs. (1988). Evaluation of the health hazard of clove cigarettes. *JAMA.* 260(24): 3641–44.

Couturier EG, Hering R, Steiner TJ. (1992). Weekend attacks in migraine patients: caused by caffeine withdrawal? *Cephalalgia.* 12(2): 99–100.

Damaj MI, Patrick GS, Creasy KR, Martin BR. (1997). Pharmacology of lobeline, a nicotinic receptor ligand. *J Pharmacol Exp Ther.* 282(1): 410–19.

Damaj MI, Slemmer JE, Carroll FI, Martin BR. (1999). Pharmacological characterization of nicotine's interaction with cocaine and cocaine analogs. *J Pharmacol Exp Ther.* 289(3): 1229–36.

Della Bella D, Carenzi A, Frigeni V, Reggiani A, Zambon A. (1985). Involvement of monoaminergic and peptidergic components in cathinone-induced analgesia. *Eur J Pharmacol.* 114(2): 231–34.

Desjardins GC, Brawer JR, Beaudet A. (1990). Distribution of mu, delta, and kappa opioid receptors in the hypothalamus of the rat. *Brain Res.* 536(1–2): 114–23.

Devine DP, Leone P, Wise RA. (1993). Mesolimbic dopamine neurotransmission is increased by administration of mu-opioid receptor antagonists. *Eur J Pharmacol.* 243(1): 55–64.

Di Chiara G, North RA. (1992). Neurobiology of opiate abuse. *Trends Pharmacol Sci.* 13(5): 185–93.

Diez-Guerra FJ, Augood S, Emson PC, Dyer RG. (1987). Opioid peptides inhibit the release of noradrenaline from slices of rat medial preoptic area. *Exp Brain Res.* 66(2): 378–84.

Dolara P, Luceri C, Ghelardini C, Monserrat C, Aiolli S, Luceri F, Lodovici M, Menichetti S, Romanelli MN. (1996). Analgesic effects of myrrh. *Nature.* 379(6560): 29.

Elliott K, Kest B, Man A, Kao B, Inturrisi CE. (1995). N-methyl-D-aspartate (NMDA) receptors, mu and kappa opioid tolerance, and perspectives on new analgesic drug development. *Neuropsychopharmacology.* 13(4): 347–56.

Evans CJ, Keith DE, Morrison H, Magendzo K, Edwards RH. (1992). Cloning of a delta opioid receptor by functional expression. *Science.* 258: 1952–55.

Farrell M. (1994). Opiate withdrawal. *Addiction.* 89(11): 1471–75.

Fennelly M, Galletly DC, Purdie GI. (1991). Is caffeine withdrawal the mechanism of postoperative headache? *Anesth Analg.* 72(4): 449–53.

Ferreira SH, Moncada S, Vane JR. (1997). Prostaglandins and the mechanism of analgesia produced by aspirin-like drugs. 1973. *Br J Pharmacol.* Feb. 120(4 suppl): 401–12.

Ferri S, Cavicchini E, Romualdi P, Speroni E, Murari G. (1986). Possible mediation of catecholaminergic pathways in the antinociceptive effect of an extract of Cannabis sativa L. *Psychopharmacology (Berlin).* 89(2): 244–47.

Feuerstein TJ, Albrecht C, Wessler I, Zentner J, Jackisch R. (1998). delta 1-Opioid receptor-mediated control of acetylcholine (ACh) release in human neocortex slices. *Int J Dev Neurosci.* 16(7–8): 795–802.

Feuerstein TJ, Gleichauf O, Peckys D, Landwehrmeyer GB, Scheremet R, Jackisch R. (1996). Opioid receptor-mediated control of acetylcholine release in human neocortex tissue. *Naunyn Schmiedebergs Arch Pharmacol.* 354(5): 586–92.

Fields HL, Heinricher MM, Mason P. (1991). Neurotransmitters in nociceptive modulatory circuits. *Ann Rev Neurosci.* 14: 219–45.

File SE, Rodgers RJ. (1979). Partial anxiolytic action of morphine sulphate following microinjection into the central nucleus of the amygdala in rats. *Pharmacol Biochem Behav.* 11(3): 313–18.

Fischer G, Etzersdorfer P, Eder H, Jagsch R, Langer M, Weninger M. (1998). Buprenorphine maintenance in pregnant opiate addicts. *Eur Addict Res.* 4(suppl 1): 32–36.

Forbes JA, Beaver WT, Jones KF, Kehm CJ, Smith WK, Gongloff CM, Zeleznock JR, Smith JW. (1991). Effect of caffeine on ibuprofen analgesia in postoperative oral surgery pain. *Clin Pharmacol Ther.* 49(6): 674–84.

Franck L, Vilardi J. (1995). Assessment and management of opioid withdrawal in ill neonates. *Neonatal Network.* 14(2): 39–48.

Fride E, Mechoulam R. (1993). Pharmacological activity of the cannabinoid receptor agonist, anandamide, a brain constituent. *Eur J Pharmacol.* 231(2): 313–4.

Gerra G, Calbiani B, Zaimovic A, Sartori R, Ugolotti G, Ippolito L, Delsignore R, Rustichelli P, Fontanesi B. (1998). Regional cerebral blood flow and comorbid diagnosis in abstinent opioid addicts. *Psychiatry Res.* 83(2): 117–26.

Ghelardini C, Galeotti N, Bartolini A. (1997). Caffeine induces central cholinergic analgesia. *Naunyn Schmiedebergs Arch Pharmacol.* 356(5): 590–95.

Gilbert PE. (1981). A comparison of THC, nantradol, nabilone, and morphine in the chronic spinal dog. *J Clin Pharmacol.* 21(8–9 suppl): 311S–19S.

Gower AJ. (1987). Effects of acetylcholine agonists and antagonists on yawning and analgesia in the rat. *Eur J Pharmacol.* 139(1): 79–89.

Groenewegen WA, Heptinstall S. (1990). A comparison of the effects of an extract of feverfew and parthenolide, a component of feverfew, on human platelet activity in-vitro. *J Pharm Pharmacol.* 42(8): 553–57.

Gromek D, Kisiel W, Stojakowska A, Kohlmunzer S. (1991). Attempts of chemical standardizing of Chrysanthemum parthenium as a prospective antimigraine drug. *Pol J Pharmacol Pharm.* 43(3): 213–17.

Grossman A. (1983). Brain opiates and neuroendocrine function. *Clin Endocrinol Metab.* 12(3): 725–46.

Gruenwald J, Brendler T, Jaenicke C. (1998). *PDR for Herbal Medicines*, 1st ed. Montvale, NJ: Medical Economics Company.

Guidotti TL, Laing L, Prakash UB. (1989). Clove cigarettes. The basis for concern regarding health effects. *West J Med.* 151(2): 220–28.

Guo A, Vulchanova L, Wang J, Li X, Elde R. (1999). Immunocytochemical localization of the vanilloid receptor 1 (VR1): relationship to neuropeptides, the P2X3 purinoceptor and IB4 binding sites. *Eur J Neurosci.* 11(3): 946–58.

Hagan RM, Hughes IE. (1984). Opioid receptor sub-types involved in the control of transmitter release in cortex of the brain of the rat. *Neuropharmacology.* 23(5): 491–95.

Hamann SR, Martin WR. (1994). Hyperalgesic and analgesic actions of morphine, U50-488, naltrexone, and (–)-lobeline in the rat brainstem. *Pharmacol Biochem Behav.* 47(1): 197–201.

Hamann W, di Vadi PP. (1999). Analgesic effect of the cannabinoid analogue nabilone is not mediated by opioid receptors. *Lancet.* 353(9152): 560.

Hampson AJ, Bornheim LM, Scanziani M, Yost CS, Gray AT, Hansen BM, Leonoudakis DJ, Bickler PE. (1998). Dual effects of anandamide on NMDA receptor-mediated responses and neurotransmission. *J Neurochem.* 70(2): 671–6.

Hanks GW, O'Neill WM, Simpson P, Wesnes K. (1995). The cognitive and psychomotor effects of opioid analgesics: II. A randomized controlled trial of single doses of morphine, lorazepam, and placebo in healthy subjects. *Eur J Clin Pharmacol.* 48(6): 455–60.

Hine B. (1985). Morphine and delta 9-tetrahydrocannabinol: two-way cross tolerance for antinociceptive and heart-rate responses in the rat. *Psychopharmacology (Berlin).* 87(1): 34–38.

Hokfelt T, Elde R, Johansson O, Terenuis L, Stein L. (1977). The distribution of enkephalin-immunoreactive cell bodies in the rat central nervous system. *Neurosci Lett.* 5: 25.

Houtsmuller EJ, Walsh SL, Schuh KJ, Johnson RE, Stitzer ML, Bigelow GE. (1998). Dose-response analysis of opioid cross-tolerance and withdrawal suppression during LAAM maintenance. *J Pharmacol Exp Ther.* 285(2): 387–96.

Hulse GK, Milne E, English DR, Holman CD. (1997). The relationship between maternal use of heroin and methadone and infant birth weight. *Addiction.* 92(11): 1571–79.

Hulse GK, Milne E, English DR, Holman CD. (1998). Assessing the relationship between maternal opiate use and neonatal mortality. *Addiction.* 93(7): 1033–42.

Huong NT, Matsumoto K, Yamasaki K, Duc NM, Nham NT, Watanabe H. (1997). Majonoside-R2, a major constituent of Vietnamese ginseng, attenuates opioid-induced antinociception. *Pharmacol Biochem Behav.* 57(1–2): 285–91.

Hwang D, Fischer NH, Jang BC, Tak H, Kim JK, Lee W. (1996). Inhibition of the expression of inducible cyclooxygenase and proinflammatory cytokines by sesquiterpene lactones in macrophages correlates with the inhibition of MAP kinases. *Biochem Biophys Res Commun.* 226(3): 810–18.

Insel PA. (1996). Analgesic-antipyretic and anti-inflammatory agents and drugs employed in the treatment of gout. In: *Goodman and Gilman's The Pharmacol-*

ogical Basis of Therapeutics. Hardman JG, Limbird LE, Molinoff PB, Ruddon RW, Goodman Gilman A, eds. New York: McGraw-Hill.

Iwamoto FT. (1989). Antinociception after nicotine administration into the mesopontine tegmentum of rats: Evidence for muscarinic actions. *J Pharmacol Exp Ther*. 251: 412–21.

Iwamoto FT. (1991). Characterization of the antinociception induced by nicotine in the pedunculopontine tegmental nucleus and the nucleus raphe magnus. *J Pharmacol Exp Ther*. 257: 120–33.

Iwamoto FJ, Marion L. (1993). Characterization of the antinociception produced by intrathecally administered muscarinic agonists in rats. *J Pharmacol Exp Ther*. 266: 329–38.

Jain NK, Kulkarni SK. (1999). Antinociceptive and anti-inflammatory effects of Tanacetum parthenium L. extract in mice and rats. *J Ethnopharmacol*. 68(1–3): 251–59.

Johnson ES, Kadam NP, Hylands DM, Hylands PJ. (1985). Efficacy of feverfew as prophylactic treatment of migraine. *Br Med J (Clin Res Ed)*. 291(6495): 569–73.

Johnson SW, North RA. (1992). Opioids excite dopamine neurons by hyperpolarization of local interneurons. *J Neurosci*. 12(2): 483–88.

Kalivas PW, Duffy P. (1987). Sensitization to repeated morphine injection in the rat: possible involvement of A10 dopamine neurons. *J Pharmacol Exp Ther*. 241(1): 204–12.

Kandel ER, Schwartz JH, Jessell TM, eds. (1991). *Principles of Neural Science*, 3rd ed. Norwalk, CT: Appleton and Lange.

Kauppila T, Mecke E, Pertovaara A. (1992). Enhancement of morphine-induced analgesia and attenuation of morphine-induced side-effects by cocaine in rats. *Pharmacol Toxicol*. 71(3): 173–78.

Kellstein DE, Malseed RT, Goldstein FJ. (1988). Opioid-monoamine interactions in spinal antinociception: evidence for serotonin but not norepinephrine reciprocity. *Pain*. 34(1): 85–92.

Kerr B, Hill H, Coda B, Calogero M, Chapman CR, Hunt E, Buffington V, Mackie A. (1991). Concentration-related effects of morphine on cognition and motor control in human subjects. *Neuropsychopharmacology*. 5(3): 157–66.

Ketter TA, Andreason PJ, George MS, Lee C, Gill DS, Parekh PI, Willis MW, Herscovitch P, Post RM. (1996). Anterior paralimbic mediation of procaine-induced emotional and psychosensory experiences. *Arch Gen Psychiatry*. 53(1): 59–69.

Khachaturian H, Lewis ME, Alessi NE, Watson SJ. (1985). Time of origin of opioid peptide-containing neurons in the rat hypothalamus. *J Comp Neurol*. 236: 538–46.

Khachaturian H, Lewis ME, Hollt V, Watson SJ. (1983). Telencephalic enkephalinergic systems in the rat brain. *J Neurosci*. 3: 844–55.

Kiefel JM, Cooper ML, Bodnar RJ. (1992a). Inhibition of mesencephalic morphine analgesia by methysergide in the medial ventral medulla of rats. *Physiol Behav.* 51: 201–5.

Kiefel JM, Cooper ML, Bodnar RJ. (1992b). Serotonin receptor subtype antagonists in the medial ventral medulla inhibit mesencephalic opiate analgesia. *Brain Res.* 597: 331–38.

Kiefel JM, Paul D, Bodnar RJ. (1989). Reduction in opioid and non-opioid forms of swim analgesia by 5-HT2 receptor antagonists. *Brain Res.* 500(1–2): 231–40.

Kiefel JM, Rossi GC, Bodnar RJ. (1993). Medullary mu and delta opioid receptors modulate mesencephalic morphine analgesia in rats. *Brain Res.* 624: 151–61.

Kieffer BL, Befort K, Gaveriaux-Ruff C, Hirth CG. (1992). The delta-opioid receptor: isolation of a cDNA by expression cloning and pharmacological characterization. *Proc Nat Acad Sci USA.* 89(24): 12048–52.

Kim HS, Oh KW, Rheu HM, Kim SH. (1992). Antagonism of U-50,488H-induced antinociception by ginseng total saponins is dependent on serotonergic mechanisms. *Pharmacol Biochem Behav.* 42(4): 587–93.

Kiritsy-Roy JA, Shyu BC, Danneman PJ, Morrow TJ, Belczynski C, Casey KL. (1994). Spinal antinociception mediated by a cocaine-sensitive dopaminergic supraspinal mechanism. *Brain Res.* 644(1): 109–16.

Kizelshteyn G, Bairamian M, Inchiosa MA Jr, Chase JE. (1992). Enhancement of bupivacaine sensory blockade of rat sciatic nerve by combination with phenol. *Anesth Analg.* 74(4): 499–502.

Kraetsch HG, Hummel T, Lotsch J, Kussat R, Kobal G. (1996). Analgesic effects of propyphenazone in comparison to its combination with caffeine. *Eur J Clin Pharmacol.* 49(5): 377–82.

Kumor KM, Haertzen CA, Johnson RE, Kocher T, Jasinski D. (1986). Human psychopharmacology of ketocyclazocine as compared with cyclazocine, morphine, and placebo. *J Pharmacol Exp Ther.* 238(3): 960–68.

Lane BW, Ellenhorn MJ, Hulbert TV, McCarron M. (1991). Clove oil ingestion in an infant. *Hum Exp Toxicol.* 10(4): 291–94.

Lapchak PA, Araujo DM, Collier B. (1989). Regulation of endogenous acetylcholine release from mammalian brain slices by opiate receptors: hippocampus, striatum, and cerebral cortex of guinea-pig and rat. *Neuroscience.* 31(2): 313–25.

Laska EM, Sunshine A, Zighelboim I, Roure C, Marrero I, Wanderling J, Olson N. (1983). Effect of caffeine on acetaminophen analgesia. *Clin Pharmacol Ther.* 33(4): 498–509.

Lichtman AH, Martin BR. (1991). Cannabinoid-induced antinociception is mediated by a spinal alpha 2-noradrenergic mechanism. *Brain Res.* 559(2): 309–14.

Lichtman AH, Martin BR. (1997). The selective cannabinoid antagonist SR 141716A blocks cannabinoid-induced antinociception in rats. *Pharmacol Biochem Behav.* 57(1–2): 7–12.

Lin Y, Morrow TJ, Kiritsy-Roy JA, Terry LC, Casey KL. (1989). Cocaine: evidence for supraspinal, dopamine-mediated, non-opiate analgesia. *Brain Res.* 479(2): 306–12.

Lindvall O, Björklund A. (1974). The organization of the ascending catecholamine neuron systems in the rat brain as revealed by the glyoxylic acid fluorescence method. *Acta Phys Scand Suppl.* 412: 1–48.

Llewelyn MB, Azami B, Grant CM, Roberts MHJ. (1981). Analgesia following microinjection of nicotine into the periaqueductal gray matter (PAG). *Neurosci Lett.* 7: S277.

London ED, Waller SB, Wamsley JK. (1985). Autoradiographic localization of [^{3}H] nicotine binding sites in the rat brain. *Neurosci Lett.* 53: 179–84.

Malec D, Michalska E. (1988). The effect of methylxanthines on morphine analgesia in mice and rats. *Pol J Pharmacol Pharm.* 40(3): 223–32.

Mantegazza P, Tammiso R, Zambotti F, Zecca L, Zonta N. (1984). Purine involvement in morphine antinociception. *Br J Pharmacol.* 83(4): 883–88.

Markowitz K, Moynihan M, Liu M, Kim S. (1992). Biologic properties of eugenol and zinc oxide-eugenol. A clinically oriented review. *Oral Surg Oral Med Oral Pathol.* 73(6): 729–37.

Marles RJ, Kaminski J, Arnason JT, Pazos-Sanou L, Heptinstall S, Fischer NH, Crompton CW, Kindack DG, Awang DV. (1992). A bioassay for inhibition of serotonin release from bovine platelets. *J Nat Prod.* 55(8): 1044–56.

Martin G, Nie Z, Siggins GR. (1997). mu-Opioid receptors modulate NMDA receptor-mediated responses in nucleus accumbens neurons. *J Neurosci.* 17(1): 11–22.

Martin WJ, Tsou K, Walker JM. (1998). Cannabinoid receptor-mediated inhibition of the rat tail-flick reflex after microinjection into the rostral ventromedial medulla. *Neurosci Lett.* 242(1): 33–36.

Mascolo N, Jain R, Jain SC, Capasso F. (1989). Ethnopharmacologic investigation of ginger (Zingiber officinale). *J Ethnopharmacol.* Nov. 27(1–2): 129–40.

Mather LE. (1987). Opioid pharmacokinetics in relation to their effects. *Anaesth Intensive Care.* 15(1): 15–22.

Matthews JC, Collins A. (1983). Interactions of cocaine and cocaine congeners with sodium channels. *Biochem Pharmacol.* 32(3): 455–60.

Mayer DJ, Price DD. (1976). Central nervous system mechanisms of analgesia. *Pain.* 2(4): 379–404.

Meadway C, George S, Braithwaite R. (1998). Opiate concentrations following the ingestion of poppy seed products—evidence for “the poppy seed defence”. *Forensic Sci Int.* 96(1): 29–38.

Meng ID, Manning BH, Martin WJ, Fields HL. (1998). An analgesia circuit activated by cannabinoids. *Nature.* 395(6700): 381–3.

Mignat C, Wille U, Ziegler A. (1995). Affinity profiles of morphine, codeine, dihydrocodeine, and their glucuronides at opioid receptor subtypes. *Life Sci.* 56(10): 793–99.

Milhorn HT Jr. (1992). Pharmacologic management of acute abstinence syndromes. *Am Fam Physician.* 45(1): 231–39.

Misra AL, Pontani RB, Vadlamani NL. (1985). Potentiation of morphine analgesia by caffeine. *Br J Pharmacol.* 84(4): 789–91.

Misra AL, Pontani RB, Vadlamani NL. (1987). Stereospecific potentiation of opiate analgesia by cocaine: predominant role of noradrenaline. *Pain.* 28(1): 129–38.

Mogil JS, Shin YH, McCleskey EW, Kim SC, Nah SY. (1998). Ginsenoside Rf, a trace component of ginseng root, produces antinociception in mice. *Brain Res.* May 11;792(2): 218–28.

Moore RY, Bloom FE. (1979). Central catecholamine neuron systems: anatomy and physiology of the norepinephrine and epinephrine systems. *Ann Rev Neurosci.* 113–68.

Moss DE, Johnson RL. (1980). Tonic analgesic effects of delta 9-tetrahydrocannabinol as measured with the formalin test. *Eur J Pharmacol.* Feb. 8;61(3): 313–15.

Mulé SJ, Casella GA. (1988). Rendering the "poppy-seed defense" defenseless: identification of 6-monoacetylmorphine in urine by gas chromatography/mass spectroscopy. *Clin Chem.* July 34: 7 1427–30.

Murillo-Rodriguez E, Sanchez-Alavez M, Navarro L, Martinez-Gonzalez D, Drucker-Colin R, Prospero-Garcia O. (1998). Anandamide modulates sleep and memory in rats. *Brain Res.* 812(1–2): 270–4.

Murphy JJ, Heptinstall S, Mitchell JR. (1998). Randomised double-blind placebo-controlled trial of feverfew in migraine prevention. *Lancet.* 2(8604): 189–92.

Musto D. (1991). Opium, cocaine, and marijuana in American history. *Sci Am.* 7: 40–47.

Nah SY, Park HJ, McCleskey EW. (1995). A trace component of ginseng that inhibits Ca2+ channels through a pertussis toxin-sensitive G protein. *Proc Natl Acad Sci USA.* 92(19): 8739–43.

Narahashi T, Frazier DT. (1971). Site of action and active form of local anesthetics. *Neurosci Res.* 4: 65–99.

Negus SS, Henriksen SJ, Mattox A, Pasternak GW, Portoghese PS, Takemori AE, Weinger MB, Koob GF. (1993). Effect of antagonists selective for mu, delta, and kappa opioid receptors on the reinforcing effects of heroin in rats. *J Pharmacol Exp Ther.* 265(3): 1245–52.

Nencini P, Ahmed AM, Anania MC, Moscucci M, Paroli E. (1984). Prolonged analgesia induced by cathinone. The role of stress and opioid and nonopioid mechanisms. *Pharmacology.* 29(5): 269–81.

Nencini P, Anania MC, Moscucci M, Pasquarelli V, Ahmed AM. (1988). Brief foot shock analgesia: long-lasting enhancement induced by cathinone, an amphetamine-like agent. *Pharmacology.* 37(2) 114–24.

Nencini P, Fraioli S, Pascucci T, Nucerito CV. (1998). (–)-Norpseudoephedrine, a metabolite of cathinone with amphetamine-like stimulus properties, enhances the analgesic and rate decreasing effects of morphine, but inhibits its discriminative properties. *Behav Brain Res.* 92(1): 11–20.

Nguyen TT, Matsumoto K, Yamasaki K, Nguyen MD, Nguyen TN, Watanabe H. (1995). Crude saponin extracted from Vietnamese ginseng and its major constituent majonoside-R2 attenuate the psychological stress- and foot-shock stress-induced antinociception in mice. *Pharmacol Biochem Behav.* 52(2): 427–32.

Nguyen TT, Matsumoto K, Yamasaki K, Nguyen MD, Nguyen TN, Watanabe H. (1996). The possible involvement of GABAA systems in the antinarcotic effect of majonoside-R2, a major constituent of Vietnamese ginseng, in mice. *Jpn J Pharmacol.* 71(4): 345–49.

Nguyen TT, Matsumoto K, Yamasaki K, Watanabe H. (1997). Involvement of supraspinal GABA receptors in majonoside-R2 suppression of clonidine-induced antinociception in mice. *Life Sci.* 61(4): 427–36.

Noyes R Jr, Brunk SF, Avery DAH, Canter AC. (1975). The analgesic properties of delta-9-tetrahydrocannabinol and codeine. *Clin Pharmacol Ther.* 18(1): 84–89.

Ohkubo T, Kitamura K. (1997). Eugenol activates Ca(2+)-permeable currents in rat dorsal root ganglion cells. *J Dent Res.* 76(11): 1737–44.

O'Neill WM, Hanks GW, White L, Simpson P, Wesnes K. (1995). The cognitive and psychomotor effects of opioid analgesics: I. A randomized controlled trial of single doses of dextropropoxyphene, lorazepam, and placebo in healthy subjects. *Eur J Clin Pharmacol.* 48(6): 447–53.

Onogi T, Minami M, Kuraishi Y, Satoh M. (1992). Capsaicin-like effect of (6)-shogaol on substance P-containing primary afferents of rats: a possible mechanism of its analgesic action. *Neuropharmacology.* 31(11): 1165–69.

Orlowski JP. (1999). Whatever happened to Reye's syndrome? Did it ever really exist? *Crit Care Med.* 27(8): 1582–87.

Pasternak GW, Standifer KM. (1995). Mapping of opioid receptors using antisense oligodeoxynucleotides: correlating their molecular biology and pharmacology. *Trends Pharmacol Sci.* 16(10): 344–50.

Pattrick M, Heptinstall S, Doherty M. (1989). Feverfew in rheumatoid arthritis: a double blind, placebo controlled study. *Ann Rheum Dis.* 48(7): 547–49.

Paul BD, Dreka C, Knight ES, Smith ML. (1996). Gas chromatographic/mass spectrometric detection of narcotine, papaverine, and thebaine in seeds of Papaver somniferum. *Planta Med.* 62(6): 544–47.

Paul D, Mana MJ, Pfaus JG, Pinel JP. (1988). Attenuation of morphine analgesia by the S2 antagonists, pirenperone and ketanserin. *Pharmacol Biochem Behav.* 31(3): 641–47.

Peng YB, Lin Q, Willis WD. (1996). Involvement of alpha-2 adrenoceptors in the periaqueductal gray-induced inhibition of dorsal horn cell activity in rats. *J Pharmacol Exp Ther.* 278: 125–35.

Pertovaara A, Tukeva T. (1990). Cocaine: effect on spinal projection neurons in the rat. *Brain Res Bull.* 25(1): 1–6.

Phillips S, Ruggier R, Hutchinson SE. (1993). Zingiber officinale (ginger)—an antiemetic for day case surgery. *Anaesthesia.* 48(8): 715–17.

Price DD. (1988). *Psychological and Neural Mechanisms of Pain.* New York: Raven Press, 1988.

Pugh G Jr, Abood ME, Welch SP. (1995). Antisense oligodeoxynucleotides to the kappa-1 receptor block the antinociceptive effects of delta 9-THC in the spinal cord. *Brain Res.* 689(1): 157–58.

Pugh G Jr, Smith PB, Dombrowski DS, Welch SP. (1996). The role of endogenous opioids in enhancing the antinociception produced by the combination of delta 9-tetrahydrocannabinol and morphine in the spinal cord. *J Pharmacol Exp Ther.* 279(2): 608–16.

Pugh WJ, Sambo K. (1988). Prostaglandin synthetase inhibitors in feverfew. *J Pharm Pharmacol.* 40(10): 743–45.

Raft D, Gregg J, Ghia J, Harris L. (1977). Effects of intravenous tetrahydrocannabinol on experimental and surgical pain. Psychological correlates of the analgesic response. *Clin Pharmacol Ther.* 21(1): 26–33.

Ramarao P, Bhargava HN. (1990). Antagonism of the acute pharmacological actions of morphine by Panax ginseng extract. *Gen Pharmacol.* 21(6): 877–80.

Rapp SE, Egan KJ, Ross BK, Wild LM, Terman GW, Ching JM. (1996). A multidimensional comparison of morphine and hydromorphone patient-controlled analgesia. *Anesth Analg.* 82(5): 1043–48.

Reche I, Fuentes JA, Ruiz-Gayo M. (1996). Potentiation of delta 9-tetrahydrocannabinol-induced analgesia by morphine in mice: involvement of mu- and kappa-opioid receptors. *Eur J Pharmacol.* 318(1): 11–16.

Reche I, Ruiz-Gayo M, Fuentes JA. (1998). Inhibition of opioid-degrading enzymes potentiates delta9-tetrahydrocannabinol-induced antinociception in mice. *Neuropharmacology.* 37(2): 215–22.

Reinscheid RK, Nothacker HP, Bourson A, Ardati A, Henningsen RA, Bunzow JR, Grandy DK, Langen H, Monsma FJ Jr, Civelli O. (1995). Orphanin FQ: a neuropeptide that activates an opioidlike G protein-coupled receptor. *Science.* 270(5237): 792–94.

Reisine T, Bell GI. (1993). Molecular biology of opioid receptors. *Trends Neurosci.* 16(12): 506–10.

Reisine T, Pasternak G. (1996). Opioid analgesics and antagonists. In: *Goodman and Gilman's The Pharmacological Basis of Therapeutics*. Hardman JG, Limbird LE, Molinoff PB, Ruddon RW, Goodman Gilman A, eds. New York: McGraw-Hill.

Robbers JE, Speedie MK, Tyler VE. (1996). *Pharmacognosy and Pharmacobiotechnology*. Baltimore: Willams and Wilkins.

Rose JS, Branchey M, Buydens-Branchey L, Stapleton JM, Chasten K, Werrell A, Maayan ML. (1996). Cerebral perfusion in early and late opiate withdrawal: a technetium-99m-HMPAO SPECT study. *Psychiatry Res.* 67(1): 39–47.

Rossi G, Pan YX, Cheng J, Pasternak GW. (1994). Blockade of morphine analgesia by an antisense oligodeoxynucleotide against the mu receptor. *Life Sci.* 54: 375–79.

Rossi GC, Pasternak GW, Bodnar RJ. (1993). Synergistic brainstem interactions for morphine analgesia. *Brain Res.* 624: 171–80.

Rossi GC, Pasternak GW, Bodnar RJ. (1994). Mu and delta opioid synergy between the periaqueductal gray and the rostro-ventral medulla. *Brain Res.* 665: 85–93.

Rossi GC, Perlmutter M, Leventhal L, Talatti A, Pasternak GW. (1998). Orphanin FQ/nociceptin analgesia in the rat. *Brain Res.* 792(2): 327–30.

Rudgley R. (1993). *Essential Substances*. New York: Kodansha International.

Saha N, Datta H, Sharma PL. (1991). Effects of morphine on memory: interactions with naloxone, propranolol, and haloperidol. *Pharmacology*. 42(1): 10–14.

Saper CB, Breder CD. (1994). The neurologic basis of fever. *N Engl J Med.* 330(26): 1880–86.

Sar M, Stumpf WE, Miller RJ, Chang KJ, Cuatrecasas P. (1978). Immunohistochemical localization of enkephalin in the rat brain and spinal cord. *J Comp Neurol.* 182: 17–37.

Sargent JD, Baumel B, Peters K, Diamond S, Saper JR, Eisner LS, Solbach P. (1988). Aborting a migraine attack: naproxen sodium v ergotamine plus caffeine. *Headache*. 28(4): 263–66.

Sawynok J. (1995). Pharmacological rationale for the clinical use of caffeine. *Drugs*. 49(1): 37–50.

Sawynok J. (1998). Adenosine receptor activation and nociception. *Eur J Pharmacol.* 347(1): 1–11.

Schlaepfer TE, Strain EC, Greenberg BD, Preston KL, Lancaster E, Bigelow GE, Barta PE, Pearlson GD. (1998). Site of opioid action in the human brain: mu and kappa agonists' subjective and cerebral blood flow effects. *Am J Psychiatry*. 155(4): 470–73.

Scoville WL. (1912). Note on capsicum. *J Am Pharm Assoc.* 1: 453.

Segal M, Dudai Y, Amsterdam A. (1978). Distribution of an alpha-bungarotoxin-binding cholinergic nicotinic receptor in rat brain. *Brain Res.* 148(1): 105–19.

Segal M, Sandberg D. (1977). Analgesia produced by electrical stimulation of catecholamine nuclei in the rat brain. *Brain Res.* 123: 369–72.

Sell AB, Carlini EA. (1976). Anesthetic action of methyleugenol and other eugenol derivatives. *Pharmacology.* 14(4): 367–77.

Servan-Schreiber D, Perlstein WM, Cohen JD, Mintun M. (1998). Selective pharmacological activation of limbic structures in human volunteers: a positron emission tomography study. *J Neuropsychiatry Clin Neurosci.* 10(2): 148–59.

Sharma JN, Srivastava KC, Gan EK. (1994). Suppressive effects of eugenol and ginger oil on arthritic rats. *Pharmacology.* 49(5): 314–18.

Shippenberg TS, Bals-Kubik R, Herz A. (1993). Examination of the neurochemical substrates mediating the motivational effects of opioids: role of the mesolimbic dopamine system and D-1 vs. D-2 dopamine receptors. *J Pharmacol Exp Ther.* 265(1): 53–59.

Shyu KW, Lin MT. (1985). Hypothalamic monoaminergic mechanisms of aspirin-induced analgesia in monkeys. *J Neural Transm.* 62(3–4): 285–93.

Sierra V, Duttaroy A, Lutfy K, Candido J, Billings B, Zito SW, Yoburn BC. (1992). Potentiation of opioid analgesia by cocaine: the role of spinal and supraspinal receptors. *Life Sci.* 50(8): 591–97.

Smith FL, Cichewicz D, Martin ZL, Welch SP. (1998). The enhancement of morphine antinociception in mice by delta9-tetrahydrocannabinol. *Pharmacol Biochem Behav.* 60(2): 559–66.

Smith FL, Fujimori K, Lowe J, Welch SP. (1998). Characterization of delta9-tetrahydrocannabinol and anandamide antinociception in nonarthritic and arthritic rats. *Pharmacol Biochem Behav.* 60(1): 183–91.

Smith PB, Martin BR. (1992). Spinal mechanisms of delta 9-tetrahydrocannabinol-induced analgesia. *Brain Res.* 578(1–2): 8–12.

Smith PB, Welch SP, Martin BR. (1994). Interactions between delta 9-tetrahydrocannabinol and kappa opioids in mice. *J Pharmacol Exp Ther.* 268(3): 1381–87.

Sopranzi N, De Feo G, Mazzanti G, Braghiroli L. (1991). [The biological and electrophysiological parameters in the rat chronically treated with Lobelia inflata L]. *Clin Ter.* 137(4): 265–68.

Spanagel R, Herz A, Shippenberg TS. (1992). Opposing tonically active endogenous opioid systems modulate the mesolimbic dopaminergic pathway. *Proc Natl Acad Sci USA.* 89(6): 2046–50.

Spinella M, Bodnar RJ. (1996). Excitatory amino acid antagonists in the rostroventral medulla inhibit mesencephalic morphine analgesia in rats. *Pain.* 64: 545–52.

Spinella M, Schaeffer LA, Bodnar RJ. (1997). Ventral medullary mediation of mesencephalic morphine analgesia by muscarinic and nicotinic cholinergic receptor antagonists in rats. *Analgesia.* 3: 119–30.

Spinella M, Znamensky V, Moroz M, Ragnauth A, Bodnar RJ. (1999). Actions of NMDA and cholinergic receptor antagonists in the rostral ventromedial medulla upon beta-endorphin analgesia elicited from the ventrolateral periaqueductal gray. *Brain Res.* 829(1–2): 151–59.

Srikiatkhachorn A, Tarasub N, Govitrapong P. (1999). Acetaminophen-induced antinociception via central 5-HT(2A) receptors. *Neurochem Int.* 34(6): 491–98.

Su YF, McNutt RW, Chang KJ. (1998). Delta-opioid ligands reverse alfentanil-induced respiratory depression but not antinociception. *J Pharmacol Exp Ther.* 287(3): 815–23.

Suekawa M, Ishige A, Yuasa K, Sudo K, Aburada M, Hosoya E. (1984). Pharmacological studies on ginger: I. Pharmacological actions of pungent constitutents, (6)-gingerol and (6)-shogaol. *J Pharmacobiodyn.* 7(11): 836–48.

Suh HW, Song DK, Kim YH. (1997). Effects of ginsenosides injected intrathecally or intracerebroventricularly on antinociception induced by morphine administrated intracerebroventricularly in the mouse. *Gen Pharmacol.* 29(5): 873–77.

Suh HW, Song DK, Lee KJ, Choi SR, Kim YH. (1996). Intrathecally injected nicotine enhances the antinociception induced by morphine but not beta-endorphin, D-Pen2,5-enkephalin and U50,488H administered intrathecally in the mouse. *Neuropeptides.* 30(4): 373–78.

Sumner H, Salan U, Knight DW, Hoult JR. (1992). Inhibition of 5-lipoxygenase and cyclooxygenase in leukocytes by feverfew. Involvement of sesquiterpene lactones and other components. *Biochem Pharmacol.* 43(11): 2313–20.

Szallasi A, Blumberg PM. (1999). Vanilloid (Capsaicin) receptors and mechanisms. *Pharmacol Rev.* 51(2): 159–212.

Taiwo YO, Levine JD. (1988). Prostaglandins inhibit endogenous pain control mechanisms by blocking transmission at spinal noradrenergic synapses. *J Neurosci.* 8(4): 1346–49.

Taylor F, Dickenson A. (1998). Nociceptin/orphanin FQ. A new opioid, a new analgesic? *Neuroreport.* 9(12): R65–70.

Tokuyama S, Wakabayashi H, Ho IK. (1996). Direct evidence for a role of glutamate in the expression of the opioid withdrawal syndrome. *Eur J Pharmacol.* 295(2–3): 123–29.

Tyler VE. (1994). *Herbs of Choice: The Therapeutic Use of Phytomedicinals.* Binghamton, NY: The Haworth Press.

Van Bockstaele EJ, Aston-Jones G, Pieribone VA, Ennis H, Shipley HY. (1991). Subregions of the periaqueductal gray topographically innervate the rostral ventral medulla in the rat. *J Comp Neurol.* 309: 305–27.

Vivian JA, Kishioka S, Butelman ER, Broadbear J, Lee KO, Woods JH. (1998). Analgesic, respiratory, and heart rate effects of cannabinoid and opioid agonists in rhesus monkeys: antagonist effects of SR 141716A. *J Pharmacol Exp Ther.* 286(2): 697–703.

Vogler BK, Pittler MH, Ernst E. (1998). Feverfew as a preventive treatment for migraine: a systematic review. *Cephalalgia.* 18(10): 704–8.

Waddell AB, Holtzman SG. (1999). Modulation of cocaine-induced antinociception by opioid-receptor agonists. *Pharmacol Biochem Behav.* 62(2): 247–53.

Walker DJ, Zacny JP. (1998). Subjective, psychomotor, and analgesic effects of oral codeine and morphine in healthy volunteers. *Psychopharmacology (Berlin).* 140(2): 191–201.

Watling KJ. (1998). *The RBI Handbook of Receptor Classification and Signal Transduction*, 3rd ed. Natick, MA: RBI.

Watson SJ, Akil H, Richard CW, Barchas JD. (1978). Evidence for two separate opiate peptide neuronal systems. *Nature.* 275: 226–28.

Weber JT, Hayataka K, O'Connor MF, Parker KK. (1997a). Rabbit cerebral cortex 5HT1a receptors. *Comp Biochem Physiol C Pharmacol Toxicol Endocrinol.* 117(1): 19–24.

Weber JT, O'Connor MF, Hayataka K, Colson N, Medora R, Russo EB, Parker KK. (1997b). Activity of Parthenolide at 5HT2A receptors. *J Nat Prod.* 60(6): 651–53.

Welburn PJ, Starmer GA, Chesher GB, Jackson DM. (1976). Effect of cannabinoids on the abdominal constriction response in mice: within cannabinoid interactions. *Psychopharmacologia.* 46(1): 83–85.

Welch SP. (1997). Characterization of anandamide-induced tolerance: comparison to delta 9-THC-induced interactions with dynorphinergic systems. *Drug Alcohol Depend.* 45(1–2): 39–45.

Welch SP, Huffman JW, Lowe J. (1998). Differential blockade of the antinociceptive effects of centrally administered cannabinoids by SR141716A. *J Pharmacol Exp Ther.* 286(3): 1301–8.

Welch SP, Stevens DL. (1992). Antinociceptive activity of intrathecally administered cannabinoids alone, and in combination with morphine, in mice. *J Pharmacol Exp Ther.* 262(1): 10–18.

Werling LL, Brown SR, Cox BM. (1987). Opioid receptor regulation of the release of norepinephrine in brain. *Neuropharmacology.* 26(7B): 987–96.

Wise RA. (1989). Opiate reward: sites and substrates. *Neurosci Biobehav Rev.* 13(2–3): 129–33.

Wood MM, Ashby MA, Somogyi AA, Fleming BG. (1998). Neuropsychological and pharmacokinetic assessment of hospice inpatients receiving morphine. *J Pain Symptom Manage.* 16(2): 112–20.

Yamamoto T, Nozaki-Taguchi N, Sakashita Y, Kimura S. (1999). Nociceptin/orphanin FQ: role in nociceptive information processing. *Prog Neurobiol.* 57(5): 527–35.

Yeung JC, Rudy TA. (1980). Multiplicative interaction between narcotic agonisms expressed at spinal and supraspinal sites of antinociceptive action as revealed by concurrent intrathecal and intracerebroventricular injections of morphine. *J Pharmacol Exp Ther.* 215: 633–42.

Yoon SR, Nah JJ, Shin YH, Kim SK, Nam KY, Choi HS, Nah SY. (1998). Ginsenosides induce differential antinociception and inhibit substance P-induced nociceptive response in mice. *Life Sci.* 62(21): PL 319–25.

Young ER, MacKenzie TA. (1992). The pharmacology of local anesthetics—a review of the literature. *J Can Dent Assoc.* 58(1): 34–42.

Zadina JE, Hackler L, Ge LJ, Kastin AJ. (1997). A potent and selective endogenous agonist for the mu-opiate receptor. *Nature.* 386(6624): 499–502.

Zagon A. (1995). Internal connection in the rostral ventromedial medulla of the rat. *J Autonomic Nerv Sys.* 53: 43–56.

Zarrindast MR, Khoshayand MR, Shafaghi B. (1999). The development of cross-tolerance between morphine and nicotine in mice. *Eur Neuropsychopharmacol.* 9(3): 227–33.

Zarrindast MR, Nami AB, Farzin D. (1996). Nicotine potentiates morphine antinociception: a possible cholinergic mechanism. *Eur Neuropsychopharmacol.* 6(2): 127–33.

Zarrindast MR, Pazouki M, Nassiri-Rad S. (1997). Involvement of cholinergic and opioid receptor mechanisms in nicotine-induced antinociception. *Pharmacol Toxicol.* 81(5): 209–13.

Zukin RS, Eghbali M, Olive D, Unterwald EM, Tempel A. (1998). Characterization and visualization of rat and guinea pig brain kappa opioid receptors: evidence for kappa 1 and kappa 2 opioid receptors. *Proc Natl Acad Sci USA.* 85(11): 4061–65.

Chapter 9

Aarons DH, Rossi GV, Orzechowski RF. (1977). Cardiovascular actions of three harmala alkaloids: harmine, harmaline, and harmalol. *J Pharm Sci.* 66(9): 1244–48.

Abdel-Fattah AF, Matsumoto K, Gammaz HA, Watanabe H. (1995). Hypothermic effect of harmala alkaloid in rats: involvement of serotonergic mechanism. *Pharmacol Biochem Behav.* 52(2): 421–26.

Abraham HD. (1983). Visual phenomenology of the LSD flashback. *Arch Gen Psychiatry.* 40(8): 884–89.

Abraham HD, Aldridge AM, Gogia P. (1996). The psychopharmacology of hallucinogens. *Neuropsychopharmacology.* 14(4): 285–98.

Abraham HD, Duffy FH. (1996). Stable quantitative EEG difference in post-LSD visual disorder by split-half analysis: evidence for disinhibition. *Psychiatry Res.* 67(3): 173–87.

Abraham HD, Mamen A. (1996). LSD-like panic from risperidone in post-LSD visual disorder. *J Clin Psychopharmacol.* June 16(3): 238–41.

Abuzzahab FS Sr, Anderson BJ. (1971). A review of LSD treatment in alcoholism. *Int Pharmacopsychiatry.* 6(4): 223–35.

Aghajanian GK. (1980). Mescaline and LSD facilitate the activation of locus coeruleus neurons by peripheral stimuli. *Brain Res.* 186(2): 492–98.

Aghajanian GK, Marek GJ. (1999). Serotonin and Hallucinogens. *Neuropsychopharmacology.* 21(2S): 16S–23S.

Ahn HS, Makman MH. (1979). Interaction of LSD and other hallucinogens with dopamine-sensitive adenylate cyclase in primate brain: regional differences. *Brain Res.* 162(1): 77–88.

Aigner TG. (1995). Pharmacology of memory: cholinergic-glutamatergic interactions. *Curr Opinion Neurobiol.* 5(2): 155–60.

Airaksinen MM, Lecklin A, Saano V, Tuomisto L, Gynther J. (1987). Tremorigenic effect and inhibition of tryptamine and serotonin receptor binding by beta-carbolines. *Pharmacol Toxicol.* 60(1): 5–8.

Akhondzadeh S, Stone TW. (1995). Induction of a novel form of hippocampal long-term depression by muscimol: involvement of GABAA but not glutamate receptors. *Br J Pharmacol.* 115(3): 527–33.

Akhondzadeh S, Stone TW. (1996). Maintenance of muscimol-induced long-term depression by neurosteroids. *Prog Neuropsychopharmacol Biol Psychiatry.* 20(2): 277–89.

Alburges ME, Hanson GR. (1999). Ibogaine pretreatment dramatically enhances the dynorphin response to cocaine. *Brain Res.* 847(1): 139–42.

Ali SF, Newport GD, Slikker W Jr, Rothman RB, Baumann MH. (1996). Neuroendocrine and neurochemical effects of acute ibogaine administration: a time course evaluation. *Brain Res.* 737(1–2): 215–20.

Anderson EF. (1996). *Peyote: The Divine Cactus.* Tuscon: University of Arizona Press.

Appel JB, Callahan PM. (1989). Involvement of 5-HT receptor subtypes in the discriminative stimulus properties of mescaline. *Eur J Pharmacol.* 159(1): 41–46.

Arbogast RE, Kozlowski MR. (1988). Quantitative morphometric analysis of the neurotoxic effects of the excitotoxin, ibotenic acid, on the basal forebrain. *Neurotoxicology* Spring. 9(1): 39–45.

Ayub N, Donaldson D, Bedford D, Alloway R, Ryalls M. (1997). Lessons to be learned: a case study approach. Hyperactivity and confusion in the presentation of hyoscine overdose. *J Royal Soc Health.* 117(4): 242–44.

Badio B, Padgett WL, Daly JW. (1997). Ibogaine: a potent noncompetitive blocker of ganglionic/neuronal nicotinic receptors. *Mol Pharmacol.* 51(1): 1–5.

Baghdoyan HA, Mallios VJ, Duckrow RB, Mash DC. (1994). Localization of muscarinic receptor subtypes in brain stem areas regulating sleep. *Neuroreport.* 5(13): 1631–34.

Barker A, Jones R, Prior J, Wesnes K. (1998). Scopolamine-induced cognitive impairment as a predictor of cognitive decline in healthy elderly volunteers: a 6-year follow-up. *Int J Geriatr Psychiatry.* 13(4): 244–47.

Bartus RT, Johnson HR. (1976). Short-term memory in the rhesus monkey: disruption from the anti-cholinergic scopolamine. *Pharmacol Biochem Behav.* 5(1): 39–46.

Batini C, Bernard JF, Buisseret-Delmas C, Horcholle-Bossavit G. (1980). [Harmaline tremor: activity of the interposito-rubral system and of the bulbo-ponto-reticular formation]. *C R Seances Acad Sci D.* 291(11): 905–7.

Baumann MH, Rothman RB, Ali SF. (1998). Neurochemical and neuroendocrine effects of ibogaine in rats: comparison to MK-801. *Ann NY Acad Sci.* 844: 252–64.

Bekar LK, Jabs R, Walz W. (1999). GABAA receptor agonists modulate K+ currents in adult hippocampal glial cells in situ. *Glia.* 26(2): 129–38.

Benwell ME, Holtom PE, Moran RJ, Balfour DJ. (1996). Neurochemical and behavioural interactions between ibogaine and nicotine in the rat. *Br J Pharmacol.* 117(4): 743–9.

Berg KA, Maayani S, Goldfarb J, Clarke WP. (1998). Pleiotropic behavior of 5-HT2A and 5-HT2C receptor agonists. *Ann NY Acad Sci.* 861: 104–10.

Beug MW, Bigwood J. (1982). Psilocybin and psilocin levels in twenty species from seven genera of wild mushrooms in the Pacific Northwest, U.S.A. *J Ethnopharmacol.* 5(3): 271–85.

Bhargava HN, Cao YJ. (1997). Effects of noribogaine on the development of tolerance to antinociceptive action of morphine in mice. *Brain Res.* 771(2): 343–46.

Bieger D. (1984). Muscarinic activation of rhombencephalic neurones controlling oesophageal peristalsis in the rat. *Neuropharmacology.* 23(12A): 1451–64.

Binienda Z, Beaudoin MA, Thorn BT, Prapurna DR, Johnson JR, Fogle CM, Slikker W Jr, Ali SF. (1998). Alteration of electroencephalogram and monoamine concentrations in rat brain following ibogaine treatment. *Ann NY Acad Sci.* 844: 265–73.

Bigwood J, Beug MW. (1982). Variation of psilocybin and psilocin levels with repeated flushes (harvests) of mature sporocarps of Psilocybe cubensis (Earle) Singer. *J Ethnopharmacol.* 5(3): 287–91.

Blackburn JR, Szumlinski KK. (1997). Ibogaine effects on sweet preference and amphetamine induced locomotion: implications for drug addiction. *Behav Brain Res.* 89(1–2): 99–106.

Blier P, Steinberg S, Chaput Y, de Montigny C. (1989). Electrophysiological assessment of putative antagonists of 5-hydroxytryptamine receptors: a single-cell study in the rat dorsal raphe nucleus. *Can J Physiol Pharmacol.* 67(2): 98–105.

Blin J, Piercey MF, Giuffra ME, Mouradian MM, Chase TN. (1994). Metabolic effects of scopolamine and physostigmine in human brain measured by positron emission tomography. *J Neurol Sci.* 123(1–2): 44–51.

Blum K, Futterman SL, Pascarosa P. (1977). Peyote, a potential ethnopharmacologic agent for alcoholism and other drug dependencies: possible biochemical rationale. *Clinical Toxicol.* 11(4): 459–72.

Bonson KR, Buckholtz JW, Murphy DL. (1996). Chronic administration of serotonergic antidepressants attenuates the subjective effects of LSD in humans. *Neuropsychopharmacology.* 14(6): 425–36,

Bonson KR, Murphy DL. (1996). Alterations in responses to LSD in humans associated with chronic administration of tricyclic antidepressants, monoamine oxidase inhibitors, or lithium. *Behav Brain Res.* 73(1–2): 229–33.

Boss V, Conn PJ. (1992). Metabotropic excitatory amino acid receptor activation stimulates phospholipase D in hippocampal slices. *J Neurochem.* 59(6): 2340–43.

Boutros NN, Bowers MB. (1996). Chronic substance-induced psychotic disorders: state of the literature. *J Neuropsychiatry Clin Neurosci.* 8(3): 262–9.

Bowen WD, Vilner BJ, Williams W, Bertha CM, Kuehne ME, Jacobson AE. (1995). Ibogaine and its congeners are sigma 2 receptor-selective ligands with moderate affinity. *Eur J Pharmacol.* 1279(1): R1–3.

Brauner-Osborne H, Nielsen B, Krogsgaard-Larsen P. (1998). Molecular pharmacology of homologues of ibotenic acid at cloned metabotropic glutamic acid receptors. *Eur J Pharmacol* 350(2–3): 311–16.

Brown JH, Taylor P. (1996). Muscarinic receptor agonists and antagonists. In: *Goodman and Gilman's The Pharmacological Basis of Therapeutics*, 9th ed. Hardman JG, Limbird LE, Molinoff PB, Ruddon RW, Goodman Gilman A, eds. New York: McGraw-Hill.

Buckholtz NS, Zhou DF, Freedman DX. (1988). Serotonin2 agonist administration down-regulates rat brain serotonin2 receptors. *Life Sci.* 42(24): 2439–45.

Buckholtz NS, Zhou DF, Freedman DX, Potter WZ. (1990). Lysergic acid diethylamide (LSD) administration selectively downregulates serotonin2 receptors in rat brain. *Neuropsychopharmacology.* 3(2): 137–48.

Burris KD, Breeding M, Sanders-Bush E. (1991). (+)Lysergic acid diethylamide, but not its nonhallucinogenic congeners, is a potent serotonin 5HT1C receptor agonist. *J Pharmacol Exp Ther.* Sept. 258(3): 891–96.

Burris KD, Sanders-Bush E. (1992). Unsurmountable antagonism of brain 5-hydroxytryptamine2 receptors by (+)-lysergic acid diethylamide and bromolysergic acid diethylamide. *Mol Pharm.* 42(5): 826–30.

Callaway JC, Grob CS. (1998). Ayahuasca preparations and serotonin reuptake inhibitors: a potential combination for severe adverse interactions. *J Psychoactive Drugs.* 30(4): 367–69.

Callaway JC, Raymon LP, Hearn WL, McKenna DJ, Grob CS, Brito GS, Mash DC. (1996). Quantitation of N,N-dimethyltryptamine and harmala alkaloids in human plasma after oral dosing with ayahuasca. *J Analytical Toxicol.* 20(6): 492–97.

Cantor M. (1990). Interviews: ibogaine treated addicts. *The Truth Seeker.* 117: 23–26.

Cao YJ, Bhargava HN. (1997). Effects of ibogaine on the development of tolerance to antinociceptive action of mu-, delta-, and kappa-opioid receptor agonists in mice. *Brain Res.* 752(1–2): 250–4.

Cappendijk SL, Dzoljic MR. (1993). Inhibitory effects of ibogaine on cocaine self-administration in rats. *Eur J Pharmacol.* 241(2–3): 261–65.

Carli M, Samanin R. (1992). Serotonin2 receptor agonists and serotonergic anorectic drugs affect rats' performance differently in a five-choice serial reaction time task. *Psychopharmacology (Berlin).* 106(2): 228–34.

Castaneda C. (1968). *The Teachings of Don Juan: A Yaqui Way of Knowledge.* Berkeley and Los Angeles: University of California Press.

Chen K, Kokate TG, Donevan SD, Carroll FI, Rogawski MA. (1996). Ibogaine block of the NMDA receptor: in vitro and in vivo studies. *Neuropharmacology.* 35(4): 423–31.

Codd EE. (1995). High affinity ibogaine binding to a mu opioid agonist site. *Life Sci.* 57(20): PL315–20.

Cohen MM, Shiloh Y. (1977–78). Genetic toxicology of lysergic acid diethylamide (LSD-25). *Mutation Res.* 47(3–4): 183–209.

Cohen RM, Gross M, Semple WE, Nordahl TE, Sunderland T. (1994). The metabolic brain pattern of young subjects given scopolamine. *Exp Brain Res.* 100(1): 133–43.

Colasanti B, Khazan N. (1975). Electroencephalographic studies on the development of tolerance and cross tolerance to mescaline in the rat. *Psychopharmacologia.* 43(3): 201–5.

Cooper JR, Bloom FE, Roth RH. (1996). *The Biochemical Basis of Neuropharmacology*, 7th ed. New York: Oxford.

Culver CM, King FW. (1974). Neuropsychological assessment of undergraduate marijuana and LSD users. *Arch Gen Psychiatry.* 31: 707–711.

Da Costa L, Sulklaper I, Naquet R. (1980). [Modification of awake-sleep equilibrium by tabernanthine and some of its derivatives in the cat]. *Rev Elec Neurophysiol Clin.* 10(1): 105–12.

Davidson MC, Cutrell EB, Marrocco RT. (1999). Scopolamine slows the orienting of attention in primates to cued visual targets. *Psychopharmacology (Berlin).* 1142(1): 1–8.

Davis M. (1987). Mescaline: excitatory effects on acoustic startle are blocked by serotonin2 antagonists. *Psychopharmacology (Berlin).* 93(3): 286–91.

Deecher DC, Teitler M, Soderlund DM, Bornmann WG, Kuehne ME, Glick SD. (1992). Mechanisms of action of ibogaine and harmaline congeners based on radioligand binding studies. *Brain Res.* 571(2): 242–47.

Deliganis AV, Pierce PA, Peroutka SJ. (1991). Differential interactions of dimethyltryptamine (DMT) with 5-HT1A and 5-HT2 receptors. *Biochem Pharmacol.* 41(11): 1739–44.

Delourme-Houde J. (1946). Contribution a l'etude de l'iboga [Tabernanthe Iboga H. Bn]. *Ann Pharm Franc.* 4: 30–36.

Demisch L, Neubauer M. (1979). Stimulation of human prolactin secretion by mescaline. *Psychopharmacology (Berlin).* 64(3): 361–63.

de Montigny C, Chaput Y, Blier P. (1990). Modification of serotonergic neuron properties by long-term treatment with serotonin reuptake blockers. *J Clin Psychiatry.* 51(suppl B): 4–8.

Dewey SL, Smith GS, Logan J, Brodie JD, Simkowitz P, MacGregor RR, Fowler JS, Volkow ND, Wolf AP. (1993). Effects of central cholinergic blockade on striatal dopamine release measured with positron emission tomography in normal human subjects. *Proc Nat Acad Sci USA.* 90(24): 11816–20.

Dhahir HI. (1971). A comparative study of the toxicity of ibogaine and serotonin. *Dissertation Abstract Int.* 32(4-B): 2311.

Doblin R. (1998). Dr. Leary's Concord Prison Experiment: a 34-year follow-up study. *J Psychoactive Drugs.* 30(4): 419–26.

Dolzhenko AT, Komissarov IV, Serdiuk SE. (1983). [Harman and 3-methylharman—blockaders of presynaptic alpha 2-adrenoreceptors]. *Farmakol Toksikol.* 46(1): 20–23.

Dorrance DL, Janiger O, Teplitz RL. (1975). Effect of peyote on human chromosomes. Cytogenetic study of the Huichol Indians of Northern Mexico. *JAMA.* 234(3): 299–302.

Du W, Aloyo VJ, Harvey JA. (1997). Harmaline competitively inhibits [3H]MK-801 binding to the NMDA receptor in rabbit brain. *Brain Res.* 770(1–2): 26–29.

Du W, Harvey JA. (1997). Harmaline-induced tremor and impairment of learning are both blocked by dizocilpine in the rabbit. *Brain Res.* 745(1–2): 183–88.

Ebert U, Kirch W. (1998). Scopolamine model of dementia: electroencephalogram findings and cognitive performance. *Eur J Clin Investigation.* 28(11): 944–49.

Ebert U, Siepmann M, Oertel R, Wesnes KA, Kirch W. (1998). Pharmacokinetics and pharmacodynamics of scopolamine after subcutaneous administration. *J Clin Pharmacol.* 38(8): 720–26.

Egan CT, Herrick-Davis K, Miller K, Glennon RA, Teitler M. (1998). Agonist activity of LSD and lisuride at cloned 5HT2A and 5HT2C receptors. *Psychopharmacology (Berlin).* 136(4): 409–14.

Ergene E, Schoener EP. (1993). Effects of harmane (1-methyl-beta-carboline) on neurons in the nucleus accumbens of the rat. *Pharmacol Biochem Behav.* 44: 4951–57.

Eugster CH, Muller GF, Good R. (1965). [The active ingredients from Amanita muscaria: ibotenic acid and muscazone]. *Tetrahedron Lett.* 23: 1813–15.

Fernández de Arriba A, Lizcano JM, Balsa MD, Unzeta M. (1994). Inhibition of monoamine oxidase from bovine retina by beta-carbolines. *J Pharm Pharmacol.* 46(10): 809–13.

File SE, Lister RG, Nutt DJ. (1982). The anxiogenic action of benzodiazepine antagonists. *Neuropharmacology.* 21(10): 1033–37.

Flicker C, Ferris SH, Serby M. (1992). Hypersensitivity to scopolamine in the elderly. *Psychopharmacology (Berlin).* 107(2–3): 437–41.

Flicker C, Serby M, Ferris SH. (1990). Scopolamine effects on memory, language, visuospatial praxis, and psychomotor speed. *Psychopharmacology (Berlin).* 100(2): 243–50.

Frances B, Gout R, Cros J, Zajac JM. (1992). Effects of ibogaine on naloxone-precipitated withdrawal in morphine-dependent mice. *Fundam Clin Pharmacol.* 6(8–9): 327–32.

Frederick DL, Gillam MP, Lensing S, Paule MG. (1997). Acute effects of LSD on rhesus monkey operant test battery performance. *Pharmacol Biochem Behav.* 57(4): 633–41.

Freedland CS, Mansbach RS. (1999). Behavioral profile of constituents in ayahuasca, an Amazonian psychoactive plant mixture. *Drug Alcohol Depend.* 54(3): 183–94.

French ED, Dillon K, Ali SF. (1996). Effects of ibogaine, and cocaine and morphine after ibogaine, on ventral tegmental dopamine neurons. *Life Sci.* 59(12): PL199–205.

Frumin MJ, Herekar VR, Jarvik ME. (1976). Amnesic actions of diazepam and scopolamine in man. *Anesthesiology.* 45(4): 406–12.

Fryer JD, Lukas RJ. (1999). Noncompetitive functional inhibition at diverse, human nicotinic acetylcholine receptor subtypes by bupropion, phencyclidine, and ibogaine. *J Pharmacol Exp Ther.* 288(1): 88–92.

Ghansah E, Kopsombut P, Malleque MA, Brossi A. (1993). Effects of mescaline and some of its analogs on cholinergic neuromuscular transmission. *Neuropharmacology.* 32(2): 169–74.

Giacomelli S, Palmery M, Romanelli L, Cheng CY, Silvestrini B. (1998). Lysergic acid diethylamide (LSD) is a partial agonist of D2 dopaminergic receptors and it potentiates dopamine-mediated prolactin secretion in lactotrophs in vitro. *Life Sci.* 63(3): 215–22.

Gitelman DR, Prohovnik I. (1992). Muscarinic and nicotinic contributions to cognitive function and cortical blood flow. *Neurobiol Aging.* 13(2): 313–18.

Glennon RA. (1990). Do classical hallucinogens act as 5-HT2 agonists or antagonists? *Neuropsychopharmacology.* 3(5–6): 509–17.

Glick SD, Gallagher CA, Hough LB, Rossman KL, Maisonneuve IM. (1992a). Differential effects of ibogaine pretreatment on brain levels of morphine and (+)-amphetamine. *Brain Res.* 588(1): 173–76.

Glick SD, Kuehne ME, Maisonneuve IM, Bandarage UK, Molinari HH. (1996a). 18-Methoxycoronaridine, a non-toxic iboga alkaloid congener: effects on morphine and cocaine self-administration and on mesolimbic dopamine release in rats. *Brain Res.* 719(1–2): 29–35.

Glick SD, Kuehne ME, Raucci J, Wilson TE, Larson D, Keller RW Jr, Carlson JN. (1994). Effects of iboga alkaloids on morphine and cocaine self-administration in rats: relationship to tremorigenic effects and to effects on dopamine release in nucleus accumbens and striatum. *Brain Res.* Sept. 19;657(1–2): 14–22.

Glick SD, Maisonneuve IS. (1998). Mechanisms of antiaddictive actions of ibogaine. *Ann NY Acad Sci.* 844: 214–26.

Glick SD, Maisonneuve IM, Pearl SM. (1997). Evidence for roles of kappa-opioid and NMDA receptors in the mechanism of action of ibogaine. *Brain Res.* 749(2): 340–43.

Glick SD, Maisonneuve IM, Visker KE, Fritz KA, Bandarage UK, Kuehne ME. (1998). 18-Methoxycoronardine attenuates nicotine-induced dopamine release and nicotine preferences in rats. *Psychopharmacology (Berlin).* 139(3): 274–80.

Glick SD, Pearl SM, Cai J, Maisonneuve IM. (1996b). Ibogaine-like effects of noribogaine in rats. *Brain Res.* 713(1–2): 294–97.

Glick SD, Rossman K, Rao NC, Maisonneuve IM, Carlson JN. (1992b). Effects of ibogaine on acute signs of morphine withdrawal in rats: independence from tremor. *Neuropharmacology.* 31(5): 497–500.

Glover V, Liebowitz J, Armando I, Sandler M. (1982). beta-Carbolines as selective monoamine oxidase inhibitors: in vivo implications. *J Neural Transm.* 54(3–4): 209–18.

Gogolák G, Jindra R, Stumpf C. (1977). Effect of harmaline on the cerebellorubral system. *Experientia.* 33(10): 1352–54.

Goldman H, Fischer R, Nicolov N, Murphy S. (1975). Lysergic acid diethylamide affects blood flow to specific areas of the conscious rat brain. *Experientia.* 31(3): 328–30.

Granon S, Poucet B, Thinus-Blanc C, Changeux JP, Vidal C. (1995). Nicotinic and muscarinic receptors in the rat prefrontal cortex: differential roles in working memory, response selection, and effortful processing. *Psychopharmacology (Berlin).* 119(2): 139–44.

Grasby PM, Frith CD, Paulesu E, Friston KJ, Frackowiak RS, Dolan RJ. (1995). The effect of the muscarinic antagonist scopolamine on regional cerebral blood flow during the performance of a memory task. *Exp Brain Res.* 104(2): 337–48.

Grech DM, Balster RL. (1997). The discriminative stimulus effects of muscimol in rats. *Psychopharmacology (Berlin).* 129(4): 339–47.

Grella B, Dukat M, Young R, Teitler M, Herrick-Davis K, Gauthier CB, Glennon RA. (1998). Investigation of hallucinogenic and related beta-carbolines. *Drug Alcohol Depend.* 50(2): 99–107.

Grinspoon L, Bakalar JB. (1986). Can drugs be used to enhance the psychotherapeutic process? *Am J Psychotherapy.* 40(3): 393–404.

Grinspoon L, Bakalar JB. (1997). *Psychedelic Drugs Reconsidered.* New York: Lindesmith Center.

Gruenwald J, Brendler T, Jaenicke C. (1998). *PDR for Herbal Medicines,* 1st ed. Montvale, NJ: Medical Economics Company.

Grob CS, McKenna DJ, Callaway JC, Brito GS, Neves ES, Oberlaender G, Saide OL, Labigalini E, Tacla C, Miranda CT, Strassman RJ, Boone KB. (1996). Human psychopharmacology of hoasca, a plant hallucinogen used in ritual context in Brazil. *J Nerv Ment Dis.* 184(2): 86–94.

Hajo N, Dupont C, Wepierre J. (1981). [Effects of tabernanthine on various cardiovascular parameters in the rat and dog]. *J Pharmacol.* 12(4): 441–53.

Hajo-Tello N, Dupont C, Wepierre J, Cohen Y, Miller R, Godfraind T. (1985). Effects of tabernanthine on calcium and catecholamine stimulated contractions of isolated vascular and cardiac muscle. *Arch Int Pharmacodyn Ther.* 276(1): 35–43.

Hall RC, Popkin MK, Mchenry LE. (1977). Angel's trumpet psychosis: a central nervous system anticholinergic syndrome. *Am J Psychiatry.* 134(3): 312–14.

Halpern JH, Pope HG Jr. (1999). Do hallucinogens cause residual neuropsychological toxicity? *Drug Alcohol Depend.* 53(3): 247–56.

Hamon G, Castillon A, Gaignault JC, Worcel M. (1985). Peripheral cardiovascular effects of tabernanthine tartrate in anaesthetized rats. *Arch Int Pharmacodyn Ther.* 276(1): 60–72.

Harder JA, Baker HF, Ridley RM. (1998). The role of the central cholinergic projections in cognition: implications of the effects of scopolamine on discrimination learning by monkeys. *Brain Res Bull.* 45(3): 319–26.

Harner, MJ. (1973). The role of hallucinogenic plants in European witchcraft. In: *Hallucinogens and Shamanism.* Harner MJ, ed. London: Oxford University Press.

Harsing LG Jr, Sershen H, Lajtha A. (1994). Evidence that ibogaine releases dopamine from the cytoplasmic pool in isolated mouse striatum. *J Neural Transm.* Gen sect. 96(3): 215–25.

Helsley S, Fiorella D, Rabin RA, Winter JC. (1997a). Effects of ibogaine on performance in the 8-arm radial maze. *Pharmacol Biochem Behav.* 58(1): 37–41.

Helsley S, Fiorella D, Rabin RA, Winter JC. (1998a). A comparison of N,N-dimethyltryptamine, harmaline, and selected congeners in rats trained with LSD as a discriminative stimulus. *Prog Neuropsychopharmacol Biol Psychiatry.* 22(4): 649–63.

Helsley S, Rabin RA, Winter JC. (1997b). The effects of noribogaine and harmaline in rats trained with ibogaine as a discriminative stimulus. *Life Sci.* 60(9): PL147–53.

Helsley S, Rabin RA, Winter JC. (1998b). The effects of beta-carbolines in rats trained with ibogaine as a discriminative stimulus. *Eur J Pharmacol.* 345(2): 139–43.

Hermle L, Funfgeld M, Oepen G, Botsch H, Borchardt D, Gouzoulis E, Fehrenbach RA, Hirsch KS, Fritz HI. (1981). Teratogenic effects of mescaline, epinephrine, and norepinephrine in the hamster. *Teratology.* 23(3): 287–91.

Hermle L, Funfgeld M, Oepen G, Botsch H, Borchardt D, Gouzoulis E, Fehrenbach RA, Spitzer M. (1992). Mescaline-induced psychopathological, neuropsychological, and neurometabolic effects in normal subjects: experimental psychosis as a tool for psychiatric research. *Biol Psychiatry.* 32(11): 976–91.

Hirsch KS, Fritz HI. (1981). Teratogenic effects of mescaline, epinephrine, and norepinephrine in the hamster. *Teratology.* 23(3): 287–91.

Holland MS. (1992). Central anticholinergic syndrome in a pediatric patient following transdermal scopolamine patch placement. *Nurse Anesth.* 3(3): 121–24.

Honore T, Krogsgaard-Larsen P, Hansen JJ, Lauridsen J. (1981). Glutamate and aspartate agonists structurally related to ibotenic acid. *Molec Cell Biochem.* 38 Spec. no. (pt 1): 123–28.

Hough LB, Pearl SM, Glick SD. (1996). Tissue distribution of ibogaine after intraperitoneal and subcutaneous administration. *Life Sci.* 58(7): PL119–22.

Huxley A. (1954). *The Doors of Perception.* New York: Harper.

Ito Y, Segawa K, Fukuda H. (1995). Functional diversity of GABAA receptor ligand-gated chloride channels in rat synaptoneurosomes. *Synapse.* 19(3): 188–96.

Itzhak Y, Ali SF. (1998). Effect of ibogaine on the various sites of the NMDA receptor complex and sigma binding sites in rat brain. *Ann NY Acad Sci.* 844: 245–51.

James W. (1902). *The Varieties of Religious Experience.* New York: Longmans, Green.

Jones HE, Balster RL. (1998). Muscimol-like discriminative stimulus effects of GABA agonists in rats. *Pharmacol Biochem Behav.* 59(2): 319–26.

Julien RM. (1998). *A Primer of Drug Action*, 8th ed. New York: W. H. Freeman.

Karler R, Calder LD, Chaudhry IA, Turkanis SA. (1989). Blockade of "reverse tolerance" to cocaine and amphetamine by MK-801. *Life Sci* 145(7): 599–606.

Kay DC, Martin WR. (1978). LSD and tryptamine effects on sleep/wakefulness and electrocorticogram patterns in intact cats. *Psychopharmacology (Berlin).* 58(3): 223–28.

Kebabian JW, Neumeyer JL. (1994). *The RBI Handbook of Receptor Classification.* Natick, MA: Research Biochemicals International.

Kesner RP, Jackson-Smith P, Henry C, Amann K. (1995). Effects of ibogaine on sensory-motor function, activity, and spatial learning in rats. *Pharmacol Biochem Behav.* 51(1): 103–9.

Khanna JM, Shah G, Weiner J, Wu PH, Kalant H. (1993). Effect of NMDA receptor antagonists on rapid tolerance to ethanol. *Eur J Pharmacol.* 230(1): 23–31.

Kikuchi M, Wada Y, Nanbu Y, Nakajima A, Tachibana H, Takeda T, Hashimoto T. (1999). EEG changes following scopolamine administration in healthy subjects. Quantitative analysis during rest and photic stimulation. *Neuropsychobiol.* 39(4): 219–26.

Klock JC, Boerner U, Becker CE. (1975). Coma, hyperthermia, and bleeding associated with massive LSD overdose, a report of eight cases. *Clin Toxicol.* 8(2): 191–203.

Kovera CA, Kovera MB, Singleton EG, Ervin FR, Williams IC, Mash DC. (1998). Decreased drug craving during inpatient detoxification with ibogaine. Poster presented at the College of Problems Drug Dependence Sixtieth Annual Scientific Meeting.

Krebs-Thomson K, Paulus MP, Geyer MA. (1998). Effects of hallucinogens on locomotor and investigatory activity and patterns: influence of 5-HT2A and 5-HT2C receptors. *Neuropsychopharmacology.* 18(5): 339–51.

Laudrup P, Klitgaard H. (1993). Metabotropic and ionotropic excitatory amino acid receptor agonists induce different behavioral effects in mice. *Eur J Pharmacol.* 250(1): 15–22.

Layer RT, Skolnick P, Bertha CM, Bandarage UK, Kuehne ME, Popik P. (1996). Structurally modified ibogaine analogs exhibit differing affinities for NMDA receptors. *Eur J Pharmacol* 309(2): 159–65.

Leal MB, Elisabetsky E. (1996). Absence of alkaloids in Psychotria carthagenensis Jacq. (Rubiaceae). *J Ethnopharmacol.* 54(1): 37–40.

Liljequist R, Mattila MJ. (1979). Effect of physostigmine and scopolamine on the memory functions of chess players. *Med Biol.* 57(6): 402–5.

Little JT, Johnson DN, Minichiello M, Weingartner H, Sunderland T. (1998). Combined nicotinic and muscarinic blockade in elderly normal volunteers: cognitive, behavioral, and physiologic responses. *Neuropsychopharmacology.* 19(1): 60–69.

Liu X, Matochik JA, Cadet JL, London ED. (1998). Smaller volume of prefrontal lobe in polysubstance abusers: a magnetic resonance imaging study. *Neuropsychopharmacology.* 18(4): 243–52.

Lorden JF, Stratton SE, Mays LE, Oltmans GA. (1988). Purkinje cell activity in rats following chronic treatment with harmaline. *Neuroscience.* 27(2): 465–72.

Lotsof HS. (1995). Ibogaine in the treatment of chemical dependence disorders: clinical perspectives. *Bull Multidisciplinary Assoc Psychedelic Stud.* 5: 16–27.

Ludwig A, Levine J, Stark L, Lazar R. (1969). A clinical study of LSD treatment in alcoholism. *Am J Psychiatry.* 126(1): 59–69.

Luciano D. (1998). Observations on treatment with ibogaine. *Am J Addict.* 7(1): 89–90.

Lutes J, Lorden JF, Beales M, Oltmans GA. (1988). Tolerance to the tremorogenic effects of harmaline: evidence for altered olivo-cerebellar function. *Neuropharmacology*. 27(8): 849–55.

Luxton T, Parker LA, Siegel S. (1996). Ibogaine fails to interrupt the expression of a previously established one-trial morphine place preference. *Prog Neuropsychopharmacol Biol Psychiatry*. 20(5): 857–72.

Mach RH, Smith CR, Childers SR. (1995). Ibogaine possesses a selective affinity for sigma 2 receptors. *Life Sci*. 57(4): PL57–62.

Madsen U, Ferkany JW, Jones BE, Ebert B, Johansen TN, Holm T, Krogsgaard-Larsen P. (1990). NMDA receptor agonists derived from ibotenic acid. Preparation, neuroexcitation, and neurotoxicity. *Eur J Pharmacol*. 189(6): 381–91.

Mah SJ, Tang Y, Liauw PE, Nagel JE, Schneider AS. (1998). Ibogaine acts at the nicotinic acetylcholine receptor to inhibit catecholamine release. *Brain Res*. 797(1): 173–80.

Maisonneuve IM, Keller RW Jr, Glick SD. (1991). Interactions between ibogaine, a potential anti-addictive agent, and morphine: an in vivo microdialysis study. *Eur J Pharmacol*. 199(1): 35–42.

Maisonneuve IM, Mann GL, Deibel CR, Glick SD. (1997). Ibogaine and the dopaminergic response to nicotine. *Psychopharmacology (Berlin)*. 129(3): 249–56.

Maisonneuve IM, Rossman KL, Keller RW Jr, Glick SD. (1992). Acute and prolonged effects of ibogaine on brain dopamine metabolism and morphine-induced locomotor activity in rats. *Brain Res*. 575(1): 69–73.

Marek GJ, Aghajanian GK. (1996). LSD and the phenethylamine hallucinogen DOI are potent partial agonists at 5-HT2A receptors on interneurons in rat piriform cortex. *J Pharmacol Exp Ther*. 278(3): 1373–82.

Markel H, Lee A, Holmes RD, Domino EF. (1994). LSD flashback syndrome exacerbated by selective serotonin reuptake inhibitor antidepressants in adolescents. *J Pediatrics*. Pt 1. 125(5): 817–19.

Mascher E. (1967). Psycholytic therapy: Statistics and indications. In: *Neuropsychopharmacology*, Brill H, ed. Amsterdam: Excerpta Medica Foundation.

Mash DC, Kovera CA, Buck BE, Norenberg MD, Shapshak P, Hearn WL, Sanchez-Ramos J. (1998). Medication development of ibogaine as a pharmacotherapy for drug dependence. *Ann NY Acad Sci*. 844: 274–92.

Mash DC, Staley JK, Pablo JP, Holohean AM, Hackman JC, Davidoff RA. (1995). Properties of ibogaine and its principal metabolite (12-hydroxyibogamine) at the MK-801 binding site of the NMDA receptor complex. *Neurosci Lett*. 192(1): 53–56.

Matossian MK. (1982). Ergot and the Salem witchcraft affair. *Am Scientist*. 70(4): 355–57.

Mayer ML, Westbrook GL. (1987). The physiology of excitatory amino acids in the vertebrate central nervous system. *Prog Neurobiol*. 28(3): 197–276.

McCall RB. (1982). Neurophysiological effects of hallucinogens on serotonergic neuronal systems. *Neurosci Biobehav Rev.* 6(4): 509–14.

McGlothlin WH, Arnold DO, Freedman DX. (1969). Organicity measures following repeated LSD ingestion. *Arch Gen Psychiatry.* 21: 704–9.

Meador KJ, Loring DW, Lee GP, Taylor HS, Hughes DR, Feldman DS. (1988). In vivo probe of central cholinergic systems. *J Gerontol.* 43(6): M158–62.

Meehan SM, Schechter MD. (1998). LSD produces conditioned place preference in male but not female fawn hooded rats. *Pharmacol Biochem Behav.* 59(1): 105–8.

Mehta AK, Ticku MK. (1989). Benzodiazepine and beta-carboline interactions with GABAA receptor-gated chloride channels in mammalian cultured spinal cord neurons. *J Pharmacol Exp Ther.* 249(2): 418–23.

Meneguz A, Betto P, Ricciarello G. (1994). Different effects of harmine on plasma concentrations of L-dopa and on cerebral dopamine metabolism in rabbits and rats. *Pharmacology.* 48(6): 360–66.

Miller RC, Godfraind T. (1983). The action of tabernanthine on noradrenaline-stimulated contractions and 45Ca movements in rat isolated vascular smooth muscle. *Eur J Pharmacol.* 96(3–4): 251–59.

Mittman SM, Geyer MA. (1991). Dissociation of multiple effects of acute LSD on exploratory behavior in rats by ritanserin and propranolol. *Psychopharmacology (Berlin).* 105(1): 69–76.

Molchan SE, Martinez RA, Hill JL, Weingartner HJ, Thompson K, Vitiello B, Sunderland T. (1992). Increased cognitive sensitivity to scopolamine with age and a perspective on the scopolamine model. *Brain Res Rev.* 17(3): 215–26.

Molchan SE, Matochik JA, Zametkin AJ, Szymanski HV, Cantillon M, Cohen RM, Sunderland T. (1994). A double FDG/PET study of the effects of scopolamine in older adults. *Neuropsychopharmacology.* 10(3): 191–98.

Molinari HH, Maisonneuve IM, Glick SD. (1996). Ibogaine neurotoxicity: a re-evaluation. *Brain Res.* 737(1–2): 255–62.

Moncrieff J. (1989). Determination of pharmacological levels of harmane, harmine, and harmaline in mammalian brain tissue, cerebrospinal fluid, and plasma by high-performance liquid chromatography with fluorimetric detection. *J Chromatogr.* 496(2): 269–78.

Morley JE, Yamada T, Walsh JH, Lamers CB, Wong H, Shulkes A, Damassa DA, Gordon J, Carlson HE, Hershman JM. (1980). Morphine addiction and withdrawal alters brain peptide concentrations. *Life Sci.* 26(26): 2239–44.

Moroz I, Parker LA, Siegel S. (1997). Ibogaine interferes with the establishment of amphetamine place preference learning. *Exp Clin Psychopharmacol.* 5(2): 119–22.

Mousah H, Jacqmin P, Lesne M. (1986). Interaction of carbolines and some GABA receptor ligands with the GABA and the benzodiazepine receptors. *J Pharmacol.* 17(4): 686–91.

Murray TF, Craigmill AL, Fischer GJ. (1977). Pharmacological and behavioral components of tolerance to LSD and mescaline in rats. *Pharmacol Biochem Behav*. 7(3): 239–44.

National Institute of Drug Abuse (1990). *National Household Survey of Drug Abuse, Main Findings*. Pub. No. 91-1788, Washington, DC. U.S. Department of Health and Human Services; Alcohol and Drug Abuse, and Mental Health Administration.

Newton RA, Phipps SL, Flanigan TP, Newberry NR, Carey JE, Kumar C, McDonald B, Chen C, Elliott JM. (1996). Characterisation of human 5-hydroxytryptamine2A and 5-hydroxytryptamine2C receptors expressed in the human neuroblastoma cell line SH-SY5Y: comparative stimulation by hallucinogenic drugs. *J Neurochem*. 67(6): 2521–31.

Obach RS, Pablo J, Mash DC. (1998). Cytochrome P4502D6 catalyzes the O-demethylation of the psychoactive alkaloid ibogaine to 12-hydroxyibogamine. *Drug Metab Dispos*. 26(8): 764–68.

O'Callaghan JP, Rogers TS, Rodman LE, Page JG. (1996). Acute and chronic administration of ibogaine to the rat results in astrogliosis that is not confined to the cerebellar vermis. *Ann NY Acad Sci*. 801: 205–16.

Ogawa M, Magata Y, Ouchi Y, Fukuyama H, Yamauchi H, Kimura J, Yonekura Y, Konishi J. (1994). Scopolamine abolishes cerebral blood flow response to somatosensory stimulation in anesthetized cats: PET study. *Brain Res*. 650(2): 249–52.

O'Hearn E, Molliver ME. (1997). The olivocerebellar projection mediates ibogaine-induced degeneration of Purkinje cells: a model of indirect, trans-synaptic excitotoxicity. *J Neurosci*. 17(22): 8828–41.

O'Hearn E, Zhang P, Molliver ME. (1995). Excitotoxic insult due to ibogaine leads to delayed induction of neuronal NOS in Purkinje cells. *Neuroreport*. 6(12): 1611–16.

Okonmah AD, Brown JW, Blyden GT, Soliman KF. (1988). Prenatal effects of acute harmaline exposure on fetal brain biogenic amine metabolism. *Pharmacology*. 37(3): 203–8.

Oliva GA, Bucci MP, Fioravanti R. (1993). Impairment of saccadic eye movements by scopolamine treatment. *Percept Motor Skills* 76(1): 159–67.

Pablo JP, Mash DC. (1998). Noribogaine stimulates naloxone-sensitive [35S]GTPgammaS binding. *Neuroreport*. Jan. 5;9(1): 109–14.

Palumbo PA, Winter JC. (1992). Stimulus effects of ibogaine in rats trained with yohimbine, DOM, or LSD. *Pharmacol Biochem Behav*. 43(4): 1221–26.

Pardanani JH, McLaughlin JL, Kondrat RW, Cooks RG. (1977). Cactus alkaloids: XXXVI. Mescaline and related compounds from Trichocereus peruvianus. *Lloydia*. 40(6): 585–90.

Parrott AC. (1987). Transdermal scopolamine: effects of single and repeated patches upon psychological task performance. *Neuropsychobiology*. 17(1–2): 53–59.

Pearl SM, Herrick-Davis K, Teitler M, Glick SD. (1995). Radioligand-binding study of noribogaine, a likely metabolite of ibogaine. *Brain Res.* 675(1–2): 342–44.

Pearl SM, Hough LB, Boyd DL, Glick SD. (1997). Sex differences in ibogaine antagonism of morphine-induced locomotor activity and in ibogaine brain levels and metabolism. *Pharmacol Biochem Behav.* 57(4): 809–15.

Pearl SM, Maisonneuve IM, Glick SD. (1996). Prior morphine exposure enhances ibogaine antagonism of morphine-induced dopamine release in rats. *Neuropharmacology.* 35(12): 1779–84.

Peden NR, Pringle SD, Crooks J. (1982). The problem of psilocybin mushroom abuse. *Hum Toxicol.* 1(4): 417–24.

Penington NJ, Reiffenstein RJ. (1986). Direct comparison of hallucinogenic phenethylamines and D-amphetamine on dorsal raphe neurons. *Eur J Pharmacol.* 122(3): 373–77.

Perouka SJ. (1996). Drugs effective in the therapy of migraine. In *Goodman and Gilman's The Pharmacological Basis of Therapeutics.* Hardman JG, Limbird LE, Molinoff PB, Ruddon RW, Goodman Gilman A, eds. New York: McGraw-Hill.

Pierce PA, Peroutka SJ. (1990a). Antagonist properties of d-LSD at 5-hydroxytryptamine2 receptors. *Neuropsychopharmacology.* 3(5–6): 503–8.

Pierce PA, Peroutka SJ. (1990b). d-Lysergic acid diethylamide differentially affects the dual actions of 5-hydroxytryptamine on cortical neurons. *Neuropharmacology.* 29(8): 705–12.

Pilotte NS, Mitchell WM, Sharpe LG, De Souza EB, Dax EM. (1991). Chronic cocaine administration and withdrawal of cocaine modify neurotensin binding in rat brain. *Synapse.* 9(2): 111–20.

Popik P. (1996). Facilitation of memory retrieval by the "anti-addictive" alkaloid, ibogaine. *Life Sci.* 59(24): PL379–85.

Popik P, Glick SD. (1996). Ibogaine, a putatively anti-addictive alkaloid. *Drugs of the Future.* 21(11): 1109–15.

Popik P, Layer RT, Fossom LH, Benveniste M, Geter-Douglass B, Witkin JM, Skolnick P. (1995). NMDA antagonist properties of the putative antiaddictive drug, ibogaine. *J Pharmacol Exp Ther.* 275(2): 753–60.

Prioux-Guyonneau M, Mocaer-Cretet E, Cohen Y, Jacquot C. (1984). Evidence for an activating effect of tabernanthine on rat brain catecholamine synthesis and elimination. *Experientia.* 40(12): 1388–89.

Prohovnik I, Arnold SE, Smith G, Lucas LR. (1997). Physostigmine reversal of scopolamine-induced hypofrontality. *Cereb Blood Flow Metab.* 17(2): 220–28.

Rabey JM, Neufeld MY, Treves TA, Sifris P, Korczyn AD. (1996). Cognitive effects of scopolamine in dementia. *J Neural Transm.* Gen sect. 103(7): 873–81.

Rabin RA, Winter JC. (1996a). Effects of ibogaine and noribogaine on phosphoinositide hydrolysis. *Brain Res.* 731(1–2): 226–29.

Rabin RA, Winter JC. (1996b). Ibogaine and noribogaine potentiate the inhibition of adenylyl cyclase activity by opioid and 5-HT receptors. *Eur J Pharmacol.* 316(2–3): 343–48.

Rasmussen K, Aghajanian GK. (1986). Effect of hallucinogens on spontaneous and sensory-evoked locus coeruleus unit activity in the rat: reversal by selective 5-HT2 antagonists. *Brain Res.* 385(2): 395–400.

Ray OS, Ksir C. (1990). *Drugs, Society, and Human Behavior.* St. Louis: Times Mirror/Mosby.

Rech RH, Commissaris RL. (1982). Neurotransmitter basis of the behavioral effects of hallucinogens. *Neurosci Biobehav Rev.* 6(4): 521–27.

Reid MS, Hsu K Jr, Souza KH, Broderick PA, Berger SP. (1996). Neuropharmacological characterization of local ibogaine effects on dopamine release. *J Neural Transm.* 103(8–9): 967–85.

Renner MJ, Dodson DL, Leduc PA. (1992). Scopolamine suppresses both locomotion and object contact in a free-exploration situation. *Pharmacol Biochem Behav.* 41(3): 625–36.

Rezvani AH, Overstreet DH, Lee YW. (1995). Attenuation of alcohol intake by ibogaine in three strains of alcohol-preferring rats. *Pharmacol Biochem Behav.* 52(3): 615–20.

Rezvani AH, Overstreet DH, Yang Y, Maisonneuve IM, Bandarage UK, Kuehne ME, Glick SD. (1997). Attenuation of alcohol consumption by a novel nontoxic ibogaine analogue (18-methoxycoronaridine) in alcohol-preferring rats. *Pharmacol Biochem Behav.* 58(2): 615–19.

Rho B, Glick SD. (1998). Effects of 18-methoxycoronaridine on acute signs of morphine withdrawal in rats. *Neuroreport.* 9(7): 1283–85.

Robbers JE, Speedie MK, Tyler VE. (1996). *Pharmacosnosy and Pharmacobiotechnology.* Baltimore: Williams and Wilkins.

Riedel W, Hogervorst E, Leboux R, Verhey F, van Praag H, Jolles J. (1995). Caffeine attenuates scopolamine-induced memory impairment in humans. *Psychopharmacology (Berlin).* 122(2): 158–68.

Robertson HA. (1980). Harmaline-induced tremor: the benzodiazepine receptor as a site of action. *Eur J Pharmacol.* 67(1): 129–32.

Rommelspacher H, Nanz C, Borbe HO, Fehske KJ, Müller WE, Wollert U. (1980). 1-Methyl-beta-carboline (harmane), a potent endogenous inhibitor of benzodiazepine receptor binding. *Naunyn Schmiedebergs Arch Pharmacol.* 314(1): 97–100.

Rosier A, Cornette L, Orban GA. (1998). Scopolamine-induced impairment of delayed recognition of abstract visual shapes. *Neuropsychobiology.* 37(2): 98–103.

Roth MT, Fleegal MA, Lydic R, Baghdoyan HA. (1996). Pontine acetylcholine release is regulated by muscarinic autoreceptors. *Neuroreport.* 7(18): 3069–72.

Rubner O, Kummerhoff PW, Haase H. (1997). [An unusual case of psychosis caused by long-term administration of a scopolamine membrane patch. Paranoid hallucinogenic and delusional symptoms]. *Nervenarzt.* 68(1): 77–79.

Rudgley R. (1993). *Essential Substances.* New York: Kodansha International.

Rupniak NM, Samson NA, Steventon MJ, Iversen SD. (1991). Induction of cognitive impairment by scopolamine and noncholinergic agents in rhesus monkeys. *Life Sci.* 48(9): 893–99.

Rusted JM. (1988). Dissociative effects of scopolamine on working memory in healthy young volunteers. *Psychopharmacology (Berlin).* 96(4): 487–92.

Rusted JM, Warburton DM. (1988). The effects of scopolamine on working memory in healthy young volunteers. *Psychopharmacology (Berlin).* 96(2): 145–52.

Sagalés T, Erill S, Domino EF. (1975). Effects of repeated doses of scopolamine on the electroencephalographic stages of sleep in normal volunteers. *Clin Pharmacol Ther.* 18(06): 727–32.

Sanders-Bush E, Burris KD, Knoth K. (1988). Lysergic acid diethylamide and 2,5-dimethoxy-4-methylamphetamine are partial agonists at serotonin receptors linked to phosphoinositide hydrolysis. *J Pharmacol Exp Ther.* 246(3): 924–28.

Savage C. (1952). Lysergic acid diethylamide (LSD-25). A clinical-psychological study. *Am J Psychiatry.* 108: 896–900.

Sbordone RJ, Wingard JA, Elliott MK, Jervey J. (1978). Mescaline produces pathological aggression in rats regardless of age or strain. *Pharmacol Biochem Behav.* 8(5): 543–46.

Schneider AS, Nagel JE, Mah SJ. (1996). Ibogaine selectively inhibits nicotinic receptor-mediated catecholamine release. *Eur J Pharmacol.* 317(2–3): R1–2.

Scholz WK. (1994). An ibotenate-selective metabotropic glutamate receptor mediates protein phosphorylation in cultured hippocampal pyramidal neurons. *J Neurochem.* 62(5): 1764–72.

Schultes RE, Hofman A. (1980). *The Botany and Chemistry of Hallucinogens,* 2nd ed. Springfield, IL: Charles C. Thomas Publishers.

Schultes RE, Hofman A. (1992). *Plants of the Gods: Their Sacred, Healing, and Hallucinogenic Powers.* Rochester, VT: Healing Arts Press.

Schwarcz R, Foster AC, French ED, Whetsell WO Jr, Köhler C. (1984). Excitotoxic models for neurodegenerative disorders. *Life Sci.* 35(1): 19–32.

Schwarcz R, Hokfelt T, Fuxe K, Jonsson G, Goldstein M, Terenius L. (1979). Ibotenic acid-induced neuronal degeneration: a morphological and neurochemical study. *Exp Brain Res.* 37(2): 199–216.

Schwartz RH. (1988). Mescaline: a survey. *Am Fam Physician.* 37(4): 122–24.

Sershen H, Harsing LG Jr, Hashim A, Lajtha A. (1992b). Ibogaine reduces amphetamine-induced locomotor stimulation in C57BL/6By mice, but stimulates locomotor activity in rats. *Life Sci.* 51(13): 1003–11.

Sershen H, Hashim A, Harsing L, Lajtha A. (1992a). Ibogaine antagonizes cocaine-induced locomotor stimulation in mice. *Life Sci.* 50(15): 1079–86.

Sershen H, Hashim A, Lajtha A. (1994a). Effect of ibogaine on serotonergic and dopaminergic interactions in striatum from mice and rats. *Neurochem Res.* 19(11): 1463–66.

Sershen H, Hashim A, Lajtha A. (1994b). Ibogaine reduces preference for cocaine consumption in C57BL/6By mice. *Pharmacol Biochem Behav.* 47(1): 13–19.

Sershen H, Hashim A, Lajtha A. (1997). Ibogaine and cocaine abuse: pharmacological interactions at dopamine and serotonin receptors. *Brain Res Bull.* 42(3): 161–68.

Shawcross WE. (1983). Recreational use of ergoline alkaloids from Agyreia nervosa. *J Psychoactive Drugs.* 15(4): 251–59.

Sheppard SG. (1994). A preliminary investigation of ibogaine: case reports and recommendations for further study. *J Subst Abuse Treat.* 11(4): 379–85.

Shiromani PJ, Fishbein W. (1986). Continuous pontine cholinergic microinfusion via mini-pump induces sustained alterations in rapid eye movement (REM) sleep. *Pharmacol Biochem Behav.* 25(6): 1253–61.

Sisko, B. (1993). Interrupting drug dependency with ibogaine: a summary four case case histories. *Multidisciplinary Association For Psychedelic Studies.* 4: 15–24.

Smith RL, Canton H, Barrett RJ, Sanders-Bush E. (1998). Agonist properties of N,N-dimethyltryptamine at serotonin 5-HT2A and 5-HT2C receptors. *Pharmacol Biochem Behav.* Nov. 61(3): 323–30.

Spanos NP. (1983). Ergotism and the Salem witch panic: a critical analysis and an alternative conceptualization. *J Hist Behav Sci.* 19(4): 358–69.

Spitzer M. (1992). Mescaline-induced psychopathological, neuropsychological, and neurometabolic effects in normal subjects: experimental psychosis as a tool for psychiatric research. *Biol Psychiatry.* 32(11): 976–91.

Staley JK, Ouyang Q, Pablo J, Hearn WL, Flynn DD, Rothman RB, Rice KC, Mash DC. (1996). Pharmacological screen for activities of 12-hydroxyibogamine: a primary metabolite of the indole alkaloid ibogaine. *Psychopharmacology (Berlin).* 127(1): 10–8.

Stanford JA, Fowler SC. (1998). At low doses, harmaline increases forelimb tremor in the rat. *Neurosci Lett.* 241(1): 41–44.

Steiner HX, McBean GJ, Kohler C, Roberts PJ, Schwarcz R. (1984). Ibotenate-induced neuronal degeneration in immature rat brain. *Brain Res.* 307(1–2): 117–24.

Strassman RJ. (1984). Adverse reactions to psychedelic drugs: a review of the literature. *J Nerv Ment Dis.* 172: 577–95.

Strassman RJ. (1995). Hallucinogenic drugs in psychiatric research and treatment. Perspectives and prospects. *J Nerv Ment Dis.* 183(3): 127–38.

Strassman RJ. (1996). Human psychopharmacology of N,N-dimethyltryptamine. *Behav Brain Res.* 73(1–2): 121–24.

Strassman RJ, Qualls CR. (1994). Dose-response study of N,N-dimethyltryptamine in humans: I. Neuroendocrine, autonomic, and cardiovascular effects. *Arch Gen Psychiatry.* 51(2): 85–97.

Strassman RJ, Qualls CR, Uhlenhuth EH, Kellner R. (1994). Dose-response study of N,N-dimethyltryptamine in humans: II. Subjective effects and preliminary results of a new rating scale. *Arch Gen Psychiatry.* 51(2): 98–108.

Sunder Sharma S, Bhargava HN. (1998). Enhancement of morphine antinociception by ibogaine and noribogaine in morphine-tolerant mice. *Pharmacology.* 57(5): 229–32.

Sunderland T, Esposito G, Molchan SE, Coppola R, Jones DW, Gorey J, Little JT, Bahro M, Weinberger DR. (1995). Differential cholinergic regulation in Alzheimer's patients compared to controls following chronic blockade with scopolamine: a SPECT study. *Psychopharmacology (Berlin).* 121(2): 231–41.

Sutin EL, Shiromani PJ, Kelsoe JR Jr, Storch FI, Gillin JC. (1986). Rapid-eye movement sleep and muscarinic receptor binding in rats are augmented during withdrawal from chronic scopolamine treatment. *Life Sci.* 39(25): 2419–27.

Sweetnam PM, Lancaster J, Snowman A, Collins JL, Perschke S, Bauer C, Ferkany J. (1995). Receptor binding profile suggests multiple mechanisms of action are responsible for ibogaine's putative anti-addictive activity. *Psychopharmacology (Berlin).* 118(4): 369–76.

Titeler M, Lyon RA, Glennon RA. (1988). Radioligand binding evidence implicates the brain 5-HT2 receptor as a site of action for LSD and phenylisopropylamine hallucinogens. *Psychopharmacology (Berlin).* 94(2): 213–16.

Trouvin JH, Jacqmin P, Rouch C, Lesne M, Jacquot C. (1987). Benzodiazepine receptors are involved in tabernanthine-induced tremor: in vitro and in vivo evidence. *Eur J Pharmacol.* 140(3): 303–9.

Trujillo KA, Akil H. (1991). Inhibition of morphine tolerance and dependence by the NMDA receptor antagonist MK-801. *Science.* 251(4989): 85–7.

Trulson ME. (1986). Dissociations between the effects of hallucinogens on behavior and raphe unit activity in behaving cats. *Pharmacol Biochem Behav.* 24(2): 351–57.

Trulson ME, Crisp T, Henderson LJ. (1983). Mescaline elicits behavioral effects in cats by an action at both serotonin and dopamine receptors. *Eur J Pharmacol.* 96(1–2): 151–54.

Tse SY, Mak IT, Dickens BF. (1991). Antioxidative properties of harmane and beta-carboline alkaloids. *Biochem Pharmacol.* 42(3): 459–64.

Tsuang MT, Simpson JC, Kronfol Z . (1982). Subtypes of drug abuse with psychosis. Demographic characteristics, clinical features, and family history. *Arch Gen Psychiatry.* 39(2): 141–47.

Tweedie DJ, Burke MD. (1987). Metabolism of the beta-carbolines, harmine and harmol, by liver microsomes from phenobarbitone- or 3-methylcholanthrene-treated mice. Identification and quantitation of two novel harmine metabolites. *Drug Metab Dispos.* 15(1): 74–81.

Vandermaelen CP, Aghajanian GK. (1983). Electrophysiological and pharmacological characterization of serotonergic dorsal raphe neurons recorded extracellularly and intracellularly in rat brain slices. *Brain Res.* 289(1–2): 109–19.

van der Zee EA, Luiten PG. (1999). Muscarinic acetylcholine receptors in the hippocampus, neocortex, and amygdala: a review of immunocytochemical localization in relation to learning and memory. *Prog Neurobiol.* 58(5): 409–71.

van Dongen PW, de Groot AN. (1995). History of ergot alkaloids from ergotism to ergometrine. *Eur J Obstet Gynecol Reprod Biol.* 160(2): 109–16.

Venault P, Chapouthier G, de Carvalho LP, Simiand J, Morre M, Dodd RH, Rossier J. (1986). Benzodiazepine impairs and beta-carboline enhances performance in learning and memory tasks. *Nature.* 321(6073): 864–66.

Vesalainen RK, Kaila TJ, Kantola IM, Tahvanainen KU, Juhani Airaksinen KE, Kuusela TA, Eckberg DL. (1998). Low-dose transdermal scopolamine decreases blood pressure in mild essential hypertension. *J Hypertens.* 16(3): 321–9.

Vitiello B, Martin A, Hill J, Mack C, Molchan S, Martinez R, Murphy DL, Sunderland T. (1997). Cognitive and behavioral effects of cholinergic, dopaminergic, and serotonergic blockade in humans. *Neuropsychopharmacology.* 16(1): 15–24.

Watts VJ, Lawler CP, Fox DR, Neve KA, Nichols DE, Mailman RB. (1995). LSD and structural analogs: pharmacological evaluation at D1 dopamine receptors. *Psychopharmacology (Berlin).* 118(4): 401–9.

Wei D, Maisonneuve IM, Kuehne ME, Glick SD. (1998). Acute iboga alkaloid effects on extracellular serotonin (5-HT) levels in nucleus accumbens and striatum in rats. *Brain Res.* 800(2): 260–68.

Wells GB, Lopez MC, Tanaka JC. (1999). The effects of ibogaine on dopamine and serotonin transport in rat brain synaptosomes. *Brain Res Bull.* 48(6): 641–7.

Welsh SE, Kachelries WJ, Romano AG, Simansky KJ, Harvey JA. (1998). Effects of LSD, ritanserin, 8-OH-DPAT, and lisuride on classical conditioning in the rabbit. *Pharmacol Biochem Behav.* 59(2): 469–75.

Wilkinson JA. (1987). Side effects of transdermal scopolamine. *J Emerg Med.* 5(5): 389–92.

Wing LL, Tapson GS, Geyer MA. (1990). 5HT-2 mediation of acute behavioral effects of hallucinogens in rats. *Psychopharmacology (Berlin).* 100(3): 417–25.

Wong DF, Lever JR, Hartig PR, Dannals RF, Villemagne V, Hoffman BJ, Wilson AA, Ravert HT, Links JM, Scheffel U, et al. (1987). Localization of serotonin 5-HT2 receptors in living human brain by positron emission tomography using N1-([11C]-methyl)-2-Br-LSD. *Synapse.* 1(5): 393–98.

Yanai K, Ido T, Ishiwata K, Hatazawa J, Takahashi T, Iwata R, Matsuzawa T. (1986). In vivo kinetics and displacement study of a carbon-11-labeled hallucinogen, N,N-[11C]dimethyltryptamine. *Eur J Nucl Med.* 12(3): 141–46.

Yeomans JS. (1995). Role of tegmental cholinergic neurons in dopaminergic activation, antimuscarinic psychosis and schizophrenia. *Neuropsychopharmacology.* 12(1): 3–16.

Yeomans JS, Mathur A, Tampakeras M. (1993). Rewarding brain stimulation: role of tegmental cholinergic neurons that activate dopamine neurons. *Behav Neurosci.* 107(6): 1077–87.

Young GB. (1998). *Consciousness, in Coma and Impaired Consciousness: A Clinical Perspective.* Young GB, Ropper AH, Bolton CF, eds. New York: McGraw-Hill.

Yu X, Imam SZ, Newport GD, Slikker W Jr, Ali SF. (1999). Ibogaine blocked methamphetamine-induced hyperthermia and induction of heat shock protein in mice. *Brain Res.* 823(1–2): 213–16.

Zaczek R, Coyle JT. (1982). Excitatory amino acid analogues: neurotoxicity and seizures. *Neuropharmacology.* 21(1): 15–26.

Zemishlany Z, Thorne AE. (1991). Anticholinergic challenge and cognitive functions: a comparison between young and elderly normal subjects. *Isr J Psychiatry Relat Sci.* 28(3): 32–41.

Zetler G, Singbartl G, Schlosser L. (1972). Cerebral pharmacokinetics of tremor-producing harmala and iboga alkaloids. *Pharmacology.* 7(4): 237–48.

Zhang L, Dyer DC. (1993). Lysergic acid diethylamide is a partial agonist at 5-HT2 receptors in ovine uterine artery of late pregnancy. *Eur J Pharmacol.* 230(1): 115–17.

Zinkand WC, Moore WC, Thompson C, Salama AI, Patel J. (1992). Ibotenic acid mediates neurotoxicity and phosphoinositide hydrolysis by independent receptor mechanisms. *Mol Chem Neuropathol.* 16(1–2): 1–10.

Ziskind AA. (1988). Transdermal scopolamine-induced psychosis. *Postgrad Med.* 84(3): 73–76.

Zoltoski RK, Velazquez-Moctezuma J, Shiromani PJ, Gillin JC. (1993). The relative effects of selective M1 muscarinic antagonists on rapid eye movement sleep. *Brain Res.* 608(2): 186–90.

Zubaran C, Shoaib M, Stolerman IP, Pablo J, Mash DC. (1999). Noribogaine generalization to the ibogaine stimulus: correlation with noribogaine concentration in rat brain. *Neuropsychopharmacology.* July 21(1): 119–26.

Chapter 10

Abel EL. (1970). Marijuana and memory. *Nature.* 227(263): 1151–52.

Abel EL. (1971). Marihuana and memory: acquisition or retrieval? *Science.* 173(4001): 1038–40.

Abel EL. (1981). Marihuana and sex: a critical survey. *Drug Alcohol Dependence.* 8(1): 1–22.

Abel EL, Dintcheff BA, Day N. (1980). Effects of marihuana on pregnant rats and their offspring. *Psychopharmacology (Berlin).* 71(1): 71–74.

Aceto MD, Scates SM, Lowe JA, Martin BR. (1995). Cannabinoid precipitated withdrawal by the selective cannabinoid receptor antagonist, SR 141716A. *Eur J Pharmacol.* 282(1–3): R1–2.

Adams IB, Compton DR, Martin BR. (1998). Assessment of anandamide interaction with the cannabinoid brain receptor: SR 141716A antagonism studies in mice and autoradiographic analysis of receptor binding in rat brain. *J Pharmacol Exp Ther.* 284(3): 1209–17.

Adams PM, Barratt ES. (1975). Effect of chronic marijuana administration of stages of primate sleep-wakefulness. *Biol Psychiatry.* 10(3): 315–22.

Ali SF, Newport GD, Scallet AC, Paule MG, Bailey JR, Slikker W Jr. (1991). Chronic marijuana smoke exposure in the rhesus monkey: IV. Neurochemical effects and comparison to acute and chronic exposure to delta-9-tetrahydrocannabinol (THC) in rats. *Pharmacol Biochem Behav.* 40(3): 677–82.

Bachman JA, Benowitz NL, Herning RI, Jones RT. (1979). Dissociation of autonomic and cognitive effects of THC in man. *Psychopharmacology (Berlin).* 61(2): 171–75.

Baker D, Pryce G, Croxford JL, Brown P, Pertwee RG, Huffman JW, Layward L. (2000). Cannabinoids control spasticity and tremor in a multiple sclerosis model. *Nature.* 404(6773): 84–87.

Baloh RW, Sharma S, Moskowitz H, Griffith R. (1979). Effect of alcohol and marijuana on eye movements. *Aviat Space Environ Med.* 50(1): 18–23.

Barnett G, Licko V, Thompson T. (1985). Behavioral pharmacokinetics of marijuana. *Psychopharmacology (Berlin).* 85(1): 51–56.

Basbaum AI, Fields HL. (1978). Endogenous pain control mechanisms: review and hypothesis. *Ann Neurol.* 4: 451–62.

Basbaum AI, Fields HL. (1984). Endogenous pain control systems: brainstem spinal pathways and endorphin circuitry. *Ann Rev Neurosci.* 7: 309–38.

Beal JE, Olson R, Laubenstein L, Morales JO, Bellman P, Yangco B, Lefkowitz L, Plasse TF, Shepard KV. (1995). Dronabinol as a treatment for anorexia associated with weight loss in patients with AIDS. *J Pain Symptom Manage.* 10(2): 89–97.

Beal JE, Olson R, Lefkowitz L, Laubenstein L, Bellman P, Yangco B, Morales JO, Murphy R, Powderly W, Plasse TF, et al. (1997). Long-term efficacy and safety of dronabinol for acquired immunodeficiency syndrome-associated anorexia. *J Pain Symptom Manage.* 14(1): 7–14.

Belgrave BE, Bird KD, Chesher GB, Jackson DM, Lubbe KE, Starmer GA, Teo RK. (1979). The effect of (–) trans-delta9-tetrahydrocannabinol, alone and in combination with ethanol, on human performance. *Psychopharmacology (Berlin).* 62(1): 53–60.

Bibra E. (1995). *Plant Intoxicants.* Rochester, VT: Healing Arts Press.

Biegon A, Joseph A. (1995). Development of HU-211 as a neuroprotectant for ischemic brain damage. *Neurol Res.* 17: 4275–80.

Bonnin A, Fernandez-Ruiz JJ, Martin M, Rodriguez de Fonseca F, Hernandez ML, Ramos JA. (1993). Delta 9-Tetrahydrocannabinol affects mesolimbic dopaminergic activity in the female rat brain: interactions with estrogens. *J Neural Trans Gen Section*. 92(2–3): 81–95.

Boutros NN, Bowers MB. (1996). Chronic substance-induced psychotic disorders: state of the literature. *J Neuropsychiatry Clin Neurosci*. 8(3): 262–69.

Brewster ME, Pop E, Foltz RL, Reuschel S, Griffith W, Amselem S, Biegon A. (1997). Clinical pharmacokinetics of escalating i.v. doses of dexanabinol (HU-211), a neuroprotectant agent, in normal volunteers. *Int J Clin Pharmacol Ther*. 35: 9361–65.

Buonamici M, Young GA, Khazan N. (1982). EEG power spectra in the rat. Effects of acute delta 9-THC administration on EEG and EEG power spectra in the rat. *Neuropharmacology*. 21(8): 825–29.

Cabral GA, Toney DM, Fischer-Stenger K, Harrison MP, Marciano-Cabral F. (1995). Anandamide inhibits macrophage-mediated killing of tumor necrosis factor-sensitive cells. *Life Sci*. 56(23–24): 2065–72.

Calhoun SR, Galloway GP, Smith DE. (1998). Abuse potential of dronabinol (Marinol). *J Psychoactive Drugs*. 30(2): 187–96.

Carta G, Nava F, Gessa GL. (1998). Inhibition of hippocampal acetylcholine release after acute and repeated Delta9-tetrahydrocannabinol in rats. *Brain Res*. 809(1): 1–4.

Casswell S, Marks DF. (1973a). Cannabis and temporal disintegration in experienced and naive subjects. *Science*. 179(75): 803–5.

Casswell S, Marks DF. (1973b). Cannabis induced impairment of performance of a divided attention task. *Nature*. 241(5384): 60–61.

Castaneda E, Moss DE, Oddie SD, Whishaw IQ. (1991). THC does not affect striatal dopamine release: microdialysis in freely moving rats. *Pharmacol Biochem Behav*. 40(3): 587–91.

Castellano C, Cabib S, Palmisano A, Di Marzo V, Puglisi-Allegra S. (1997). The effects of anandamide on memory consolidation in mice involve both D1 and D2 dopamine receptors. *Behav Pharmacol*. 8(8): 707–12.

Chait LD. (1990). Subjective and behavioral effects of marijuana the morning after smoking. *Psychopharmacology (Berlin)*. 100(3): 328–33.

Chait LD, Perry JL. (1994). Effects of alcohol pretreatment on human marijuana self-administration. *Psychopharmacology (Berlin)*. 113(3–4): 346–50.

Chan GC, Hinds TR, Impey S, Storm DR. (1998). Hippocampal neurotoxicity of Delta9-tetrahydrocannabinol. *J Neurosci*. 18(14): 5322–32.

Charalambous A, Marciniak G, Shiue CY, Dewey SL, Schlyer DJ, Wolf AP, Makriyannis A. (1991). PET studies in the primate brain and biodistribution in mice using (−)-5′-18F-delta 8-THC. *Pharmacol Biochem Behav*. 40(3): 503–7.

Childers SR, Breivogel CS. (1998). Cannabis and endogenous cannabinoid systems. *Drug Alcohol Dependence*. 51(1–2): 173–87.

Chiu P, Olsen DM, Borys HK, Karler R, Turkanis SA. (1979). The influence of cannabidiol and delta 9-tetrahydrocannabinol on cobalt epilepsy in rats. *Epilepsia.* 20(4): 365–75.

Clark LD, Hughes R, Nakashima EN. (1970). Behavioral effects of marihuana. Experimental studies. *Arch Gen Psychiatry.* 23(3): 193–98.

Colasanti BK, Lindamood C 3d, Craig CR. (1982). Effects of marihuana cannabinoids on seizure activity in cobalt-epileptic rats. *Pharmacol Biochem Behav.* 16(4): 573–78.

Collins DR, Pertwee RG, Davies SN. (1994). The action of synthetic cannabinoids on the induction of long-term potentiation in the rat hippocampal slice. *Eur J Pharmacol.* 259(3): R7–8.

Colombo G, Agabio R, Diaz G, Lobina C, Reali R, Gessa GL. (1998). Appetite suppression and weight loss after the cannabinoid antagonist SR 141716. *Life Sci.* 63(8): PL113–17.

Cone EJ, Johnson RE, Moore JD, Roache JD. (1986). Acute effects of smoking marijuana on hormones, subjective effects and performance in male human subjects. *Pharmacol Biochem Behav.* 24(6): 1749–54.

Consroe P, Kennedy K, Schram K. (1991). Assay of plasma cannabidiol by capillary gas chromatography/ion trap mass spectroscopy following high-dose repeated daily oral administration in humans. *Pharmacol Biochem Behav.* 40(3): 517–22.

Consroe P, Musty R, Rein J, Tillery W, Pertwee R. (1997). The perceived effects of smoked cannabis on patients with multiple sclerosis. *Eur Neurol.* 38(1): 44–48.

Cook SA, Lowe JA, Martin BR. (1998). CB1 receptor antagonist precipitates withdrawal in mice exposed to Delta9-tetrahydrocannabinol. *J Pharmacol Exp Ther.* 285(3): 1150–56.

Cooler P, Gregg M. (1977). Effect of delta-9-tetrahydrocannabinol on intraocular pressure in humans. *Southern Med J.* 70(8): 951–54.

Corcoran ME, McCaughran JA Jr, Wada JA. (1978). Antiepileptic and prophylactic effects of tetrahydrocannabinols in amygdaloid kindled rats. *Epilepsia.* 19(1): 47–55.

Cutler MG, Mackintosh JH. (1984). Cannabis and delta-9-tetrahydrocannabinol. Effects on elements of social behaviour in mice. *Neuropharmacology.* 23(9): 1091–97.

Dalterio S, Bartke A, Mayfield D. (1985a). Effects of delta 9-tetrahydrocannabinol on testosterone production in vitro: influence of Ca++, Mg++, or glucose. *Life Sci.* 37(15): 1425–33.

Dalterio S, Mayfield D, Bartke A, Morgan W. (1985b). Effects of psychoactive and non-psychoactive cannabinoids on neuroendocrine and testicular responsiveness in mice. *Life Sci.* 36(13): 1299–306.

Dalterio S, Steger R, Peluso J, de Paolo L. (1987). Acute delta 9-tetrahydrocannabinol exposure: effects on hypothalamic-pituitary-testicular activity in mice. *Pharmacol Biochem Behav.* March 26(3): 533–37.

Darley CF, Tinklenberg JR, Roth WT, Vernon S, Kopell BS. (1977). Marijuana effects on long-term memory assessment and retrieval. *Psychopharmacology (Berlin)*. May 9;52(3): 239–41.

Das SK, Paria BC, Chakraborty I, Dey SK. (1995). Cannabinoid ligand-receptor signaling in the mouse uterus. *Proc Natl Acad Sci USA*. 92(10): 4332–36.

Davidson, K. (1999). *Carl Sagan: A Life*. NY: John Wiley and Sons.

Devane WA, Axelrod J. (1994). Enzymatic synthesis of anandamide, an endogenous ligand for the cannabinoid receptor, by brain membranes. *Proc Natl Acad Sci USA*. 91(14): 6698–701.

Devane WA, Hanus L, Breuer A, Pertwee RG, Stevenson LA, Griffin G, Gibson D, Mandelbaum A, Etinger A, Mechoulam R. (1992). Isolation and structure of a brain constituent that binds to the cannabinoid receptor. *Science*. 258(5090): 1946–49.

Diana M, Melis M, Gessa GL. (1998a). Increase in meso-prefrontal dopaminergic activity after stimulation of CB1 receptors by cannabinoids. *Eur J Neurosci*. Sept. 10(9): 2825–30.

Diana M, Melis M, Muntoni AL, Gessa GL. (1998b). Mesolimbic dopaminergic decline after cannabinoid withdrawal. *Proc Natl Acad Sci USA*. Aug. 18;95(17): 10269–73.

Diaz S, Specter S, Coffey RG. (1993). Suppression of lymphocyte adenosine 3′:5′-cyclic monophosphate (cAMP) by delta-9-tetrahydrocannabinol. *Int J Immunopharmacol*. 15(4): 523–32.

Di Marzo V. (1998). 2-Arachidonoyl-glycerol as an "endocannabinoid": limelight for a formerly neglected metabolite. *Biochemistry (Moscow)*. 63(1): 13–21.

Dittrich A, Battig K, von Zeppelin I. (1973). Effects of (−) delta-9-tetrahydrocannabinol (delta-9-THC) on memory, attention, and subjective state. *Psychopharmacologia*. 33: 369–76.

Domino EF. (1981). Cannabinoids and the cholinergic system. *J Clin Pharmacol*. 21(8–9 suppl): 249S–55S.

Dornbush RL, Fink M, Freedman AM. (1971). Marijuana, memory, and perception. *Am J Psychiatry*. 128(2): 194–97.

Drewnowski A, Grinker JA. (1978). Food and water intake, meal patterns, and activity of obese and lean Zucker rats following chronic and acute treatment with delta9-tetrahydrocannabinol. *Pharmacol Biochem Behav*. 9(5): 619–30.

Duffy A, Milin R. (1996). Case study: withdrawal syndrome in adolescent chronic cannabis users. *J Am Acad Child Adolesc Psychiatry*. 35(12): 1618–21.

Egertova M, Giang DK, Cravatt BF, Elphick MR. (1998). A new perspective on cannabinoid signalling: complementary localization of fatty acid amide hydrolase and the CB1 receptor in rat brain. *Proc Royal Soc London B Biol Sci*. 265(1410): 2081–85.

Eldridge JC, Landfield PW. (1990). Cannabinoid interactions with glucocorticoid receptors in rat hippocampus. *Brain Res*. 534(1–2): 135–41.

Eldridge JC, Murphy LL, Landfield PW. (1991). Cannabinoids and the hippocampal glucocorticoid receptor: recent findings and possible significance. *Steroids*. 56(5): 226–31.

Engelsman EL. (1989). Dutch policy on the management of drug-related problems. *Br J Addict*. 84(2): 211–18.

Evans MA, Harbison RD, Brown DJ, Forney RB. (1976). Stimulant actions of delta9-tetrahydrocannabinol in mice. *Psychopharmacology (Berlin)*. 50(3): 245–50.

Feinberg I, Jones R, Walker JM, Cavness C, March J. (1975). Effects of high dosage delta-9-tetrahydrocannabinol on sleep patterns in man. *Clin Pharmacol Ther*. 17(4): 458–66.

Feinberg I, Jones R, Walker J, Cavness C, Floyd T. (1976). Effects of marijuana extract and tetrahydrocannabinol on electroencephalographic sleep patterns. *Clin Pharmacol Ther*. 19(6): 782–94.

Fletcher JM, Page JB, Francis DJ, Copeland K, Naus MJ, Davis CM, Morris R, Krauskopf D, Satz P. (1996). Cognitive correlates of long-term cannabis use in Costa Rican men. *Arch Gen Psychiatry*. 53(11): 1051–57.

Foy MR, Teyler TJ, Vardaris RM. (1982). delta 9-THC and 17-beta-estradiol in hippocampus. *Brain Res Bull*. 8(4): 341–45.

French ED, Dillon K, Wu X. (1997). Cannabinoids excite dopamine neurons in the ventral tegmentum and substantia nigra. *Neuroreport*. 8(3): 649–52.

Fride E. (1995). Anandamides: tolerance and cross-tolerance to delta 9-tetrahydrocannabinol. *Brain Res*. 697(1–2): 83–90.

Fride E, Mechoulam R. (1993). Pharmacological activity of the cannabinoid receptor agonist, anandamide, a brain constituent. *Eur J Pharmacol*. 231(2): 313–14.

Fried PA. (1995a). Prenatal exposure to marihuana and tobacco during infancy, early and middle childhood: effects and an attempt at synthesis. *Arch Toxicol*. 17: 233–60.

Fried PA. (1995b). The Ottawa Prenatal Prospective Study (OPPS): methodological issues and findings—it's easy to throw the baby out with the bath water. *Life Sci*. 56(23–24): 2159–68.

Gallily R, Yamin A, Waksmann Y, Ovadia H, Weidenfeld J, Bar-Joseph A, Biegon A, Mechoulam R, Shohami E. (1997). Protection against septic shock and suppression of tumor necrosis factor alpha and nitric oxide production by dexanabinol (HU-211), a nonpsychotropic cannabinoid. *J Pharmacol Exp Ther*. 283(2): 918–24.

Garrett ER, Hunt CA. (1977). Pharmacokinetics of delta9-tetrahydrocannabinol in dogs. *J Pharm Sci*. 66(3): 395–407.

Gessa GL, Casu MA, Carta G, Mascia MS. (1998). Cannabinoids decrease acetylcholine release in the medial-prefrontal cortex and hippocampus, reversal by SR 141716A. *Eur J Pharmacol*. 355(2–3): 119–24.

Golub MS, Sassenrath EN, Chapman LF. (1982). An analysis of altered attention in monkeys exposed to delta-9-tetrahydrocannabinol during development. *Neurobehav Toxicol Teratol.* 4(4): 469–72.

Goparaju SK, Ueda N, Taniguchi K, Yamamoto S. (1999). Enzymes of porcine brain hydrolyzing 2-arachidonoylglycerol, an endogenous ligand of cannabinoid receptors. *Biochem Pharmacol.* 57(4): 417–23.

Goparaju SK, Ueda N, Yamaguchi H, Yamamoto S. (1998). Anandamide amidohydrolase reacting with 2-arachidonoylglycerol, another cannabinoid receptor ligand. *FEBS Letters.* 422(1): 69–73.

Graceffo TJ, Robinson JK. (1998). Delta-9-tetrahydrocannabinol (THC) fails to stimulate consumption of a highly palatable food in the rat. *Life Sci.* 62(8): PL85–88.

Grinspoon L. (1999). *Marihuana Reconsidered,* 2nd ed. Oakland, CA: Quick American Archives. Orig. published Cambridge: Harvard University Press, 1977.

Grinspoon L, Bakalar JB. (1992). Marihuana. In: *Substance Abuse: A Comprehensive Textbook*, 2nd ed. Lowinson JH, Ruiz P, Millman RB, eds. Baltimore: Williams and Wilkins, pp 236–46.

Hamann W, di Vadi PP. (1999). Analgesic effect of the cannabinoid analogue nabilone is not mediated by opioid receptors. *Lancet.* 353(9152): 560.

Hampson AJ, Grimaldi M, Axelrod J, Wink D. (1998). Cannabidiol and (–)Delta9-tetrahydrocannabinol are neuroprotective antioxidants. *Proc Natl Acad Sci USA.* 95(14): 8268–73.

Harclerode J. (1984). Endocrine effects of marijuana in the male: preclinical studies. *NIDA Res Monogr.* 44: 46–64.

Heishman SJ, Arasteh K, Stitzer ML. (1997). Comparative effects of alcohol and marijuana on mood, memory, and performance. *Pharmacol Biochem Behav.* 58(1): 93–101.

Heishman SJ, Stitzer ML, Yingling JE. (1989). Effects of tetrahydrocannabinol content on marijuana smoking behavior, subjective reports, and performance. *Pharmacol Biochem Behav.* 34(1): 173–79.

Herkenham M, Lynn AB, Johnson, MR, Melvin LS, de Costa BR, Rice KC. (1991). Characterization and localization of cannabinoid receptors in the rat brain: a quantitative in vitro autoradiographic study. *J Neurosci.* 11: 563–83.

Heyser CJ, Hampson RE, Deadwyler SA. (1993). Effects of delta-9-tetrahydrocannabinol on delayed match to sample performance in rats: alterations in short-term memory associated with changes in task specific firing of hippocampal cells. *J Pharmacol Exp Ther.* 264(1): 294–307.

Hoffman DI, Brunemann KD, Gori GB, Wynder EL. (1975). On the carcinogenicity of marijuana smoke. *Recent Adv Phytochemistry.* 9: 45–48.

Hooker WD, Jones RT. (1987). Increased susceptibility to memory intrusions and the Stroop interference effect during acute marijuana intoxication. *Psychopharmacology (Berlin).* 91(1): 20–24.

Howlett AC. (1984). Inhibition of neuroblastoma adenylate cyclase by cannabinoid and nantradol compounds. *Life Sci.* 35(17): 1803–10.

Hunt CA, Jones RT. (1980). Tolerance and disposition of tetrahydrocannabinol in man. *J Pharmacol Exp Ther.* 215(1): 35–44.

Hutcheson DM, Tzavara ET, Smadja C, Valjent E, Roques BP, Hanoune J, Maldonado R. (1998). Behavioural and biochemical evidence for signs of abstinence in mice chronically treated with delta-9-tetrahydrocannabinol. *Br J Pharmacol.* 125(7): 1567–77.

Jentsch JD, Andrusiak E, Tran A, Bowers MB Jr, Roth RH. (1997). Delta 9-tetrahydrocannabinol increases prefrontal cortical catecholaminergic utilization and impairs spatial working memory in the rat: blockade of dopaminergic effects with HA966. *Neuropsychopharmacology.* 16(6): 426–32.

Johansson E, Agurell S, Hollister LE, Halldin MM. (1988). Prolonged apparent half-life of delta 1-tetrahydrocannabinol in plasma of chronic marijuana users. *J Pharm Pharmacol.* 40(5): 374–75.

Johansson E, Halldin MM, Agurell S, Hollister LE, Gillespie HK. (1989). Terminal elimination plasma half-life of delta 1-tetrahydrocannabinol (delta 1-THC) in heavy users of marijuana. *Eur J Clin Pharmacol.* 37(3): 273–77.

Joranson DE, Ryan KM, Gilson AM, Dahl JL. (2000). Trends in medical use and abuse of opioid analgesics. *JAMA.* 283(13): 1710–14.

Joy JE, Watson SJ, Benson JA, eds. (1999). *Marijuana and Medicine: Assessing the Science Base.* Institute of Medicine. Washington, DC: National Academy Press.

Kaminski NE, Abood ME, Kessler FK, Martin BR, Schatz AR. (1992). Identification of a functionally relevant cannabinoid receptor on mouse spleen cells that is involved in cannabinoid-mediated immune modulation. *Mol Pharmacol.* 42(5): 736–42.

Karler R, Calder LD, Sangdee P, Turkanis SA. (1984). Interaction between delta-9-tetrahydrocannabinol and kindling by electrical and chemical stimuli in mice. *Neuropharmacology.* 23(11): 1315–20.

Karler R, Calder LD, Turkanis SA. (1986). Prolonged CNS hyperexcitability in mice after a single exposure to delta-9-tetrahydrocannabinol. *Neuropharmacology.* 25(4): 441–46.

Karler R, Turkanis SA. (1981). The cannabinoids as potential antiepileptics. *J Clin Pharmacol.* 21(8–9 suppl): 437S–48S.

Koe BK, Milne GM, Weissman A, Johnson MR, Melvin LS. (1985). Enhancement of brain [^{3}H]flunitrazepam binding and analgesic activity of synthetic cannabimimetics. *Eur J Pharmacol.* 109(2): 201–12.

Kondo S, Kondo H, Nakane S, Kodaka T, Tokumura A, Waku K, Sugiura T. (1998). 2-Arachidonoylglycerol, an endogenous cannabinoid receptor agonist: identification as one of the major species of monoacylglycerols in various rat tissues, and evidence for its generation through CA2+-dependent and -independent mechanisms. *FEBS Lett.* 429(2): 152–56.

Kouri E, Pope HG Jr, Yurgelun-Todd D, Gruber S. (1995). Attributes of heavy vs. occasional marijuana smokers in a college population. *Biol Psychiatry*. 38(7): 475–81.

Leweke M, Kampmann C, Radwan M, Dietrich DE, Johannes S, Emrich HM, Munte TF. (1998). The effects of tetrahydrocannabinol on the recognition of emotionally charged words: an analysis using event-related brain potentials. *Neuropsychobiology*. 37(2): 104–11.

Liu X, Matochik JA, Cadet JL, London ED. (1998). Smaller volume of prefrontal lobe in polysubstance abusers: a magnetic resonance imaging study. *Neuropsychopharmacology*. 18(4): 243–52.

Lukas SE, Mendelson JH, Benedikt R. (1995). Electroencephalographic correlates of marihuana-induced euphoria. *Drug Alcohol Dependence*. 37(2): 131–40.

MacCoun R, Reuter P. (1997). Interpreting Dutch cannabis policy: reasoning by analogy in the legalization debate. *Science*. 278(5335): 47–52.

Mallet PE, Beninger RJ. (1998). The cannabinoid CB1 receptor antagonist SR141716A attenuates the memory impairment produced by delta9-tetrahydrocannabinol or anandamide. *Psychopharmacology (Berlin)*. 140(1): 11–19.

Marks DF, MacAvoy MG. (1989). Divided attention performance in cannabis users and non-users following alcohol and cannabis separately and in combination. *Psychopharmacology (Berlin)*. 99(3): 397–401.

Martin BR. (1985). Structural requirements for cannabinoid-induced antinociceptive activity in mice. *Life Sci*. 36(16): 1523–30.

Mathew RJ, Wilson WH, Coleman RE, Turkington TG, DeGrado TR. (1997). Marijuana intoxication and brain activation in marijuana smokers. *Life Sci*. 60(23): 2075–89.

Mathew RJ, Wilson WH, Humphreys D, Lowe JV, Weithe KE. (1993). Depersonalization after marijuana smoking. *Biol Psychiatry*. 33(6): 431–41.

Mathew RJ, Wilson WH, Turkington TG, Coleman RE. (1998). Cerebellar activity and disturbed time sense after THC. *Brain Res*. 797(2): 183–89.

Matsuzaki M, Casella GA, Ratner M. (1987). delta 9-Tetrahydrocannabinol: EEG changes, bradycardia, and hypothermia in the rhesus monkey. *Brain Res Bull*. 19(2): 223–29.

Mattes RD, Engelman K, Shaw LM, Elsohly MA. (1994). Cannabinoids and appetite stimulation. *Pharmacol Biochem Behav*. 49(1): 187–95.

McMillan DE, Snodgrass SH. (1991). Effects of acute and chronic administration of delta 9-tetrahydrocannabinol or cocaine on ethanol intake in a rat model. *Drug Alcohol Dependence*. 27(3): 263–74.

Mendelson JH, Mello NK, Ellingboe J, Skupny AS, Lex BW, Griffin M. (1986). Marihuana smoking suppresses luteinizing hormone in women. *J Pharmacol Exp Ther*. 237(3): 862–66.

Munro S, Thomas KL, Abu-Shaar M. (1993). Molecular characterization of a peripheral receptor for cannabinoids. *Nature*. 365(6441): 61–65.

Murillo-Rodriguez E, Sanchez-Alavez M, Navarro L, Martinez-Gonzalez D, Drucker-Colin R, Prospero-Garcia O. (1998). Anandamide modulates sleep and memory in rats. *Brain Res.* 812(1–2): 270–74.

Murphy LL, Gher J, Steger RW, Bartke A. (1994). Effects of delta 9-tetrahydrocannabinol on copulatory behavior and neuroendocrine responses of male rats to female conspecifics. *Pharmacol Biochem Behav.* 48(4): 1011–17.

Murphy LL, Newton SC, Dhali J, Chavez D. (1991). Evidence for a direct anterior pituitary site of delta-9-tetrahydrocannabinol action. *Pharmacol Biochem Behav.* 40(3): 603–7.

Murray JB. (1986). Marijuana's effects on human cognitive functions, psychomotor functions, and personality. *J Gen Psychol.* 113(1): 23–55.

Musty RE, Kaback L. (1995). Relationships between motivation and depression in chronic marijuana users. *Life Sci.* 56(23–24): 2151–58.

Nahas G, Latour C. (1992). The human toxicity of marijuana. *Med J Aust.* 156(7): 495–97.

Navarro M, Fernandez-Ruiz JJ, De Miguel R, Hernandez ML, Cebeira M, Ramos JA. (1993). Motor disturbances induced by an acute dose of delta 9-tetrahydrocannabinol: possible involvement of nigrostriatal dopaminergic alterations. *Pharmacol Biochem Behav.* 45(2): 291–98.

Navarro M, Rubio P, de Fonseca FR. (1995). Behavioural consequences of maternal exposure to natural cannabinoids in rats. *Psychopharmacology (Berlin).* 122(1): 1–14.

Nelson K, Walsh D, Deeter P, Sheehan F. (1994). A phase II study of delta-9-tetrahydrocannabinol for appetite stimulation in cancer-associated anorexia. *J Palliative Care.* 10(1): 14–18.

Noyes R Jr, Brunk SF, Avery DAH, Canter AC. (1975). The analgesic properties of delta-9-tetrahydrocannabinol and codeine. *Clin Pharmacol Ther.* 18(1): 84–89.

O'Brien CP. (1996). Drug Addiction and Abuse. In: *Goodman and Gilman's The Pharmacological Basis of Therapeutics.* Hardman JG, Limbird LE, Molinoff PB, Ruddon RW, Goodman Gilman A, eds. New York: McGraw-Hill.

Paria BC, Wang XN, Dey SK. (1994). Effects of chronic treatment with delta-9-tetrahydrocannabinol on uterine growth in the mouse. *Life Sci.* 55(9): 729–34.

Parker ES, Birnbaum IM, Weingartner H, Hartley JT, Stillman RC, Wyatt RJ. (1980). Retrograde enhancement of human memory with alcohol. *Psychopharmacology (Berlin).* 69(2): 219–22.

Patrick G, Straumanis JJ, Struve FA, Fitz-Gerald MJ, Manno JE. (1997). Early and middle latency evoked potentials in medically and psychiatrically normal daily marihuana users: a paucity of significant findings. *Clin Electroencephalogr.* 28(1): 26–31.

Patrick G, Straumanis JJ, Struve FA, Nixon F, Fitz-Gerald MJ, Manno JE, Soucair M. (1995). Auditory and visual P300 event related potentials are not altered in medically and psychiatrically normal chronic marihuana users. *Life Sci.* 56(23–24): 2135–40.

Paule MG, Allen RR, Bailey JR, Scallet AC, Ali SF, Brown RM, Slikker W Jr. (1992). Chronic marijuana smoke exposure in the rhesus monkey: II. Effects on progressive ratio and conditioned position responding. *J Pharmacol Exp Ther.* 260(1): 210–22.

Perez-Reyes M, Hicks RE, Bumberry J, Jeffcoat AR, Cook CE. (1988). Interaction between marihuana and ethanol: effects on psychomotor performance. *Alcohol Clin Exp Res.* 12(2): 268–76.

Pertwee RG, Browne SE, Ross TM, Stretton CD. (1991). An investigation of the involvement of GABA in certain pharmacological effects of delta-9-tetrahydrocannabinol. *Pharmacol Biochem Behav.* 40(3): 581–85.

Pertwee RG, Ross TM. (1991). Drugs which stimulate or facilitate central cholinergic transmission interact synergistically with delta-9-tetrahydrocannabinol to produce marked catalepsy in mice. *Neuropharmacology.* 30(1): 67–71.

Peters BA, Lewis EG, Dustman RE, Straight RC, Beck EC. (1976). Sensory, perceptual, motor, and cognitive functioning and subjective reports following oral administration of delta9-tetrahydrocannabinol. *Psychopharmacologia.* 47(2): 141–48.

Petro DJ, Ellenberger C Jr. (1981). Treatment of human spasticity with delta 9-tetrahydrocannabinol. *J Clin Pharmacol.* 21(8–9 suppl): 413S–16S.

Pfefferbaum A, Darley CF, Tinklenberg JR, Roth WT, Kopell BS. (1977). Marijuana and memory intrusions. *J Nerv Ment Dis.* 165(6): 381–86.

Plasse TF, Gorter RW, Krasnow SH, Lane M, Shepard KV, Wadleigh RG. (1991). Recent clinical experience with dronabinol. *Pharmacol Biochem Behav.* 40(3): 695–700.

Pope HG Jr, Yurgelun-Todd D. (1996). The residual cognitive effects of heavy marijuana use in college students. *JAMA.* 275(7): 521–27.

Rafaelsen L, Christrup H, Bech P, Rafaelsen OJ. (1973). Effects of cannabis and alcohol on psychological tests. *Nature.* 242(5393): 117–18.

Raft D, Gregg J, Ghia J, Harris L. (1977). Effects of intravenous tetrahydrocannabinol on experimental and surgical pain. Psychological correlates of the analgesic response. *Clin Pharmacol Ther.* 21(1): 26–33.

Ray O, Ksir C. (1990). *Drugs, Society, and Human Behavior.* St. Louis: Times Mirror/Mosby College Publishing.

Reichman M, Nen W, Hokin LE. (1987). Effects of delta 9-tetrahydrocannabinol on prostaglandin formation in brain. *Mol Pharmacol.* 32(5): 686–90.

Rettori V, Wenger T, Snyder G, Dalterio S, McCann SM. (1988). Hypothalamic action of delta-9-tetrahydrocannabinol to inhibit the release of prolactin and growth hormone in the rat. *Neuroendocrinology.* 47(6): 498–503.

Robbers JE, Speedie MK, Tyler VE. (1996). *Pharmacognosy and Pharmacobiotechnology.* Baltimore: Willams and Wilkins.

Rodriguez de Fonseca F, Carrera MRA, Navarro M, Koob GF, Weiss F. (1997). Activation of corticotropin-releasing factor in the limbic system during cannabinoid withdrawal. *Science.* 276(5321): 2050–54.

Rodriguez de Fonseca F, Cebeira M, Ramos JA, Martin M, Fernandez-Ruiz JJ. (1994). Cannabinoid receptors in rat brain areas: sexual differences, fluctuations during estrous cycle, and changes after gonadectomy and sex steroid replacement. *Life Sci.* 54(3): 159–70.

Romero J, de Miguel R, García-Palomero E, Fernández-Ruiz JJ, Ramos JA. (1995). Time-course of the effects of anandamide, the putative endogenous cannabinoid receptor ligand, on extrapyramidal function. *Brain Res.* 694(1–2): 223–32.

Rudgley R. (1993). *Essential Substances.* New York: Kodansha International.

Ruh MF, Taylor JA, Howlett AC, Welshons WV. (1997). Failure of cannabinoid compounds to stimulate estrogen receptors. *Biochem Pharmacol.* 53(1): 35–41.

Scallet AC. (1991). Neurotoxicology of cannabis and THC: a review of chronic exposure studies in animals. *Pharmacol Biochem Behav.* 40(3): 671–76.

Schultes RE, Hofman A. (1992). *Plants of the Gods.* Rochester, VT: Healing Arts Press.

Shen M, Thayer SA. (1999). Delta9-tetrahydrocannabinol acts as a partial agonist to modulate glutamatergic synaptic transmission between rat hippocampal neurons in culture. *Mol Pharmacol.* 55(1): 8–13.

Sherwood RA, Keating J, Kavvadia V, Greenough A, Peters TJ. (1999). Substance misuse in early pregnancy and relationship to fetal outcome. *Eur J Pediatr.* 158(6): 488–92.

Shook JE, Burks TF. (1989). Psychoactive cannabinoids reduce gastrointestinal propulsion and motility in rodents. *J Pharmacol Exp Ther.* 249(2): 444–49.

Sofia RD, Solomon TA, Barry H 3rd. (1976). Anticonvulsant activity of delta9-tetrahydrocannabinol compared with three other drugs. *Eur J Pharmacol.* 35(1): 7–16.

Stapleton JM, Guthrie S, Linnoila M. (1986). Effects of alcohol and other psychotropic drugs on eye movements: relevance to traffic safety. *J Stud Alcohol.* 47(5): 426–32.

Stark P, Dews PB. (1980). Cannabinoids: I. Behavioral effects. *J Pharmacol Exp Ther.* 214(1): 124–30.

Stella N, Schweitzer P, Piomelli D. (1997). A second endogenous cannabinoid that modulates long-term potentiation. *Nature.* 388(6644): 773–78.

Striem S, Bar-Joseph A, Berkovitch Y, Biegon A. (1997). Interaction of dexanabinol (HU-211), a novel NMDA receptor antagonist, with the dopaminergic system. *Eur J Pharmacol.* 338(3): 205–13.

Struve FA, Patrick G, Straumanis JJ, Fitz-Gerald MJ, Manno J. (1998). Possible EEG sequelae of very long duration marihuana use: pilot findings from topographic quantitative EEG analyses of subjects with 15 to 24 years of cumulative daily exposure to THC. *Clin Electroencephalogr.* 29(1): 31–36.

Struve FA, Straumanis JJ, Patrick G. (1994). Persistent topographic quantitative EEG sequelae of chronic marihuana use: a replication study and initial discriminant function analysis. *Clin Electroencephalogr.* 25(2): 63–75.

Struwe M, Kaempfer SH, Geiger CJ, Pavia AT, Plasse TF, Shepard KV, Ries K, Evans TG. (1993). Effect of dronabinol on nutritional status in HIV infection. *Ann Pharmacother.* 27(7–8): 827–31.

Taylor HG. (1998). Analysis of the medical use of marijuana and its societal implications. *J Am Pharm Assoc (Washington).* 38(2): 220–27.

Thomas BF, Wei X, Martin BR. (1992). Characterization and autoradiographic localization of the cannabinoid binding site in rat brain using [^{3}H]11-OH-delta 9-THC-DMH. *J Pharmacol Exp Ther.* 263(3): 1383–90.

Thorat SN, Bhargava HN. (1994). Effects of NMDA receptor blockade and nitric oxide synthase inhibition on the acute and chronic actions of delta 9-tetrahydrocannabinol in mice. *Brain Res.* 667(1): 77–82.

Tinklenberg JR, Melges FT, Hollister LE, Gillespie HK. (1970). Marijuana and immediate memory. *Nature.* 226(251): 1171–72.

Tramposch A, Sangdee C, Franz DN, Karler R, Turkanis SA. (1981). Cannabinoid-induced enhancement and depression of cat monosynaptic reflexes. *Neuropharmacology.* 20(6): 617–21.

Tripathi HL, Vocci FJ, Brase DA, Dewey WL. (1987). Effects of cannabinoids on levels of acetylcholine and choline and on turnover rate of acetylcholine in various regions of the mouse brain. *Alcohol Drug Res.* 7(5–6): 525–32.

Tunving K. (1985). Psychiatric effects of cannabis use. *Acta Psychiat Scand.* 72: 209–17.

Turkanis SA, Karler R. (1981). Electrophysiologic properties of the cannabinoids. *J Clin Pharmacol.* 21(8–9 suppl): 449S–63S.

Turkanis SA, Smiley KA, Borys HK, Olsen DM, Karler R. (1979). An electrophysiological analysis of the anticonvulsant action of cannabidiol on limbic seizures in conscious rats. *Epilepsia.* 20(4): 351–63.

Tyrey L. (1984). Endocrine aspects of cannabinoid action in female subprimates: search for sites of action. *NIDA Res Monogr.* 44: 65–81.

Ungerleider JT, Andrysiak T, Fairbanks L, Goodnight J, Sarna G, Jamison K. (1982). Cannabis and cancer chemotherapy: a comparison of oral delta-9-THC and prochlorperazine. *Cancer.* 50(4): 636–45.

Varma VK, Malhotra AK, Dang R, Das K, Nehra R. (1988). Cannabis and cognitive functions: a prospective study. *Drug Alcohol Dependence.* 21(2): 147–52.

Vaupel DB, Morton EC. (1982). Anorexia and hyperphagia produced by five pharmacologic classes of hallucinogens. *Pharmacol Biochem Behav.* 17(3): 539–45.

Vincent BJ, McQuiston DJ, Einhorn LH, Nagy CM, Brames MJ. (1983). Review of cannabinoids and their antiemetic effectiveness. *Drugs.* 25(suppl 1): 52–62.

Volkow ND, Gillespie H, Mullani N, Tancredi L, Grant C, Ivanovic M, Hollister L. (1991). Cerebellar metabolic activation by delta-9-tetrahydrocannabinol in human brain: a study with positron emission tomography and 18F-2-fluoro-2-deoxyglucose. *Psychiatry Res.* 40(1): 69–78.

Voth EA, Schwartz RH. (1997). Medicinal applications of delta-9-tetrahydrocannabinol and marijuana. *Ann Int Med.* May 126(10): 791–98.

Wada JA, Osawa T, Corcoran ME. (1975). Effects of tetrahydrocannabinols on kindled amygdaloid seizures and photogenic seizures in Senegalese baboons, Papio papio. *Epilepsia.* 16(3): 439–48.

Wada JA, Wake A, Sato M, Corcoran ME. (1975). Antiepileptic and prophylactic effects of tetrahydrocannabinols in amygdaloid kindled cats. *Epilepsia.* 16(3): 503–10.

Walker A, Rosenberg M, Balaban-Gil K. (1999). Neurodevelopmental and neurobehavioral sequelae of selected substances of abuse and psychiatric medications in utero. *Child Adolesc Psychiatr Clin North Am.* 8(4): 845–67.

Waskow IE, Olsson JE, Salzman C, Katz MM. (1970). Psychological effects of tetrahydrocannabinol. *Arch Gen Psychiatry.* 22(2): 97–107.

Weidenfeld J, Feldman S, Mechoulam R. (1994). Effect of the brain constituent anandamide, a cannabinoid receptor agonist, on the hypothalamo-pituitary-adrenal axis in the rat. *Neuroendocrinology.* 59(2): 110–2.

Welch SP. (1997). Characterization of anandamide-induced tolerance: comparison to delta 9-THC-induced interactions with dynorphinergic systems. *Drug Alcohol Dependence.* 45(1–2) 39–45.

Wert RC, Raulin ML. (1986). The chronic cerebral effects of cannabis use: I. Methodological issues and neurological findings. *Int J Addict.* 21(6): 605–28.

Westlake TM, Howlett AC, Ali SF, Paule MG, Scallet AC, Slikker W Jr. (1991). Chronic exposure to delta 9-tetrahydrocannabinol fails to irreversibly alter brain cannabinoid receptors. *Brain Res.* 544(1): 145–49.

Williams CM, Rogers PJ, Kirkham TC. (1998). Hyperphagia in pre-fed rats following oral delta9-THC. *Physiol Behav.* 65(2): 343–46.

Wilson WH, Ellinwood EH, Mathew RJ, Johnson K. (1994). Effects of marijuana on performance of a computerized cognitive-neuromotor test battery. *Psychiatry Res.* 51(2): 115–25.

Wu TC, Tashkin DP, Rose JE, Djahed B. (1988). Influence of marijuana potency and amount of cigarette consumed on marijuana smoking pattern. *J Psychoactive Drugs.* 20(1): 43–46.

Zhuang S, Kittler J, Grigorenko EV, Kirby MT, Sim LJ, Hampson RE, Childers SR, Deadwyler SA. (1998). Effects of long-term exposure to delta9-THC on expression of cannabinoid receptor (CB1) mRNA in different rat brain regions. *Brain Res Mol Brain Res.* 62(2): 141–49.

Recommended Reading

This is a list of texts and key articles that are especially valuable in the study of psychoactive plant drugs. They are highly recommended for those seeking further reading on the respective topics.

General Neuroscience

Carlson NR. (2001). *Physiology of Behavior*, 7th ed. Boston: Allyn and Bacon.

Cooper JR, Bloom FE, Roth RH. (1996). *The Biochemical Basis of Neuropharmacology*, 7th ed. New York: Oxford University Press.

DeArmond SJ, Fusco MM, Dewey MM. (1989). *Structure of the Human Brain*, 3rd ed. New York: Oxford University Press.

Hall ZW. (1992). *Introduction to Molecular Neurobiology*. Sunderland, MA: Sinauer.

Hille B. (1992). *Ionic Channels of Excitable Membranes*, 2nd ed. Sunderland, MA: Sinauer Associates.

Kandel E, Schwartz JH, Jessel TM, eds. (2000). *Principles of Neural Science*, 4th ed. New York: McGraw-Hill.

Waitling KJ. (1998). *The RBI Handbook of Receptor Classification*, 3rd ed. Natick, MA: Research Biochemicals International.

Parent A. (1996). *Carpenter's Human Neuroanatomy*, 9th ed. Baltimore: Williams and Wilkins.

Siegel GJ, Agranoff BW, Albers RW, Molinoff PB, eds. (1994). *Basic Neurochemistry: Molecular, Cellular, and Medical aspects*, 6th ed. New York: Lipincott–Raven.

Neuropsychology

Heilman KM, Valenstein E. (1993). *Clinical Neuropsychology*, 3rd ed. New York: Oxford University Press.

Lezak, MD. (1995). *Neuropsychological Assessment.* New York: Oxford University Press.

Spreen O, Strauss E. (1998). *A Compendium of Neuropsychological Tests*, 2nd ed. New York: Oxford University Press.

Pharmacology

Hardman JG, Gilman AG, Limbird LE, eds. (1996). *Goodman and Gilman's The Pharmacological Basis of Therapeutics*, 9th ed. New York: McGraw-Hill.

Clark WG, Brater DC, Johnson AR. (1992). *Goth's Medical Pharmacology*, 12th ed. St. Louis: Mosby, 1988.

Pharmacognosy

Blumenthal M, ed. (1998). *The Complete German Commission E Monographs: Therapeutic Guide to Herbal Medicines.* Integrative Medicine Communications.

Gruenwald J, Brendler T, Jaenicke C. (1998). *PDR for Herbal Medicines*, 1st ed. Montvale, NJ: Medical Economics.

Robbers JE, Speedie MK, Tyler VE. (1996). *Pharmacognosy and Pharmacobiotechnology.* Baltimore: Willams and Wilkins.

Tyler V. (1994). *Herbs of Choice.* New York: The Haworth Press. 1999.

History/Ethnopharmacology

Rudgley R. (1993). *Essential Substances.* New York: Kodansha International.

Rudgley R. (1998). *The Encyclopaedia of Psychoactive Substances.* NY: St. Martin Press.

Escohotado A. (1999). *A Brief History of Drugs: From the Stone Age to the Stonedl Age.* Symington KA, trans. Rochester, VT: Park Street Press.

Herb Cultivation

Sturdivant L, Blakely T. (1999). *Medicinal Herbs in the Garden, Field, and Marketplace.* Friday Harbor, WA: San Juan Naturals.

Herbal Sedatives and Anxiolytics

Lebot V, Merlin M, Lindstrom L. (1997). *Kava—The Pacific Elixir: The Definitive Guide to Its Ethnobotany, History, and Chemistry.* Rochester, VT: Healing Arts Press. [Originally published: New Haven: Yale University Press, c1992.]

Houghton PJ. (1988). The biological activity of Valerian and related plants. *J Ethnopharmacol.* 22(2): 121–42.

Stimulant Plants

Balfour DJ. (1994). Neural mechanisms underlying nicotine dependence. *Addiction.* 89(11): 1419–23.

Bolla KI, Cadet JL, London ED. (1998). The neuropsychiatry of chronic cocaine abuse. *J Neuropsychiatry Clin Neurosci.* 10(3): 280–89.

Elmi AS. (1983). The chewing of khat in Somalia. *J Ethnopharmacol.* 8(2): 163–76.

Kalix P. (1988). Khat: a plant with amphetamine effects. *J Subst Abuse Treat.* 5(3): 163–69.

Leshner AI, Koob GF. (1999). Drugs of abuse and the brain. *Proc Assoc Am Physicians.* 111(2): 99–108.

Pomerleau OF. (1992). Nicotine and the central nervous system: biobehavioral effects of cigarette smoking. *Am J Med.* 93(1A): 2S–7S.

Snyder SH, Sklar P. (1984). Behavioral and molecular actions of caffeine: focus on adenosine. *J Psychiatr Res.* 18(2): 91–106.

Stolerman IP, Shoaib M. (1991). The neurobiology of tobacco addiction. *Trends Pharmacol Sci.* 12(12): 467–73.

Woolverton WL, Johnson KM. (1992). Neurobiology of cocaine abuse. *Trends Pharmacol Sci.* 13(5): 193–200.

Cognitive Enhancers

Itil T, Martorano D. (1995). Natural substances in psychiatry (Ginkgo biloba in dementia). *Psychopharmacol Bull.* 31(1): 147–58.

Itil TM, Eralp E, Ahmed I, Kunitz A, Itil KZ. (1998). The pharmacological effects of Ginkgo biloba, a plant extract, on the brain of dementia patients in comparison with tacrine. *Psychopharmacol Bull.* 34(3): 391–97.

Field B, Vadnal R. (1998). Ginkgo biloba and memory: an overview. *Nutr Neurosci.* 1: 2565–67.

Oken BS, Storzbach DM, Kaye JA. (1998). The efficacy of Ginkgo biloba on cognitive function in Alzheimer disease. *Arch Neurol.* 55(11): 1409–15.

Schneider LS, Olin JT. (1994). Overview of clinical trials of Hydergine in dementia. *Arch Neurol.* 51: 787–97.

Warburton DM. (1992). Nicotine as a cognitive enhancer. *Prog Neuropsychopharmacol Biol Psychiatry.* 16(2): 181–91.

Psychotherapeutic Herbs

Kim HL, Streltzer J, Goebert D. (1999). St. John's wort for depression: a meta-analysis of well-defined clinical trials. *J Nerv Ment Dis.* 187(9): 532–38.

Linde K, Ramirez G, Mulrow CD, Pauls A, Weidenhammer W, Melchart D. (1996). St. John's wort for depression—an overview and meta-analysis of randomised clinical trials. *BMJ.* 313(7052): 253–58.

Gaster B, Holroyd J. (2000). St John's wort for depression: a systematic review. *Arch Intern Med.* 160(2): 152–56.

Analgesics and Anesthetics

Basbaum AI, Fields HL. (1984). Endogenous pain control systems: brainstem spinal pathways and endorphin circuitry. *Annu Rev Neurosci.* 7: 309–38.

Price DD. (1988). *Psychological and Neural Mechanisms of Pain.* New York: Raven Press.

Pasternak GW. (1993). Pharmacological mechanisms of opioid analgesics. *Clin Neuropharmacol.* 16(1): 1–18.

Hallucinogens

Anderson, EF. (1996). *Peyote: The Divine Cactus.* Tuscon: University of Arizona Press.

Harner MJ, ed. (1973). *Hallucinogens and Shamanism.* New York: Oxford University Press.

Schultes RE, Hofman A. (1992). *Plants of the Gods: Their Sacred, Healing, and Hallucinogenic Powers.* Rochester, VT: Healing Arts Press.

Schultes RE, Hofman A. (1980). *The Botany and Chemistry of Hallucinogens,* 2nd ed. Springfield, IL: Charles C. Thomas Publishers.

Grinspoon L, Bakalar JB. (1997). *Psychedelic Drugs Reconsidered.* New York: The Lindesmith Center.

Cannabis

Childers SR, Breivogel CS. (1998). Cannabis and endogenous cannabinoid systems. *Drug Alcohol Department.* 51(1–2): 173–87.

Fletcher JM, Page JB, Francis DJ, Copeland K, Naus MJ, Davis CM, Morris R, Krauskopf D, Satz P. (1996). Cognitive correlates of long-term cannabis use in Costa Rican men. *Arch Gen Psychiatry.* 53(11): 1051–57.

Grinspoon L, Bakalar JB. (1997). *Marihuana, the Forbidden Medicine.* New Haven: Yale University Press.

Joy JE, Watson SJ, Benson JA, eds. (1999). *Marijuana and Medicine: Assessing the Science Base*. Institute of Medicine. Washington, DC: National Academy Press.

Mechoulam R, Fride E, Di Marzo V. (1998). Endocannabinoids. *Eur J Pharmacol.* 359(1): 1–18.

Murray JB. (1986). Marijuana's effects on human cognitive functions, psychomotor functions, and personality. *J Gen Psychol.* 113(1): 23–55.

Taylor HG. (1998). Analysis of the medical use of marijuana and its societal implications. *J Am Pharm Assoc (Washington)*. 38(2): 220–27.

Index